Clinical Trials
A Methodologic Perspective

Steven Piantadosi, M.D., Ph.D.

Johns Hopkins Oncology Center

A Wiley-Interscience Publication
JOHN WILEY & SONS, INC.
New York • Chichester • Weinheim • Brisbane • Singapore • Toronto

This text is printed on acid-free paper.

Library of Congress Cataloging in Publication Data:

Piantadosi, Steven.
  Clinical trials: a methodologic perspective/ Steven Piantadosi.
     p.   cm. — (Applied probability and statistics ; 1346)
  "A Wiley-Interscience publication."
  Includes bibliographical references and index.
  ISBN 0-471-16393-7 (cloth : alk. paper)
  1. Clinical trials—Statistical methods.   I. Series: Wiley series in probability and statistics. Applied probability and statistics ; 1346.
  [DNLM: 1. Research—methods.   2. Clinical Trials—methods.
3. Statistics—methods.   W 20.5 P581c 1997]
  R853.C55P53   1997
  610'.72—DC21
  DNLM/DLC
  for Library of Congress   96-46311
                                                                          CIP

Printed in the United States of America
10 9 8 7 6 5 4

This book is dedicated to:

Pippy, Wooster, Moogie, Champ, Lulu, and Monkey

Contents

Preface

In recent years, a great deal has been written about clinical trials and closely related areas of biostatistics, biomathematics, biometry, epidemiology, and clinical epidemiology. The motive for writing this book is that there still seems to be a need among both physicians and biostatisticians for direct, relevant accounts of basic statistical methods in clinical trials. The need for both trialists and clinical investigators to learn about good methodology is particularly acute in oncology, where investigators search for treatment advances of great clinical importance, but modest size relative to the variability and bias which characterize studies of human disease. A similar need with the same motivation exists in many other diseases.

On the medical side of clinical trials, the last few years have seen a sharpened focus on training of clinical investigators in research methods. Training efforts have ranged from short intensive courses to research fellowships lasting years and culminating in a postgraduate degree. The evolution of teaching appears to be toward defining a specialty in clinical research. The material in this book should be of interest to those who take this path. The technical subjects may seem difficult at first, but the clinician should soon become comfortable with them.

On the biostatistical side of clinical trials, there has been a near explosion of methods in recent years. However, this is not a book on statistical theory. Readers with a good foundation in biostatistics should find the technical subjects practical and quite accessible. It is my hope that such students will see some cohesiveness to the field, fill in gaps in their knowledge, and be able to explore areas such as ethics and misconduct that are important to clinical trials.

There are some popular perceptions about clinical trials to which this book does not subscribe. For example, some widely used terminology regarding trials is unhelpful and I have attempted to counteract it by proposing alternatives. Also, noncomparative trial designs (e.g., early developmental studies) are often inappropriately excluded from discussions of methods. I have tried to present concepts that unify all designed studies rather than ideas that artificially distinguish them. Dealing with pharmacokinetic-based designs tends to complicate some of the mathematics, but the concepts are essential for understanding these trials.

The book is intended to provide at least enough material for the core of a one-half-semester course on clinical trials. In research settings where trials are used, the audience for such a course will likely have varying skills and directions. However, with a background of basic biostatistics, an introductory course in clinical trials or research methods, and appropriate didactic discussion, the material presented here should be useful to a heterogeneous group of students.

Acknowledgments

Many individuals have contributed to this book in indirect, but significant ways. I am reminded of two colleagues, now deceased, who helped to shape my thinking about clinical trials. David P. Byar, M.D. nurtured my early academic and quantitative interest in clinical trials in the early 1980s at the National Institutes of Health. After I joined the Johns Hopkins School of Medicine, Brigid G. Leventhal, M.D. showed me a mature, compassionate, and rigorous view of clinical trials from a practitioner's perspective. I hope the thoughts in this book reflect some of the good attitudes and values of these fine scholars. Other colleagues have taught me many lessons regarding clinical trials through their writings, lectures, conversations, and willingness to answer many questions. I would particularly like to thank Mitchell H. Gail, M.D., Ph.D. and Curtis L. Meinert, Ph.D. for much valuable advice and good example over the years. One of the most worthwhile experiences that a trial methodologist can have is to review and influence the designs of clinical trials while they are being developed. My colleagues at Johns Hopkins have cooperated in this regard through the Oncology Center's Clinical Research Committee, especially Hayden Braine, M.D., who has chaired the Committee wisely for many years.

Through long-standing collaborations with the Lung Cancer Study Group, I met many clinical scholars with much to say and teach about trials. I would like to thank them, especially E. Carmack Holmes, M.D., John R. Ruckdeschel, M.D., and Robert Ginzberg, M.D. for showing me a model of interdisciplinary collaboration and friendship, which continued to outlive the financial arrangements. Recent collaborations with colleagues in the New Approaches to Brain Tumor Therapy Consortium have also enhanced my appreciation and understanding of early developmental trials.

In recent months, many colleagues have assisted me by reading and offering comments on drafts of the chapters that follow. For this help, I would like to thank Lina Asmar, Ph.D., Tatiana Barkova, Ph.D., Jeanne DeJoseph, Ph.D., C.N.M., R.N., Suzanne Dibble, D.N.Sc., R.N., James Grizzle, Ph.D., Curt Meinert, Ph.D., Mitch Gail, M.D., Ph.D., Barbara Hawkins, Ph.D., Steven Goodman, M.D., Ph.D., Cheryl Enger, Ph.D., Guanghan Liu, Ph.D., J. Jack Lee, Ph.D., Claudia Moy, Ph.D., John O'Quigley, Ph.D., Thomas F. Pajak, Ph.D., Charles Rohde, Ph.D., Barbara Starklauf, M.A.S., Manel C. Wijesinha, Ph.D., and Marianna Zahurak, M.S. Many of the good points belong to them – the errors are mine.

Students in my classes on the *Design and Analysis of Clinical Trials* and *Design of Experiments* at the Johns Hopkins School of Hygiene and Public Health have contributed to this book by working with drafts, making helpful comments, working problems, or just discussing particular points. I would especially like to thank Maria Deloria, Kathleen Weeks, Ling-Yu Ruan, and Jeffrey Blume for their input. Helen Cromwell and Patty Hubbard have provided a great deal of technical assistance with the preparation of the manuscript. Gary D. Knott, Ph.D., Barry J. Bunow, Ph.D., and the staff at Civilized Software, Bethesda, Maryland (www.civilized.com) furnished me with MLAB software, without which many tasks in the following pages would be difficult.

This book was produced in LaTeX using *Scientific Workplace* version 2.5. I am indebted to Kathy Watt of TCI Software Research in Las Cruces, New Mexico, (www.tcisoft.com) for assistance in preparing the style. A special thanks goes to Irene Roach for editing an early draft of the manuscript and to Sean Roach for collecting and translating hard-to-find references.

It is not possible to write a book without stealing a large amount of time from one's family. Bonnie, Anne L., and Steven T. not only permitted this to happen, but also were supportive, helpful, and understood why I felt it was necessary. I am most grateful to them for their patience and understanding throughout this project.

STEVEN PIANTADOSI

Baltimore, Maryland
March 1997

Clinical Trials

CHAPTER 1

Preliminaries

1.1   Introduction

The best time to contemplate the quality of evidence from a clinical trial is before it begins. Conceptualizing and designing good clinical trials is never an accident, but results from careful planning. Therefore, this book attempts to acquaint investigators with ideas of design methodology that are also helpful in conducting, analyzing, and assessing clinical trials. From this early planning perspective, I deal with a number of relevant subjects; some that find general agreement and some that are contentious. It is unlikely that a reader experienced with clinical trials will agree with all that I say or emphasize, but my perspective should be mainstream, internally consistent, and useful for learning.

This book is not intended to be an introduction to the subject. It is part of a 1- or 2-quarter structured postgraduate *second* course in clinical trials for an audience with quantitative skills and a biological focus. It has evolved from the merging of two courses: one in experimental design and one in clinical trials. Specifically, the book assumes a working knowledge of basic biostatistics and some familiarity with clinical trials, either didactic or practical. It is also helpful if the reader understands some more advanced statistical concepts, especially lifetables, survival models, and likelihoods. I recognize that clinicians often lack this knowledge. However, many contemporary researchers are seeking it through training in clinical investigation methods or experimental therapeutics. No clinical knowledge is needed to understand the concepts in this book, although it will be helpful throughout.

Many readers of this book will find the discussion to be somewhat uneven. In some places, the content will seem basic, while in others, it appears technically complex. This is the result of covering the interdisciplinary practice of clinical trials and trying to address a population of students with varying backgrounds. The material in this book is intended to be supplemented with lecture and discussion. The reader who does not have an opportunity for formal classroom dialogue may need to explore the references more carefully. Some exercises and discussion questions are provided at the end of each chapter. These are intentionally left open-ended, with a suggestion that the student answer them in the form of a one- or two-page memorandum, as though providing an expert opinion to less-experienced investigators.

The study of clinical trials can be approached from a number of perspectives: 1) quantitative or biostatistical, 2) administrative or managerial, 3) clinical, and/or 4) ethical. The emphasis in this book will be on the quantitative perspective, because it generalizes readily to all of the disciplines in which trials are conducted. However, the discussion does not neglect the other viewpoints, because they are also essential to understanding trials. Many examples will relate to cancer, because that is the primary field in which I work, but the concepts will generalize to other areas.

Scientists who specialize in clinical trials might be called "trial methodologists" or "trialists", although they are frequently dubbed "statisticians". I will use all these terms interchangeably with the following warning regarding rigor. Statistics is an old and broad profession. There is not a one-to-one correspondence between statisticians or biostatisticians and knowledge of clinical trials. However, trial methodologists, whether statisticians or not, are likely to know a lot about biostatistics and will be accustomed to working with statistical experts. In many cases, trial methodologists are not statisticians at all, but evolve from epidemiologists or clinicians with a strongly quantitative orientation.

1.1.1 Scope of this book

Whenever possible, the discussion in this book pertains to all types of trials: developmental, safety, comparative, and large-scale studies, although there is an emphasis on comparative designs. The context will inform the reader how general the discussion is intended to be. There are many important aspects of clinical trials not covered here in any detail. These include administration, funding, conduct, quality control, and the considerable infrastructure necessary to conduct trials. These are all vitally important, but fall outside of the scope of this book. Fortunately, there are excellent sources for this material.

No book can be a substitute for regular interaction with a trial methodologist during both the planning stages of a clinical investigation and its analysis. I do not suggest passive reliance on such consultations, but intend to facilitate disseminating knowledge from which true collaborations between clinicians and trialists will result. Although many clinicians think of bringing their final data to a statistician, a collaboration will be most valuable during the design phase of a study when an experienced trialist may prevent serious methodologic errors, help streamline a study, or suggest ways to avoid costly mistakes.

The wide availability of computers is a mixed benefit for clinical research methodology. Although it facilitates accurate and timely keeping of data, modern computing also permits or encourages researchers to produce "statistical" reports without much attention to study design and without fully understanding assumptions, methods, limitations, and pitfalls of the procedures being employed. The ideas in this book are intended to counteract these tendencies. Good design inhibits potential errors by involving a statistical expert in the study as a collaborator from the beginning. Most aspects of the study will improve as a result including resource utilization, quality assurance, precision, and the scope of analyses. Good design can also simplify analyses by reducing bias and variability and removing the influence of complicating factors. In this way, number crunching becomes less important than sound statistical reasoning.

The student of clinical trials should also understand that the field is growing and changing in response to both biological and statistical developments. A picture of good methodology today may be inadequate in the near future. This is probably more true of analytic methods than design, where the fundamentals will change more slowly. Analysis methods often will depend on new statistical developments or theory. These in turn depend on 1) computing hardware, 2) reliable and accessible software, 3) training and re-training of trialists in the use of new methods, 4) acceptance of the procedure by the statistical and biological communities, and 5) sufficient time for the innovations to diffuse into practice.

Good trial design requires a willingness to examine many alternatives within the confines of reliably answering the basic biological question. The most common errors related to trial design are devoting insufficient resources or time to the study, rigidly using standard types of designs when better (e.g., more efficient) designs are available, or undoing the benefits of a good design with a poorly planned (or executed) analysis. I hope that the reader of this book will come to understand where there is much flexibility in the design and analysis of trials and where there is not.

1.1.2   Other sources of knowledge

The periodical literature related to clinical trials is large. I have attempted to provide current useful references for accessing it in this book. Aside from individual study reports, there are at least two journals strongly related to trials. The first is *Controlled Clinical Trials*, which is the official journal of the Society for Clinical Trials (mostly a U.S. organization). The journal was begun in 1980 and is devoted to trial methodology. The Society was founded in 1981 and its 1500 members meet yearly. A second helpful periodical source is *Statistics in Medicine*, which frequently has articles of interest to the trialist. It began publication in 1982 and is the official publication of the International Society for Clinical Biostatistics (mostly a European organization). These two societies have begun joint meetings every few years.

Many papers of importance to clinical trials and related statistical methods appear in various other applied statistical and clinical journals. One journal of particular interest to drug development researchers is the *Journal of Biopharmaceutical Statistics*. A useful general reference source is the journal *Biostatistica*, which contains abstracts from diverse periodicals. Statistical methodology for clinical trials appears in several journals. The topic was reviewed with an extensive bibliography by Simon [1991]. A more extensive bibliography covering trials broadly has been given by Hawkins [1991].

In addition to journals, there are a number of books and monographs dealing with clinical trials. The text by Meinert [1986] is a practical view of the infrastructure and administrative supports necessary to perform quality trials, especially randomized controlled trials. Freedman, Furberg, and DeMets [1982] and Pocock [1996] also discuss many conceptual and practical issues in their excellent books, which do not require extensive statistical background. There is a relatively short and highly readable book by Silverman [1985] with many real-world examples. In the field of cancer trials, Buyse, Staquet, and Sylvester [1984] is an excellent source. The book by Leventhal and Wittes [1988] is useful for a strong clinical orientation.

In the field of AIDS, a useful source is Finkelstein and Schoenfeld [1995]. The serious student should also be familiar with the classic papers by Peto et al. [1977a; 1977b]. Spilker [e.g., 1993] has written a large volume of material about clinical trials, much of it oriented toward pharmaceutical research and not statistical methods. Another useful reference with an industry perspective is Wooding [1994]. Data management is an important subject for investigators, but falls outside the scope of this book. The subject is probably made more complex by the fact that vastly more data are routinely collected during developmental trials than is needed to meet the objectives. Good sources of knowledge concerning data management include the book edited by Rondel, Varley, and Webb [1993] and an issue of *Controlled Clinical Trials* (April 1995) devoted to data management. Books on other relevant topics will be mentioned in context later.

Even in a very active program of clinical research, a relatively short exposure to the practical side of clinical trials cannot illustrate all of the important lessons. This is because it may take years for any single clinical trial, and many such studies, to yield all of their information useful for learning about methodology. Even so, the student of clinical trials will learn some lessons more quickly by being involved in an actual study, compared with simply studying theory. In this book, I illustrate many concepts with published trials. In this way, the reader can have the benefit of observing studies from a long-term perspective, which would otherwise be difficult to acquire.

1.1.3   Review of notation and terminology is helpful

Galileo said:

> The book of the universe is written in mathematical language, without which one wanders in vain through a dark labyrinth.

Statisticians light their dark labyrinth using abstract symbols (e.g., Greek letters) as a shorthand for important mathematical quantities and concepts. I will also use these symbols when appropriate in this book, because many ideas are troublesome to explain without good notation. However, because this book is not oriented primarily toward statistical theory, the use of symbols will be minimal and tolerable, even to non-mathematical readers. A review and explanation of common usage of symbols consistent with the clinical trials literature is given in Chapter 20. Because some statistical terms may be unfamiliar to some readers, definitions and examples are also provided. A list of abbreviations used in the book is also provided.

The terminology of clinical trials is not without its ambiguities. A recent firm effort has been made to standardize definitions in a dictionary devoted to clinical trial terminology [Meinert, 1996]. Most of the terms within this book are used in a way consistent with such definitions. A notable exception is that I propose and use explanatory alternatives to the widely used, uninformative, inconsistent, and difficult-to-generalize "phase I, II, III, and IV" designations for clinical trials. This topic is discussed in Chapter 4.

This book does not and cannot provide all of the technical statistical background that is needed to understand clinical trial design and analysis thoroughly. Fortunately, help is available in the form of good practical references. Examples are the books by Armitage and Berry [1994] and Marubini and Valsecchi [1995]. More concise summaries are given by Campbell and Machin [1990] and Everitt [1989]. More specialized references will be mentioned later.

1.1.4   Examples, data, and programs are provided

It is not possible to learn all the important lessons about clinical trials from classroom instruction or reading, nor is it possible for every student to be involved with actual trials as part of a structured course. This problem is most correctable for topics related to the analysis of trial results, where real data can be provided. For some examples used in this book, the data are provided in Chapter 19. Throughout the book, I have made a concerted effort to provide examples of trials that are instructive but small, so as to be digestible by the student. Also, computerized data files and programs to read and analyze them are provided on the Program and Data Disk, which accompanies the book. The same disk contains some sample size and related programs that can minimize certain design calculations. More powerful sample size (and other) design software that is available commercially is discussed in Chapter 7.

1.2   Summary

The premise of this book is that well-designed experimental research is an appropriate basis for clinical care. The purpose of this book is to address issues in the methodology of clinical trials in a format accessible to interested clinician scientists. The audience is intended to be practicing clinicians, statisticians, trialists, and others with a need for good clinical research methodology. The text attempts to relate to the clinical trials literature and offers examples with data and computer programs for some topics. A review of notation and terminology is also provided.

Chapter References

Armitage, P., and Berry, G. (1994). Statistical Methods in Medical Research, 3rd Edition. Oxford: Blackwell.

Buyse, M.E., Staquet, M.J., and Sylvester, R.J. (Eds.) (1984). Cancer Clinical Trials. Methods and Practice. Oxford: Oxford University Press.

Campbell, M.J., and Machin, D. (1990). Medical Statistics. Chichester: John Wiley & Sons.

Everitt, B.S. (1989). Statistical Methods for Medical Investigations. New York: Oxford University Press.

Finkelstein, D.M., and Schoenfeld, D.A. (Eds.) (1995). AIDS Clinical Trials. New York: Wiley-Liss.

Freidman, L.M., Furberg, C.D., and DeMets, D.L. (1985). Fundamentals of Clinical Trials, Second Edition. Littleton, Mass.: PSG Publishing.

Hawkins, B.S. (1991). Controlled clinical trials in the 1980s: A bibliography. Controlled Clin. Trials 12: 5-272.

Leventhal, B.G., and Wittes, R.E. (1988). Research Methods in Clinical Oncology. New York: Raven Press.

Marubini, E., and Valsecchi, M.G. (1995). Analysing Survival Data from Clinical Trials and Observational Studies. Chichester: John Wiley & Sons.

Meinert, C.L. (1986). Clinical Trials: Design, Conduct, and Analysis. Oxford: Oxford University Press.

Meinert, C.L. (1996). A Dictionary of Clinical Trials. Baltimore: Johns Hopkins Center for Clinical Trials.

Peto, R., Pike, M.C., Armitage, P., Breslow, N.E., Cox, D.R., Howard, S.V., Mantel, N., McPherson, K., Peto, J., and Smith, G. (1977a). Design and analysis of randomized clinical trials requiring prolonged observation of each patient. I. Introduction and design. Br. J. Cancer. 34: 585-612.

Peto, R., Pike, M.C., Armitage, P., Breslow, N.E., Cox, D.R., Howard, S.V., Mantel, N., McPherson, K., Peto, J., and Smith, G. (1977b). Design and analysis of randomized clinical trials requiring prolonged observation of each patient. II. Analysis and examples. Br. J. Cancer. 35: 1-39.

Pocock, S.J. (1996). Clinical Trials: A Practical Approach. New York: John Wiley & Sons.

Rondel, R.K., Varley, S.A., and Webb, C.F. (Eds.) (1993). Clinical Data Management. Chichester: John Wiley & Sons.

Silverman, W.A. (1985). Human Experimentation: A Guided Step Into the Unknown. Oxford: Oxford University Press.

Simon, R. (1991). A decade of progress in statistical methodology for clinical trials. Statistics in Med. 10: 1789-1817.

Spilker, W.A. (1991). Guide to Clinical Trials. New York: Raven Press.

Wooding, W.M. (1994). Planning Pharmaceutical Clinical Trials. New York: John Wiley & Sons.

CHAPTER 2

Clinical Trials and Research

2.1   Introduction

Just over 100 years ago, medicine was in a state of therapeutic nihilism. Nineteenth-century science had discovered that many diseases spontaneously improved without therapy, and that many popular treatments, such as certain natural products and blood letting, were ineffective. However, when scientists showed that diseases like pellagra and diabetes could have their effects relieved with medicinals, belief in treatment began to return. Following the discovery of penicillin and sulfanilamide in the twentieth century, the period of nihilism ended [Thomas, 1977].

More recently, discovery of the effectiveness of drugs for the treatment of cancer and high blood pressure, new antibiotics, and antipsychotics have demonstrated the value of treatment. The search for effective treatments, sorting out the benefits of competing therapies, and establishing optimum treatment combinations illustrate the importance of clinical investigation methods. The role of experimental design and analysis has become more important because of the greater detail in modern biological theories and the complexities in treatments of disease. The clinician is usually interested in small, but biologically important, treatment effects that can be obscured by non-rigorous studies. These interests push well-performed clinical trials to the very center of clinical research today, although it also creates problems for all aspects of clinical research [Ahrens, 1992].

2.1.1   Clinical reasoning requires generalizing

The word *clinical* is derived from the Greek *kline,* which means bed. In modern usage, *clinical* not only refers to the bedside, but is used more generally in referring to the care of human patients. Historically, the quantum unit of clinical reasoning has been the case history and the primary focus of clinical inference has been the individual patient. Before the widespread use of experimental trials, clinical methods of generalizing from the individual to the population were informal. The concepts of person-to-person variability and its sources were also described informally. Medical judgement can not be captured in a set of rules. Instead, it is a form of "tacit knowledge" [Polanyi, 1957].

Useful clinical observations are made against this background of reliable experience. Many valid generalizations have been made through incremental improvement of existing ideas. This process explains many advancements made in medicine and biology up to the twentieth century. Incremental improvement is a reliable, though slow method, which can optimize many complex processes. For example, the writing of this book proceeded largely by slightly improving earlier drafts. However, there was a foundation of design which greatly facilitated the entire process. In many circumstances, clinical trials can provide a similar foundation of design for clinical inference, greatly amplifying the benefits of careful observation.

2.1.2   Statistical reasoning emphasizes inference based on designed data production

The word *statistics* is derived from the Greek *statis* and *statista,* which mean *state.* The exact origin of the modern usage of the term *statistics* is obscured by the fact that the word was used mostly in a political context to describe territory, populations, trade, industry and related characteristics of countries from the 1500s until about 1850. A brief review of this history was given by Kendall, who stated that scholars began using data in a reasoned way around 1660 [Kendall, 1960]. The word *statistik* was used in 1748 to describe a particular body of analytic knowledge by the German scholar Gottfried Achenwall (1719-1772) in *Vorbereitung zur Staatswissenschaft* [Achenwall, 1748; Hankins, 1930]. The context seems to indicate that the word was already used in the way we use it now, but some later writers suggest that he originated it [Fang, 1972; Lilencron, 1967].

Today, statistics is the theoretical science or formal study of the inferential process, especially the planning and analysis of experiments, surveys, or observational studies. It has become a distinct field of study only in the twentieth century [Stigler, 1986]. Although based largely on probability theory, statistics is not, strictly speaking, a branch of mathematics. Even though the same methods of axioms, formal deductive reasoning, and logical proof are used in both statistics and mathematics, the fields are distinct in origin, theory, practice, and application.

Making reasonable and accurate inferences from data in the presence of uncertainty is an important and far-reaching intellectual skill. The application of this skill is not merely a collection of *ad hoc* tricks and techniques, an unfortunate view occasionally held by clinicians. The failure to master statistical concepts can lead to numerous errors and biases in medical research, a compendium of which is given by Andersen [1990]. Statistics is a way of thinking or an approach to everyday problems. It relies heavily on aspects of designed data production. Data alone are not sufficient and not all observations should be given equal weight for inferences.

Statistical reasoning is characterized by the following criteria:

1. Establishing an objective framework for conducting an investigation,
2. Placing of data and theory on an equal scientific footing,

3. Designing data production through experimentation,
4. Quantifying of the influence of chance,
5. Estimating systematic and random effects, and
6. Combining theory and data using formal methods.

Reasoning using these tools permits efficient use of information, time, and resources.

2.1.3 Clinical and statistical reasoning converge in research

Because of their different origins and purposes, clinical and statistical reasoning could be viewed as fundamentally incompatible by scientists who do not look further. In fact, the introduction of numerical comparisons and statistical methods into assessments of therapeutic efficacy has been resisted by medical practitioners at nearly every opportunity in the last 200 years [Matthews, 1995]. But the force that combines these different types of reasoning is research. The clinical researcher is one who investigates formal hypotheses arising from work in the clinic [Frei, 1982; Frei and Freireich, 1993].

Biological research requires two interdependent tasks that statistics does well: generalizing observations from few to many, and combining empirical and theory-based knowledge. In the science of clinical research, empirical knowledge comes from observation and data, while theory-based knowledge comes from either established biology or hypothesis. In statistics, the empirical knowledge comes from data or observations, while the theory-based knowledge is that of probability and determinism, formalized in mathematical models. Models specifically, and statistics in general, are the most efficient and useful way to make combinations of theory and observation.

This explains both the successful application of statistics to many diverse areas and the difficulty that some clinicians have in understanding and applying statistical modes of thought. In purely clinical tasks, there is relatively little need for statistical modes of reasoning. The best use and interpretation of diagnostic tests is one interesting exception. Clinical research is a different matter entirely and demands critical and quantitative views of research designs and data. To perform, report, and interpret clinical research studies requires statistical modes of reasoning. Nearly all important biological problems have a significant biometric component. Carter, Scheaffer, and Marks [1986] focused on this point appropriately when they said

> Statistics is unique among academic disciplines in that statistical thought is needed at every stage of virtually all research investigations, including planning the study, selecting the sample, managing the data, and interpreting the results.

The historical development of clinical trials has depended mostly on biological and medical advances, as opposed to applied mathematical or statistical developments. A broad survey of mathematical advances in the biological and medical sciences supports this interpretation [Lancaster, 1994]. For example, the experimental method was known to the Greeks, especially Strato of Lampsacus (c. 250 B.C.E.)

[Magner, 1979]. Gavarret gave a formal specification of the principles of medical statistics in 1840 [Gavarett, 1840]. In the 1920s, R. A. Fisher demonstrated and advocated the use of true experimental designs, especially randomization, in studying biological problems [Fisher, 1935; Box, 1980].

Yet it was the mid 1900s before the methodology of clinical trials began to be applied earnestly. The delay in applying existing quantitative methods to clinical problem solving was probably a consequence of many factors, including inaccurate models of disease, lack of drugs and other therapeutic options being developed, physician resistance, an authoritarian medical system that relied heavily on expert opinion, and the absence of the infrastructure needed to support clinical trials. An excellent historical review of statistical developments behind clinical trials is given by Gehan and Lemak [1994]. Broader discussions of the history of trials are given by Bull [1959], Meinert [1986], and Pocock [1996]. It is interesting to read early discussions of trial methods [e.g., Herdan, 1953] to see issues of concern that persist today.

Since the 1940s, clinical trials have seen a widening scope of applicability. This increase is a consequence of many factors, including the questioning of medical dogma, notable success in applying experimental designs in both the clinical and basic science fields, governmental funding priorities, regulatory oversight of drugs and medical devices with its more stringent demands, and development of applied statistical methods. In addition, the public, governmental, industrial, and academic response to important diseases like cardiovascular disease, cancer, and AIDS has increased the willingness of, and necessity for, clinicians to engage in structured experiments to answer important questions reliably [Gehan and Schneiderman, 1990; Greenhouse, 1990; Halperin, DeMets, and Ware, 1990]. Finally, the correct perception that well-done clinical trials are robust, i.e., insensitive to deviations from many underlying assumptions, has led to their wider use. Health professionals who wish to conduct and evaluate clinical research need to become competent in this field.

2.1.4   Clinical trials can be rigorously defined

An *experiment* is a series of observations made under conditions controlled by the scientist. A *clinical trial* is an experiment testing medical treatments on human subjects. The clinical investigator controls factors that contribute to variability, bias, the application of the treatment, ascertainment of outcome, and analysis. Experiments attempt to resolve an uncertainty that has been explicitly specified by isolating both the control variable (i.e., treatment) and the outcome from extraneous influences. *Design* is the process or structure that isolates the factors of interest.

Using the word "experiment" can make some observers of clinical trials uncomfortable. Terminology can convey values, especially to patients considering participating in a clinical trial. The informal definition of "experiment" often implies ignorance, and it can be used pejoratively to indicate that the experimenter lacks respect for the study participants. For example, consider this article from a national daily newspaper:

> Patients are not always fully informed that they are guinea pigs in medical research studies authorized by the Food and Drug Administration, *The* (Cleveland) *Plain Dealer* said. The newspaper analysis of FDA files found that in 4,154 inspections of researchers testing new drugs on humans, the FDA cited more than 53% for failing to fully disclose the experimental nature of the work [USA Today, 1996].

This was the full article, which aside from other errors, tends to equate being "guinea pigs", with "experiment", and deception. However, the use of the word "experiment" in a scientific context to describe clinical trials has a tradition [Beecher, 1970; Fleiss, 1986; Freund, 1972; Fried, 1974; Hill, 1963; Katz, 1972; McNeill, 1993; Silverman, 1985]. The usage of this term in this book will always be according to the definition above, as in *conducting an experiment,* rather than indicating disrespect for, or *experimenting on,* study participants.

The definition of "clinical trial" does not require that a comparison of therapies be made, although this is true of an important class of study designs. A clinical trial requires only the formal structure of an experiment, particularly control over treatment assignment by the investigator. Definitions aside, Sir Austin Bradford Hill [1963] stated it quite well:

> In the assessment of a treatment, medicine always has proceeded, and always must proceed, by way of experiment. The experiment may merely consist in giving the treatment to a particular patient or series of patients, and of observing and recording what follows – with all the difficulty of interpretation, of distinguishing the *propter hoc* from the *post hoc*. Nevertheless, even in these circumstances and in face of the unknown a question has been asked of Nature, and it has been asked by means of trial in the human being. There can be no possible escape from that. This is *human* experimentation – of one kind at least. *Somebody* must be the first to exhibit a new treatment in man. *Some patient*, whether for good or ill, must be the first to be exposed to it.

In addition to being true experiments, clinical trials possess important general characteristics of the scientific method. These include: *instumentalizing perception* or *measurement,* which enhances repeatability and quantification; *externalizing plans and memory* in a written record, to facilitate reference and defense; *control of extraneous factors* as part of the study design (e.g., using internal controls and methods to control bias); and submitting completed work to *external recognition, verification, or disproof.* Well-designed studies also provide evidence that can falsify theory, a hallmark of the scientific method [Popper, 1959]. All of these fundamental and general characteristics of scientific inquiry are integrated in the modern practice of clinical trials.

Sometimes investigations that superficially appear to be clinical trials are not. Examples are so-called "seeding trials", occasionally conducted by pharmaceutical companies as marketing tools, because they encourage physicians to prescribe a new drug [Kessler et al., 1994]. The distinction between such efforts and true clinical trials can be made by examining the purposes and design of the study. Warning signs for seeding trials include 1) a design that cannot support the research goals, 2) investigators are recruited because of their prescribing habits rather than scientific expertise, 3) the sponsor provides unrealistically high reimbursements for participation, 4) minimal data or those of little scientific interest are collected, 5) the study is conducted through the sponsor's marketing program rather than research division, and 6) the agent being tested is similar to numerous therapeutic alternatives.

2.1.5 Trials and statistical methods fit within a spectrum of clinical research

Clinical experiments do not originate and reveal their findings in isolation. Trials co-exist with clinical and pre-clinical research of all types, some of which is supportive of their findings and some of which is not. The following categorization of clinical research, adapted from Ahrens [1992], shows how designed experiments fit within the spectrum of clinical research. Based on scientific objectives, sponsor funding, and technical skills and training of investigators, clinical research can be divided into seven areas. These are:

1. Studies of disease mechanisms. The studies may be either descriptive or analytic but require laboratory methods and clinical observations under controlled conditions. Examples are metabolic and pharmacologic studies.

2. Studies of disease management. These studies involve evaluations of developing treatments, modalities, or preventive measures and have outcomes with direct clinical relevance. Often, internal controls and true experimental designs will be used. Most **clinical trials** fit within this category.

3. In vitro studies on materials of human origin. These are studies using observational designs and blood, tissue, or other samples that attempt to show associations thought to be clinically important. Series of surgical or pathologic studies are often this type.

4. Models of human health and disease processes. These studies include animal and theoretical (e.g., mathematical) models of disease, often used to guide laboratory and clinical investigations.

5. Field surveys. These are descriptive or analytic studies of risk factors or disease correlates in populations. Examples include epidemiologic and genetic studies.

6. Technology development. This type of research includes development and mechanistic testing of new diagnostic and therapeutic methods.. Examples of technology developed in these types of studies include imaging devices and methods, diagnostics, vaccines, and applied analytic methods such as biostatistical methods.

7. Health care delivery. These studies focus on economic and social effects of health care practice and delivery. Examples include studies of education and training, cost effectiveness, health care access, and financing.

Any one or several of these types of clinical research studies can relate directly to clinical trials. For example, they may be precursor, follow-up, or parallel studies essential to the design and interpretation of a clinical trial. In any case, experimental designs have a central role in the spectrum of clinical research studies.

2.2   Differences in Statistical Perspectives

2.2.1   Philosophy of inference divides statisticians

At least two philosophies of statistical inference coexist today. The view and practice held by a majority of statisticians is "frequentist", a name derived from the definition of probability in terms of frequencies of outcomes or long-run behavior. This school of thought makes use of tools familiar to many clinicians, such as significance tests, confidence intervals, and unbiased estimators. An alternative view or method of inference is called "Bayesian", named for the English clergyman Thomas Bayes. The Bayesian school uses ideas loosely associated with Bayes' posthumous publication from 1763 [Bayes, 1763; 1958]. A characteristic of the Bayesian method is its formal incorporation of information from prior knowledge or from outside the experiment. This often necessitates accepting subjective notions of probability or degree of belief. Examples are given later. The use of subjective probabilities is one of the major sources of controversy about Bayesian methods.

Bayesian methods offer some potential advantages for the design and analysis of clinical trials. Once the investigator describes uncertainty through a probability distribution, the Bayesian method offers a formal and consistent process for solving inferential problems. Bayesian methods are coherent, which means that they do not violate logical axioms of uncertainty. Non-Bayesian methods violate such axioms in some circumstances. A large body of knowledge from outside the study may be important in designing, analyzing, and interpreting it. Frequentist methods cannot account for this information in a formal way. Bayesian methods yield probability statements about the unknowns from which inferences can be made.

In many cases, Bayesian approaches lead to the same or similar procedures as those employed by frequentist statisticians. In other cases, the procedures and results are different, fueling a debate as to how the approaches can be justified. Discussion of Bayesian inference and approaches can be found in Cornfield [1969], O'Hagan [1994], Lindley [1965], Barnett [1982], or Spiegelhalter, Freedman, and Parmar [1994]. The contrast between Bayesian and frequentist views of clinical trials can be seen succinctly in papers (and the accompanying discussion) by Berry [1993] and Whitehead [1993]. For an in-depth discussion of a Bayesian perspective in a real-world clinical trial, see Kadane [1996]. A concise and practical discussion of some issues related to confidence intervals is given by Burton [1994].

An approach to the statistical aspects of clinical trials must depend partly on practical grounds. Because of computational difficulties, Bayesian methods have not been widely accessible or used by statisticians until recently. Reflecting this, the approaches to clinical trial design and analysis outlined in this book are predominantly frequentist in origin. This is not so much an endorsement of that philosophical perspective as an acquiescence to simplicity and the preponderance of techniques likely to be encountered in the clinical trials literature. Frequentist techniques have been presented essentially without alternatives to clinicians for 50 years.

In some places in this book, a Bayesian perspective is sketched alongside the frequentist one. In other circumstances, Bayesian methods exist but have not been discussed. Whenever possible, the student of clinical trials should investigate related Bayesian methods to see if they might be better suited than traditional methods to the problem at hand. One area where the approaches yield substantially different results is in monitoring and interim analyses of trials, discussed in Chapter 10. It is my sense that many clinicians, given the chance, might naturally prefer inference based on Bayesian thinking, except that the techniques are often mathematically more complex than frequentist procedures and have not had as many advocates in the statistical profession.

Although differences between frequentist and Bayesian methods are consequential, there are more important methodologic concerns in clinical trials. For example, it is important to use methods to increase precision and eliminate bias when designing studies. The proper counting of events and emphasis on estimation is essential when conducting analyses. When reporting results, objectivity and thoroughness are the keys. Each of these issues is probably of more practical importance than the philosophical differences between frequentists and Bayesians.

2.2.2   Statistical procedures are not standardized

All clinical trials reflect features of true experimental designs. Statistical reasoning is essential in designing the architecture of the trial, choosing a sample size, deciding to stop an ongoing study early, and in analyzing and interpreting trial results. Even with this common backdrop, there are many issues and approaches to clinical trials that are not standardized. Some lack of standardization is a consequence of making study designs and analyses responsive to the needs of a specific biological question. Nuances in the scientific question may drive substantial differences in design. An example is the use of placebos in comparative trials. It may not be ethical or scientifically appropriate to use placebo controls when standard treatments are known to provide benefit for a serious illness. In self-limited diseases, or those with no known treatments, a trial with a placebo group could be the most appropriate and informative.

Lack of standardization also reflects the fact that study designs and statistical methods of analysis are not fixed consequences of the research question or data collected. To understand this, it is important to distinguish between *standards* and *standardization*. Having standards implies a minimal acceptable quality or depth of sophistication in design and analysis of trials. This is usually considered a good idea. Standardization implies uniformity, which is almost never the best idea for clinical investigations.

Different researchers could perform different analyses, possibly yielding different inferences. When this occurs, it is often the result of selecting one statistical approach instead of another, although both may be perfectly appropriate for a given research question. Also, the same data may be relevant to different clinical, biological, or analytic issues. However, the same situation arises because of fundamental philosophical differences of opinion about the correct quantitative approach to the bio-logical question. In these and other ways, clinical trials are as subject to differences of opinion as other areas of scientific inquiry.

Example

There are several different frequentist approaches to design, data monitoring, analysis, inference, and reporting used by clinical trialists. Important differences between the approaches can be obscured by the complexities inherent in clinical research. However, it is essential to understand the basic properties and strengths and weaknesses of each approach, because they affect other methods employed in trials. The main approaches could be labeled 1) estimation, 2) hypothesis testing, and 3) significance testing.

Estimation is oriented toward providing reliable and valid estimates of a statistically defined quantity (parameter). Aside from being clinically important, the parameter characterizes a convenient statistical model that provides a framework for estimation and determining the precision of the estimate. A simple example is a population average (or difference in averages) which can often be characterized by the mean and variance of a Gaussian distribution.

Hypothesis testing is a tool useful for making certain structured decisions. In this approach, we either reject a (null) hypothesis, or fail to reject it, according to a predefined criterion, which can be quantified as a p-value. The chance of rejecting the null hypothesis when it is, in fact, correct is fixed by the criterion. The p-value is inconsequential except to observe if it is larger or smaller than the criterion. In contrast, significance testing attempts to evaluate the strength of evidence against a hypothesis by using the magnitude of the p-value. Unfortunately, the p-value is not fully capable of this task. All of these approaches are employed routinely in analyzing clinical trials, sometimes even within the same analysis and report. Each will be discussed in an appropriate place later in this book.

2.2.3   Practical controversies exist

Philosophical differences aside, there are many practical issues about clinical trials that generate disagreement. For a condensed discussion, see Byar, Simon, Friedewald, et al. [1976]. Lack of uniformity in a developing discipline can be good, because it stimulates creativity and questioning of assumptions. But non-uniformity can also imply that incorrect or suboptimal procedures are being applied in some clinical trials. This could be a problem if such errors are not evident from the published reports or if other investigators are not knowledgeable enough to detect the mistakes. In a number of areas of trial design and conduct, there is no general agreement about the best standard to recommend. Some of these, listed below, are actively evolving, and others are likely to remain somewhat contentious.

The use of *randomization* is sometimes controversial. It raises some ethical concerns (discussed in Chapter 3), and may be inconvenient or unnecessary in some circumstances. However, the advantages of randomization are considerable and it is not very controversial when properly applied. Details are discussed in Chapter 9.

Intention-to-treat is the idea that subjects in a randomized clinical trial should be analyzed according to the treatment group to which they were assigned, even if they did not receive the intended treatment or received only a portion of it. This perspective is usually supported by statisticians, because it yields desirable properties for testing the null hypothesis of no treatment difference. Many clinicians and other investigators often favor analyses based on treatment actually received, an approach which is advertised as more accurately estimating the true biological effect of the treatment. Their claim may not be true. This is an important topic and will be covered in depth in Chapter 11.

Even in randomized trials, imbalances between the treatment groups can occur by chance. Randomization theory permits us to ignore such imbalances when testing treatment differences, although pragmatic concerns often lead to the use of *adjustment* procedures through statistical modeling. These methods essentially view the trial as a database (although perhaps an exceptionally high-quality one) and yield estimates of treatment effect "controlled" for covariate imbalances. Trialists do not agree on the need to perform these types of analyses or what factors should be used for adjustment. This topic is discussed in Chapter 13.

An approach to eliminating the need for adjusted analyses is to ensure that the treatment groups are balanced with respect to influential prognostic variables. One method for inducing balance is to use *stratification* with blocked treatment assignments, which forces exact balance of the stratification variables frequently during the trial. Although theoretically unnecessary as suggested above, debates about whether or not to use stratification routinely are a minor issue in trial design. Additional details are discussed in Chapter 9.

The expense and complexities of clinical trials limit their wide applicability. However, there is a broad need for reliable and unbiased inferences like those that usually result from well-performed randomized comparisons. This tension has led to *large-scale trials* (LST), discussed in Chapter 4, which test the worth of interventions in large populations without the extensive data collection and other infrastructure needed for many trials. The idea of conducting LSTs is not especially controversial but establishing the best methods for doing so and defining relaxed notions of treatment and eligibility in such studies can be a problem.

In spite of high-profile instances of enhanced inferences arising from their use, *overviews* or *meta-analyses* remain a somewhat controversial tool for assessing evidence from multiple clinical trials. Sources of difficulty that can limit the utility of overviews include the fact that each study included may have a slightly different design, and the possibility that not all relevant studies or the underlying data are accessible to the persons performing the overview. This could be a problem if only the published literature is used as a source of information about trials performed. Overviews are discussed in Chapter 17.

There are other areas that create controversy among trialists but are not primarily statistical in nature. These include aspects of reporting, quality control of trial data, and political intrusions into and regulation of trials. Although each of these topics is important, they will not be covered here.

2.3 Use of Trials

2.3.1 Clinical trials are ubiquitous

The statistical concepts on which trial methods are based are usually well grounded and very reliable, often having been of service to agriculture, industrial quality control, and reliability testing. Today, trials are used to develop and test interventions in nearly all areas of medicine and public health [Office of Technology Assessment, 1983]. Some of the specialties most active in using trials are cancer, cardiovascular disease, and AIDS. These areas share a need to evaluate new drugs, drug combinations, and other treatment modalities. However, trial methods can also be used to assess *treatment algorithms* as compared with isolated interventions, making them suitable to a wide array of therapeutic and prevention questions.

Many medical *devices* have not been subject to the same comparative testing as drugs. For example, recent problems surrounding the use of silicone breast implants might have been prevented or anticipated and lessened if more structured methods of evaluation had been used in their development. This points to another force supporting the use of trials as reliable evaluation tools: regulatory agencies such as the Food and Drug Administration. For clarifying safety and efficacy concerns about new treatments prior to marketing approval, randomized controlled trials are excellent and irreplaceable tools [Leber, 1991].

Learning about the full scope and numbers of clinical trials in any field is probably impossible. In the field of cancer, details regarding many clinical trials are available through the Physician Data Query (PDQ) system. PDQ was begun in 1984 and reflects an effort to make physicians treating cancer patients aware of the studies being performed, expert opinion about the trials, and a sketch of the treatment protocol [Hubbard, Martin, and Thurn, 1995]. Currently, there are 1500 cancer clinical trials listed in PDQ and these are updated monthly. Both on-line computer access and paper copy is available [Pyros Education Group, 1996]. Similar resources in other fields, such as heart disease and AIDS, where clinical trials are numerous and important, do not seem to be available.

The potential use of clinical trials in developing surgical treatments and some medical devices is similar to that in medical disciplines. However, unlike drugs and many medical devices, surgical interventions are often developed at low cost by individuals or small groups, are usually not oriented toward disease prevention, are usually undertaken with patients having a good prognosis, and are often not amenable to blinded methods of assessment. Also, surgical treatments often increase short-term risks to higher levels than most medical interventions. Small developmental trials may not always capture all of the experience-based knowledge of the surgeon with regard to a particular procedure. These differences do not prevent surgical therapies from being evaluated by controlled clinical trials. Most clinical trial methods can extend directly to the evaluation of surgical treatments.

2.3.2   Trials can provide confirmatory evidence

Aside from testing novel ideas, clinical trials are frequently used to test or reinforce findings from earlier studies that may be unconvincing. There are a variety of reasons why two or more trials might be performed while studying essentially the same research question (usually by different sets of investigators). In some circumstances, this may happen inadvertently. For example, in pharmaceutical studies, the onset or planning of a trial may be confidential and could be undertaken simultaneously by different companies using slightly different treatments. In retrospect, these trials may be seen as confirmatory. The same situation may arise in different countries for scientific or political reasons.

Confirmatory trials may also be planned. When the results of a new trial seems to contradict prevailing biological theory, many researchers or practitioners may be unconvinced by the findings, particularly if there are methodological problems with the study design, as there frequently are. This could be true, for example, when there is relatively little supporting evidence from preclinical experiments or epidemiologic studies. Confirmatory trials may be needed to establish the new findings as being correct and convince researchers to modify their theories. When the magnitude of estimated treatment effects is disproportionate to what one might expect biologically, a similar need for confirmatory studies may arise.

There are numerous types of design flaws, methodologic errors, problems with study conduct, or analysis and reporting mistakes that can render clinical trials less than convincing. We would expect the analysis and reporting errors to be correctable if the design of the study is good, but they are frequently accompanied by more serious shortcomings. In any case, trials with obvious flaws are open to criticism, which may limit their widespread acceptance. Such skepticism may motivate a confirmatory study.

Finally, there is a tendency for studies with positive results to find their way preferentially into the literature (publication bias). Some of these errors are the result of chance, data-driven hypotheses, or emphasis on analyses of subsets rather than the entire comparison groups. Readers of trials seem to protect themselves instinctively from uncritically accepting results as final until the findings have been verified independently. The way in which practitioners use the information from clinical trials seems to be very complex. An interesting perspective on this is given by Henderson [1995] in the context of breast cancer clinical trials. Medicine is a conservative science and behavior usually does not change on the basis of one study. Thus, confirmatory trials of some type may be necessary to provide a firm basis for changing clinical practice.

2.3.3   Clinical trials are unwieldy and messy

Like many scientific endeavors, clinical trials are constrained by fiscal and human resources, ethical concern for the participants, and the current scientific and political milieu. Trials are unwieldy and expensive to conduct. They require collaborations between patients, physicians, nurses, data managers, and methodologists. They are subject to extensive review and oversight at the institutional level, by funding agencies, and by regulators. Trials consume significant time and resources and, like all experiments, can be in error. Multi-institutional trials may cost from millions up to hundreds of millions of dollars and often take more than five years to complete. Clinical trials studying treatments for prevention of disease are among the most important but cumbersome, expensive, and lengthy to conduct.

Certain studies may be feasible at one time, given all these constraints, but infeasible a few months or years later (or earlier). In other words, many studies have a "window of opportunity" during which they can be accomplished and during which they are more likely to have an impact on clinical practice. For comparative trials, this window often exists relatively early after the process of development of a therapy. Later, clinicians' opinions about the treatment solidify, even without good data, and economic incentives can favor or disfavor a new treatment. Then, many practitioners are reluctant to undertake or participate in a comparative clinical trial. The issues surrounding a trial of extracorporeal membrane oxygenation (ECMO) in infants with respiratory failure illustrate, in part, the window of opportunity. This trial is discussed in Chapters 3 and 9.

Clinical trials are frequently messier than we would like. A highly experienced and respected basic science researcher tells the story of an experiment he instructed a lab technician to perform by growing tumors in laboratory rats:

> Once we decided to set up an immunologic experiment to study host defenses. I was out of town, and I had a new technician on board, and I asked him to order 40 rats. When I returned, I discovered we had a mixture of Sprague-Dawley, Wistar, and Copenhagen rats. Furthermore, their ages ranged from 3 months to 2 years. I had asked him to inject some tumor cells and was horrified to find out that he had used three tumor lines of prostate cancer cells and administered 10^3 to 10^8 cells in various parts of the animals and on different days during a period of 2 weeks. Unfortunately, 20% of the animals escaped during the experiment so we could present data only on age-matched controls [Coffey, 1978].

At this point, we might begin to lose confidence in the findings of this experiment as a controlled laboratory trial. However, these circumstances might well describe a clinical trial under normal circumstances, and it could be a useful one because of the amount of structure used successfully. These types of complications are common in clinical trials, not because of the investigator's laxity, but because of the nature of working with sick humans. Alternatives to clinical trials are usually messier than trials themselves.

Trials are more common now than ever before, because they are the most reliable means of making correct inferences about treatments in certain commonly encountered clinical circumstances. For example, when treatment differences are about the same size as patient-to-patient variability and/or the bias from flawed research designs, a rigorous clinical trial is the only reliable way to separate the treatment effect from the noise. Physicians are often genuinely interested in treatments that improve standard therapy only moderately. We can be sure that patients are always interested in even small to moderate treatment benefits. The more common or widespread a disease is, the more important even modest improvements in outcome will be. Thus, clinical trials may often be necessary to control for the effects of bias and variability, which can obscure small but important treatment effects.

Well-performed clinical trials offer other advantages over most uncontrolled studies. These include a complete and accurate specification of the study population at base line, rigorous definitions of treatment, bias control, and active ascertainment of endpoints. These features will be discussed later.

2.3.4   Other methods are valid for making clinical inferences

Historically, many medical advances have been made without the formal methods of comparison found in controlled clinical trials; in particular, without randomization, statistical design, and analysis. For example, vitamins, insulin, and many drugs and antimicrobials (e.g., penicillin), vaccines, and tobacco smoke have had their effects convincingly demonstrated without using controlled clinical trials. Studies that demonstrated these effects were epidemiological, historically controlled, or, in some cases, uncontrolled. Thus, true experimental designs are not the only path to advancing medical knowledge.

Recently, ganciclovir was approved by the U.S. Food and Drug Administration for the treatment of retinitis caused by cytomegalovirus in patients with human immunodeficiency virus (HIV) infection. The evidence in favor of ganciclovir efficacy consisted of a relatively small but well-performed study using historical controls [Jabs et al., 1989]. The treatment benefit was large, supported by other data, and the toxicity profile of the treatment was acceptable. (However, it took a clinical trial to establish that another drug, foscarnet, was associated with longer survival and similar visual outcome as ganciclovir.)

In contrast, consider the difficulty in inferring the benefit of zidovudine (AZT) treatment in prolonging the survival of HIV positive patients from retrospective studies [e.g., Moore, Hidalgo, and Sugland, 1991]. Although AZT appeared to prolong survival in this study, the control group had a shorter survival than untreated patients earlier in the epidemic. Sicker patients did not live long enough to receive AZT, making the treatment appear beneficial. This illustrates the difficulty in defining treatment in retrospect. Some issues related to using observational data for assessing AIDS treatments are discussed by Gail [1996].

Studies based on nonexperimental comparative designs can provide valid and convincing evidence of treatment efficacy. Using nonexperimental designs to make reliable treatment inferences requires five things: 1) the treatment of interest must occur naturally, 2) the study subjects have to provide valid observations for the biological question, 3) the natural history of the disease with standard therapy, or in the absence of the intervention, must be well-known, 4) the effect of the treatment or intervention must be large enough to overshadow random error and bias, and 5) evidence of efficacy must be consistent with other biological knowledge. These constraints are sometimes difficult to satisfy, because they point to factors that are beyond the investigator's control, particularly the need to have a large treatment effect.

Nonexperimental designs

There are at least three types of nonexperimental designs that can yield convincing evidence of treatment differences when the above assumptions are met: epidemiologic studies, historically controlled trials, and databases. Epidemiologic designs are an efficient way to study rare events and can control some important sources of random error and bias. They represent a lower standard of evidence for treatment studies, because, without randomization, the investigator cannot control unknown confounders. Nevertheless, they are a valuable source of evidence. These strengths and weaknesses are typified by case-control designs, which compare exposures (determined retrospectively) in subjects with a condition versus "controls" without the condition. The design is not useful for studying the effects of treatment because of the reasons cited and because it is difficult to define "treatment" retrospectively.

Jenks and Volkers [1992] outlined a number of factors possibly associated with increased cancer risk. Some were biologically plausible while others seem to be based only on statistical associations. Apparent increases in cancer risks for factors such as electric razors and height could be due to bias (or chance). In any case, small increases in risk are at the limit of resolution of observational study designs. Many provocative associations between human disease and environmental exposures or other factors are not amenable to study by clinical trial designs, because the exposures or factors are not under the experimenter's control. A good example of this is the question of right- versus left-handedness and its relationship to longevity [Halpern and Coren, 1991].

Historically controlled studies can also provide convincing evidence. Although improvements in supportive care, temporal trends, or different methods of evaluation for the same disease can render these studies uninterpretable, there are circumstances in which they are valid and convincing. An example might be the study of promising new treatments in advanced diseases with a uniformly poor prognosis. A specific example of this is genetically engineered tumor vaccines, tested in patients with advanced cancer. Large beneficial treatment effects could show themselves by prolonging survival far beyond that which is known to be possible using conventional therapy. However, consider how unreliable treatment inferences based on historical controls would be in a disease like AIDS, where supportive care and treatment of complications have improved so much in the last 10–15 years. Silverman [1985] gives some striking examples of time trends in infectious disease mortality. Stroke mortality has also shown clinically significant secular trends [Bonita and Beaglehole, 1996; Brown et al., 1996]. Similar problems can be found with historical controls in many diseases [Dupont, 1985].

Database studies are sometimes suggested as a valid way of making treatment inferences. Such studies are convenient when the data are available, inexpensive to conduct, and may be based on a very large number of patients. For example, patients treated at a single institution may be followed with the help of a database that facilitates both clinical management and asking research questions. In such situations, treatment selection is partly an outcome and partly a predictor of how the patient is doing. Therefore, treatment comparisons are suggestive, but not definitive tests of relative efficacy. All of these study designs will be discussed in more detail in Chapter 4.

2.3.5 Trials are difficult to apply in some circumstances

Aside from valid methods of inference other than trials, designed experiments may be difficult to apply in some settings. In oncology, there are many conditions requiring multiple therapies or modalities for treatment. Although the number of factors is theoretically manageable by study design, practical limitations can prevent the use of traditional clinical trials to evaluate systematically treatment combinations and interactions. Similarly, when minor changes in a complex therapy are needed, a trial may be an impractical or inappropriate thing to do. In very early developmental studies, such as for medical devices or surgery, when the technique or treatment is changing significantly or rapidly, formal trials may be unhelpful and could slow the developmental process.

Trials may be difficult to apply when studying treatments that depend on proficiency. Technical skills, such as treatment timing, dosage, or modifications might be required for some treatments. Proficiency may require that specific ancillary treatments be given. These problems could arise in complex diagnostic or therapeutic procedures, such as surgery. Well-designed trials can often isolate the therapeutic component of interest, but this may not always be the case. When treatments are difficult to study because they depend on proficiency, they may also be of lesser interest because they are hard to generalize to clinical practitioners at large.

Comparative trials may have limited applicability, because of human factors, such as ethical considerations, or strongly held beliefs of practitioners. Logistical difficulties prevent many trials which could otherwise theoretically be appropriate. For example, the AIDS epidemic motivated trialists to examine many basic assumptions about how studies were designed and conducted [Byar, Schoenfeld, Green et al., 1990]. Time and money may prevent the implementation of some trials. Trials are also not the right tool for studying rare outcomes in large cohorts or some diagnostic modalities. However, in all these cases, the methods used to gather data or otherwise to design methods to answer the biological question can benefit from quantification, structure, and statistical modes of thought. Bailar et al. [1984] suggest a framework for evaluating studies without internal controls. This provides additional support for the value of studying trial methodology.

Clinical trials can be difficult to understand unless the model of disease and the treatment mechanism fit conventional knowledge. A controversial illustration of this is a recent randomized clinical trial, funded by the Uniformed Services University of the Health Sciences (USUHS), studying the effect of therapeutic touch on pain and infection in burn victims. A brief description of the intervention is:

> The idea behind the practice of Therapeutic Touch is that the human energy field is abundant and flows in balanced patterns in health but is depleted and/or unbalanced in illness or injury. The Therapeutic Touch practitioner assesses the patient's energy field patterns with his/her hands to identify areas of depleted, congested, blocked, or unbalanced energy. Then, the Therapeu-

tic Touch treatment consists of a series of techniques implemented to replenish, clear, modulate and rebalance the patient's energy field patterns [Turner, 1994].

In this study, one group of patients was treated by a nurse trained in therapeutic touch, while the other was treated by a nurse who was trained to mimic the treatment. Because the patients had first, second, or third degree burns on 5 to 70 percent of their bodies, the practitioners did not actually touch the study subjects, but only moved their hands over them. Care was taken to train the mimics so their hand movements appeared real. This study was severely criticized by Selby and Scheiber [1996], because of the unconventional model of disease, the fact that patients were not actually touched, and the mimic or sham treatment control group. The results of the study have not been published as of this writing.

In a few circumstances, biological knowledge may suggest that trials would be futile. For example, suppose a disease can result from a defect in any one of several metabolic or genetic pathways, and that the population is heterogeneous with respect to such defects. Treatments that target only one of the pathways are not likely to be effective in everyone. Therefore, clinical trials of such treatments will probably not be informative, unless they are done in a restricted population.

2.3.6   Randomized studies can be initiated early

While comparative clinical trials may not be the method of choice for making treatment inferences in some circumstances, there are many situations where it is advantageous to implement trials early in the process of developing a new therapy. Some clinical trials methodologists have called for "randomization from the first patient" to reflect these circumstances [Chalmers, 1975a, 1975b; Spodick, 1983]. The window of opportunity for performing a randomized trial may only exist early and can close as investigators gather more knowledge of the treatment. Many disincentives to experimentation such as practitioner bias, economic factors, and ethical constraints can arise later.

Reasons why very early initiation of randomized trials are desirable include: 1) the ethical climate is conducive to, or even requires it, 2) high-quality scientific evidence may be most useful early, 3) early trials delay or prevent widespread adoption of ineffective therapies, and 4) non-randomized designs used later may yield useful evidence. These points may be particularly important when no or few treatments are available for a serious disease (consider the history of AIDS) or when the new therapy is known to be safe (e.g., some disease-prevention trials). Many times, randomized trials yield important information about ancillary or secondary endpoints that would be difficult to obtain in other ways.

There are also reasons why randomization from the first patient may be difficult or impossible to apply. These include: 1) the best study design and protocol may depend on information that is not available early (e.g., the correct dose of a drug), 2) adequate resources may not be available, 3) investigators may be unduly influenced by a few selected case reports, 4) patients, physicians, and sponsors may be biased, 5) the trial may not accrue well enough to be feasible, and 6) sample size and other design parameters may be impossible to judge without preliminary trials. When safe and effective treatments are already available, there may not be much incentive to conduct randomized trials early. For examples of randomized trials initiated early, see Chalmers [1975b], Garceau et al. [1964], and Resnick et al. [1968].

2.4   Summary

Clinical and statistical thinking are not incompatible, but complementary. The goal of both types of reasoning is generalization. The clinical approach generalizes primarily on a biological basis, while statistical modes of reasoning generalize primarily on the basis of data. Research broadly and clinical trials specifically require a combination of clinical and statistical reasoning. This leads to a formal definition of a clinical trial as a designed experiment.

There is no approach to inference upon which all statisticians agree. The two most common schools of inference, frequentist and Bayesian, have different approaches to using information from within and outside the experiment. The differences can be consequential for the design and analysis of clinical trials. Even within the frequentist school, methods are not universal.

Although trials can be unwieldy because of their size, complexity, duration, and cost, they are applied in many areas of medicine and public health. While not the only method for making valid inferences, clinical trials are suited to situations where it is important to learn about treatment effects or differences that are about the same magnitude as the random error and bias that invariably characterize medical studies. Investigators should be alert to circumstances where the window of opportunity to conduct randomized trials occurs early.

2.5   Questions for Discussion

1. Are there situations in which it would be difficult or inefficient to perform clinical trials? Discuss.

2. Are there circumstances or examples of clinical trials that do not have all the characteristics of the scientific method? Give specific examples if you can.

3. Historically, statistical methods have been stimulated by gambling, astronomy, agriculture, manufacturing, economics, and medicine. Briefly sketch the importance of these for developing statistical methods. Within medicine, what fields have stimulated clinical trials methods the most? Why?

4. Discuss reasons why and why not randomized prevention trials, particularly those employing treatments like diet, trace elements, and vitamins, should be conducted without "developmental" trials.

Chapter References

Achenwall, G. (1748). Vorbereitung zur Staatswissenschaft. This became the introduction to: Staatsverfassung der heutigen vornehmsten europäischen Reiche und Völker im Grundrisse. Göttingen, 1749.

Ahrens, E.H. (1992). The Crisis in Clinical Research: Overcoming Institutional Obstacles. New York: Oxford University Press.

Andersen, B. (1990). Methodological Errors in Medical Research. Oxford: Blackwell Scientific Publications.

Barnett, V. (1982). Comparative Statistical Inference, 2nd edition. New York: John Wiley & Sons.

Bailar, J.C.I., Louis, T.A., Lavori, P.W., and Polansky, M. (1984). Studies without internal controls. New Engl. J. Med. 311: 156-162.

Bayes, T. (1763). An essay towards solving a problem in the doctrine of chances. Phil. Trans. Roy. Soc. Lond. 53: 370-418.

Bayes, T. (1958). Reprint of the 1763 paper. Biometrika 45: 298-315.

Beecher, H.K. (1970). Research and the Individual: Human Studies. Boston: Little, Brown and Company.

Berry, D.A. (1993). A case for Bayesianism in clinical trials. Statistics in Med. 12: 1377-1393.

Bonita, R., and Beaglehole, R. (1996). The enigma of the decline in stroke deaths in the United States. Stroke 27: 370-372.

Box, J.F. (1980). R. A. Fisher and the design of experiments, 1922-1926. Am. Statistician 34: 1-7.

Brown, R.D., Whisnant, J.P., Sicks, J.D., O'Fallon, W.M., and Wiebers, D.O. (1996). Stroke incidence, prevalence, and survival: Secular trends in Rochester, Minnesota, through 1989. Stroke 27: 373-380.

Bull, J.P. (1959). The historical development of clinical therapeutic trials. J. Chron. Dis. 10: 218-248.

Burton, P.R. (1994). Helping doctors to draw appropriate inferences from the analysis of medical studies. Statistics in Med. 13: 1699-1713.

Byar, D.P., Simon, R.M., Friedewald, W.T., et al. (1976). Randomized clinical trials. Perspectives on some recent ideas. New Engl. J. Med. 295: 74-80.

Byar, D.P., Schoenfeld, D.A., Green, S.B., et al. (1990). Design considerations for AIDS trials. New Engl. J. Med. 323: 1343-1348.

Carter, R.L., Scheaffer, R.L., and Marks, R.G. (1986). The role of consulting units in statistics departments. Am. Stat. 40: 260-262.

Chalmers, T.C. (1975a). Ethical aspects of clinical trials. Am. J. Ophthalmol. 79: 753-758.

Chalmers, T.C. (1975b). Randomization of the first patient. Med. Clin. North Am. 59: 1035-1038.

Coffey, D.S. (1978). General summary remarks (regarding the Workshop in Genitourinary Cancer Immunology, Iowa City, 1976). Department of Health, Education, and Welfare. National Cancer Institute Monograph 49. Publication No. (NIH) 78-1467.

Cornfield, J. (1969). The Bayesian outlook and its application. Biometrics 25: 617-657.

Dupont, W.D. (1985). Randomized vs. historical clinial trials: Are the benefits worth the cost? Am. J. Epid. 122: 940-946.

Fang, J. (1972). Mathematicians from Antiquity to Today. Hauppage, NY: Paideia Press.

Fisher, R.A. (1935). The Design of Experiments. Edinburgh: Oliver and Boyd.

Fleiss, J.L. (1986). The Design and Analysis of Clinical Experiments. New York: John Wiley & Sons.

Frei, E. III (1982). Clinical cancer research: An embattled species. Cancer 50: 1979-1992.

Frei, E. III, and Freireich, E. (1993). The clinical cancer researcher – still an embattled species. J. Clin. Oncol. 11: 1639-1651.

Freund, P.A. (1972). Experimentation with Human Subjects. Great Britain: Clarke Doble and Brendon Ltd.

Fried, C. (1974). Medical experimentation: Personal integrity and social policy. Vol. 5, [A.G. Bearn, D.A.K. Black, and H.H. Hiatt (Eds.)]. Amsterdam: North-Holland.

Gail, M.H. (1996). Use of observational data, including surveillance studies, for evaluating AIDS therapies. Statistics in Medicine 15: 2273-2288.

Garceau, A.J., Donaldson, R.M., O'Hara, E.T., Callow, A.D., Muench, H., Chalmers, T.C., and the Boston Inter-Hospital Liver Group. (1964). A controlled trial of prophylactic porta-caval shunt surgery. N. Engl. J. Med. 270: 496-500.

Gavarret, J. (1840). Principes Généraux de Statistique Médicale, ou, Dévelopement des Règles Qui Doivent Présider à Son Emploi. Bechet jeune et Labé, Paris.

Gehan, E.A., and Lemak, N.A. (1994). Statistics in Medical Research: Developments in Clinical Trials. New York: Plenum.

Gehan, E.A. and Schneiderman, M.A. (1990). Historical and methodological developments in clinical trials at the National Cancer Institute. Statistics in Med. 9: 871-880.

Greenhouse, S.W. (1990). Some historical and methodological developments in early clinical trials at the National Institutes of Health. Statistics in Med. 9: 893-901.

Halperin, M., DeMets, D.L., and Ware, J.H. (1990). Early methodological developments for clinical trials at the National Heart, Lung, and Blood Institute. Statistics in Med. 9: 881-892.

Halpern, D.F. and Coren, S. (1991). Handedness and life span (letter). New Engl. J. Med. 324: 998. See also letters in 325: 1041-1043.

Hankins, F.H. (1930). Gottfried Achenwall. In E.R.A. Seligman and A. Johnson (Eds.), Encyclopaedia of the Social Science, New York: Macmillan.

Hill, A.B. (1963). Medical ethics and controlled trials. British Med. J. April 20: 1043-1049.

Henderson, I.C. (1995). Using clinical trial information in the practice of medicine. Cancer Journal 1: 101-103.

Herdan, G. (1955). Statistics of Therapeutic Trials. Amsterdam: Elsevier.

Hubard, S.M., Martin, N.B., and Thurn, A.L. (1995). NCI's cancer information systems – bringing medical knowledge to clinicians. Oncology 9: 302-314.

Jabs, D., Enger, C. and Bartlett, J.G. (1989). Cytomegalovirus retinitis and acquired immunodeficiency syndrome. Arch. Ophthal. 107: 75-80.

Jenks, S. and Volkers, N. (1992). Razors and refirigerators and reindeer – oh my! J. National Cancer Institute 84: 1863.

Kadane, J.B. (Ed.) (1996). Bayesian Methods and Ethics in a Clinical Trial Design. New York: John Wiley & Sons.

Katz, J. (1972). Experimentation with Human Beings. New York: Russell Sage Foundation.

Kendall, M.G. (1960). Where shall the history of statistics begin? Biometrika 47: 447-449.

Kessler, D.A., Rose, J.L., Temple, R.J., Schapiro, R., and Griffin, J.P. (1994). Therapeutic-class wars – drug promotion in a competitive marketplace. New Engl. J. Med. 331: 1350-1353.

Lancaster, H.O. (1994). Quantitative Methods in Biological and Medical Sciences: A Historical Essay. New York: Springer-Verlag.

Leber, P. (1991). Is there an alternative to the randomized controlled trial? Psychopharm. Bull. 27: 3-8.

Lilencron, F. von (Ed.). (1967). Achenwall, in Allgemeine Deutsche Biographie, Second Edition. Berlin: Duncker & Humblot.

Lindley, D.V. (1965). Introduction to Probability and Statistics from a Bayesian View Point. Cambridge: Cambridge University Press.

Magner, L.N. (1979). A History of the Life Sciences. New York-Basel: Marcel Dekker.

Matthews, J.R. (1995). Quantification and the Quest for Medical Certainty. Princeton: Princeton University Press.

McNeill, P.M. (1993). The Ethics and Politics of Human Experimentation. Cambridge: Press Syndicate of the University of Cambridge.

Meinert, C.L. (1986). Clinical Trials: Design, Conduct, and Analysis. Oxford: Oxford University Press.

Moore, R.D., Hidalgo, J., and Sugland, B.W. (1991). Zidovudine and the natural history of the acquired immunodeficiency syndrome. New Engl. J. Med. 324: 1412-1416.

Office of Technology Assessment (1983). Factors affecting the impact of RCTs on medical practice, in The Impact of Randomized Clinical Trials on Health Policy and Medical Practice. Washington, DC: Government Printing Office, OTA-BP-H-22.

O'Hagan, A. (1994). Kendall's Advanced Theory of Statistics, Volume 2B, Bayesian Inference. London: Edward Arnold.

Pocock, S.J. (1996). Clinical Trials: A Practical Approach. New York: John Wiley & Sons.

Polanyi, M. (1957). Personal Knowledge. Chicago: University of Chicago Press.

Popper, K.R. (1959). The Logic of Scientific Discovery. London: Hutchinson & Co.

Pyros Education Group (1996). Current Clinical Trials: Oncology. Green Brook, N.J.: Thomas J. Timko.

Resnick, R.H., Ishihara, A., Chalmers, T.C., Schimmel, E.M., and the Boston Inter-Hospital Liver Group. (1968). A controlled trial of colon bypass in chronic hepatic encephalopathy. Gastroenterology 54: 1057-1069.

Selby, C. and Scheiber, B. (1996). Science or pseudoscience? Pentagon grant funds alternative health study. Skeptical Inquirer 20: 15-17.

Silverman, W.A. (1985) Human Experimentation: A Guided Step Into the Unknown. Oxford: Oxford University Press.

Spiegelhalter, D.J., Freedman, L.S., and Parmar, M.K.B. (1994). Bayesian approaches to randomized trials. J. R. Statist. Soc. A 157: 357-416.

Spodick, D.H. (1983). Randomize the first patient: Scientific, ethical, and behavioral bases. Am. J. Cardiol. 51: 916-917.

Stigler, S. (1986). The History of Statistics. Cambridge, Mass.: Belknap Press.

Thomas, L. (1977). Biostatistics in medicine. (Editorial). Science 198(4318): 675.

Turner, J.G. (1994). The Effect of Therapeutic Touch on Pain and Infection in Burn Patients (N94-020A1). Grant No. MDA 905-94-Z-0080, Uniformed Services University of the Health Sciences.

USA Today (1996). Nationline: Full Disclosure. Monday, December 16.

Whitehead, J. (1993). The case for frequentism in clinical trials. Statistics in Med. 12: 1405-1413.

CHAPTER 3

Ethical Considerations

3.1   Introduction

Clinical trials are ethically appropriate, necessary, and some would say, required in many circumstances of medical uncertainty. Resolving every uncertainty does not require a designed experiment, and some scientifically valid designs are ethically inappropriate. Because of this, ethical issues surrounding clinical trials are important and pervasive. In many respects, they are as important as the science, which explains why trials have been examined so critically from an ethical perspective. Patients place a great deal of trust in clinical investigators and often participate in trials when the chance of personal benefit is low. Altruism is a common motive for this behavior. The clinical investigator must continue to earn this trust by demonstrably protecting patient interests. Furthermore, ethical considerations have a strong impact on study design.

For these reasons, I will discuss ethical issues in clinical trials "up front" so that they can be seen in a larger context and their impact on the design and conduct of trials can be appreciated. There are many thoughtful and detailed discussions of ethics related to medicine broadly [Reich, 1995] and clinical trials specifically [Beauchamp and Childress, 1979; Fried, 1974; Freund, 1972; Katz, 1972; Levine, 1986; Ramsey, 1974]. Special problems related to cancer treatments are discussed in depth and from a modern perspective in Williams [1992]. A broad international view is given by McNeill [1993]. The discussion here has a more restricted focus on design of clinical trials, but should provide a perspective on important concerns such as ethical principles, informed consent, trial monitoring, and randomization.

Clinical trials highlight the potential conflict of obligations that physicians and other health care practitioners have between their current patient and those yet to be encountered. Discussions of this issue have been taking place in the literature for over 25 years [Gilbert, McPeek, and Mosteller, 1977; Herbert, 1977; Hill, 1963; Tukey, 1977]. Schafer [1982] points out the conflict of obligations, stating:

> In his traditional role of healer, the physician's commitment is exclusively to his patient. By contrast, in his modern role of scientific investigator, the physician engaged in medical research or experimentation has a commitment to promote the acquisition of scientific knowledge.

The tension between these two roles exists in clinical trials, but also in other areas of medicine. For example, epidemiologists recognize the need for protection of their research subjects and have proposed ethical guidelines for studies [Coughlin, 1995; Fayerweather, Higginson, and Beauchamp, 1991]. Quantitative medical decision making methods can also highlight ethical dilemmas [Brett, 1981].

Although clinical trials highlight legitimate ethical concerns [Hellman and Hellman, 1991], advocates for trials sometimes respond to challenges by reiterating important discoveries supported by experiments [Passamani, 1991]. This type of discourse neither clearly displays realistic alternatives to trials nor effectively counters criticisms. The importance of the scientific issue or the knowledge gained is not a counterweight to ethical concerns. Instead, we must explore the uses of a true experimental approach to clinical questions balanced with ethical considerations.

3.2   Overview

Clinical trials are something of a lightning rod for ethical concerns, because they bring into sharp focus two seemingly opposed roles of the physician in modern medicine [Levine, 1992]. Competing demands on the physician have been present throughout history and are not created uniquely by clinical trials. Before the age of clinical trials, Ivy [1948] suggested that the patient is always an experimental subject. Shimkin [1953] also took this view. Today, the roles of patient advocate and researcher are not the only two points of conflict for the physician. For example, the desires for academic and financial success compete with both patient care and research. Thus, the practitioner is faced with numerous potential ethical conflicts.

Some discussions about ethical concerns in clinical trials are mainly relevant to randomized designs. However, the most fundamental issues do not depend on the method of selecting treatments for study, only on the fact that the experimentalist does not commit exclusively to a patient. The discussion here is intended to relate to trials of all types. The term "physician" will be used to indicate health care practitioners broadly.

3.2.1   Trials are ethical in the setting of uncertainty

To begin the discussion, a preview of the conclusions is helpful. No modern or historical ethical guidelines proscribe either the advocacy of clinical trials by physicians or the role of physicians as experimentalists. When properly set, designed, and conducted, a clinical trial is an ethically appropriate way to acquire new knowledge. Although many ethically appropriate treatment decisions are based on knowledge acquired outside the scope of definitive clinical trials, ignorance can be unethical. For example, clinical decisions based only on weak evidence, opinion, or dogma, without the benefit of rigorous scientific support, raise their own ethical questions. The practitioner has an ethical obligation to acknowledge uncertainty honestly and take steps to avoid continued ignorance.

Well-designed and conducted clinical trials are ethically more acceptable than some alternatives, such as acquiring knowledge ineffectively, by tragic accident, or failing to learn from seemingly unavoidable but serious clinical errors. Thus, there are imperatives to conduct medical research [Eisenberg, 1977]. In some circumstances, both the practitioner and patient are unsure of the best treatment to select. In others, the usual treatments are known to be incompletely effective. In these cases, encouraging the patient to participate in a clinical trial and possibly gaining some individual or collective benefit, may be the most ethical stance.

Medical interventions of all types, including clinical trials, can be poorly applied in specific instances or for certain patients. When discussing ethics, we must distinguish between the *methodology of trials* and the *characteristics of a particular trial*. When this is done, we can see that clinical trials are not inherently unethical. Unethical aspects of a trial, if they exist, are a consequence of the details of the scientific question or the design and conduct of a specific trial in a specific circumstance. When sponsors of research and investigators follow the basic principles of ethics for human subjects experiments that have evolved over the last 50 years, the resulting studies are likely to be appropriate.

3.2.2   Research and practice are not separable

One of the principal difficulties in thinking about ethical issues in clinical trials arises from an artificial distinction between *research* and *practice* in medicine. (Actually, the word *practice* implies uncertainty, but it is most often used in a context of certainty.) Some activities of the physician seem to be done primarily for the good of the individual patient and we place these in the domain of practice. Other actions seem to be performed for the collective good or to acquire generalizable knowledge, and we label these as research. This distinction is often convenient for discussion purposes, but is artificial. An appropriate description is that physician behavior is nearly always both research and practice. Before the wide use of clinical trials, Guttentag [1953] acknowledged this duality and suggested that research and practice for the same patient might need to be conducted by different physicians.

A more accurate distinction could be based on the physician's degree of certainty. When the physician is certain of the outcome from a specific therapy for a particular patient, applying the treatment might be described as *practice*. When the physician is unsure of the outcome, applying the treatment could be considered *research*, at least in part. Thinking about the issue in terms of the continuum of degrees of certainty illustrates the artificial nature of the research-practice dichotomy.

Sometimes physician behavior can be labeled as practice in one setting, but when part of a larger structure, the same behavior becomes research. Comparison of two standard therapies in a randomized trial is an example. The distinction between practice and research seems to be a result of the settings in which the actions take place, which in turn, is a possible consequence of the motives of the physician. The dichotomy, if it exists, is largely a consequence of the specific circumstances in which treatments are used.

There are very few actions which the physician can carry out for the benefit of the individual patient that cannot yield some knowledge applicable to the general good. Likewise, nearly all knowledge gained from research can be of some benefit to individual patients. It is possible for patients to be misinformed about, or harmed by, either inappropriate practice actions or improper research activities. Both activities can have large or small risk-benefit ratios.

In modern academic medical centers, the research-practice duality of medicine is clearly evident. In these settings, physicians are trained not only to engage in good practice but also to maintain a mind set that encourages learning both from clinical practice and from formal experimentation. Even with strong financial incentives to separate them, it is clear that research and clinical practice are one and the same in many of these institutions. Not surprisingly, these academic settings are the places most closely associated with performing clinical trials. However, academic medicine is a recent development. In the past, many medical advances were made in mostly traditional practice settings, precisely because physicians both took advantage of, and created, research opportunities.

Double standards

The artificial distinction between research and practice can create double standards regarding ethical conduct. The *practitioner* is free to represent his or her treatment preferences for the patient with relatively informal requirements for explaining alternatives, rationale, risks, and benefits. Similarly, a second practitioner who prefers a different treatment may have minimal requirements to offer alternatives. However, the *investigator* studying a randomized comparison of the two standard treatments to determine which one is superior will likely incur ethical obligations well beyond either practitioner. A perspective on this point is given by Lantos [1993; 1994].

A second, and more far-reaching double standard can be seen in cases where individuals have been injured as a result of treatments that were not thoroughly studied during development. Thalidomide for sedation during pregnancy is one example. Physicians cannot expect to provide any individual with health care that is in his or her best interest without knowing the detailed properties of that therapy, including risks and benefits. This knowledge often comes most efficiently from clinical trials. A discussion of the sources and potential problems arising from this double standard is given by Chalmers and Silverman [1987].

A third source of double standards arises in considering different cultural expectations regarding medical care, patient information, and research. Some cultures place fewer restrictions on research practices in humans than those in the U.S., or perhaps the individuals in the population have a greater expectation that these types of studies will be done. One cannot make value judgments from this fact. For example, there are considerable differences in the expectations regarding informed consent for research studies between the U.S., Europe, Africa, and Asia. These differences are a consequence of many factors, including the structure and economics of health care, physician attitudes, patient expectations, attitudes toward litigation, the nature

of threats to the public health, and cultural norms, especially regarding risk acceptance and consent.

Other practices

Research and practice are not the only categories of physician activity. Levine [1986]
also distinguishes "nonvalidated practices" and "practice for the benefit of others".
Nonvalidated or investigational practices are those that have not been convincingly
shown to be effective. The reasons for this might be that the therapy is new or that
its efficacy was never rigorously shown in the first place. Practice for the benefit of
others includes organ donation, vaccination, and quarantine. Ethical issues related
to these are complex and cannot be covered here.

3.2.3 Practice based on unproven treatments is not ethical

Despite knowledge, skill, and empathy for the patient, the practitioner sometimes
selects treatments without being certain about their effectiveness. Some unproven
practices are sensible and are not likely to cause harm, such as meditation, exercise,
relaxation, and visualization. These and related activities may be life-styles as much
as they are therapies. They may improve a patient's quality of life, especially when
applied to self-limited conditions and normally do not replace treatments of established benefit. The discussion here does not pertain to such adjunctive treatments.

Ethical questions arise when unproven therapies replace proven ones, particularly
for chronic or fatal illnesses. Ignorance about the relative merits of a treatment cannot
carry ethical legitimacy for the physician, even in a purely "practice" setting. To
summarize:

> A physician's moral obligation to offer each patient the best available treat-
> ment cannot be separated from the twin clinical and ethical imperatives to
> base that choice of treatment on the best available and obtainable evidence.
> The tension between the interdependent responsibilities of giving personal
> and compassionate care, as well as scientifically sound and validated treat-
> ment, is intrinsic to the practice of medicine today . . . Controlled clinical tri-
> als – randomized when randomization is feasible, ethically achievable, and
> scientifically appropriate – are an integral part of the ethical imperative that
> physicians should know what they are doing when they intervene into the
> bodies, psyches, and biographies of vulnerable, suffering human beings [Roy,
> 1986].

Lack of knowledge can persist purely as a consequence of the newness of a therapy. We are familiar with the use of clinical trials in this circumstance to gain experience with and acquire knowledge about the treatment. However, ignorance can
remain even in the light of clinical experience with a therapy if the experience is
outside of a suitably structured environment or setting that permits learning. This
can happen when the proponents of the treatment have not made sufficient efforts

to evaluate it objectively, even though they are clinically qualified and have good intentions.

There are popular unproven therapies for many conditions including AIDS, cancer, arthritis, diabetes, musculoskeletal conditions, skin diseases, and lupus. The Office of Alternative Medicine at the National Institutes of Health defines "alternative" therapies to be those that are unproven and has taken steps to investigate many of them. There is a wide spectrum of such therapies, even if one restricts focus to a single disease like cancer [Aulas, 1996; Bridgen, 1995; Casselith and Chapman, 1996; Office of Technology Assessment, 1990].

The American Cancer Society (ACS) investigates and summarizes scientific evidence concerning some unproven cancer treatments through its Committee on Questionable Methods of Cancer Management. They have researched cancer practices related to "metabolic therapy" in Tijuana and other Mexican border clinics [ACS, 1990]. Although heterogeneous, metabolic therapies rely on 1) detoxification, 2) strengthening the immune system, and 3) special methods to attack the cancer. Other methods have been classified as nutritional therapies [ACS, 1993].

These methods sound reasonable for cancer treatment, but none has been shown to be safe and effective using structured evaluation tools like clinical trials. Thus, the evidence about them is unconvincing in spite of the "clinical experience" that proponents have accumulated. As many as 5 percent of cancer patients abandon traditional therapies in favor of alternative methods and 10-50 percent of cancer patients employ some alternative therapy [McGinnis, 1990]. Unconventional therapy is used by a sizeable fraction of people in the U.S. [Eisenberg, et al., 1993].

According to the ACS, a number of other practices for treating cancer fall into a similar category. These include fresh cell therapy, the Revici method, Livingston-Wheeler therapy, macrobiotic diets, Laetrile, immuno-augmentative therapy, psychic surgery, the Gerson method, the Greek cancer cure of Hariton Alivizatos, cancell / entelev, and others. Although many or all of these treatments have professional advocates and have been associated with anecdotes of benefit, they are most often used in an environment that inhibits rigorous evaluation. See Barrett [1993] for a review of this and related subjects. Efforts by the National Institutes of Health to study some unconventional treatments have been subject to controversy [e.g., Marshall, 1994]. No doubt, unproven treatments for other diseases have proponents and can be found in similar settings that discourage objective evaluation. In any case, strongly held opinion cannot ethically substitute for experimental testing.

3.2.4   There are legitimate ethical concerns about clinical trials

Although well-designed and conducted clinical trials fit within modern ethical guidelines (discussed below), these studies highlight important concerns and create the potential to violate the rights of research subjects. Although there is a chance for investigators to move away from the best interests of the individual patient, clinical trials do not *require* it. While the tensions discussed above exist, they can be managed through scrupulous attention to the ethical design of each element of the research process such as randomization, informed consent, study monitoring, and the use of placebos. Other concerns highlighted by clinical trials include treatment preference, demonstration trials, and the "personal care principle".

Many of these points can be illustrated by recent randomized trials of extracorporeal membrane oxygenation (ECMO) for neonates with respiratory failure. This series of studies has been discussed at length in the pediatric and clinical trials literature. Some issues related to treatment allocation and the ECMO trials are discussed in Chapter 9. For a recent review with useful references from an ethical perspective, see Miké, Krauss, and Ross [1993].

Randomization

Is it ever appropriate for a physician to support selecting a patient's treatment by chance alone? Some physicians and patients will answer "no" to this question, while many others can sketch circumstances which allow (or even encourage) it. It is simple to imagine circumstances in which randomization could be used inappropriately. Some may feel that it is an obligation of the physician to have a preference on behalf of the individual patient, even when the evidence does not favor any particular treatment.

The justification of randomization follows from a state of relative ignorance called "equipoise" by some authors [Freedman, 1987]. If equipoise cannot exist, as some critics of clinical trials claim, then randomization is not justified. Because of changes in individual and collective equipoise during a trial, concerns about the ethical climate for continuing a trial can be aided by a Data Safety Monitoring Committee [Baum, Houghton, and Abrams, 1994]. These are discussed in Chapter 10.

Treatment preference

Treatment preference presents another potential problem for both participants and investigators in clinical trials. If patients strongly prefer a particular treatment, should they be dissuaded from it to participate in a trial? If a physician has a preference for a particular treatment, either in general or for a particular patient, can he or she recommend that patients participate in a comparative trial? The answer to both questions is "no". Patients and physicians with firm preferences, even those based on weak evidence, are not eligible to participate in trials, even if the best judgment suggests that it is the right thing to do. If patients or physicians with preferences are coaxed into participating in a trial, they may bring reservations with them that will make them more likely to withdraw from the study or lead to strong dissatisfaction with their treatment result.

One could argue that knowledgeable physicians should *always* have a preference which would guide a treatment choice for an individual patient. Because individualized treatment assignment is lost in a trial, at least for the initial selection, the physician is ignoring any obligation to form a preference. This is not a real problem. There are many instances where knowledgeable physicians are unable to form a preference for any particular treatment, especially when they have counterbalancing risks and benefits. Sometimes a new but unproven therapy seems to offer a potential for improvement that goes beyond well-known mediocre treatments. For this reason, many experienced physicians often seem to be willing to participate in evaluating new therapies.

Informed consent

Informed consent is a vital concern in clinical trials. There are numerous examples of studies where patients have been exposed to potentially or definitively harmful treatments without being fully apprised of the risk. Some possible examples from tests of radioactive substances from 1945 to 1975 recently came to light [U.S. Congress, 1980]. Presumably, patients would not voluntarily accept some of the risks inherent in those studies.

When this problem occurs, it is a result of error, not because ethically appropriate consent is never possible to obtain. Sick or dying patients and their families are vulnerable, and it is questionable how much technical information about new treatments they can truly understand, especially when it is presented to them quickly. This problem arises when using treatments already known to be effective as well as when testing experimental ones. It is interesting that informed consent procedures, originally developed to protect research subjects from exploitation, are now viewed by many practitioners as devices to protect them from litigation.

Monitoring

During the conduct of a comparative study, evidence may become available that one treatment is superior. It may be safer or have a more favorable effect on the disease. What should be done to protect patients enrolled in the trial who are receiving the inferior treatment? Trial designs frequently incorporate procedures, analyses, and guidelines to deal with this situation. If investigators find the evidence convincing, they should recommend stopping the study or offering the better treatment to all patients. This can present some problems if the trial has important secondary endpoints which would only become evaluable after continued treatment. This too is not a unique problem to clinical trials. Consider what happens when practitioners become convinced that any new treatment is superior to one being used. Nevertheless, it is especially of concern in comparative experiments.

Active versus placebo controls

Assigning patients to a placebo treatment is not always ethical. It may not be justified when effective therapy exists. Some clinical trials continue to be performed using experimental therapy versus placebo in questionable situations. Rothman and Michels [1994] discussed this problem with some examples. Depending on the nature and strength of physicians' belief, the issue of what constitutes an appropriate control can be a matter of opinion.

Problems using placebo controls cannot be fixed by informing patients that they might not receive effective treatment and obtaining their consent, or by suggesting that a period on placebo will not cause harm. A better approach might be to evaluate the new treatment against standard therapy without compromising the safety of the patients.

There are circumstances in which investigators and patients might be comfortable refusing to use standard therapy and comparing a new treatment to a placebo.

This might happen, for example, if the standard treatment is associated with high morbidity and the new treatment being tested has low morbidity. In fact, such a situation has nothing to do with the trial, because patients could sensibly refuse to take any treatment where the risk/benefit ratio is high. Also, placebo controls might be scientifically and ethically justified when evidence arises suggesting that standard therapy is ineffective.

Demonstration trials

When ample evidence already exists, or investigators are already convinced, that a particular treatment is best, it may be unethical to conduct a trial to convince colleagues of its superiority. Such studies are sometimes termed "demonstration trials". There are situations where not all practitioners are convinced by the same evidence or same standard of evidence. This happens often in different countries and/or depending on strength of prior belief and local standards of practice. Ethical standards are also local and some studies are acceptable to certain physicians in one place but viewed as inappropriate in another. In any case, most practitioners would discourage comparative trials performed only to strengthen evidence.

Sometimes the standard of care contains procedures or treatments that are unnecessary. Electronic fetal monitoring during labor may be an example. In such situations, a demonstration trial may be appropriate. More generally, demonstration trials to show equivalence are ethically less of a problem than those intended to show a difference.

Personal care

The "personal care principle" (PCP) has been raised by some critics of clinical trials as an important ethical guideline that randomized studies can violate. The PCP appears to have roots in the Hippocratic oath and states that physicians have an obligation to act always in the best interests of the individual patient [Fried, 1974]. The PCP does not support the lack of knowledge or opinion that often motivates making treatment choices as part of a structured experiment, particularly by random assignment. If the PCP were, in fact, a minimal standard of conduct (or ethical principle), it could create serious problems for conducting randomized clinical trials [e.g., Royall, 1991], except that patients could always agree to participate in trials despite their practitioners' opinions. A helpful discussion of issues surrounding the PCP is given by Markman [1992], Freedman [1992], and Royall [1992].

In a sense, physicians are taught to believe in, and endorse, the personal care ideal. Many accept the notion that they should always make the "best" recommendation based on the knowledge available and the patient's wishes. This does not mean that such recommendations are always based on scientific fact or well-formed opinion. Sometimes physician preferences are based on important non-rational factors. Other times, preferences are based on unimportant factors. An insightful physician will probably recognize that many treatment "preferences" are artificial and carry no ethical legitimacy. More to the point, *the PCP is not a defining ethical principle* but an ideal for which the practitioner strives.

In its simplest form, the PCP makes the physician–patient relationship analogous to the attorney–client relationship. A such, it appears to be a product of, and contribute to, an adversarial relationship between society and the patient, making the sick person in need of physician protection. Although physicians and patients are partners, the environment is not usually adversarial. If we pursue this analogy slightly further than it should go, one could consider research to be an adversarial circumstance for the patient, and clinical trials would be a sort of "plea bargain" where the patient compromises to have an overall best outcome.

There are more fundamental problems with the PCP than this analogy suggests. For example, the PCP does not encourage patients and physicians to take full advantage of genuine and widespread uncertainty or differences of opinion that motivate randomization. It does not acknowledge the lack of evidence when treatments are being developed. It raises moral and ethical questions of its own, by discouraging or removing an objective evaluation tool that can correct for economic and other biases that enter decisions about treatment selection. All of these issues are illustrated by the history of Laetrile, discussed briefly on page 67. The ascendancy of a personal care ideal may have been an artifact of a time when medical resources were very abundant. In any case, the PCP is violated in many instances that have nothing to do with randomization or clinical trials, as discussed below.

3.2.5   Physicians always have two roles

There are many circumstances besides clinical trials in which physicians' obligations extend beyond the individual patient or are otherwise conflicting. In some circumstances, significant obligations extend to other members of society or to patients yet to be encountered. In other cases, the physician may have conflicting obligations to the same patient (e.g., care of the terminally ill patient). Dual roles for the physician are evident when he or she has extended obligations.

The examples listed below are circumstances consistent with both tradition and current ideas about "good" health care. They illustrate the somewhat mythical nature of acting only in the best interests of the individual patient. Although clinical trials highlight dual obligations, medical practitioners encounter and manage conflicts of commitment in other places.

Examples

The first example is *teaching and training* of new physicians and health care professionals. This is necessary for the well-being of future patients, but it is not always in the best interests of the current patient to participate. It is true that, with adequate supervision of trainees, the risks to patients from teaching are small. In some ways, the patient derives benefit from being on a teaching service. However, the incremental risks attributable to inexperienced practitioners are not zero and there may be few benefits for the patient. Even if safe, teaching programs often result in additional inconvenience to the patient. Aside from outright errors, teaching programs may perform more physical exams, diagnostic tests, and procedures than are strictly necessary. Thus, the safest and most convenient strategy for the individual patient would be to have an experienced physician and to permit no teaching around his or her bedside.

Vaccination is another example for which the physician advocates, and with the individual patient, accepts risks for the benefit of other members of society. With a communicable disease like polio, diphtheria, or pertussis and a reasonably safe vaccine, the most *practical* strategy for the individual is to be vaccinated. However, the *optimal* strategy for the individual patient is to have everyone *else* vaccinated so that he or she can derive the benefit without any risk. For example, almost all cases of polio between 1980 and 1994 were caused by the oral polio vaccine [Centers for Disease Control, 1997]. A strategy avoiding vaccination is impractical for the patient because the behavior of others cannot be guaranteed. This is not a workable policy for the physician to promote either, because it can be applied only to a few individuals, demonstrating the obligation of the physician to all patients.

Triage, whether in the emergency room, battlefield hospital, or domestic disaster, is a classic example of the physician placing the interests of some patients above those of others and acting for the collective good. It is a form of *rationing of health care*, a broader circumstance in which the interests of the individual are not paramount. Although in the U.S. we are not accustomed to rationing (at least in such stark terms), constrained health care resources produce it, and may increasingly do so in the future. For example, physicians working directly for profit-making companies and managed health plans, rather than being hired by the individual patient, could create competing priorities and highlight the dual obligations of the physician.

Abortion is another circumstance in which the physician has obligations other than to the individual patient. No stand on the moral issues surrounding abortion is free of this dilemma. Whether the fetus or the mother is considered the patient, potential conflicts arise. This is true also of other special circumstances such as the separation of conjoined twins or *in utero* therapy for fatal diseases in which there is no obvious line of obligation. For a discussion of the many problems surrounding fetal research, see Ramsey [1975].

Organ donation is almost never in the best medical interests of the donor, especially when the donor gives a kidney, bone marrow, blood, or other organ while still alive and healthy. It is true that donors have little risk in many of these situations, especially ones from which they recover quickly, such as blood donation, but the risk is not zero. Even in the case of the donor being kept alive only by artificial means, it seems that no medical benefit can be derived by donating organs, except to people other than the donor. However, it is clear that physicians endorse and facilitate altruistic organ donation, again illustrating their dual roles.

The dual obligations of the physician can be found in requirements for *quarantine, reporting,* or *contact tracing* of certain diseases or conditions. Circumstances requiring this behavior include infectious diseases, sexually transmitted diseases, suspected child abuse, and gunshot wounds. Although these requirements relate, in part, to non-medical interests, reporting and contact tracing highlights dual obligations and seems to stretch even the principle of physician confidentiality. The fact that required reporting of infectious diseases compromises some rights of the patient is evidenced by government and public unwillingness to require it for HIV positive and AIDS diagnoses in response to concerns from those affected.

Treatments to control epidemics (aside from quarantine) can present ethical conflicts between those affected and those at risk. For example, in the summer of 1996 there was an epidemic of food poisoning centered in Sakai, Japan, caused by the O157 strain of *E. coli*. At one point in the epidemic, almost 10,000 people were affected and the number of cases was growing by 100 per day. At least seven people died and nearly all those infected were schoolchildren. As a means to stop or slow the epidemic, Sakai health officials considered treating with antibiotics 400 individuals who were apparently in their week-long incubation period. The treatment was controversial because, while it kills O157 *E. coli*, endotoxin would be released which could make the individuals sick. The obligations of health providers in such a situation cannot be resolved without ethical conflicts.

A final example of dual obligations can be found in *market-driven health care financing*. In this system, employers contract with insurance companies for coverage and reimbursement. Both the patient and physician are effectively removed from negotiating important aspects of clinical care. If the physician is employed by a health care provider rather than the patient, competing obligations are possible [Levinsky, 1996].

These examples of the competing obligations of the physician are no more or less troublesome than clinical trials. Like clinical trials, each has reasons why, and circumstances in which, they are appropriate and ethical. We are familiar with many of them and have seen their place in medical practice more clearly than the relatively recent arrival of clinical trials. However, the dual obligations of the physician are present and have always been with us. Obligations to individuals as well as to "society" can be compassionately and sensibly managed in most circumstances. This inevitable duality of roles that confronts the physician investigator is not a persuasive argument against performing clinical trials.

3.2.6   Ethical considerations are important determinants of design

Clinical trials incorporate design characteristics to accommodate ethical concerns. This is true on at least two levels. The first is when the practitioner assesses the risks and benefits of treatment for the individual patient on an ongoing basis. The physician always has an obligation to terminate experimental therapy when it is no longer in the best interests of an individual patient. Second, the physician must be constantly aware of information from the study and decide if the evidence is strong enough to require a change in clinical practice, either with regard to the participants in the trial or to new patients. In many trials, this awareness comes from a Data Safety Monitoring Committee, discussed in Chapter 10. Both of these perspectives require substantive design features.

Consider early pharmacologic oriented studies in humans as an example. The initial dose of drug employed, while based on evidence from animal experiments, is conservatively chosen. It is unlikely that low doses will be of benefit to the patient, particularly with drugs used in life-threatening diseases like cancer or AIDS. Ethical concern over risk of harm requires these designs to test low doses ahead of high doses. Such studies often permit the patient to receive additional doses of drug later, perhaps changing their risk/benefit ratio.

In the next stage of drug development, when a therapeutic dosage has been established, staged designs, or those with "stopping rules", are frequently used to minimize exposing patients to ineffective drugs, and to detect large improvements quickly. Similar designs are used in comparative trials. These designs, developed largely in response to ethical concerns, are discussed in more depth in Chapter 10. In these and other circumstances, ethical concerns drive modifications to the clinically, statistically, or biologically optimal designs.

3.3   Historical Perspective

Before discussing modern views of biomedical ethics, it is helpful to understand the path that biomedical experimentation has taken to reach its current state. A concise discussion is offered by Reiser [1993]. The landmarks that have shaped our current view are few, but highly visible. Many are a consequence of improper treatment of research subjects. A concise review is given by McNeill [1993, chapter 1].

3.3.1   The Hippocratic tradition does not proscribe clinical trials

The Hippocratic Oath has been one component of modern-day ethical guidelines for the practice of medicine. It represents an ideal which has been extensively modified by modern medical practice, scientific discovery, cultural standards, and patient expectations. Many physicians no longer repeat the full oath upon graduation from medical school and some have rarely (or never) seen it. Most clinical trial statisticians have not studied it and occasionally, someone will imply that the oath is inconsistent with experimentation. To examine its actual implications for clinical trials, it is useful to examine the full text. This translation comes from *Dorland's Medical Dictionary* [1994]:

> I swear by Apollo the physician, by Æsculapius, Hygeia, and Panacea, and I take to witness all the gods, all the goddesses, to keep according to my ability and my judgment the following Oath:
> To consider dear to me as my parents him who taught me this art; to live in common with him and if necessary to share my goods with him; to look upon his children as my own brothers, to teach them this art if they so desire without fee or written promise; to impart to my sons and the sons of the master who taught me and the disciples who have enrolled themselves and have agreed to the rules of the profession, but to these alone, the precepts and the instruction. I will prescribe regimen for the good of my patients according to my ability and my judgment and never do harm to anyone. To please no one will I prescribe a deadly drug, nor give advice which may cause his death. Nor will I give a woman a pessary to procure abortion. But I will preserve the purity of my life and my art. I will not cut for stone, even for patients in whom the disease is manifest; I will leave this operation to be performed by practitioners (specialists in this art). In every house where I come I will enter only

for the good of my patients, keeping myself far from all intentional ill-doing and all seduction, and especially from the pleasures of love with women or men, be they free or slaves. All that may come to my knowledge in the exercise of my profession or outside of my profession or in daily commerce with men, which ought not to be spread abroad, I will keep secret and will never reveal. If I keep this oath faithfully, may I enjoy my life and practice my art, respected by all men and in all times; but if I swerve from it or violate it, may the reverse be my lot.

It is easy to see why the oath is not often repeated in full and not taken literally by modern physicians. It contains components which are sexist, proscriptive, celibate, and superstitious. The three specific clinical proscriptions (i.e., abortion, surgery for urinary stones, and the use of "deadly" drugs) have long since fallen, as has the pledge for free instruction. Principles that have found widespread acceptance or are reflected in the ethics of today's medical practice are "doing no harm", prescribing for "the good of my patients", confidentiality, and an obligation to teach. Even confidentiality in modern medicine is open to some question [Siegler, 1982], particularly in the situations described above surrounding reportable diseases.

One could not expect the Hippocratic oath to mention clinical trials, even implicitly, because the concept did not exist when it was written. However, the use of plural "patients" is noteworthy because one might interpret it to imply a collective obligation as well as an individual one. We cannot make too much of this, in any case. The oath is primarily a traditional idealization and not a required code of conduct for all circumstances. These limitations also apply to our modern ethical principles.

3.3.2   Nuremberg contributed an awareness of the worst problems

The term "experimentation", especially related to human beings, was given a dreadful connotation by the events of World War II. The evidence of criminal and unscientific behavior of physicians in the concentration camps of Nazi Germany became evident worldwide during the 1946–1947 Nuremberg trials. There were numerous incidents of torture, murder, and experimentation atrocities committed by Nazi physicians. In fact, 20 physicians and three others were tried for these crimes at Nuremberg [Annas and Grodin, 1992]. Sixteen individuals were convicted and given sentences ranging from imprisonment to death. Four of the seven individuals executed for their crimes were physicians.

At the time of the trial, there were no existing international standards for the ethics of experimentation with human subjects. The judges presiding at Nuremberg outlined ten principles that are required to satisfy ethical conduct for human experimentation. This was the Nuremberg Code, adopted in 1947. The Code established principles for each of the following points:

1.   The study participants must give voluntary consent.
2.   There must be no reasonable alternative to conducting the experiment.

3. The anticipated results must have a basis in biological knowledge and animal experimentation.
4. The procedures should avoid unnecessary suffering and injury.
5. There is no expectation for death or disability as a result of the trial.
6. The degree of risk for the patient is consistent with the humanitarian importance of the study.
7. The subjects are protected against even a remote possibility of death or injury.
8. The study must be conducted by qualified scientists.
9. The subject can stop participation at will.
10. The investigator has an obligation to terminate the experiment if injury seems likely.

The Nuremberg code has been influential in United States and international law to provide groundwork for standards of ethical conduct.

3.3.3   The Helsinki Declaration is widely adopted

In 1964, the 18th World Medical Association (WMA) meeting in Helsinki, Finland, adopted a formal code of ethics for physicians engaged in clinical research [World Medical Association, 1964]. This became known as the Helsinki Declaration, which has been revised by the WMA in 1975 (Tokyo), 1983 (Venice), and 1989 (Hong Kong). This declaration is intended to be reviewed and updated periodically. Fewer than half of the world's countries are members of the WMA, in part apparently, because it did not take a stand against apartheid in South Africa.

The exact provisions of the Helsinki Declaration contain some elements which are potentially conflicting. For example, it begins by stating "It is the mission of the physician to safeguard the health of the people". However, in the next paragraph it endorses the Declaration of Geneva of the World Medical Association, which states regarding the obligations of physicians, "the health of my patient will be my first consideration" and the International Code of Medical Ethics which states "a physician shall act only in the patient's interest when providing medical care which might have the effect of weakening the physical and mental condition of the patient". Later, it states "Medical progress is based on research which ultimately must rest in part on experimentation involving human subjects".

It is noteworthy that the principle of acting only in the individual patient's interest seems to be qualified and that the declaration presupposes the ethical legitimacy of biomedical and clinical research. Among other ideas, it outlines principles stating that research involving human subjects must conform to generally accepted scientific principles, be formulated in a written protocol, be conducted only by qualified individuals, and include written informed consent from the participants.

3.3.4   Other international guidelines have been proposed

The United Nations General Assembly adopted the International Covenant on Civil and Political Rights in 1976, which states (Article 7): *No one shall be subjected to torture or to cruel, inhuman or degrading treatment or punishment. In particular, no one shall be subjected without his free consent to medical or scientific experimentation.* In 1982, the World Health Organization (WHO) and the Council for International Organizations of Medical Sciences (CIOMS) issued a document, *Proposed International Guidelines for Biomedical Research Involving Human Subjects,* to help developing countries apply the principles in the Helsinki Declaration and the Nuremberg Code. The guidelines were extended in a second document in 1991 dealing with epidemiologic studies, in part, in response to needs arising from field trials testing AIDS vaccines and drugs. The second document was called *International Guidelines for Ethical Review of Epidemiologic Studies.* In 1992, the Guidelines were revised at a meeting in Geneva, resulting in the *International Ethical Guidelines for Biomedical Research Involving Human Subjects.* Some areas of medical research are not mentioned in the guidelines, including human genetic research, embryo and fetal research, and research using fetal tissue. [Council for International Organizations of Medical Sciences, 1993].

Guideline 11 of these regulations states: *As a general rule, pregnant or nursing women should not be subjects of any clinical trials except such trials as are designed to protect or advance the health of pregnant or nursing women or fetuses or nursing infants, and for which women who are not pregnant or nursing would not be suitable subjects.* This Guideline is directly opposite current thinking by many women's advocacy groups in the U.S., the FDA, and NIH, which have relaxed or removed such restrictions in favor of allowing pregnant women more self-determination regarding participation in clinical research of all types.

3.3.5   High-profile mistakes were made in the U.S.

Despite the events at Nuremberg, a persistent ethical complacency in the United States followed. In the late 1940s and early 1950s, the American Medical Association (AMA) was keenly aware of Nuremberg and felt that its own principles were sufficient for protecting research subjects [Ivy, 1948; Judicial Council of the AMA, 1946]. The principles advocated by the AMA at that time were 1) patient consent, 2) safety as demonstrated by animal experiments, and 3) investigator competence. A few examples of ethically inappropriate studies are sketched here. Some others are given by Beecher [1966].

In 1936, the U.S. Public Heath Service had started a study of the effects of untreated syphilis in Tuskegee, Alabama. Three-hundred-ninety-nine men with advanced disease were studied along with 201 controls. The study continued long after effective treatment for the disease was known, coming to public attention in 1972 [Brandt, 1978; Department of Health Education, and Welfare, 1973; Jones, 1981]. In fact, there had been numerous medical publications relating the findings of the study, some after the development of penicillin [e.g., Schuman et al., 1955]. The study had no written protocol.

Another study at the Jewish Chronic Diseases Hospital in Brooklyn in 1963 saw cancer cells injected into 22 debilitated elderly patients without their knowledge to see if they would immunologically reject the cells [Katz, 1972]. Consent was said to have been obtained orally, but records of it were not kept. The hospital's Board of

Trustees was informed of the experiment by several physicians who were concerned that the patients did not give consent. The Board of Regents of the State University of New York reviewed the case and concluded that the investigators were acting in an experimental rather than therapeutic relationship, requiring patient consent.

At Willowbrook State Hospital in New York, retarded children were deliberately infected with viral hepatitis as part of a study of its natural history [Katz, 1972]. Some subjects were fed extracts of stool from those with the disease. Investigators defended the study because nearly all residents of the facility could be expected to become infected with the virus anyway. However, even the recruitment was ethically suspect, because overcrowding prevented some patients from being admitted to the facility unless their parents agreed to the study.

3.4   Modern Perspective

3.4.1   Institutional review boards provide ethical oversight

In response to events like those described above, Congress established the National Commission for the Protection of Human Subjects of Biomedical and Behavioral Research through the 1974 National Research Act. Interestingly, it was the first national commission to function under the new Freedom of Information Act of 1974 so that all of its deliberations were public and fully recorded. The Act required the establishment of Institutional Review Boards (IRB) for all research funded in whole or in part by the federal government. In the form of the 1978 Belmont Report, this Commission provided a set of recommendations and guidelines for the conduct of research with human subjects and established Institutional Review Boards [National Commission for Protection of Human Subjects of Biomedical and Behavioral Research, 1978].

In 1981, the federal regulations were modified to require IRB approval for all drugs or products regulated by the FDA. This requirement does not depend on the funding source, the research volunteers, or the location of the study. Regulations permitting compassionate use of experimental drugs were disseminated in 1987 and 1991. IRBs must have at least five members with expertise relevant to safeguarding the rights and welfare of patients participating in biomedical research. At least one member of the IRB should be a scientist, one a non-scientist, and at least one should be unaffiliated with the institution. The IRB should be made up of individuals with diverse racial, gender, and cultural backgrounds. Individuals with a conflict of interest may not participate in deliberations. The scope of the IRB includes, but is not limited to, consent procedures and research design.

The Belmont Report outlined ethical principles and guidelines for the protection of human subjects. A major component of this report was the nature and definition of informed consent in various research settings. In the Belmont report, three basic ethical principles relevant to research involving human subjects were identified. The report recognized that "these principles cannot always be applied so as to resolve beyond dispute particular ethical problems". These principles are discussed in the next section.

IRBs approve human research studies that meet specific prerequisites. The criteria are 1) the risks to the study participants are minimized, 2) the risks are reasonable in relation to the anticipated benefits, 3) the selection of study participants is equitable, 4) informed consent is obtained and appropriately documented for each participant, 5) there are adequate provisions for monitoring data collected to ensure the safety of the study participants, and 6) the privacy of the participants and confidentiality of the data are protected.

Informed consent is a particularly important aspect of these requirements. The consent procedures and documents must indicate that the study involves research, describe reasonable foreseeable risks and discomfort, and describe potential benefits and alternatives. In addition, the consent document must describe the extent to which privacy of data will be maintained, treatment for injuries incurred, and who to contact for questions. Finally, the consent indicates that participation is voluntary and no loss of benefits will occur if the patient does not enter the study.

3.4.2   Ethical principles permit clinical trials

The ethical principles to which physicians aspire probably cannot be universally applied. In other words, one cannot *deduce* an ethical course of action in all circumstances, even after accepting a set of principles. However, there are three ethical ideals which are widely accepted in modern medical practice: respect for persons (individual autonomy), beneficence, and justice [Levine, 1986; National Commission for Protection of Human Subjects of Biomedical and Behavioral Research, 1978]. Taken together, they provide guidance for ethically appropriate behavior when conducting human experimentation. The National Commission addressed the ethics of human research specifically in outlining the principles and acknowledged the conflicts that can occur in specific circumstances and even between the principles themselves.

Respect for Persons (Autonomy)

Autonomy is the right of self-governance and means that patients have the right to decide what should be done for them during their illness. Because autonomy implies decision, it requires information for the basis of a decision. Autonomous patients need to be informed of alternatives, including no treatment when appropriate, and the risks and benefits associated with each.

The principle of autonomy is not restricted to clinical trial settings, but is broadly applicable in medical care. Practitioners who prefer a particular treatment usually recognize that realistic alternatives are possible and that the individual needs to make informed selections. In situations where the patient is incapacitated or otherwise unable to make informed decisions, the principle of autonomy extends to those closest to the patient. This may mean that patients without autonomy (e.g., children or incapacitated patients) should not be allowed to participate in research.

Clinical trials often ask that patients surrender some degree of autonomy. For example, in a trial, the patient may not be able to choose between two or more appropriate treatments (randomization may do it) or the patient may be asked to undergo inconvenient or extensive evaluations to comply with the study protocol. In a masked clinical trial, the patient may be made aware of risks and benefits of each treatment, but be unable to apply that information personally with certainty. However, to some extent, the patient's autonomy is retrievable. When clinical circumstances require it or when reliable information becomes available, the patient can be more fully informed or trial participation can be ended. The "re-consent" process is an example of this.

Temporarily giving up autonomy is not unique to clinical trials, but is a feature of many medical circumstances. Consider the patient who undergoes surgery using a general anesthetic. Although informed beforehand of the risks and benefits, the patient is not autonomous during the procedure, particularly if the surgeon encounters something unexpected.

Respect for persons is an idea that incorporates two ethical convictions. The first is autonomy, as discussed above, and second, that persons with diminished autonomy need protection from potential abuses. Some individuals, especially those who have illnesses, mental disability, or circumstances that restrict their personal freedom, have diminished autonomy. People in these categories may need protection, or even exclusion, from certain research activities. Other individuals may need only to acknowledge that they undertake activities freely and are aware of potential risks.

A circumstance in which application of this principle is problematic occurs in using prisoners for research purposes. One could presume that prisoners should have the opportunity to volunteer for research. However, prison conditions could be coercive on individuals who appear to volunteer for research activities. This is especially true if there are tangible benefits or privileges to be gained from participation in this research. Consequently, as the Belmont Report states, it is not clear whether prisoners should be allowed to volunteer or should be protected in such circumstances.

Beneficence and Nonmaleficence

Beneficence is a principle that reflects the patient's right to receive advantageous or favorable consideration, i.e., derive benefit. Nonmaleficence is the physician's duty to avoid harm (*primum non nocere*) and to minimize the risk of harm. We can refer to these principles jointly as beneficence. Because physicians also have a duty to benefit others when possible, the principle of beneficence has the potential to conflict with itself. For example, knowledge of what provides benefit and causes harm comes from research. Therefore, investigators are obliged to make practical and useful assessments of the risks and benefits involved in research. This necessitates resolving the potential conflict between risk to participants and benefit to future patients.

Research can create more than minimal risk without immediate direct benefit to the research subject. In some cases, such research will not be permitted by oversight committees. However, in other cases, it may be justified. For example, many arguments have been made by patients infected with HIV that unproven but potentially beneficial treatments should be available to them. Some of these treatments carry the possibility of harm with a low potential for benefit. The use of baboon bone marrow transplantation in AIDS may be an example.

The assessment of risks and benefits requires that research studies be scientifically valid and therefore properly designed. However, valid studies do not automatically have value or significance for science, the participants, or future patients. In addition to validity, the study must investigate an important question and have an appropriate risk/benefit ratio for the participants. Investigators should probably establish the scientific validity of a proposed study prior to considering the ethical question of whether or not is has value or significance. The principle of beneficence can be satisfied only when both components are favorable.

Justice

The principle of justice addresses the question of fairly distributing the benefits and burdens of research. Compensation for injury during research is a direct application of this principle. Injustice occurs when benefits are denied without good reason or when the burdens are unduly imposed on particular individuals. In the early part of this century, burdens of research fell largely upon poor patients admitted to the public wards of the hospital. In contrast, benefits of improvements learned at their expense often accrued to private patients. The injustice of denying treatment to men in the Tuskegee Syphilis Study has already been discussed.

There are some circumstances in which distinctions based on experience, competence, age, and other criteria justify differential treatment. For reasons already mentioned, research should be conducted preferentially on adults rather than children. Institutionalized patients and prisoners should be involved in research only if it relates directly to their conditions and there are not alternative subjects with full autonomy.

3.4.3   Ethical principles have practical implications

Modern principles of biomedical ethics imply three formal requirements for the ethical conduct of research [Wells, 1992]. The first is informed consent of the participants. The second is assessment and disclosure of the risks and benefits. The third requires the appropriate selection of research subjects. The practical application of these ideas requires several components including optimal study design, investigator competence, a balance of risk and benefit for study participants, patient privacy, and impartial oversight of consent procedures [Sieber, 1993]. These are discussed next.

Good study design

Good study design means that patients on a trial are contributing to answering a scientific question that is important and that has a high chance of being answered by the experiment being undertaken. Research designs which are grossly flawed or those that cannot answer the biological question are not ethical. Similarly, those that ask unimportant questions are unethical, even if they pose minimal risk. As Rutstein [1969] said:

It may be accepted as a maxim that a poorly or improperly designed study involving human subjects ... is by definition unethical. Moreover, when a study is in itself scientifically invalid, all other ethical considerations become irrelevant.

Investigator competence

There are two components to investigator competence: technical and humanistic. Technical competence is assessed by education, knowledge, certification, and experience. In addition to technical competence, the investigator must have research competence. This means, for example, that the investigator has performed a competent systematic review of current knowledge and previous trials to be certain that the planned study is justified. When the clinical trial is completed, an accurate and complete description of the results should be published to insure dissemination of the knowledge [Herxheimer, 1993].

Humanistic competence requires compassion and empathy. These cannot be taught in the same way that technical competence can, but the proper clinical and research environment and good research mentoring facilitate it.

Balance of harm and benefit

The assessments of risk and benefits implies that the research is properly designed and has been reviewed from this perspective by the investigators. Occasionally, alternative ways of providing benefits to the patient might be available without involving research. In any case, investigators must take care to distinguish between the probability of harm and the severity of the effect. These distinctions can be obscured when terms like "high" or "low risk" are used. For example, if a life-threatening or fatal side effect is encountered with low frequency, is this high risk? Similarly, benefits have magnitudes and probabilities associated with them. Furthermore, risks or benefits may not accrue only to the research subject. In some cases, the risks or benefits may affect patient families or society at large.

Physicians engaged in a clinical trial must exclude patients from the study if they are at undue risk or are otherwise vulnerable [Weijer and Fuks, 1994]. Having the study reviewed by the IRB or other ethics board, satisfying eligibility criteria, and using informed consent do not eliminate this duty. Patients may be found to have an unexpectedly high risk as a result of errors in judgement about their risk, atypical reactions or side effects from the treatment, or for unknown reasons. In any case, the individuals affected and others like them should be excluded from further participation.

Privacy

Patient rights to privacy has a long tradition. This right must be protected and has been made ascendent even in circumstances such as the AIDS epidemic, where certain benefits to society could be gained by restricting the right to privacy (e.g., contact tracing and AIDS screening). It is maintained by appropriate precautions regarding written records and physician conduct. In the information age, extra care is required to maintain privacy on computerized records or other electronic media that can be easily shared with colleagues and widely disseminated.

Maintaining privacy requires steps such as patient consent, restricting the collection of personal information to appropriate settings, ensuring security of records, and preventing disclosure. These and other privacy principles have been crafted into a comprehensive set of guidelines in Australia [Cooper, 1991], and are relevant broadly.

Institutional review

Review of proposed and ongoing research studies is performed by institutions through at least two mechanisms. In the U.S., the first is the Institutional Review Board (IRB) which is responsible for the ethical oversight of all Public Health Service sponsored investigation. In other countries, this role is covered by an Independent Ethics Committee (IEC) (Australia), a Local Research Ethics Committee (LREC) (England), or a Research Ethics Board (Canada). For convenience, I will refer to all such committees as IRBs. IRB committees are typically composed of medical practitioners, bioethicists, lawyers, and community representatives. They review planned trials from an ethical perspective, including consent documents and procedures. Increasingly, IRBs are being asked also to review the scientific components of research studies. This can be helpful when the expertise is available and a hindrance when it is not.

A second method by which institutions or collaborative clinical trial groups review studies is by using a Data and Safety Monitoring Committee (DSMC). These committees oversee ongoing clinical trials with regard to treatment efficacy and safety. If convincing evidence about efficacy is provided by the trial before its planned conclusion, the DSMC will recommend early termination. Similarly, if serious unforeseen toxicities or side effects are discovered, the trial might be halted. Designing and executing this aspect of a trial can be complex and is discussed in Chapter 10.

Informed consent

Informed consent is a complex but important aspect of the practice and regulation of clinical trials. The requirement for consent is grounded in moral and legal theory and clinical practice. A perspective on this and historical developments in informed consent is given by Faden and Beauchamp [1986]. Broad reviews of issues surrounding informed consent are given by Appelbaum, Lidz, and Meisel [1987], and Rozovsky [1990]. In the context of AIDS, a useful review has been written by Gray, Lyons, and Melton [1995].

Elements of informed consent include information provided to the patient, comprehension of that information by the patient and his or her family, and an assessment of the voluntary nature of the consent. The information required in a consent document generally includes the nature of the research procedure, its scientific purpose, and alternatives to participation in the study. Patient comprehension is facilitated by careful attention to the organization, style, and reading level of consent forms. When children are subjects of research, it is frequently necessary to obtain informed consent from the legal guardian and obtain assent from the child. To verify that consent is given voluntarily, the conditions under which it is obtained must be free of coercion and undue influence. Conditions should not permit overt threats or undue influence to affect the individual's choice.

A problem area for consent is in conducting research on emergency medical treatments. It is instructive to review the problems with consent in the emergency room setting as a microcosm of consent issues [Biros et al., 1995]. The principal difficulty is in being able to obtain valid consent from critically ill patients to test promising new treatments with good research designs. Some patients may be unconscious, relatives may be unavailable, or there may not be sufficient time to meet the same standards of informativeness and consent as in ordinary hospital or clinic settings.

In 1996, the FDA and NIH proposed new measures for the protection of research subjects in emergency settings. The new FDA rules and NIH policies on emergency consent waiver make it easier to study drugs and devices in patients with life-threatening conditions who are unable to give informed consent. The new regulations permit enrolling patients in research studies without their consent provided the following criteria are met:

1. An independent physician and an IRB agree to the research and that it addresses a life-threatening situation,
2. The patient is in a life-threatening situation,
3. Conventional treatments are unproven or unsatisfactory,
4. The research is necessary to determine the safety and efficacy of the treatment and it cannot be carried out otherwise,
5. Informed consent cannot feasibly be obtained from the patient or legal representative,
6. The risks and potential benefits of the experimental procedure are reasonable compared with those for the underlying medical condition of the patient and standard treatments,
7. Additional protections are in place such as consultations with the community, advance public disclosure of the study design and risks, public disclosure of the study results, and FDA review of the study protocol.

The merits and weaknesses of these specialized rules will be evident in the next few years as they are applied in specific research projects.

Data monitoring

As indicated above, safety monitoring of data collected during a clinical trial is a requirement of ethical oversight. Adverse events should be reported to sponsors and regulators promptly. Efficacy monitoring is not an explicit requirement, although it is frequently conducted according to predetermined structured plans. Both of these concerns may be dealt with by a Data and Safety Monitoring Committee (DSCMC). This aspect of trial design and conduct is discussed in Chapter 10.

3.4.4   Investigators must maintain objectivity

The Code of Federal Regulations (42 CFR 50) specifies rules to ensure objectivity in research sponsored by the Public Health Service. Investigators must disclose significant financial interests defined as equity exceeding $10,000 or five percent or more ownership that would reasonably appear to affect the design, conduct, or reporting of research supported by the PHS. Personal financial interests as well as those of a spouse and dependent children are included.

Significant financial interest is defined as anything of monetary value including salary, consulting fees, honoraria, equity such as stocks or other types of ownership, and intellectual property rights such as patents, copyrights, and royalties. Significant financial interest does not include income from seminars, lectures, or teaching sponsored by public or not-for-profit organizations below the thresholds cited above.

Management of financial interests that could create bias may require investigators to reduce or eliminate the holdings, recognition and oversight by the research institution, public disclosure, or modification of the research plan. Investigators can anticipate such problems and disqualify themselves from participation in studies that present the opportunity for bias. Many experienced investigators have potential conflicts, often of a minor or indirect nature. An example is when their university or institution benefits directly from a particular study, although they do not. Such cases can often be managed simply by public disclosure.

Research misconduct or fraud is an extreme example of loss of objectivity. This important subject is discussed in Chapter 18. Misconduct can have many contributing factors, but a lack of objectivity about the role of the investigator is often one cause.

Although often unrecognized, competing research interests are a potential source of lack of objectivity. Consider the investigator who has multiple research opportunities, or a mix of research and "practice" options, available to patients. For example, there might be competing clinical trials with the same or similar eligibility criteria. This can lead to the physician acting as an investigator for some patients, a different investigator for others, and as a practitioner for still others. If treatment or research preferences are driven partly by financial concerns, reimbursement issues, ego, research prowess, or other pressures, the potential for conflicting interests is high.

Although this situation is common in academic medical centers where many studies are available, investigators often do not recognize it as a source of conflict. A solution to such problems is facilitated by non-overlapping investigations, a clear priority for any competing studies, and not concurrently conducting research and practice in the same patient population. This may mean, for example, that when conducting a clinical trial, ineligible patients or those declining participation because of a treatment preference might be best referred to a trustworthy colleague not participating in the study.

3.5   Professional Statistical Ethics

In recent years, professional societies have examined ethical issues surrounding the practice of statistical methods. Both the American Statistical Association (ASA) and the Royal Statistical Society (RSS) have published guidelines for the conduct of their members. The two sets of guidelines are similar in content [ASA, 1995; RSS, 1993].

The ASA is the oldest professional society in the United States. Its Committee on Professional Ethics perceives the potential benefit and harm from the use of statistical methods in science and public policy. Circumstances where statistical thinking can be misused include not only clinical trials and other areas of medicine, but also statistical findings presented as evidence in courts of law, and some political issues. The ASA's position on ethical matters follows closely those of W. E. Deming, one of its most prominent members [Deming, 1986]. Although the Society for Clinical Trials is more directly concerned and involved with clinical trials and has many statisticians as members, they have not dealt directly with professional ethics of statisticians in this context.

The ASA and RSS guidelines do not articulate fundamental professional ethical principles directly in the way that has been done for patients' rights in medical research, nor do they deal directly with clinical trials. However, the message implicit in the guidelines has several components similar in spirit to those outlined earlier in this chapter and is relevant to statistical practice surrounding clinical trials. These include 1) investigator competence, 2) disclosure of potential conflicts, 3) confidentiality, 4) documentation of methods, and 5) openness. Both sets of guidelines are summarized and abstracted here.

3.5.1   General

Statisticians have a public duty to maintain integrity, particularly where private interests can inappropriately affect the development or application of statistical knowledge. Statisticians should follow several general guidelines:

- Maintain professional competence and keep abreast of developments,
- Have constant regard for human rights,
- Present findings and interpretations honestly and objectively,
- Avoid untrue, deceptive, or undocumented statements,
- Disclose financial or other interests that may affect or appear to affect their professional statements,
- Seek to advance public knowledge and understanding, and
- Encourage and support fellow members in their professional development.

3.5.2   Data collection

Collecting data for inquiries can present a burden for patients or other respondents. It may be seen as an invasion of privacy and often raises concerns about confidentiality. Therefore, statisticians should do the following:

- Collect only the data needed for the purposes of the inquiry,
- Inform each respondent about the nature and sponsorship of the project and the intended uses of the data,
- Establish the intentions and ability of the sponsor to protect confidentiality,
- Inform respondents of the strengths and limitations of confidentiality protections,
- Process the data collected according to the intentions and remove respondent identifying information where appropriate, and
- Ensure that when data are transferred to other persons or organizations, confidentiality is maintained through written agreement if necessary.

3.5.3   Openness

Statistical work must be open to assessment of quality, assumptions, methods, and data processing. Statisticians should, therefore, do the following:

- Delineate the scope of the inquiry and inferences that can be derived from it,
- Emphasize the essential nature of statistical components in the investigation,
- Document data sources and known inaccuracies, steps taken to refine the data, and the procedures and assumptions applied,
- Make the data available with appropriate protections of privacy,
- Recognize the role of judgment and possibility for disagreement in the selection of statistical procedures, and
- Refer criticism to the investigation and not to the individuals conducting the study.

3.5.4   Client relationships

Clients and sponsors may be unfamiliar with statistical practice and procedures. The statistician should provide information as shown below:

- Make their qualifications to undertake the inquiry clear,
- Inform clients or sponsors of all factors that conflict with the statistician's impartiality,
- Accept no contingency fee arrangements,
- Fulfill all commitments and obligations,
- Apply methods without regard for a desirable outcome,
- Outline clearly and concisely alternate approaches along with the methods used, and
- Maintain confidentiality with regard to other clients or sponsors.

3.5.5   Extensions

The ethical guidelines of the ASA are intended to be open-ended and to permit modification. Some changes may be necessary in the future, depending on specific circumstances. For example, specialized areas such as medicine and law may require further ethical delineations. Similarly, publication of statistical reports and related documents may raise special issues not covered in the current guidelines. Finally, resolving differences of opinion or disputes may require further procedures or ethical guidelines.

3.6   Summary

Clinical trials highlight some of the competing obligations that physicians and patients face in health care today. There is potential for clinical trials to be poorly planned or conducted, compromising the ethical treatment of research subjects. This potential exists in many areas of medical practice and must be counterbalanced by safeguards and standards of ethical conduct. Features of some clinical trials such as randomization and the use of placebos illustrate clearly competing obligations. However, trials do not necessarily generate unique ethical concerns or make them unsolvable.

The history of medical experimentation in the twentieth century illustrates the potential for infringing on the rights of patients and an evolving standard for conducting medical research of all types. Protections for patients are based on international agreements and guidelines, governmental regulations, institutional standards and review, and the ethical principles of autonomy, beneficence, and justice. Careful practical implementation of these protections usually yields clinical trials that are ethically acceptable. Ethical norms, especially those for clinical trials, appear to be culturally dependent.

There are circumstances where the most ethical course of action for the physician is to recommend participation in a clinical trial. This may be the case when the physician is genuinely uncertain about the benefit of a treatment or the difference between alternative treatments. Opinions about treatments based on evidence of poor quality are not ethically legitimate, even if they are firmly held. Opinions based on scientifically weak evidence are subject to influence by financial, academic, or personal pressures.

Clinical trial statisticians are also held to standards of professional conduct. These standards require competence, confidentiality, impartiality, and openness.. Like other investigators, the statistician must demonstrate an absence of conflicts of interest.

3.7   Questions for Discussion

1. Financial and academic pressures appear not to be the primary ethical conflict in clinical trials. Is this accurate or not? Discuss how these pressures can compromise the rights of the research subject.
2. Some clinical trials aren't conducted in the U.S., either because of ethical concerns or lack of patient acceptance. Trials are sometimes more feasible in other countries even when conducted by U.S. sponsors. An example is

the pertussis vaccine trial [Greco et al., 1994; Leary, 1994; Marwick, 1994]. Comment on the ethics of this practice.

3. Are risks and benefits evenly distributed between trial participants and future patients? Discuss your point of view.

4. In recent years, there has been heightened concern over potential differences in treatment effects between men and women, especially if a trial enrolled patients of only one sex. In some cases, trials have been essentially repeated by sex, e.g., the Physicians Health Study [Steering Committee of the Physicians' Health Study Research Group, 1989] and the Womens Physicians' Health Study [Meyers et al., 1995]. When is this practice ethical and when is it not? Are there ethical concerns about resource utilization?

5. There is a need for physicians to conduct research in some settings where patients (and their families) can neither be informed nor give consent in the conventional manner. An example might be in the emergency department for cardiopulmonary resuscitation or head injury. Discuss whether or not clinical trials can be conducted ethically in such circumstances.

6. Developing interventions and conducting clinical trials in specific disease areas like medical devices, biological agents, surgery, AIDS, cytotoxic drugs, and disease prevention can be quite different. Discuss how clinical trials in these various areas raise different ethical issues.

Chapter References

American Cancer Society (ACS) (1990). Questionable cancer practices in Tijuana and other Mexican border clinics. Statement approved by the Committee on Questionable Methods of Cancer Management.

American Cancer Society (1993). Questionable methods of cancer management: "nutritional" therapies. CA Cancer Journal for Clinicians 43(5): 309-319.

Annas, G.J., and Grodin, M.A. (1992). The Nazi Doctors and the Nuremberg Code: Human Rights in Human Experimentation. New York: Oxford University Press.

Appelbaum, P.S., Lidz, C.W., and Meisel, A. (1987). Informed Consent: Legal Theory and Clinical Practice. New York: Oxford University Press.

ASA (1995). Ethical Guidelines for Statistical Practice.

Aulas, J.J. (1996). Alternative cancer treatments. Scientific American 275(3): 162-163.

Barrett, S. (1993). "Alternative" Cancer Treatment. Chapter 6 in S. Barrett and W.T. Jarvis (Eds.). The Health Robbers. Buffalo, NY: Prometheus Books.

Baum, M., Houghton, J., and Abrams, K. (1994). Early stopping rules – clinical perspectives and ethical considerations. Statistics in Medicine 13: 1459-1469.

Beauchamp, T.L., and Childress, J.F. (1989). Principles of Biomedical Ethics. 3rd Ed.., New York: Oxford University Press.

Beecher, H.K. (1966). Ethics and clinical research. New Engl. J. Med. 274: 1354-1360.

Biros, M.H., Lewis, R.J., Olson, C.M., et al. (1995). Informed consent in emergency research. JAMA 273: 1283-1287.

Brandt, A.M. (1978). Racism and research: The case of the Tuskegee syphilis study. Hastings Center Report 8: 21-29.

Brett, A.S. (1981). Sounding board – hidden ethical issues in clinical decision analysis. New Engl. J. Med. 5: 1150-1152.

Bridgen, M.L. (1995). Unproven (questionable) cancer therapies. Western J. Med. 163(5): 463-469.

Casselith, B.R. and Chapman, C.C. (1996). Alternative cancer medicine: A ten-year update. Cancer Invest. 14(4): 396-404.

Centers for Disease Control. (1997). Paralytic poliomyelitis – United States, 1980-1994. MMWR 46(4): 79-83.

Chalmers, I., and Silverman, W.A. (1987). Professional and public double standards on clinical experimentation. Controlled Clin. Trials 8: 388-391.

Cooper, J.E. (1991). Balancing the scales of public interest: Medical research and privacy. Med. J. Austr. 155: 556-560.

Coughlin, S.S. (Ed.) (1995). Ethics in Epidemiology and Clinical Research. Newton, MA: Epidemiology Resources.

Council for International Organizations of Medical Sciences (CIOMS) (1993). International Ethical Guidelines for Biomedical Research Involving Human Subjects. Geneva.

Deming, W.E. (1986). Principles of professional statistical practice. In S. Kotz, N.L. Johnson, and C.B. Read (Eds.) Encyclopedia of Statistical Sciences. New York: John Wiley & Sons.

Department of Health, Education, and Welfare (1973). Final Report of the Tuskegee Syphilis Study Ad Hoc Advisory Panel. Washington, DC: GPO.

Dorland's Medical Dictionary, 28th Edition (1994). Philadelphia: W. B. Saunders.

Eisenberg, D.M., Kessler, R.C., Foster, C., Norlock, F.E., Calkins, D.R. and Delbanco, T.L. (1993). Unconventional medicine in the United States: Prevalence, costs, and patterns of use. New Engl. J. Med. 328(4): 246-252.

Eisenberg, L. (1977). The social imperatives of medical research. Science 198: 1105-1110.

Faden, R.R., and Beauchamp, T.L. (1986). A History and Theory of Informed Consent. New York: Oxford University Press.

Fayerweather, W.E., Higginson, J., and Beauchamp, T.L. (Eds.) (1991). Ethics in Epidemiology. Journal of Clinical Epidemiology (suppl.) 44: 1S-151S.

Freedman, B. (1987). Equipoise and the ethics of clinical research. N. Eng. J. Med. 317: 141-145.

Freedman, B. (1992). A response to a purported ethical difficulty with randomized clinical trials involving cancer patients. J. Clinical Ethics 3(3): 231-234.

Freund, P.A. (1972). Experimentation with Human Subjects. Great Britain: Clarke Doble and Brendon.

Fried, C. (1974). Medical experimentation: Personal integrity and social policy. Vol. 5 [A.G. Bearn, D.A.K. Black, and H.H. Hiatt (Eds.)], Amsterdam: North-Holland.

Gilbert, J.P., McPeek, B., and Mosteller, F. (1977). Statistics and ethics in surgery and anesthesia. Science 198: 684-689.

Gray, J.N., Lyons, P.M., Jr., and Melton, G.B. (1995). Ethical and Legal Issues in AIDS Research. Baltimore: Johns Hopkins University Press.

Greco, D., Salinaso, S., and Mastrantonio, P. (1994). The Italian pertussis vaccine trial: Ethical issues (letter). JAMA 272: 1898-1899.

Guttentag, O.E. (1953). The problem of experimentation on human beings: II. The physician's point of view. Science 117: 207-210.

Hellman, S., and Hellman, D.S. (1991). Of mice but not men: Problems of the randomized clinical trial. New Eng. J. Med. 324: 1585-1589.

Herbert, V. (1977). Acquiring new information while retaining old ethics. Science 198: 690-693.

Herxheimer, A. (1993). Clinical trials: Two neglected ethical issues. J. Med. Ethics 19: 211-218.

Hill, Sir A.B. (1963). Medical ethics and controlled trials. BMJ April: 1043-1049.

Ivy, A.C. (1948). The history and ethics of the use of human subjects in medical experiments. Science 108: 1-5.

Jones, J.H. (1981). Bad blood: The Tuskegee Syphilis Experiment. New York: Free Press.

Judicial Council of the American Medical Association (1946). Supplementary Report. J. Am. Medical Assoc. 132: 1090.

Katz, J. (1972). Experimentation with Human Beings. New York: Russell Sage Foundation.

Lantos, J. (1993). Informed consent. The whole truth for patients? Cancer (suppl.) 72: 2811-2815.

Lantos, J. (1994). Ethics, randomization, and technology assessment. Cancer (suppl.) 74: 2653-2656.

Leary, W.E. (1994). Critics question ethics of U.S.-sponsored vaccine tests in Italy and Sweden. New York Times (Sunday, March 13).

Levine, R.J. (1986). Ethics and Regulation of Clinical Research. Second Edition, New Haven, Conn. and London: Yale University Press.

Levine, R.J. (1992). Clinical trials and physicians as double agents. Yale J. Biology Med. 65: 65-74.

Levinsky, N.G. (1996). Social, institutional, and economic barriers to the exercise of patients' rights. New Engl. J. Med. 334: 532-534.

Markman, M. (1992). Ethical difficulties with randomized clinical trials involving cancer patients: Examples from the field of gynecologic oncology. J. Clinical Ethics 3(3): 193-195.

Marshall, E. (1994). The politics of alternative medicine. Science 265: 2000-2002.

Marwick, C. (1994). Ethicist faults human research protection. JAMA 271: 1228-1229.

McGinnis, L.S. (1990). Alternative therapies, 1990. Cancer 67: 1788-1792.

McNeill, P.M. (1993). The Ethics and Politics of Human Experimentation. Cambridge: Press Syndicate of the University of Cambridge.

Meyers, A.H., Rosner, B., Abbey, H., Willet, W., Stampfer, M.J., and Bain, C. (1995). The Women Physicians' Health Study: Background, objectives, and methods. J. Am. Med. Womens Assoc. 50: 64-66.

Miké, V., Krauss, A.N., and Ross, G.S. (1993). Neonatal extracorporeal membrane oxygenation (ECMO): Clinical trials and the ethics of evidence. J. Med. Ethics 19: 212-218.

National Commission for Protection of Human Subjects of Biomedical and Behavioral Research (1978). The Belmont Report: Ethical Principles and Guidelines for the Protection of Human Subjects of Research. Washington, DC: DHEW Publication Number (OS) 78-0012. Appendix I, DHEW Publication No. (OS) 78-0013; Appendix II, DHEW Publication No. (OS) 78-0014.

Office of Technology Assessment (1990). Unconventional Cancer Treatments. OTA-H-405. Washington, DC: U.S. Government Printing Office.

Passamani, E. (1991). Clinical trials – Are they ethical? New Eng. J. Med. 324: 1589-1592.

Ramsey, P. (1975). The ethics of fetal research. New Haven, CT and London: Yale University Press.

Reich, W.T. (Ed.) (1995). Encyclopedia of Bioethics. New York: Simon & Schuster/Macmillan.

Reiser, S.J. (1993). The ethics movement in the biological sciences: A new voyage of discovery. Overview in R.E. Bulger, E. Heitman, and S.J. Reiser (Eds.), The Ethical Dimensions of the Biological Sciences. Cambridge: Cambridge University Press.

Rothman, K.J., and Michels, K.B. (1994). The continuing unethical use of placebo controls. New Engl. J. Med. 331: 394-398.

Roy, D.J. (1986). Controlled clinical trials: An ethical imperative. J. Chron. Dis. 39: 159-162.

Royall, R.M. (1991). Ethics and statistics in randomized clinical trials. Statistical Science 6: 52-88.

Royall, R.M. (1992). Ignorance and altruism. Journal of Clinical Ethics 3(3): 229-230.

Rozovsky, F.A. (1990). Consent to Treatment, A Practical Guide. Boston: Little Brown & Co.

RSS (1993). The Royal Statistical Society: Code of Conduct.

Rutstein, D. (1969). Daedalus 98: 523.

Schaefer, A. (1982). The ethics of the randomized clinical trial. N. Engl. J. Med. 307: 719-724.

Schuman, S.H., Olansky, S., Rivers, E., Smith, C.A., and Rambo, D.S. (1955). Untreated syphilis in the male negro. J. Chron. Dis. 2: 543-558.

Shimkin, M.B. (1953). The problem of experimentation on human beings: I. The research worker's point of view. Science 117: 205-207.

Sieber, J.E. (1993). Ethical considerations in planning and conducting research on human subjects. Academic Medicine (suppl.) 68: S9-S13.

Siegler, M. (1982). Confidentiality in medicine – A decrepit concept. New Eng. J. Med. 307: 1518-1521.

Steering Committee of the Physicians' Health Study Research Group (1989). Final report on the aspirin component of the ongoing Physicians' Health Study. New Engl. J. Med. 321: 129-135.

Tukey, J.W. (1977). Some thoughts on clinical trials, especially problems of multiplicity. Science 198: 670-684.

U.S. Congress (Aug., 1980). The Forgotten Guinea Pigs; A Report on the Health Effects of Low Level Radiation Sustained as a Result of the Nuclear Weapons Testing Program Conducted by the United States Government. Washington, DC: Government Printing Office.

Weijer, C., and Fuks, A. (1994). The duty to exclude: Excluding people at undue risk from research. Clin. Invest. Med. 17: 115-122.

Williams, C.J. (Ed.) (1992). Introducing New Treatments for Cancer: Practical, Ethical, and Legal Problems. Chichester: John Wiley & Sons.

Wells, F. (1992) Good Clinical Research Practice. Chapter 19 in Introducing New Treatments for Cancer: Practical, Ethical, and Legal Problems, edited by C.J. Williams. New York: John Wiley & Sons.

World Medical Association (1964). Declaration of Helsinki: recommendations guiding medical doctors in biomedical research involving human subjects. (Revised 1975, 1983, and 1989.) Helsinki: World Medical Association. See also British Med. J. 2: 177, 1964.

CHAPTER 4

Clinical Trials as Experimental Designs

4.1 Introduction

Formal definitions for *experiment, clinical trial,* and *design* were offered in Section 2.1.4. We can view an experiment as a series of carefully collected observations made under conditions controlled or arranged by the investigator [Stebbing, 1961]. The essential focus of control and design of a clinical trial is the assignment of study subjects to the treatment groups. True experimental designs have features to control systematic error, reduce random variation, increase precision, and assess treatment interactions. By removing systematic error and breaking apart natural correlations, the effects of interest can often be isolated and estimated with a high degree of precision. Proper design and analysis allows the investigator to attribute observed differences reliably either to the factors under control or to random error.

The study of experimental designs has developed around agricultural trials, industrial and laboratory experiments, and animal studies [Cochran and Cox, 1957; Cox, 1958; Haaland, 1989; Heiberger, 1989; Hinklemann and Kempthorne, 1994; Lorenzen and Anderson, 1993; Winer, 1962]. In these non-clinical settings, investigators have the greatest degree of control over the structure and size of the study and the experimental subjects. Clinical trials is a relatively new science to draw upon this body of knowledge [Fleiss, 1986]. In fact, the field of clinical trial design has not drawn as much strength as it could from classic experimental design until recently. An interesting area of overlap is factorial experiments, discussed in Chapter 15.

Although they have the characteristics of true experimental designs, clinical trials lack some important features of studies on inanimate objects, plants, or animals, which have been the focus of classic experimental designs. First, human responses to medical treatments tend to be more variable than those from genetically identical plants or animals or from tightly controlled physical and chemical processes.

The clinical investigator is not usually able to control as many sources of variability through design, as can the laboratory or industrial experimenter. This leads clinical experiments to have a relatively large number of subjects assigned to each treatment to provide control over random variation.

Second, experiments on non-human subjects are subject to relatively few constraints compared with clinical trials. The study can often be made as large as scientifically necessary apart from economic considerations. Ethical issues, if they exist, are not usually internal to the experiment. In contrast, clinical trials are constrained by cost and respect for research subjects. Also, some important biological questions cannot be answered because patients with the needed characteristics simply do not exist.

Third, the clinical investigator usually cannot test all subjects simultaneously, as might be done in an agricultural or industrial trial. This leads to long study durations while patients are accrued and followed. Some outcomes in clinical trials require long periods of follow-up to manifest themselves (e.g., survival or disease progression). This also prolongs study duration and creates opportunities for data to be lost. Lengthy clinical trials may allow additional sources of variability to be introduced into the treatment assessment. Changes in the health care system, new methods of supportive or ancillary care, adjuvant therapies, or other factors not anticipated in the initial design can affect the treatment estimate or comparison.

Fourth, in therapeutic trials it is often impossible to test multiple treatments in the same patient because of overlapping side effects. A focus of agricultural, industrial, and animal experiments is usually to study more than one effect. Two possible exceptions to this general difference are trials of diagnostic tests and disease prevention studies, where the interventions are usually very low risk for the study participants. These settings may be conducive to studying more than one treatment in the same patient.

Fifth, the use of uncertainty to motivate clinical trials is more formal and fundamental than in studies on inanimate objects or animals. There is always an epistemological importance to uncertainty in medicine and it can be an important tool in experimentation. The degree of uncertainty that motivates a clinical trial is likely to be higher than that underlying many experiments in agriculture, industry, or the laboratory. A high degree of certainty in the outcome results in "demonstration trials" which may be appropriate (and common) in fields other than clinical trials.

4.1.1   Study design is critical for inference

Students of clinical trials tend to approach the subject with a focus on performing correct analyses. Although there are many pitfalls for the inexperienced or uncritical data analyst, good trial design and conduct is considerably more important than analysis. Skillful analyses can almost never correct design faults. Furthermore, good designs are usually simple to analyze correctly. When a trial is well designed and properly performed, analyses can be conducted, modified, and corrected until they reveal the evidence needed from the study. We hope that all this will take place prior to publication, but the data can be assessed again later if new analytic methods are required.

Two serious shortcomings of poorly designed and implemented trials are not amenable to correction with analysis. These are systematic error, such as selection bias, and imprecision in the estimate of the treatment effect. Bias reduction is a consequence of design efforts like using objective endpoints, active ascertainment of outcomes, no *post hoc* exclusions based on outcome, and impartial treatment assignment (e.g., randomization in comparative studies). High precision is mainly a consequence of having employed an adequate sample size. If investigators have failed to use good design features for these or other important aspects of the trial, there are no analysis methods that will allow them to recover convincingly from the error.

Careful attention to design yields several benefits that cannot be guaranteed by any analysis. Proper design:

1. Allows investigators to satisfy ethical constraints;
2. Permits efficient use of scarce resources;
3. Isolates the treatment effect of interest from confounders;
4. Controls precision;
5. Reduces bias;
6. Minimizes and quantifies random error or uncertainty;
7. Simplifies and validates the analysis; and
8. Increases the external validity of the trial.

These advantages should provide sufficient reason for investigators to place an emphasis on design rather than on analysis.

4.1.2   Essentials provide for a good study

The most critical and difficult prerequisite for a good study is to select an important feasible question to answer. Accomplishing this is a consequence primarily of biological knowledge:

> The best of science doesn't consist of mathematical models and experiments, as textbooks make it seem. Those come later. It springs fresh from a more primitive mode of thought, wherein the hunter's mind weaves ideas from old facts and fresh metaphors and the scrambled crazy images of things recently seen. To move forward is to concoct new patterns of thought, which in turn dictate the design of the models and experiments [Wilson, 1992].

Apart from such insights, good experimental design and avoiding methodological errors will facilitate asking the right question.

The purpose of most trials is to estimate the magnitude of effects (or differences) in treatments that have been carefully specified. Like all rigorous experimental designs, trials are most necessary and effective when the treatment effects under ordinary conditions are likely to be masked by random and/or systematic fluctuations in the measured responses. To accomplish its goals, a trial should:

1. Quantify and reduce errors resulting from chance;

2. Reduce or eliminate bias;
3. Yield clinically relevant estimates of effects and precision;
4. Be simple in design and analysis;
5. Provide a high degree of credibility, reproducibility, and external validity; and
6. Influence future clinical practice.

Conceptual simplicity in design and analysis is a very important feature of good trials. Some investigators worry that clinical trials themselves, their infrastructure, and the statistical machinery needed to design and analyze them, are too complex to be reliable. It is true that clinical trials fall outside the range of experience of many medical practitioners and that they are by no means the only way of making valid clinical inferences. However, simple ideas often lead to simple solutions only after encountering complexities along the way. Fortunately, the complexities in clinical trials are usually logistical rather than conceptual. This is analogous to the way in which surgical treatments are often conceptually straightforward but technically complex.

When trials cannot be made simple, they should be made parsimonious. This means that they should be designed to be as simple as possible given the complexities of the research question, treatment algorithm, assessment method, and analysis. Even in complex contexts, the effect of interest can usually be isolated by the study design. Sometimes simple research questions lead to complicated statistical analyses such as those needed to model longitudinal data. In these circumstances, the study designs and analytic methods should be parsimonious, if not simple.

It is interesting that "good" clinical trials do not always influence clinical practice, at least not immediately. This may not be a shortcoming of the study, but could be a consequence of practitioners' habit or dogma, and/or seeming inconsistencies with prior knowledge. In the long run, well-performed trials may be verified (apart from outright errors of chance) and improve clinical practice.

4.2   Design Concepts

As mentioned earlier, experimental design is a way to advance knowledge efficiently and reliably. There are ways to increase knowledge that don't rely heavily on design. These include taking advantage of chance and using incremental improvements based on experience. Using chance or "natural experiments" is a powerful but inefficient method for advancing knowledge. Incremental improvements are also reliable but slow, and may reach a local rather than a global optimum. Both of these ways of acquiring new knowledge can incorporate theory, but they subordinate it to observation. In contrast, the results of experiments carry more information because they put theory on an equal footing with data.

Man can do a great deal by observation and thinking, but with them alone he cannot unravel the mysteries of Nature. Had it been possible the Greeks would have done it; and could Plato and Aristotle have grasped the value of experiment in the progress of human knowledge, the course of European history might have been very different [Osler, 1910].

4.2.1 The foundations of design are observation and theory

Medical investigations, like all science, are based on careful observation. However, there is more to science than observation alone. Theory is required to help structure, interpret, and guide observation. Without theory, we could not separate passive experience from generalizable inference (active experience). Medical investigations can be classified and distinguished from one another on the basis of the quantity and quality of both observation and theory. In particular, true experiments test theory by controlling treatment assignments, endpoint ascertainment, and analysis, whereas nonexperimental designs lack one or more of these characteristics.

Several types of clinical observations have historically been used and might, in some circumstances, provide convincing evidence about treatments. *Case reports* usually constitute the weakest clinical evidence, because they demonstrate only that an event of some interest is possible. A single such observation, if sufficiently far outside of common experience, can yield important evidence. But most often, case reports can only generate hypotheses rather than test them, because they are roughly consistent with everyday experience. The investigator does not control treatment assignment, endpoint ascertainment, or confounders in case reports, and no formal statistical analysis is possible. As an example of the information in case reports, consider that even a life-threatening disease like cancer is not uniformly fatal. There are numerous individual case reports and case series of spontaneous remission of cancer in the medical literature [Cole, 1976; Challis and Stam, 1990; O'Regan and Hirshberg, 1993]. These are sufficient to prove that spontaneous remission happens, and generate interesting clinical hypotheses, but not convincing evidence of the efficacy of any particular treatment associated with the cases.

Case series are more helpful than case reports because they carry the weight of some experience in proportion to their size and quality. However, they also only generate hypothesis rather than test it. Although some minimal statistical analysis may be possible for extensive case series, the investigator does not control treatment assignment, selection bias, confounders, or endpoint ascertainment. For example, consider the inferential importance of the small series of patients who received Jarvik-7 artificial hearts [Fox and Swazey, 1992]. Beginning with Barney Clark at the University of Utah Medical Center, five patients were given these artificial hearts by two different surgeons at three different institutions between December 2, 1982 and April 14, 1985. Patients lived between 10 and 620 days. Despite the heterogeneity, limited number of patients, and duration of follow-up, important and convincing clinical information was obtained from the case series, suggesting that the device was not ready for wider use.

Database analyses are similar to case series but usually larger in scope and often include attempts to evaluate treatment differences. However, database analyses often have shortcomings that prevent convincing comparison of treatments. Problems include selection bias, the possibility that endpoints have been ascertained passively or in a biased way, and unidentifiable confounders secondary to unknown rationale for treatment selection [Byar, 1991; Green and Byar, 1984]. Consequently, rather than being used for treatment comparisons, databases are best used for 1) storing and retrieving information about an individual patient to help clinical management or case reporting, 2) to find or describe a group of similar patients (a cohort), or 3) to study patterns in the data with descriptive models or other statistical methods (e.g., prognostic factor studies).

Observational (e.g., epidemiologic) studies yield evidence about treatment (exposure) differences and usually control endpoint ascertainment and analysis. They lack the key design strength of experiments, which is control over treatment assignment. In actual epidemiological settings, the exposure information may be determined retrospectively (i.e., remembered by the subjects) and could therefore be affected by recall bias. This might not be a problem for treatments that are documented in a medical record. However, such studies are subject to other biases because of factors confounded with treatment selection [Green and Byar, 1984].

Comparative clinical trials control all the key components of true experimental designs. When properly designed and conducted, they yield a strong expectation that bias has been controlled. Also, the precision of a trial can be increased by studying more subjects, a conceptually simple maneuver. The credibility of comparative trials is enhanced with *independent replication* or other verification. Byar [1978] called this progression from case reports to confirmed randomized clinical trials a "hierarchy of strength of evidence" (Table 4.1). Recently, Olkin [1995] has suggested that meta-analyses with original data be taken as the highest level of credibility. Meta-analyses are discussed in Chapter 17.

4.2.2 Trials are true experimental designs

In classical terms, clinical trials tend to be rather simple experimental designs. Unlike animal and agricultural studies, however, clinical trial subjects are more heterogeneous and autonomous and tend to follow the experimental protocols less closely. A consequence of heterogeneity is a requirement for larger trials than one typically finds in highly focused laboratory experiments. A consequence of autonomy is that subjects do not always receive the treatment assigned by the protocol. Clinical trials cannot guarantee investigators a valid test of treatment received.

In any case, like smaller and more focused experiments, clinical trials use important methodological hallmarks. First, the study population is well defined. Baseline data are obtained to characterize it quantitatively. Often the study cohort can be viewed as a random sample from a larger population to which the trial results will generalize. Second, treatment assignments are made using a mechanism to reduce patient selection bias. Even if there is only a single treatment group, the investigator surrenders some opinion and choice about treatments once the eligibility criteria are satisfied.

Third, the treatments employed are standardized and carefully documented, especially deviations from protocol specifications. Fourth, experimental subjects are actively followed to ascertain endpoints. The investigator does not rely only on the

Table 4.1 Strength of Evidence Provided by Types of Medical Studies (from Byar, 1978)

Case report:	A demonstration only that some event of clinical interest is possible.
Case series:	A demonstration of certain possibly related clinical events but subject to large selection biases.
Database analysis:	Treatment is not determined by experimental design but by factors such as physician or patient preference. The data are unlikely to have been collected specifically to evaluate efficacy.
Observational study:	The investigator takes advantage of "natural" exposures or treatment selection and chooses a comparison group by design.
Controlled clinical trial:	The treatment assignment is by design. Endpoint ascertainment is actively performed and analyses are planned in advance.
Replicated clinical trials:	Independent verification of treatment efficacy estimates.

patient's compliance with scheduled appointments to determine outcomes. Fifth, the study endpoints are defined in advance and their occurrences are documented in the research record. Finally, the data arising from clinical trials and the process by which they are recorded can be verified and the errors can be reduced using quality and process control methods. In many cases, the verified data are stored in accessible archives for future use. These characteristics make clinical trials valuable scientific and experimental resources.

Example 1 *The consequences of a lack of true experimental design can be seen in the history of Laetrile from the 1970s and 1980s. Laetrile gained widespread acceptance by the public as an effective cancer treatment despite a lack of controlled evaluations and considerable skepticism by the medical establishment. Although as many as 70,000 cancer patients received the drug, the environments in which it was typically used discouraged rigorous and impartial assessments. In a review of the drug's possible efficacy, investigators from the NCI were able to evaluate only 93 cases with sufficient data, of which 6 may have had objective responses [Ellison et al., 1978]. Moertel et al. [1983] studied 178 patients who received the drug in a trial without a control group and concluded that there was no evidence of efficacy.*

Design components

In classical experimental designs, there are three components of design that support the analysis and inference: treatment design, error control design, and sampling and observation design. These components are present in well-designed clinical trials, although the exact architecture of the study depends on its specific purpose. There are three general types of experiments. The first type intends to observe a quantity which is a "constant of nature" and is not associated with variability (except for measurement error). Clinical trials are seldom of this type.

A second type of trial estimates a quantity that characterizes a population. Developmental trials are often of this type. For example, the safety of a drug, device, or vaccine might be estimated by administering it to a sample from the target population. Safety could be reflected in the probability of side effects, average number of adverse events, or level of risk in the sample. Sampling variability, measurement error, and external validity are concerns in such a study.

A third type of trial intends to compare treatment effects in a target population. Although sampling variability is present, bias is often more of a concern in this type of study. Studies with this objective often use randomization to control bias. External validity may not be a major concern, because treatment *differences* are more likely to generalize outside the trial than absolute treatment effects are.

Experimental and observational units

Treatment is applied to the "experimental units" and measurements are made on the "observational units". When studying plants or industrial processes, the experimental units are likely to be groups of things. However, in most clinical trials, both the experimental unit and the observational unit are almost always the individual patient.

Community intervention trials apply treatment to more than one person as part of the experimental unit. Similarly, they also often take measurements from aggregates of individuals. Reasons why this clustering might be necessary include lower cost, political and social constraints and because some interventions naturally affect or target all members of a group [Cornfield, 1978]. These designs are being applied in studies of disease prevention and therapies in developing countries [Chowdhury et al., 1991; Kassaye, Larson, and Carlson, 1994; Mahfouz et al., 1995; Meyer et al., 1991; Sommer, et al., 1986; Whitworth et al., 1992]. The design of such studies is discussed by Gail, et al. [1996].

Example 2 *Suppose we study the transmission of a communicable disease where family members of each case are at highest risk. For practical reasons, the different interventions tested might have to be given to families as the experimental unit. The observational unit might still be the individual patient. Treatments could be compared based on the overall proportion of new cases in the treatment groups. Similarly, suppose we were testing strategies to reduce cigarette smoking. One intervention might be tried as a campaign in several cities and another in a different group of cities. Here the experimental unit is the city and the observational unit might also be the city with smoking quit rates as the outcome. A prevention clinical trial, where large groups of individuals are the experimental units, is a smoking cessation trial [COMMIT 1995a, 1995b].*

In some clinical trials, the experimental and observational unit is neither the individual nor a group of individuals. An example of such a study might be an ophthalmologic trial. One or both eyes could be entered in the trial. This presumes that the treatment can be isolated to one eye, if necessary, as might be the case for surgery.

Treatments and factors

In the classical experimental design literature, treatments are often called "factors". An industrial or agricultural experiment may involve questions about several factors, each at more than one level. For example, temperature and pressure may be factors determining the yield of a chemical reaction. Each could be tested at several levels in an attempt to maximize the overall yield of product. The need for testing multiple factors and levels is common, because many agricultural or manufacturing and other industrial processes typically involve complex processes.

Clinical trials seldom employ more than two or three treatments (factors) and, when they do, the treatments are often at a single dose (level) each. Even when trials use three or more arms, the treatment groups usually consist of either different levels of the same treatment (e.g., dose levels) or single levels of different treatments (e.g., different drugs at fixed dose levels). Thus, the simplest sorts of one-factor analyses could be applied routinely (e.g., analyses of variance) if it were not for special endpoints in clinical trials. Endpoints are discussed in Chapter 6.

Nesting

Nesting occurs when a factor or effect lies entirely within another factor or effect in a hierarchical arrangement. For example, in the usual two-group (or parallel or independent groups) clinical trial, patients are nested within treatments. In contrast, in cross-over trials, each patient eventually receives both treatments and so patients are not nested within treatment. Such non-nested designs are discussed in Chapters 15 and 16. Some non-nested designs allow greater efficiency in estimating treatment effects. However, they usually require stronger assumptions to support the applicability of the design.

Randomization

Randomization is used to remove systematic error and to justify type I error probabilities. Although applied first to agricultural experiments by R. A. Fisher, it has also become an important tool in clinical trials after the pioneering work by Hill and Doll in Great Britain. Randomization has been used so successfully in comparative studies that using it seems to imply a formal hypothesis test. However, it does not always motivate an explicit comparison and may be used merely to remove selection bias. In contrast, formal treatment comparisons in clinical trials are sometimes based on quasi-random allocation methods such as "minimization", where patient assignments are made to induce prognostic factor balance between the groups. These and other ideas related to treatment allocation are discussed in Chapter 9.

Blocking

Blocking is used to control unwanted variation. For example, suppose we are comparing two manufacturing processes, A and B, over a three-day period and we can

Table 4.2 Latin Square Layout with Four Treatments or Factors

A	B	C	D
C	D	A	B
D	A	B	C
B	C	D	A

The row and column categories represent treatments or levels of factors to be controlled.

switch easily between them. We could sequence the process in the following way: day 1, $ABAB$; day 2, $BAAB$; day 3, $BABA$. Then, each day is a block. Within each day, we can obtain a valid comparison of A and B and eliminate the day-to-day variability by averaging the $A - B$ difference over three days. Formally, a block is a set of experimental units (the number of units equals a multiple of the number of treatments) chosen so that, if the treatments are equivalent, the responses will be nearly equivalent. The order of the treatments is randomly assigned within each block. This arrangement eliminates the effect of variation between blocks.

In comparative clinical trials, the same idea is used, except that the investigator is not free to compose the blocks at will, because the exact characteristics of the individual study subjects cannot be known in advance. Instead, treatment allocation might be stratified, where the strata are defined based on expected outcome in the absence of a treatment effect (e.g., high versus low risk). Within each stratum, the assignments are randomized in blocks to induce balance between the treatments. Thus, this arrangement also controls unwanted variation between the strata. These ideas are discussed in more detail in Chapter 9.

An extension of the idea of blocking is used in Latin Square designs. The utility of these designs is best understood by considering the need for two-way elimination of heterogeneity or two factors that must be controlled when studying several treatments. The treatments can be laid out as shown in Table 4.2 with a treatment occurring exactly once in each row and each column. In agricultural experiments, the rows and columns might be plots of land, but need not have any particular shape. In industrial experiments, the plots might be different runs of a process with different control variables, where the rows and columns represent different locations in time (e.g., week and day within week). These designs are infrequently used in clinical trials.

Placebos

Even ineffective treatments can appear to produce improvements in disease processes because of random fluctuations and because patients *expect* benefit [Beecher, 1955; Roberts et al., 1993]. This is particularly true of outcomes requiring subjective assessments, either by the patient or physician. This "placebo effect" is a constant concern in clinical trials and they should be designed to remove it whenever possible. This can be done, for example, by comparing a treatment to a placebo treatment rather than to no treatment. A true placebo is an inert or inactive treatment, for example, a pill containing an inactive substance. Placebos may be most appropriate in studies of drugs in self-limited conditions or those with long durations. Testing new drugs for relief of mild pain is one example.

In many circumstances, placebos are not ethically appropriate as, for example, when an accepted treatment already exists for a serious illness. A placebo group in a comparative trial could expose some patients to the risk of not having an effective treatment. If the disease is mild and self-limited or no treatment is the standard of practice, then a placebo might be appropriate.

In some circumstances, wise use of a placebo can facilitate comparisons that might be hard to interpret otherwise. This can happen when comparing treatments that require different routes of administration. For example, suppose we wish to compare an oral medication with a different drug given intravenously for severe nausea. One treatment group might consist of oral medication followed by an intravenous placebo. The second group might receive a placebo pill followed by the intravenous drug. This scheme would make the treatments more directly comparable than if no placebos were used.

Treatment masking

Treatment masking, or blinding as it is sometimes called, is an effective way to increase the objectivity of the person(s) observing experimental outcomes. When the treatments are masked, the bias or expectations of the observer are not likely to influence the measurements taken. For example, animal testing of a cytotoxic drug might consist of longitudinal measurements of tumor diameter. If the observer knows which animals have received drug and which were given placebo, the measurements could partially reflect his or her bias about the treatment. In contrast, if the observer is masked, the measurements are less likely to be affected by prejudice. Masking is particularly important in clinical trials that require self-reporting or self-assessments by the patients.

Investigators often underestimate the value of treatment and assessment masking. There is a tendency to believe that biases are small in relation to the magnitude of treatment effects (when, in fact, the converse is usually true), or that practitioners can compensate for their prejudice and subjectivity. An interesting counter-example is provided by Noseworthy et al. [1994] in their randomized trial of cyclophosphamide and plasma exchange for multiple sclerosis. In this trial, all clinical outcome assessments were made by both masked and unmasked neurologists. The results demonstrated a significant treatment effect, as measured by unmasked neurologists, but not by masked ones. The investigators concluded that masking prevented a type I error, with clear implications for other trials.

4.3   Bayesian View

The Bayesian approach to statistical design and inference contains some elements which are different from those just discussed [Spiegelhalter, Freedman, and Parmar, 1994]. The differences are critical to understanding the strengths and weaknesses of this method. In the Bayesian view, uncertainty about unknown quantities is described by a probability distribution. Uncertainty is described in terms of observed data, x, and an unknown parameter, θ, which indexes the family of possible distributions of the data. The purpose of the investigation is to make inferences about the distribution of θ, given the data, x. For the Bayesian, all inferences are based on probability calculations.

Evidence obtained before the experiment concerning the treatment effect, θ, is summarized quantitatively in the form of a probability distribution, $f(\theta)$, called the "prior distribution". Both subjective and objective sources of information may contribute to construction of the prior distribution. The next step in Bayesian inference is to describe the distribution of the data in terms of one or more unknown parameters and a probability model for data generation. The evidence from the experiment is summarized in this "likelihood function", denoted by $\mathcal{L}(x|\theta)$. Frequentist analyses also employ the likelihood function. Finally, the prior distribution is combined with the likelihood to yield a "posterior distribution", $g(\theta|x)$, from which probability statements about the parameter of interest can be made. The posterior distribution is calculated from Bayes theorem as

$$g(\theta|x) = \frac{\mathcal{L}(x|\theta)f(\theta)}{\int \mathcal{L}(x|\theta)f(\theta)d\theta}.$$

For discrete distributions of θ, the integral in the denominator will be replaced by a sum. For complicated priors and/or likelihoods, calculating the posterior distribution can be difficult.

4.3.1   Choice of a prior distribution is a source of contention

Before the trial begins, the Bayesian summarizes knowledge (or opinion or belief) about the treatment effect in the form of a probability distribution. In fact, the prior distribution could change during the early part of the study if new information becomes available from outside sources. The prior distribution requires viewing the treatment effect as a random variable, about which probability statements can be made. There are theoretical and practical problems with this.

From a theoretical point of view, the use of subjective probability is controversial. This issue cannot be covered comprehensively in this book. Background and discussions are given by Martz and Waller [1982], O'Bryan and Walter [1979], Lindley [1965], and Savage [1954]. Aside from the notion of subjective probability, it is not obvious that representing knowledge (or ignorance) in the form of a probability distribution is the correct approach, although in the case of Bayesian inference, it is a powerful convenience. When prior information is available in the form of a probability distribution, Bayesian methods are not controversial. For example, this can happen when making inferences about probability distributions themselves.

There are some practical difficulties implementing Bayesian methods. Because clinical researchers do not automatically represent their knowledge in the form of a probability distribution, getting them to put information in this form can be a problem. This process is often called "eliciting a prior" and requires skill and planning on the part of the trial methodologist. Different clinical investigators are likely to provide different prior distributions for the same parameter, because of the subjectivity involved. Groups of investigators may not agree on a single prior, even if they agree on the need for a clinical trial. Finally, the inference, or posterior distribution, that is the basic product of the Bayesian approach depends on the prior. Therefore, different investigators may arrive at different conclusions from the same experimental data, depending on their choices of prior distributions.

Example 3 *Assume that a prior distribution can be chosen without contention. Suppose we can represent the prior information about treatment effect by a distribution of the form*

$$f(\Delta) = \phi\left(\Delta \mid \Delta_0, \frac{\sigma^2}{m}\right),$$

where $\phi(\cdot)$ is the Gaussian distribution function, Δ is the true treatment effect, and Δ_0 is the value of Δ considered most likely by the investigators. The variance of the prior distribution, σ^2/m, (σ^2 is assumed to be known) illustrates that the existing knowledge is equivalent to having observations on m previous subjects with a mean of Δ_0.

Bayesian statisticians discuss various types of prior distributions corresponding to qualitatively and quantitatively different opinions about the external data. The evidence for prior distributions can be based on previous randomized trials, nonrandomized studies, preclinical data, or investigator opinion. *Reference* priors are intended to represent a minimal amount of prior information. Some of them are "improper" probability distributions, which essentially spread belief over the entire real line. Although inference using these types of priors can yield conclusions equivalent to some frequentist inferences, these prior distributions may be unrealistic because they give equal weight to all possible values of the parameter.

Clinical priors are intended to represent the opinions and beliefs of particularly well-informed scientists about the treatment effect. Because clinicians are usually not Bayesian statisticians, eliciting this information in a quantitative form can be difficult. *Skeptical* prior distributions are those that attempt to quantify the belief that large treatment effects are unlikely. They might be appropriate for use by regulatory officials. A skeptical prior might be equivalent to assuming that a certain fraction of the trial has been completed without seeing a treatment effect. *Enthusiastic* priors are those that attempt to quantify the urge to continue a clinical trial, even when the results support the null hypothesis. These might be used in circumstances where adopting a particular promising treatment, even if it is not as effective as hoped, has few drawbacks.

4.3.2   Likelihoods are not a subject of controversy

The second component in the chain of Bayesian inference, the formation of the like-lihood function, is usually not a source of contention. Likelihoods may be used as a source of inference themselves without appealing to prior distributions or hypothesis tests [Edwards, 1972]. In most cases, the probability of observing the outcome in one subject is independent of that for other subjects on a study. The likelihood is formed by using the fact that the joint probability of observing the data is the product of independent probabilities for each event.

Example 4   *To follow the example above, suppose the experiment performed includes n subjects and the data can be summarized in a statistic Z_n, which has the form of a normal (Gaussian) likelihood*

$$\mathcal{L}(Z_n) = \phi\left(Z_n \mid \Delta, \frac{\sigma^2}{n}\right).$$

The assumption of a normal likelihood can encompass a variety of treatment effects, including mean values, hazard ratios, and differences of proportions.

4.3.3   Posterior distributions yield inferences

The posterior distribution is formed from the prior and the likelihood using Bayes' rule. A relevant form for this rule is the following. If B_1, B_2, ... B_n are disjoint events and A is any other event, we have

$$\Pr\{B_i \mid A\} = \frac{\Pr\{A \mid B_i\}\Pr\{B_i\}}{\sum_{j=1}^{n}\Pr\{A \mid B_j\}\Pr\{B_j\}}.$$

A similar form can be obtained for continuous distributions.

Example 5   *Following the example above, denote the posterior distribution by $g(\cdot)$ and we have*

$$
\begin{aligned}
g(\Delta) \;&\propto\; \mathcal{L}(Z_n \mid \Delta) \times f(\Delta) \\
&=\; \phi\left(\Delta \mid \frac{m\Delta_0 + nZ_n}{m+n}, \frac{\sigma^2}{n+m}\right).
\end{aligned}
$$

The mean of this distribution, which, in this case, is the weighted mean of the two Δ's, is an estimate of the treatment effect. Credible intervals, which are similar to confidence intervals, are regions under the distribution $g(\cdot)$ with a specified probability. For example, a $100(1 - \alpha)\%$ credible interval is the region R, which satisfies

$$R = \left\{\Delta \mid g(\Delta) > c, \int_R g(\Delta)\, d\Delta = 1 - \alpha\right\}.$$

In other words, R supports $100(1 - \alpha)\%$ of the distribution. It is customary, but not required, that these credible intervals are taken to be symmetric around the mean.

4.3.4 Bayesian inference is different

Even this brief sketch should highlight some of the important differences between the Bayesian and frequentist approaches to designing clinical trials. A major component of Bayesian design is deciding on the prior distribution which represents knowledge (or belief) about the treatment effect before the start of the trial. This can be a controversial way to proceed when it requires subjective probability, i.e., summarizing degree of belief in the form of a probability distribution. Also, an implicit Bayesian assumption is that a probability distribution is the way to represent investigator knowledge. Despite these problems, for every frequentist procedure, there is an equivalent Bayesian one. In other words, the Bayesian can view frequentist procedures as having implicitly chosen a prior distribution, which, if used as described above, would yield essentially the same inference.

Apart from questions about prior distributions, the Bayesian paradigm provides a consistent and understandable mechanism for solving inferential problems. This is a considerable strength. Furthermore, it makes inferences in the form of probability statements about the unknown parameter or treatment effect. This is intuitively appealing and broadly useful for solving clinical problems. Bayesian approaches could be crafted for all the trial types discussed in the next section.

The design considerations discussed above are also important to the Bayesian method. For example, if preliminary data about a treatment effect arise from biased studies, one would not use them uncritically to form a prior distribution for a subsequent comparative trial. Similarly, the Bayesian seeks the same control over random error and bias in comparative trials as the frequentist does. However, randomization alone does not form a basis for Bayesian inference as it can for certain frequentist procedures (see Chapter 9).

4.4 Trial Design Types

It is difficult to define or classify types of clinical trials universally. Medical disciplines often view their own issues as being unique, which tends to create specific terminology within each specialty. To facilitate explaining and discussing important design concepts, it is helpful to have terminology that is independent of the application. In this section I will review basic categories of trials and attempt to provide a broad terminology for types of designs. After descriptions and definitions, the discussion will pertain largely to trials of pharmacologic therapy.

4.4.1 Four types of clinical trial designs are commonly described

In therapeutic drug (especially cytotoxic drug) development, clinical trials are often classified simply as phase I, II, III, and IV. This terminology is inadequate for universal application, but I will review it here because it is so widely used. *Phase I studies are pharmacologically oriented* and usually attempt to find the best dose of drug to employ. *Phase II trials look for preliminary evidence of efficacy* and side effects at a fixed dose. Phases I and II are not hypothesis driven in the sense that formal comparisons to other treatments do not usually determine the experimental design.

In phase III, new treatments are compared with standard therapy, no therapy, or placebo. Investigators would not undertake the greater expense and effort of phase III comparative testing unless there was preliminary evidence from phase I and II that a new treatment was safe and effective. *Phase IV is post-marketing surveillance* and may occur after regulatory approval of a new treatment or drug to look for uncommon side effects. This type of study design is also used for purposes other than safety and efficacy, e.g., for marketing purposes.

Although this terminology was developed in, and is applied widely to, cancer treatment, some of the definitions are different in cancer prevention. In cancer prevention trials, phase II is divided into IIa and IIb. Phase IIa trials are small-scale feasibility studies using intermediate endpoints, such as cancer precursor lesions or biomarkers. (Intermediate endpoints are defined and discussed in Chapter 6). Phase IIb trials are randomized comparative studies using intermediate endpoints. Phase III cancer prevention trials are comparative designs (like IIb) using definitive clinical endpoints such as cancer incidence [Kelloff, Johnson, Crowell, et al., 1995]. Some cancer prevention investigators have used the term "phase IV" to mean a defined population study [Greenwald, 1985; Greenwald and Cullen, 1985]. The same authors define phase V to be demonstration and implementation trials. The differences in terminology, even within the field of cancer, illustrate the problem with this terminology.

4.4.2   Improved terminology is broader and recognizes more types of trials

Most non-pharmacologic therapies are developed in stages that do not fit drug development terminology. A more general description of designs would take into account the goals of trials, independently of the treatment being studied. This section will propose such a terminology and relate it to the more widely used pharmacologic terms. Although versatile, the following descriptions are unconventional and will, therefore, be used in parallel with traditional ways of labeling clinical trials. In this book, phase I, II, III, or IV will refer specifically to drug trials. When the discussion is intended to be broader than drug development, the following terminology will be used.

Early development

Nearly all early developmental studies have a similar goal. The common purpose is testing *treatment mechanism*. To the biomedical engineer, treatment mechanism has a conventional interpretation in terms of device function. To the clinical pharmacologist, treatment mechanism means bioavailability of the drug; to the surgeon, it means the operative procedure or technique; to the gene therapist, it means the function of the cells or engineered gene; and so on. Even diagnostic and screening trials have *treatment mechanisms* in this expanded sense of the word. We could refer to these earliest developmental studies as treatment mechanism (TM) trials. Treatment mechanism is not equivalent with clinical outcome, which is tested in later and larger clinical trials.

Early drug studies are often concerned with more than treatment mechanism. They also frequently employ *dose-finding* strategies. For example, when testing new drugs or disease prevention strategies we might be interested in the minimum effective dose. In developing cytotoxic drugs for oncology, a focus is usually the maximum tolerated dose, because of the belief that it will provide the best therapeutic effect. All types of dose-finding studies can be called DF trials. Thus, phase I (drug) studies are TM and DF trials, but the converse is not true.

Another characteristic of TM and DF studies is their close connection to biological models. For treatments based on drug action, the biological models are usually pharmacokinetic or dose response models. Other treatments may be based on more complex models of normal function or disease. In any case, the outcome of TM and DF studies is usually best described in terms of such a model. In later developmental trials, the model of the treatment and its interaction with the disease process or clinical outcome is less important. Even if a plausible model has not been formulated, later developmental studies can provide convincing empirical evidence of efficacy.

Middle development

Most middle developmental studies ask questions related to clinical outcome and address treatment "tolerability". Tolerability has three components: feasibility, safety, and efficacy. Because treatment tolerance is often verified earlier in development, *safety and efficacy* determination is a primary purpose of such studies, regardless of the treatment being tested. In this stage of development, investigators would like an estimate of the probability that patients will benefit from the therapy (or have serious side effects from it). These estimates will be compared with knowledge about conventional treatment to determine if additional (larger) trials are needed. Unsafe or ineffective treatments will be discarded if better alternatives exist. In some cases, improved supportive care may make treatments with serious side effects feasible for life-threatening conditions. This is common in oncology. We can refer to these studies as safety and efficacy (SE) trials.

In oncology, phase II studies are SE trials. Safety is assessed by organ system toxicity measured according to defined criteria. Evidence of efficacy is usually assessed by the surrogate outcome "response", which is a measure of tumor shrinkage. In some phase II oncology trials, efficacy can be estimated from more definitive clinical outcomes such as disease recurrence, progression, or duration of survival. In cancer prevention, phase IIa studies are SE trials that employ surrogate or intermediate outcomes.

Some middle development trials have objectives different from those just outlined. These studies can be designed to select a treatment from a small set of possibilities based on performance criteria such as success rate. Randomization might be useful for trials of this kind (discussed below) and the design might be appropriate for deciding on the best dose of drug, route, or schedule of administration. Such designs operationally choose a path for continued development of the therapy and also provide information regarding safety and efficacy.

Comparative studies

Later developmental trials usually have definitive clinical endpoints and address questions of *comparative treatment efficacy*. They employ a concurrent control group that receives either standard therapy, placebo, or an appropriate alternative treatment. Such studies are designed to provide precise and valid estimates of differences in clinical outcome attributable to the treatments or interventions. Studies that are designed to show the equivalence of a new treatment to standard therapy also fit this description. These studies could be called comparative treatment efficacy (CTE) trials and correspond to phase III. Tests of the equivalence of two treatments are also CTE trials.

In cancer prevention, both phase IIb and III studies are CTE trials. Phase IIb studies are CTE trials that employ intermediate endpoints. Thus they are not definitive unless the intermediate endpoint has been validated. Phase III cancer prevention studies are CTE trials directly analogous to treatment trials because they use definitive endpoints such as disease incidence or progression.

CTE trials are sometimes performed on an exceptionally *large scale*. For example, a typical CTE trial conducted in oncology by a multi-center collaborative group might randomize a few hundred patients. In comparison, some trials in oncology, cardiovascular disease, and prevention randomize thousands of patients. The purpose of such studies might be to assess a small treatment difference or to provide empirical evidence of external validity by employing a large heterogenous study cohort similar to the disease population. Some investigators have advocated simple methods of treatment definition and data collection to minimize the cost of these trials, giving rise to the term "large simple trials" [Yusuf, Collins, and Peto, 1984]. I will refer to such studies as large-scale (LS) trials, acknowledging the fact that they are frequently not simple. See also Freedman [1989] and Souhami [1992] for a discussion of these types of studies.

Late development

When treatments are beginning to be widely applied, as is often the case after regulatory approval, there is still an opportunity to learn about uncommon side effects, interactions with other therapies, or unusual complications. Even uncommon events may affect the use or indication of the treatment if they are serious enough. Furthermore, some treatments may become widely used after being administered to relatively few patients in CTE trials, as in the case of a few AIDS drugs, orphan drugs, or those rapidly approved. An *expanded safety* study, or ES trial, may provide important information that was not gathered earlier in development.

Some phase IV or post-marketing surveillance studies are ES trials. However, most phase IV studies capture only serious side effects and may not precisely ascertain the number of patients who have received the treatment. Furthermore, some phase IV studies are mostly intended to be marketing research, for example, to uncover new product indications that may protect patients or yield other financial benefits. A true ES trial will be designed to provide a reliable estimate of the incidence of serious side effects.

Other late development trials may recapitulate designs discussed above but be applied to subsets or defined populations of patients. Such studies may investigate or target patients thought to be the most likely to benefit from the treatment and may be driven by hypotheses generated during earlier development. These types of late developmental trials should be governed by methodologic and design concerns similar to those discussed in this book.

4.4.3 Phase I (DF) drug studies are dose-finding

Phase I clinical trials are the first studies in which a new drug is administered to human subjects. The primary purpose of phase I studies of new drugs is to establish a safe dose and schedule of administration. Other purposes are to determine the types of side effects and toxicity and organ systems involved, to assess evidence for efficacy, and to investigate basic clinical pharmacology of the drug. Not all of these goals can be met completely in any phase I trial, in part because the number of patients treated is small. However, well-conducted phase I studies can achieve substantial progress toward each of these goals. Phase I trials are not synonymous with dose response studies, but they have many characteristics in common. For a discussion of dose response designs, see Ruberg [1995a; 1995b] or Wong and Lachenbruch [1996]. Some statistical and ethical issues are discussed by Ratain et al. [1993].

Sometimes investigators say that phase I studies are not "clinical trials" because there is no treatment comparison being made. Treatment *comparisons* are not a prerequisite for experiments. Because phase I trials rely on investigator controlled treatment administration and subsequent structured observations, they are clinical trials.

In the development of cytotoxic drugs in oncology, dose-finding usually means establishing a "maximum tolerated dose" (MTD). This is the dose associated with serious but reversible side effects in a sizeable proportion of patients and the one that offers the best chance for a favorable therapeutic ratio. Side effects from cytotoxic drugs tend to be serious and are referred to as toxicities. Investigators are interested not only in the organ systems involved, but also in the duration, reversibility, and probability of specific toxicities. In this setting, evidence of efficacy is usually weak or non-existent, because many patients receive what turn out to be sub-therapeutic doses of the drug.

Ideal design

The "ideal" experimental design for a phase I dose-finding study in humans might look like the following. The investigator would employ a range of doses, $D_1 \ldots D_k$, one of which is optimal. Trial participants would be randomly assigned to one of the dose levels and each dose level would be tested in n patients. At the completion of the experiment, the probabilities of response (or toxicity) would be calculated as $p_1 = r_1/n_1, \ldots, p_k = r_k/n_k$, where r_i is the number of responses at the ith dose. Then, the dose response curve could be modeled with an appropriate mathematical form, fit to the observed probabilities, and the probability of response (or toxicity) at any desired dose level (e.g., between doses actually used) could be estimated. Estimating the MTD would not depend strongly on the specific dose-response model used.

To implement this design, one would have only to choose an appropriate sample size, mathematical form for the dose response model, and range of doses. In fact, designs such as this are used in quantitative bioassay [Govindarajulu, 1988]. Because experimental subjects would be randomly assigned to doses, there would be no confounding of dose with time, as would occur if doses were tested in increasing or decreasing order. One could even use permuted dose blocks of size k (or a multiple of k) containing one of each dose level.

One of the advantages of using such an ideal design is the ability to estimate reliably and without bias the dose of drug associated with a specific probability of response. For example, suppose investigators are interested in using a dose of drug that yields a 50% chance of having serious but reversible side effects. One could estimate this from the dose-toxicity (dose-response) function after it is fitted to the data described above. Suppose the probability of toxicity as a function of dose, d, is $f(d; \boldsymbol{\theta})$, where $\boldsymbol{\theta}$ is a vector of parameters that characterize the dose-toxicity function, and the target dose is d_0, such that $0.5 = f(d_0; \widehat{\boldsymbol{\theta}})$, where $\widehat{\boldsymbol{\theta}}$ is an estimate of $\boldsymbol{\theta}$ obtained by curve fitting, maximum likelihood, Bayesian methods, or some other appropriate method. In other words,

$$d_0 = f^{-1}(0.5; \widehat{\boldsymbol{\theta}}),$$

where $f^{-1}(p; \boldsymbol{\theta})$ is the inverse function of $f(d; \boldsymbol{\theta})$ and p is the probability of response. For suitable choices of $f(d; \boldsymbol{\theta})$, the inverse will be simple and an ideal design will assure a good estimate of $\boldsymbol{\theta}$.

For example, for a logistic dose-response function

$$f(d; \boldsymbol{\theta}) = \frac{1}{1 + e^{-\lambda(d-\mu)}},$$

where $\boldsymbol{\theta}' = \{\lambda, \mu\}$. In this parameterization, μ is the dose associated with a response probability of $\frac{1}{2}$. The inverse function is

$$f^{-1}(p; \lambda, \mu) = \mu + \frac{1}{\lambda} \log\left(\frac{p}{1-p}\right).$$

Designs in use

The "ideal" phase I design is not feasible in human studies, because ethical considerations require us to treat patients at lower doses before administering higher doses. Also, we do not want to treat many patients at either a low, ineffective dose or at an excessively high, toxic dose. In practice, a starting dose is chosen, usually based on preclinical data, and the remaining set of doses to be administered is specified in advance of the study. This pre-specification of a small set of doses to try is a feature common to many phase I designs.

Rather than treating a fixed number of patients at every dose, as was suggested above, phase I study designs are adaptive. This means that the decision to use a next higher dose depends upon the results observed at the current dose. If unacceptable side effects or toxicity are seen, higher doses will not be used. Conversely, if no

Table 4.3 Fibonacci Dose Escalation Scheme (with Modification) for DF Trials

Step	Ideal Dose	Actual Dose	Percent Increment
1	D	D	–
2	$2 \times D$	$2 \times D$	100
3	$3 \times D$	$3.3 \times D$	67
4	$5 \times D$	$5 \times D$	50
5	$8 \times D$	$7 \times D$	40
6	$13 \times D$	$9 \times D$	29
7	$21 \times D$	$12 \times D$	33
8	$34 \times D$	$16 \times D$	33

D represents the starting dose employed and is selected based on pre-clinical information.

evidence of dose limiting toxicities or side effects are seen after treating a sufficient number of patients, the next higher dose will be employed.

Investigators select the set of doses in a way that will reveal the MTD without requiring an excessive number of dose levels to be tried. The starting dose chosen depends on pre-clinical or animal toxicologic studies. For example, one method for choosing a starting dose is based on one-tenth of the dose that causes 10% mortality in rodents – the so-called LD_{10}.

A common technique for specifying the dose steps to be tried is the "modified Fibonacci" scheme. Fibonacci (Leonardo of Pisa) was a 13th-century Italian number theorist, for whom the sequence of numbers,

$$1, \ 1, \ 2, \ 3, \ 5, \ 8, \ 13, \ 21, \ldots$$

was named, where each term is the sum of the preceding two terms. The ratio of successive terms approaches $\frac{\sqrt{5}-1}{2} = .61803\ldots$ – the so-called golden ratio, which has some optimal properties with regard to mathematical searches [Wilde, 1964]. To my knowledge, this is the most direct application of a number theory concept to clinical trials. An example of how this scheme might be used to construct dose levels in a phase I trial is shown in Table 4.3. The ideal doses from the Fibonacci sequence are modified to increase less rapidly with decreasing increments.

A classic design using this method was proposed by Dixon and Mood [1948]. Their specific method is not used routinely, however. In most dose escalation designs, investigators do not fit the probit (cumulative normal) dose-response model as originally proposed and patients are often treated in groups of 3 rather than individually before deciding to change the dose. This grouped design was suggested by Wetherill [1963] and a widely used modification by Storer [1989]. Bayesian methods have been suggested [Gatsonis and Greenhouse, 1992] as have those that use graded responses [Gordon and Wilson, 1992]. Some recent suggestions for improving the statistical performance of dose escalation designs based on the continual reassessment method will be discussed in Chapter 7 [O'Quigley, 1992; O'Quigley, Pepe, and Fisher, 1990; Piantadosi and Liu, 1996].

4.4.4   Phase I data have other uses

For all phase I studies, learning about basic clinical pharmacology is important and includes measuring drug uptake, metabolism, distribution, and elimination. This information is vital to the future development and use of the drug, and is helpful in determining the relationship between blood levels and side effects, if any. These goals indicate that the major areas of concern in designing phase I trials will be selection of patients, choosing a starting dose, rules for escalating dose, and methods for determining the MTD or safe dose.

If basic pharmacology were the only goal of a phase I study, the patients might be selected from any underlying disease and without regard to functioning of specific organ systems. However, phase I studies are usually targeted for patients with the specific condition under investigation. For example, in phase I cancer trials, patients are selected from those with a disease type targeted by the new drug. Because the potential risks and benefits of the drug are unknown, patients often are those with relatively advanced disease. It is usually helpful to enroll patients with a normal cardiac, hepatic, and renal function. Because bone marrow suppression is a common side effect of cytotoxic drugs, it is usually helpful to have normal hematologic function as well when testing new drugs in cancer patients. In settings other than cancer, the first patients to receive a particular drug might have less extensive disease or even be healthy volunteers.

4.4.5   Can randomization be used in phase I or TM trials?

Early developmental trials are not comparative and selection bias is not much of a problem when using primarily treatment mechanism and pharmacologic endpoints. Randomization seems to have no role in such studies. However, consider the development of new biological agents, which are expensive to manufacture and administer and may have large beneficial treatment effects. An example of such a treatment might be genetically engineered tumor vaccines, which stimulate immunologic reactions to tumor cells and can immunize laboratory animals against their own tumors. DF study objectives for these agents are to determine the largest number of cells (dose) that can be administered and to test for side effects of the immunization.

Because these treatments give live (but lethally irradiated) tumor cells with new genes to the patient, side effects could arise from two sources: the new genes in the transfected tumor cells or the cells themselves. One way to establish the safety of the transfected cells is to compare their toxicity with that from untransfected cells. This can be done during DF trials using a randomized design. Such considerations led one group of investigators to perform a randomized dose escalation trial in the gene therapy of renal cell carcinoma [Simons, Jaffe, Weber et al., 1997]. An advantage of this design was that the therapy had the potential for large beneficial effects, which might have been evident (or convincing) from such a design.

4.4.6 SE (phase II) trials determine feasibility and estimate treatment effects

SE clinical trials use a fixed dosage of a drug (or treatment modality) and attempt to determine if the treatment should be used in large-scale comparative studies. The decision to use a new treatment in larger, more expensive clinical trials depends upon two types of information gathered at this stage of development. The first is the feasibility of the treatment, a concept which includes side effects or toxicity, the logistics of administering the treatment, and cost. The second component is treatment efficacy. A favorable balance between efficacy and feasibility suggests that it is worthwhile to test a treatment in large-scale studies. Therefore, SE trials help to prioritize treatments for comparative testing. A third purpose of SE trials is to estimate the frequency of toxicities, side effects, and benefit of the treatment. Finally, for drugs, SE studies provide additional information about the pharmacology of the agent.

Most commonly, SE studies do not employ formal comparative designs. That is, they do not use parallel treatment groups. Nevertheless, comparisons are sometimes implied by both the design and the results of SE studies. For example, estimated treatment effects can be compared with those known from using standard treatment in similar patients, to decide if a new treatment is worth pursuing. The comparison that is implicit in conducting SE trials is done outside of the framework of the experimental design. Furthermore, similar implicit comparisons might be used to estimate the proper sample size for a SE trial.

Side effects and toxicities of treatments are usually assessed on an ordinal scale and are judged to be present or absent according to predefined criteria. The proportion of patients having side effects of a certain degree is then calculated. Efficacy outcomes might be summarized in a similar fashion. The simplest way to assess efficacy in these studies is to estimate the proportion of patients who benefit in a predefined way from the treatment.

A variety of methods are used to estimate the sample size for SE studies. Typically, these trials involve between 25 and 100 patients, because resources are seldom available to study more patients, and the gain in precision that would be obtained by doing so is usually not worth the cost. The design can be fixed sample size, staged, or fully sequential. Staged designs are those conducted in groups with an option to terminate the trial after each group of patients is assessed. Fully sequential designs monitor the treatment effect after each study subject (Chapter 10). An excellent review of phase II (SE) design types is given by Herson [1984]; sample size is discussed in Chapter 7.

Design purposes

SE and CTE clinical trials are conducted in a variety of developmental areas, including drugs, drug combinations, biological and gene therapy, surgery, radiotherapy, and devices. Each of these areas can require different designs. For example, when studying drug derivatives or combinations, a good standard therapy may already exist. This means we would favor a replacement only if it appears to be substantially more effective than standard, or if it has fewer side effects. For certain types of biological agents like vaccines or gene therapies, we might expect large treatment effects. Thus, designs in high-risk populations or those with less rigorous comparison groups might be serviceable. Surgical therapies, devices, and prevention agents are often developed without formal early-phase clinical trials. Studies of treatment adjuvants require flexible designs that permit appropriate timing of the adjuvant.

Randomized SE studies

The role of randomization as a bias reducing method in comparative trials was mentioned earlier. Sometimes in SE studies, randomization is also useful [Simon, Wittes, and Ellenberg, 1985]. For example, suppose a series of similar treatments needs to be tested in patient populations, all with essentially the same eligibility criteria. The best treatment will be selected for CTE trials. Two choices arise. We could test the treatments in sequence, waiting for each trial to end before beginning the next one. Alternatively, we could conduct the studies in parallel (i.e., simultaneously), randomizing eligible patients to one of the treatments. At the conclusion of the study, instead of a formal hypothesis test, we would simply select the "best" treatment for continued testing. Randomization has been used often in this setting to remove selection bias and to permit a parallel-groups design to control temporal trends.

Some special practical circumstances are required to implement randomization in SE trials. In particular, the accrual rate must be sufficient to complete a parallel-groups design while the question is still timely. Also, the decision to conduct studies of some of the treatments cannot be a consequence of the results in other treatments. If so, the parallel design may be unethical, wasteful, or not feasible.

Randomized SE studies may be particularly well suited for selecting the best of several treatment schedules for drugs or drug combinations, because these questions imply that the same population of patients will be under study. Similarly, when addressing questions about sequencing of different modes of treatment, such as radiotherapy with chemotherapy for cancer, randomized SE studies may be good designs for treatment development.

4.4.7   CTE (phase III) trials are pivotal

CTE trials are definitive steps in the evaluation of new treatments. Their purposes are to determine the effectiveness of the new treatment relative to standard therapy and to compare the incidence and severity of side effects relative to standard therapy. In a regulatory context, such well-controlled trials are called *pivotal*. (In a treatment development context, SE trials are pivotal.) For some diseases, there may be no known effective standard therapy, in which case CTE trials might use a placebo treated control group. Most often, we think of comparative clinical trials as those employing a concurrent (perhaps randomized) control group. However, CTE trials could also be designed to compare estimated treatment effects with historical controls. The credibility of these latter types of trials may depend heavily on the magnitude of the estimated treatment effect. That is, such trials will be convincing only when they demonstrate large benefits that cannot be explained by chance or bias.

The simplest types of CTE studies are those that employ a single modality treatment. Single modality treatments are applicable in many clinical circumstances and the results of such trials are likely to be easily interpretable. However, in many chronic diseases, combined modality treatments such as drugs, surgery, radiotherapy, immunotherapy, endocrine therapy, and gene therapy might be employed in various combinations. Testing combined modality treatments requires that the investigators consider the sequencing and timing of the various treatments. The design must permit isolating the effect of the treatment(s) under investigation without confounding by other modalities.

A third type of comparative trial uses adjuvant or supplemental therapy. Adjuvant trials are combined modality studies, in which one of the treatments is given before or after the primary treatment in an attempt to enhance its effect. An example is the use of systemic chemotherapy following (or preceding) surgery for resection of tumors. Selecting the right combination of drugs and their timing relative to surgery is a challenge for CTE clinical trials.

Like SE studies, CTE trials can employ fixed sample sizes, staged designs, or fully sequential methods. Because of the size and complexity of the studies, most designs are either fixed sample size or staged. There are other important considerations in comparative trials that lead to the use of cross-over designs or factorial designs. These are discussed in Chapter 16.

Another distinguishing feature of comparative trials is that they are frequently performed using the resources of several institutions or hospitals simultaneously. This is necessary because most single institutions do not accrue a sufficient number of patients to complete comparative testing of therapies in a reasonable length of time. Thus, the logistics and organization of these studies can be complex. Furthermore, the potential heterogeneity that arises from using patients in various institutions may be a consideration in the design, analysis, and interpretation of these studies.

For many diseases, fairly effective treatments are already available and widely used. Developing new treatments in this setting presents special problems for comparative trial design. For example, suppose we wish to demonstrate that a new anti-inflammatory agent is as effective for chronic arthritis as an agent already in widespread use. Such a clinical trial would not be designed necessarily to show the superiority of the new treatment. Rather, it might be designed to demonstrate the equivalence of the new treatment with standard therapy, at least as far as pain relief and mobility are concerned. The new agent might also have a lower incidence of side effects. These designs, often called "equivalence trials", are important, but sometimes difficult to implement.

4.4.8   ES (phase IV) studies look for uncommon effects of treatment

Many researchers have described a final step in the evaluation of new therapies. This step uses large-scale ES studies, commonly termed phase IV trials. Usually the development, approval, and marketing of a new treatment is based on relatively small numbers of patients. In the case of treatments for chronic disease, acceptance may be gained after studying only a few hundred individuals. When newly developed treatments are applied to large populations, the potential for encountering rare, but serious side effects is great, motivating the need for ES studies.

A situation in which ES studies are useful is in post-marketing surveillance for side effects and toxicity of a new drug. There have been several circumstances in which these types of studies have resulted in removal of new drugs from the market because of side effects that were not thought to be a problem during development. Since 1974, at least ten drugs have been removed from the market in the U.S. because of safety concerns. The rate is higher in some other countries [Bakke et al., 1995]. In other circumstances, performing such studies would have been of benefit to both the patients and the manufacturers. An example of this is the recent problems attributed to silicone breast implants.

One of the difficulties in interpreting these large-scale post-marketing safety studies is being able to attribute complications or uncommon side effects to the treatment in question reliably, rather than to other factors associated with the underlying disease process, or to unrelated factors. This is even more of a problem when events occur at long intervals after the initial treatment. A second problem arises because many ES studies do not determine how many individuals have received the treatment, only the number who experience adverse events. An incidence rate for adverse events cannot be calculated unless the number of individuals "at risk" can be estimated. In some other countries, closer tracking of drug use after marketing permits true incidence rates to be estimated.

Because investigators are potentially interested in very uncommon side effects, especially those which are life threatening or irreversible, ES clinical trials generally employ large sample sizes. However, these studies need not be conducted only in a setting of post-marketing surveillance. For example, similar questions arise in the application of a "standard" treatment in a common disease. Even single institutions can perform studies of this type to estimate long-term complication rates and the frequency of uncommon side effects.

4.5   Other Considerations

4.5.1   Some treatments are not developed like drugs

Many treatments are not developed the way that drugs are. Examples include: trials of hardware, surgical techniques, vaccines, and biologicals; tests of adjuvants and treatment combinations; diagnostic agents; and disease prevention interventions. We could refer to developmental stages for these types of studies descriptively as discussed above. A brief sketch of some issues in these types of trials is given below.

Prevention studies

Three types of prevention interventions, at least in the field of oncology, have been described [Bertram, Kolonel, and Meyskens, 1987]. Primary prevention attempts to prevent the disease or condition from ever arising in healthy individuals. An example is diet and life-style change to prevent cancer or cardiovascular disease. Secondary prevention attempts treatments or interventions in individuals with precursors of the disease, or with early stage disease, to prevent progression or sequelae. An example would be lowering of blood pressure to prevent stroke or myocardial infarction. Tertiary prevention attempts to prevent recurrences of the disease in individuals who have already had one episode. An example is the use of vitamins to prevent or delay second malignancies in patients who have already had a primary cancer.

Like biological agents and gene therapies, disease prevention trials often present unique design characteristics. First, preventive agents are usually not developed with the same structured early phases as drugs. Instead, the suggested efficacy of prevention agents often comes from epidemiologic or other observational studies. Because many prevention agents are virtually non-toxic (e.g., low fat diet, vitamins, some trace elements), the early phase safety and dose-finding studies are less critical and may not be oriented toward pharmacokinetics.

Comparative trials with prevention agents are typically performed in disease-free, but high-risk, populations. These populations are "healthy" in the sense that they do not have overt disease. However, health is not merely the absence of disease. Populations are not truly "healthy" if they have greatly elevated risk of disease. In any case, the frequency of endpoints in such a population is likely to be lower than that in people with chronic disease, requiring larger sample sizes and longer study durations for prevention trials. The cost of such studies is proportionately higher, sometimes being in the hundreds of millions of dollars.

Because of the nature of disease prevention and the long study duration that is typical, poor adherence and delayed onset of treatment effectiveness may diminish or distort the treatment effect. Special trial designs and methods of analysis that are insensitive to these problems are needed.

Finally, many prevention treatments have a low incidence of, and non-overlapping of, side effects, making them suitable for simultaneous or combined administration in factorial designs (discussed in Chapter 15). This type of administration can permit greater efficiency in design and/or estimation of treatment interactions. While the design tools used in prevention trials are similar to those used in treatment trials, the size, complexity, and cost of prevention studies often makes them unique.

Vaccine, biological, and gene therapies

For biological agents, the treatment effects are often large, there may be little or no acute toxicity, and intermediate endpoints may be most important. Examples of clinically important intermediate endpoints are blood counts or serum levels, blood pressure, and pathological precursors of neoplasia like polyps or dysplasia. Dose-finding or pharmacology may not play a prominent role in the development of biological agents.

The phases of research for vaccine trials are also somewhat different from those sketched above for drug development. In particular, TM and DF refer to the first introduction of a vaccine into humans to determine safety and immunogenicity. There may be "dose-finding" and tests of different routes of administration. SE tests immunogenicity and efficacy in a limited number of subjects. CTE vaccine trials also test efficacy and safety and usually involve multiple study centers with control patients.

Vaccine efficacy studies may also need to estimate residual susceptibility, duration of protection, and residual infectiousness in addition to, or instead of, direct protection. Estimating these quantities might require different designs or phases of investigation. If a vaccine reduces infectiousness, even without providing direct protection, it may be useful in reducing the impact of an epidemic. Investigating important questions such as these does not lead to trial types that fit neatly into the phases described above.

Diagnostic or screening trials

Diagnostic trials are those that assess the relative effectiveness of two or more diagnostic tests in detecting a disease or condition. Often, one test will be a diagnostic "gold standard" and the other will be a new, less expensive, more sensitive, or less invasive alternative. Although not strictly required, the diagnostic procedures are often both applied to the same experimental subjects, leading to a pairing of the responses, which requires special methods for analysis.

Diagnostic tests are often not developed in as structured a fashion as drugs and other therapeutic modalities. This is the case because the risks of diagnostic procedures is often low. They may be applied in apparently healthy populations, as in screening programs, and may therefore require exceptional sensitivity and specificity to be useful. Developing better diagnostic modalities presupposes that effective treatment for the disease is available. Otherwise, there is little benefit to learning about it as early as possible.

Diagnostic trials can also be affected by biases that do not trouble treatment trials. Suppose that a disease is potentially detectable by screening during a window of time between its onset (or sometime thereafter) and the time when it would ordinarily become clinically manifest. The "lead time" is the interval from the screening detection to the usual clinical onset. Because of person-to-person variability, those with a longer window are more likely to be screened in the window. Consequently, they will be overrepresented in the population detected with the disease. This produces so-called "length-biased sampling". See Walter and Day [1983] or Day and Walter [1984] for a discussion of this problem.

Surgical trials

Clinical trials involving surgical therapies and other skill-dependent activities like medical devices (discussed below) usually have important differences from those employing drugs or biologicals. Many surgical studies and inferences appear to rely on case series. For a practical discussion related to this point, see Horton [1996] and the studies he discusses [Casey et al., 1996; Cuschieri et al., 1996; Majeed et al., 1996; Marubini et al., 1996].

One essential difference between surgical therapies and other types of treatment is the developmental phase, where trialists must distinguish between the operative procedure or technique (or device function) and patient outcome. Unlike drugs, surgical procedures are often developed by single or small groups of investigators at relatively little cost. Surgical procedures have a high degree of determinism associated with them and often work on physical principles, unlike pharmacologic agents. Sometimes, but not always, in an individual patient, investigators can equate success of the procedure with a favorable outcome. However, from a methodologic point of view, we cannot substitute trials demonstrating successful completion of the procedure for those demonstrating improved patient outcome.

When studying patient outcomes, there is a tendency for surgical studies to be confounded by patient selection factors and effects related to subtle differences in techniques that are hard to measure. Historically, many surgeons have been reluctant to apply rigorous trial design techniques, like randomization to studies of patient outcomes, tending to make comparisons of surgical methods more difficult. Nevertheless, clinical trials of all types have been applied to surgical questions and have produced important information in areas like vascular, thoracic, and oncologic surgery. For a review of the role of statistical thinking in (thoracic) surgery, see Piantadosi and Gail [1995]. McPeek, Mosteller, and McKneally [1989] discuss general issues regarding randomized trials in surgery. A broad discussion of statistical methods in surgical research is given by Murray [1991].

In general, surgical treatments are not amenable to evaluation versus placebo. Apart from the "placebo effect" and selection factors favoring those patients well enough to undergo surgery, a true surgical placebo such as sham surgery is nearly always ethically problematic. However, there have been trials in which sham surgery was justified.

Example 6   *Sham surgery was used in the NIH sponsored study of fetal tissue transplants for the treatment of Parkinson's disease. The intracranial surgical approach was through two small drill holes in the frontal bone. Because of the subjective nature of evaluations for the severity of Parkinson's disease and the fact that patients communicate their experiences in detail to one another, a placebo was considered essential. The ideal placebo would have been transplantation of an inactive cell suspension. However, the investigators could not justify the risk attributable to actually passing needles into the brain of placebo patients. Instead, patients were taken to the operating room and the low-risk portions of the procedure were carried out. This included two small incisions in the skin of the forehead and drill holes in the frontal bone after sedation. The dura was not penetrated and other aspects of the procedure were simulated so that the patient, who would be awake, would have similar experiences to anyone having the full operation. The surgeons felt strongly that this sham procedure was virtually no risk and would eliminate a placebo effect of surgery.*

In many areas surgical trials have yielded valuable information. These include studies of adjuvant therapy in lung cancer, breast sparing surgery for cancer, and studies of the benefits of coronary artery bypass grafting. Even so, the paradigm of how new surgical therapies are developed is somewhat different from that for drugs. A surgical problem might be solved by one or more of four routes: drugs, materials, devices, or technique. By technique, I mean improvements in existing surgical methods rather than replacement of non-surgical therapies with an operation. New drugs and materials may give rise to side effects or toxicities and, therefore, need a different development path from devices or techniques. They will invariably need to be studied in preclinical models. However, there is usually no concept of "dose" for materials. Adverse effects, if any, may be evident only after a long time.

Developing surgical techniques does not necessarily fit any of the phases discussed above. Techniques tend to evolve slowly and are often amenable to improvement, even while being studied, to the point of becoming individualized to certain surgeons or institutions. In principle, new surgical techniques could be readily and quickly compared with standard methods in formal clinical trials soon after being shown to be feasible. However, in spite of the relatively relaxed need for developmental testing prior to a CTE trial, new surgical techniques seem to be infrequently compared formally with old techniques.

Hardware or device trials

Like surgical treatments, medical devices tend to be developed inexpensively by small groups of investigators. At some point in development, we must distinguish between device function and clinical outcome. Case histories or case series with selected patients may tend to confuse the independent questions. One cannot substitute a study demonstrating good device function for one showing beneficial patient outcome. Trials that test differences in patient outcome attributable to a device need to be as large and rigorous as those for drugs.

Because of the informality of the early developmental process and selection of favorable case reports, devices can sometimes gain widespread use without rigorous testing of clinical outcome. Investigators may require more extensive follow-up to observe device failures than the amount of time required to see side effects from drugs or other systemically acting agents. Examples where this may have been a problem, because complications became evident only after a long time, include prosthetic heart valves found years later to be catastrophically failing, some intrauterine birth control devices, and silicone breast implants, which have been implicated in a variety of ailments. Rigorous developmental trials, long-term animal studies, and postmarketing surveillance studies might have prevented each of these problems from becoming widespread.

There are reasons why *in vivo* developmental studies of devices may not need to be as rigorous as those for drugs and biological agents. First, the action of most devices is physiologically localized rather than systemic. This leads to a greater determinism in how they work, how they might fail, and the possible manifestations of failure. Examples are catheters or implantable electrodes, which have a small set of possible side effects or complications compared with drugs and biologicals. Second, devices are often constructed of materials that have been tested in similar biological contexts and whose properties are well-known. Again, this effectively rules out, or reduces the probability of, certain complications. Examples of this are biologically inert materials, such as some metals and synthetics.

Third, devices typically operate on physical, chemical, or electronic principles that are known to be reliable, because of previous testing or evaluation outside the subject. Based on these characteristics, investigators may know much more about a device at a given point in its development than is known about a drug or biological at a comparable stage. These characteristics may contribute to less of a need for extensive developmental testing of devices compared with drugs in humans, but not less rigorous testing overall.

4.5.2 Hybrid designs may be needed for resolving special questions

Although many trial designs fit into the types discussed above, there are occasional circumstances in which other designs are more appropriate. For example, a drug study might combine dose-finding with estimation of response and toxicity rates, particularly if the basic pharmacology has already been worked out. Similarly, if one or more SE trials have already been finished, additional studies might focus more on efficacy rather than safety. These are sometimes called phase IIA and phase IIB trials. If several SE agents are being tested in the same population, a randomized design might be employed, where the least efficacious appearing treatments are dropped in favor of an expanded comparison of the remaining ones.

While these and many other hybrid designs are possible and have found some use, investigators should not sacrifice the goals and objectives of the drug or treatment development to a seemingly faster but more error-prone design. Although some savings in sample size or development time might be achieved with these and other hybrids, the costliest errors are those that cause us to pursue ineffective treatments, wasting time and resources, or those that cause us to miss improvements. These errors can only be controlled by having adequate information on which to base decisions regarding further development. Good study design, appropriate to the level of development, is the best way to provide the information needed.

4.5.3 Clinical trials cannot meet some objectives

All clinical trials are performed in the presence of significance constraints. Some of these constraints are based on ethical concerns, others are a consequence of practical issues such as available resources, and still others are the result of scientific limitations. Because clinical trials, especially comparative ones, are reliable tools for evaluating treatment effects, it is understandable that the method and approach might be employed to answer other types of questions. However, inappropriately broad use of this methodology can lead to problems of the type that are described next.

Demonstration trials

One inappropriate use of clinical trials is to attempt to demonstrate treatment effects that are already known to exist. This presents ethical problems, particularly if patients assigned to receive an inferior treatment could suffer permanent harm. Investigators cannot endorse accruing patients to a clinical trial if they believe that convincing evidence is already available concerning the superiority of one of the treatments.

Economic evaluations

Another potentially problematic use of clinical trials is for economic evaluations. In many settings, it is worthwhile and important to include cost considerations in the evaluation of new treatments. However, two problems can arise when such evaluations are performed early in treatment development. First, treatments may not be produced or applied in their most economical fashion when first tested. A seemingly high-cost therapy may prove to be less expensive with more refinement. Similarly, it could become more cost effective if refinements improve its efficacy.

Second, there is often little uncertainty associated with the cost of particular interventions, making them unsuitable as outcome measures. The cost might be essentially fixed and could be calculated directly from a protocol or regimen specification and compared directly with an alternative. In other words, the variability associated with cost can be relatively small and may not require an experimental structure to study it. Cost effectiveness does depend on the magnitude of the treatment benefit and is subject to variation. While such questions are important, they are not always best answered as part of an efficacy evaluation.

Overviews

In recent years, formal methods have been proposed and adopted for combining evidence from many clinical trials, each of which may have been too small to convincingly demonstrate a subtle treatment effect. These "overviews" or "meta-analyses" are popular ways of looking for consistency in trial results and can be very helpful for making clinically relevant inferences. They are subject to other kinds of error and biases, as discussed in Chapter 17. In any case, the primary purpose of clinical trials is not to serve as building blocks for overviews. Investigators should not routinely conduct clinical trials with low power, anticipating that a later overview will yield the correct answer about treatment efficacy.

Non-specific therapy

Another purpose for which clinical trials have been suggested is to evaluate treatments defined in a non-specific way. For example, one might ask a question like "Is chemotherapy for advanced stage lung cancer beneficial?". A clinical trial could be proposed to answer such a question. In this hypothetical trial, supportive care might be compared with chemotherapy of *any type*. The reasons for not specifying the treatment more explicitly are that individual practitioners may have differences of opinion about the appropriate therapy to use and might be unwilling to participate in a clinical trial which *requires* the use of specific agents. We might expect to overcome this problem with a trial that permits a non-specific treatment definition and employs a sufficiently large sample size. Trials such as this may not yield useful information, because any outcome will immediately raise questions about heterogeneity in the treatment group. What if certain regimens appear to be helpful and others appear to be harmful? It is unlikely that the non-specific question will continue to be of interest after the data are collected.

4.6   Importance of the Research Protocol

A protocol is the document that specifies the research plan for a clinical trial. The most difficult parts of writing a protocol are: 1) formulating and developing an important, feasible scientific question, and 2) being certain that resources (funds, patients, time) are available to answer the question. These aspects of clinical investigation cannot be dealt with here. However, given an important question and the resources to answer it, developing the written research protocol is the crucial next step in planning a clinical trial.

A useful first step in preparing a complete research protocol is developing a "concept sheet", a one- or two-page document describing the essential scientific and clinical features of the proposed study. Aside from helping to structure the final document, the concept sheet can be used to communicate the scientific aspects of the trial and gather feedback. This is particularly helpful in a collaborative group setting and for study sponsors. Changes in concepts can be made before the investigator invests in a complete protocol.

"Protocol" also has a second meaning – it is the *logical plan* or prescription for the study apart from the written document. It is important to have a high degree of fidelity between the written document and the intended logical plan. If the two do not agree closely, circumstances with individual patients will almost certainly arise that result in differences of interpretation.

There are many documents besides the research protocol that are essential for conducting a clinical trial. Examples include an Investigator's Brochure, which describes the investigational product or device, documentation of ethical review, case report or data forms, and numerous other regulatory documents. For studies that will be part of regulatory approval applications, the necessary list of documents is extensive and must be obtained from the appropriate regulatory agency. Examples of such agencies are the FDA and the Health Protection Branch (HBP) in some other countries. The International Conference on Harmonisation of Technical Requirements for Registration of Pharmaceuticals for Human Use (ICH) has outlined in detail required documents and guidelines for regulatory approval in cooperating countries [ICH, 1994].

4.6.1   Protocols have many functions

The protocol is the single most important quality control tool for all aspects of a clinical trial, because it contains a complete specification for both the research plan and treatment for the individual patient. The written protocol is also the only effective method for communicating research ideas and plans in detail to other investigators. The protocol is a peer review document because, in the planning stages, a scientific study cannot be reviewed and critiqued without the protocol. For collaborative groups and the NIH, the protocol is the quantum unit of research. For the FDA and other regulatory bodies, the protocol is a legal document in addition to its other important functions. The protocol also specifies all aspects of the statistical design of a clinical trial and, therefore, the quantitative conclusions of the study are conditional upon it. The protocol and associated consent forms also have medical-legal and ethical implications and will be examined in this light by institutional review committees.

Some investigators have suggested publication or registration of clinical trial protocols in periodicals to make the fact of a planned experiment known to the scientific community at large. For some important, high-profile, or controversial trials, the protocol rationale is published (e.g., NSABP Breast Cancer Prevention Trial [NSABP, 1992]). Although publication does not usually take place, it emphasizes the importance of the research plan. Investigators who need more motivation for careful preparation of research protocols should probably not be conducting clinical research!

4.6.2 Deviations from protocol specifications are common

In spite of the general importance of the study protocol, investigators must be mindful that, to varying degrees, the details of the trial plans are not followed precisely in all patients. This can happen, for example, because of differences in interpretation. More frequently, protocol deviations are a consequence of unanticipated events and corresponding clinical judgment about what good medical practice requires for a particular patient. Some deviations from the protocol are inconsequential, while others are substantive and could affect the validity of the trial.

The importance of deviations depend on how they affect the inferences from the trial, not on the magnitude of the errors. For example, many studies require that patients have laboratory evidence of normal major organ system function at study entry. Permitting patients with small differences in these "normal values" to enter the study will rarely affect the validity of the trial. In this situation, these deviations are minor and might be ignored. However, if we intend to study treatment effects in patients with a particular diagnosis or condition, permitting those with the wrong diagnosis to enter the trial could affect the validity of the conclusions. In this situation, these might be considered major deviations. Even so, in randomized trials, this problem would have to occur frequently or affect the treatment groups differentially to have consequences for the study validity.

Protocol deviations, even major ones, are not necessarily a sign of a poor quality study, even though some regulatory agencies take a dim view of them. Some regulators view the protocol rigidly, as a virtual *contract* to perform a study in a particular fashion in every patient. To a strong regulatory mind set, deviations are evidence of sloppiness or, if frequent enough, scientific misconduct. In my opinion, this view is inappropriate and unfortunate. The protocol represents a plan or intent, not a guarantee that every clinical circumstance will fit the mold. Furthermore, it is not obvious to what extent the protocol can or should refer to the individual patient as opposed to an idealized research subject. Human patients are autonomous and many medical decisions supercede the scientific objectives of the trial.

This is an argument in favor of a balanced view of protocol deviations. On the one hand, the protocol is a design specification and the investigators should adhere to the plans as closely as possible. On the other hand, the design exists in an environment that changes from patient to patient and some deviations are likely. The more detailed and rigid the specifications are, the more likely it is that deviations will occur. Therefore, the protocol should require only those things that are essential to the scientific and ethical integrity of the trial.

Design validity versus biological validity

When assessing a trial with a protocol that has not been followed perfectly, investigators should distinguish between *design validity* and *biological validity*. A technically well-designed and conducted trial can address a weak, meaningless, or inappropriate biological question. In contrast, a flawed design or imperfectly executed trial could provide valid and convincing biological evidence. Efforts to achieve design validity by coping with protocol deviations may not be needed if the study already provides biological validity.

The best recent example of this situation is the National Surgical Adjuvant Breast and Bowel Project (NSABP) misconduct case (see Chapter 18), in which eligibility criteria were fabricated by one investigator for a small proportion of study participants. The resulting trial, even including the ineligible patients, almost certainly had biological validity. However, many people agonized excessively over design validity and sought to increase it by discarding various fractions of the data. This raised questions about the entire trial, which prompted worries about the cooperative group, the treatment, the principal investigator, and the sponsor.

Consider that nonexperimental (retrospective) study designs can sometimes yield convincing evidence of treatment efficacy, even though patients were treated without a protocol. The problems in making reliable efficacy assessments from these designs arise because: 1) it is difficult to define retrospectively who received treatment, 2) investigators may be unable to control confounders convincingly, and 3) outcomes may not be assessed in a systematic fashion. Problems with inferences from nonexperimental designs do not occur principally because individuals didn't all follow the same protocol exactly. Prospective clinical trials correct these deficiencies by defining the treatment group clearly and by controlling bias and random error. Thus, protocol deviations in a trial that do not affect these features of the design will not diminish the validity of the study to a large degree.

4.6.3   Protocols are structured, logical, and complete

There is no way to describe a universal trial protocol, except to say that it contains detailed accurate information from which knowledgeable investigators can review or conduct a study. Usually protocols omit details about the considerable infrastructure required to perform a trial, such as administrative procedures. Even without such details, protocols are important and useful documents. This section contains a sketch of the depth and breadth of a typical trial protocol. Additional details, at least with respect to oncology protocols, can be found in Leventhal and Wittes [1988].

This outline and brief discussion is intended to assist investigators in drafting, reviewing, and improving the quality of their own clinical trials. The emphasis of this outline is on comparative trials performed in a collaborative setting. However, almost all studies would benefit from having their protocols address most of the topics below. The headings presuppose a pharmacologic therapy, but there should be little difficulty in adapting it to trials using other treatment modalities. The total length of a protocol will usually be 20 typed pages or more, written in a structured formal style with page numbers and references, and containing most of the following sections.

1. **Title Page** (essential for all protocols). The title page should include: a) study title, b) date of last revision, c) principal investigator and phone number, d) other study collaborators, and e) administrative office and phone number. When developing protocols in a collaborative setting, the revision date can prevent much confusion. Some sponsors, such as pharmaceutical companies, omit naming a principal investigator. This diffusion of responsibility is unacceptable.

2. **Contents or Index** (optional).

3. **Protocol Synopsis** (optional). A one-page description of complicated and lengthy protocols can be a great help.

4. **Schema** (essential for complex SE and CTE protocols). Patient flow with major relevant landmarks such as study entry, evaluations and treatments, and randomization are presented in diagrammatic form. The basic architecture of the study design will be evident from the schema alone. Doses, schedules, and other details regarding therapy should be deleted from the schema to prevent using it for treatment without consulting the full protocol.

5. **Objectives of the Study** (essential for all protocols). The objectives pose important scientific questions addressed by the trial. The objectives should be stated clearly, concisely, and quantitatively, and correspond with the hypotheses to be tested by the study. It is also helpful to indicate the relevant endpoints. This section is usually quite brief and is formatted as an outline with details.

6. **Introduction and Background** (essential for all protocols). This section provides the introduction and scientific background/rationale for the study and should be an adequate introduction to the subject for other investigators and reviewers. Summaries of similar or background studies will provide justification for the stated objectives. If a new treatment is being tested in SE or CTE trials, pilot data may be required to justify the larger study. Keep in mind that some readers and potential critics of the protocol will not be as expert in the science as the authors. References must be included and it should be written in a narrative style. Supporting or recent historical data that justify the design of the study need to be included.

7. **Drug Information** (essential for studies employing drugs). All drugs used in the study need to be described in alphabetical order with respect to human toxicity, pharmaceutical data, administration, storage and stability, and supplier. The investigator should list the National Service Center (NSC) number, Investigational New Drug (IND) number, if relevant, and any other standard names for the drug.

8. **Staging Criteria** (essential for all studies). This section lists the criteria or system by which extent of disease will be established. In cancer studies, extent of disease may be determined by stage, the assessment of which is often standardized. For some other diseases, extent of disease may be less standardized, or even controversial. Therefore, the criteria used to establish extent may need to be listed explicitly.

9. **Patient Eligibility Criteria** (essential for all protocols). This section is a detailed, specific, and quantitative description of eligibility requirements and exclusions. For example, eligibility criteria may depend on sub-category of disease, prior therapy, measurability of disease extent or response, performance status or disease severity, and required organ function. Exclusionary criteria should also be outlined in the same way. Criteria for exclusions should be named on the basis of knowledge obtained prior to the assessment of response or study outcome. Exclusions should not be permitted on the basis of information that only becomes known after the initiation of treatment. Any competing studies or factors that will interfere with accrual should be listed here or in a separate section.

10. **Registration or Randomization Procedures and Stratification** (essential for all protocols). Phone numbers and contacts for placing a patient on the study are provided. This should include information required for central eligibility checks. In many cases, the individuals responsible for the mechanistic parts of placing a patient on study are not physicians or persons otherwise knowledgeable about the subtleties of the study. They may require detailed procedural specifications here to avoid confusion or entry of ineligible patients later. Stratification factors may affect the randomized assignment or treatment and need to be available at the time a treatment assignment or registration is requested.

11. **Treatment Program** (essential for all protocols). This includes details of required therapy such as chemotherapy dosage, biopsies, and masking procedures. For TM studies, the dose escalation will be detailed. For studies employing more than one treatment modality, details of each need to be provided in separate sections. Within the treatment specification, secondary registrations or randomizations should be indicated. This section should also list criteria for discontinuing protocol treatment, e.g., completion of therapy, disease progression, unacceptable side effects, or patient preference.

12. **Dosage Modification/Side Effects** (essential for all protocols). This includes details of required dose modifications and reductions when toxicities or side effects are encountered. The side effects or toxicities to be monitored should be listed. Dose modifications should address the following concerns: baseline conditions that necessitate changes in the initial dose; criteria for multiple courses of treatment; dose decrements or increments to be employed; criteria for substituting treatment delays for dose reductions; an investigator to contact concerning dose modification questions; and reporting requirements for unexpected side effects.

13. **Agent Information** (essential for all agents). This section explains details of drug preparation, storage, dilution, and stability. For experimental agents availability and drug-specific background data should be given. The drug brochure for investigational agents should accompany the protocol.

14. **Treatment Evaluation** (essential for all protocols). This section provides the details for the methods of evaluation and for determining endpoints and toxicities. In studies like SE trials of cytotoxic agents in oncology, the methods

for assessing tumor response are critical to the evaluation and generalizability of the trial. Scoring, intensity, or other evaluation criteria should be listed.

15. **Serial Measurements/Study Calendar** (essential for SE and CTE studies). This lists the study parameters and milestones and the time at which they are to be determined while the patient is on protocol treatment. This should include a listing of baseline measurements. In addition, this section specifies the actions to be taken in response to specific study complications, such as steps for removing a patient from the treatment protocol because of side effects or toxicity. This section should cross reference the data forms and their submission schedule.

16. **Statistical Considerations** (essential for DF, SE, and CTE studies, optional for TM studies). This section addresses the following relevant points: recap of study objectives; required sample size, power, and the way it was estimated, precision of the design for determining major study endpoints, projected accrual rate and duration of the study, and analysis methods. Also, plans for interim analyses and guidelines for early stopping must be included. The statistical section should also outline the quantitative properties of the study with respect to secondary objectives. A sketch of the final analysis is also useful. In some cases, the analysis plan may need to be specified in considerable detail.

17. **External Collaborations or Reviews** (essential for all multi-institutional studies). This section describes arrangements and procedures with investigators outside of the parent institution. For example, the details of how to obtain pathological specimen or imaging review should be given. Names, addresses, and phone numbers should be listed for outside investigators if not given on the title page. In the event that extensive or critical portions of the study depend on collaborations outside the parent institution, supplementary protocols may need to be submitted (e.g., extensive pathologic review).

18. **Data Recording, Management, and Monitoring** (essential for all protocols). This section provides details for the collection and review of data while the study is in progress. It includes the contact person with names and addresses for submission of data forms or related collection instruments. This will include addresses and phone numbers for questions, emergencies, and the reporting of fatal, life-threatening, or unexpected reactions. The submission schedule for data forms must be outlined. In addition, the membership of a safety monitoring committee should be outlined.

19. **Special Instructions**. This section contains instructions to study managers for obtaining and mailing specimens for special laboratory tests or analyses. Any special data or data forms required by the study sponsor should be listed with instructions on how they should be handled.

20. **Communication and Publication of Data** (essential for all studies which involve collaborations, especially data management, outside of the institution, particularly pharmaceutical company sponsored studies). This section outlines agreements regarding the communication and publication of study data. Any limitation or restrictions of investigator access to the study data must

be detailed. This section should also specify prior approvals, if required, for publishing the data. The format of this section is narrative.

21. **Peer Review** (this section is optional). This section outlines the peer review procedures that the protocol may have already passed. For example, for cooperative group protocols, peer review may include the group mechanism, and NIH.

22. **Patient Consent** (essential for all protocols). This section may be submitted as an appendix with patient consent forms. The reading level of the patient consent document should be eighth grade or lower. An appropriate language should be used if there is a plan to enroll patients whose primary language is not English, and "back-translation" or other method should be used to be certain that important concepts are translated properly.

23. **References** (essential for all protocols). Include publications based on the trial (if any) and copies of important references from the protocol.

24. **Data (Case Report) Forms** (optional). Investigators are encouraged to submit proposed data forms for the study. Ideally, the forms should be self-coding for computer entry. The forms will be reviewed for capturing of items required to meet study objectives. Data forms may be submitted as an appendix.

25. **Protocol Amendments** (essential for all protocols if any amendments exist). This section includes a summary of all protocol modifications that affect patient treatment arranged in chronological order. A brief explanation of each amendment is also useful.

26. **Other Appendices** (optional). These may include ethics review documentation, toxicity criteria, flow sheets, etc.

27. **Glossary** (optional). Include definitions of special or unfamiliar terms. This section might be useful for psychosocial research terminology, new drugs, etc.

4.7 Summary

Clinical trials are true experimental designs and can be distinguished from nonexperimental studies by specific design features that help meet the scientific objectives. Controlled trials and verified comparative trials provide the strongest evidence about treatment effects, while nonexperimental designs provide the weakest. Effort spent achieving an optimal design is more efficient than trying to correct deficiencies when the data from a trial are analyzed. A good trial design will be simple, measure important clinical parameters, be precise (reduce errors of chance), eliminate bias, and provide external validity.

Most clinical trial designs require patients to be nested within treatments. Parallel or independent groups designs that use this nested structure can be improved by using randomization, blocking, and placebo treatments when feasible. Bayesian methods permit the formal incorporation information about the treatment effect from outside the trial. In this formulation, opinion or degree of belief takes an equal footing with objective prior information such as data. This feature of Bayesian inference often produces controversy.

Many clinical trials fit into one of four types. Treatment mechanism (e.g., phase I) studies are the earliest developmental drug trials with human subjects. Their objectives are usually dose-finding and studying pharmacokinetics. SE studies employ a fixed treatment dose or schedule and look for evidence of treatment feasibility, efficacy, and side effects. CTE (phase III) studies compare seemingly effective treatments to standard therapy or other treatments. Expanded safety (phase IV) studies are undertaken after a new treatment comes into wide use and are intended to observe uncommon side effects of treatment. Although widely used, this terminology originated with cytotoxic drug development and may be inadequate to describe all trials performed in other areas.

The research protocol is a written scientific plan for a clinical trial. While it does not usually describe the considerable infrastructure necessary to carry out a trial, the protocol provides enough information about the study to serve developmental and peer review purposes. In particular, protocols specify eligibility and exclusion criteria, treatment plans and modifications, endpoint assessments and other evaluations, statistical plans, and informed consent procedures and documents. Minor deviations from the protocol specifications are common and do not undermine the integrity of the trial. Frequently occurring major deviations may affect the validity of the trial or be a sign of other problems with the investigators.

4.8   Questions for Discussion

1. Many methodologic problems in trials can be avoided reliably by proper design features but not by analyses. List and discuss as many as you can think of.

2. What are circumstances in which epidemiologic designs would be preferred over comparative clinical trials for judging treatment efficacy?

3. Interventions to prevent disease often do not undergo TM and SE testing. What type of evidence can replace the information from such developmental trials?

4. In device, surgical, and biologic trials, what is meant by "device function"? Compare and contrast questions about "device function" with questions of clinical outcome.

5. Any of the following may be the experimental unit in a comparative trial: treatment course, patient, family, physician practice, village, or city. Sketch examples of where each might be used.

6. Suppose investigators conduct an SE trial evaluating response to treatment as the endpoint. The study is stopped due to loss of funding. Months later, the same study is re-instituted by the same investigators after additional support is found. Is this one or two trials? Can the data be combined and, if so, how?

7. Suppose drug A is an established treatment administered at a fixed dose. Investigators wish to study the combination of drugs A and B, but are unsure of the best dose of either one in the presence of the other. What type of design would permit studying this question? Compare it with a typical phase I trial. What if the correct doses are known but the order of A and B is in question?

8. A randomized CTE trial has five treatment arms: A, B, C, $A+B$, and $B+C$. What issues would you expect to be discussed in the analysis plan of the statistics section in the protocol? What if only the first three groups were involved?

Chapter References

Bakke, O.M., Manocchia, M., de Abajo, F., Kaitin, K.I., and Lasagna, L. (1995). Drug safety discontinuations in the United Kingdom, the United States, and Spain from 1974 through 1993: A regulatory perspective. Clin. Pharmacol. Ther. 58(1): 108-117.

Beecher, H.K. (1955). The powerful placebo. J.A.D.A. 159: 1602-1606.

Bertram, J.F., Kolonel, L.N., and Meyskens, F.L. Jr. (1987). Strategies and rationale for chemoprevention of cancer in humans. Cancer Research 47: 3012-3031.

Byar, D.P. (1978). On combining information: Historical controls, overviews, and comprehensive cohort studies.. Recent Results in Cancer Research 111: 95-98.

Byar, D.P. (1991). Problems with using observational databases to compare treatments. Statistic in Med. 10: 663-666.

Casey, A.T.H., Crockard, H.A., Bland, J.M. et al. (1996). Surgery on the rheumatoid cervical spine for the non-ambulant myelopathic patient – too much, too late? Lancet 347: 1004-1007.

Challis, G.B. and Stam, H.J. (1990). The spontaneous regression of cancer: A review of cases from 1900 to 1987. Acta Oncologica 29: 545-550.

Chowdhury, A.M., Karim, F., Rohde, J.E., Ahmed, J. and Abed, F.H. (1991). Oral rehydration therapy: A community trial comparing the acceptability of homemade sucrose and cereal-based solutions. Bull. World Health Organ. 69: 229-234.

Cochran, W.G. and Cox, G.M. (1957). Experimental Designs, 2nd Edition. New York: John Wiley & Sons.

Cole, W.H. (1976). Opening address: Spontaneous regression of cancer and the importance of finding its cause. NCI Monograph No. 44: 5-9.

COMMIT (1995a). Community intervention trial for smoking cessation (COMMIT): I. Cohort results from a four-year community intervention. Am. J. Public Health 85: 183-192.

COMMIT (1995b). Community intervention trial for smoking cessation (COMMIT): II. Changes in adult cigarette smoking prevalence. Am. J. Public Health 85: 193-200.

Cornfield, J. (1978). Randomization by group: A formal analysis. Am J Epidem. 108: 100-102.

Cox, D.R. (1992). Planning of Experiments. New York: John Wiley & Sons.

Cuschieri, A., Fayers, P., Fielding, J. et al. (1996). Postoperative morbidity and mortality after D_1 and D_2 resections for gastric cancer: Preliminary results of the MRC randomised controlled surgical trial. Lancet 347: 995-999.

Day, N.E. and Walter, S.D. (1984). Simplified models of screening for chronic disease: Estimation procedures from mass screening programmes. Biometrics 40: 1-14.

Dixon, W.J. and Mood, A.M. (1948). A method for obtaining and analyzing sensitivity data. J. Am. Statist. Assoc. 43: 109-126.

Edwards, A.W.F. (1972). Likelihood. Cambridge: Cambridge University Press.

Ellison, N.M., Byar, D.P., and Newell, G.R. (1978). Special report on Laetrile: The NCI Laetrile review. New Engl. J. Med. 229: 549-552.

Fleiss, J.L. The Design and Analysis of Clinical Experiments. New York: John Wiley & Sons.

Fox, R.C. and Swazey, J.P. (1992). Spare Parts: Organ Replacement in American Society. New York: Oxford University Press.

Freedman, L.S. (1989). The size of clinical trials in cancer research: What are the current needs? Br. J. Cancer 59: 396-400.

Gail, M.H., Mark, S.D., Carroll, R.J., Green, S.B., and Pee, D. (1996). On design considerations and randomization-based inference for community intervention trials. Statistics in Med. 15: 1069-1092.

Gatsonis, C. and Greenhouse, J.B. (1992). Bayesian methods for phase I clinical trials. Statistics in Med. 11: 1377-1389.

Goodman, S.N., Zahurak, M.L., and Piantadosi, S. (1995). Some practical improvements in the continual reassessment method for phase I studies. Statistics in Med. 14: 1149-1161.

Gordon, N.H. and Wilson, J.K. (1992). Using toxicity grades in the design and analysis of cancer phase I clinical trials. Statistics in Medicine 11: 2063-2075.

Govindarajulu, Z. (1988). Statistical Techniques in Bioassay. Basel: Karger.

Green, S.B., and Byar, D.P. (1984). Using observational data from registries to compare treatments: The fallacy of omnimetrics. Statistics in Med. 3: 361-370.

Greenwald, P. (1985). Prevention of Cancer. Chapter 10 in V.T. DeVita, S. Hellman, and S.A. Rosenberg (Eds.) Cancer: Principles and Practice of Oncology. 2nd edition. Philadelphia: J.B. Lippincott.

Greenwald, P. and Cullen, J.W. (1985). The new emphasis in cancer control. J. Nat. Cancer Inst. 74: 543-551.

Haaland, P.D. (1989). Experimental Design in Biotechnology. New York: Marcel Dekker.

Heiberger, R.M. (1989). Computation for the Analysis of Designed Experiments. New York: John Wiley & Sons.

Herson, J. (1984). Statistical Aspects in the Design and Analysis of Phase II Clinical Trials, Chapter 15, in M.J. Buyse, M.J. Staquet, and R.J. Sylvester (Eds.), Cancer Clinical Trials. Oxford: Oxford University Press.

Hinkelmann, K., and Kempthorne, O. (1994). Design and Analysis of Experiments: Vol. I: Introduction to Experimental Design. New York: Johns Wiley & Sons.

Horton, R. (1996). Surgical research or comic opera: Questions, but few answers. Lancet 347: 984.

International Conference on Harmonisation (1994). Good Clinical Practice Guideline for Essential Documents for the Conduct of a Clinical Trial. Geneva: ICH Secretariat (c/o IFPMA).

Kassaye, M., Larson, C., and Carlson, D. (1994). A randomized community trial of prepackaged and homemade oral rehydration therapies. Arch. Ped. Adolesc. Med. 148: 1288-1292.

Kelloff, G.J., Johnson, J.R., Crowell, J.A., et al. (1995). Approaches to the development and marketing approval of drugs that prevent cancer. Cancer Epidemiol. Biomarkers & Prevention 4: 1-10.

Leventhal, B.G. and Wittes, R.E. (1988). Research Methods in Clinical Oncology. New York: Raven Press.

Lindley, D.V. (1965). Introduction to Probability and Statistics from a Bayesian Viewpoint. Cambridge: Cambridge University Press.

Lorenzen, T.J. and Anderson, V.L. (1993). Design of Experiments. New York: Marcel Dekker.

Mahfouz, A.A., Abdel-Moneim, M., al-Erian, R.A. and al-Amari, O.M. (1995). Impact of chlorination of water in domestic storage tanks on childhood diarrhoea: A community trial in the rural areas of Saudi Arabia. J. Trop. Med. Hyg. 98: 126-130.

Majeed, A.W., Troy, G., Nicholl, J.P. et al. (1996). Randomised, prospective, single-blind comparison of laparoscopic versus small-incision cholecystectomy. Lancet 347: 989-994.

Martz, H.F. and Waller, R.A. (1982). Bayesian Reliability Analysis. New York: John Wiley & Sons.

Marubini, E., Mariani, L., Salvadori, B. et al. (1996). Results of a breast-cancer-surgery trial compared with observational data from routine practice. Lancet 347: 1000-1003.

McPeek, B., Mosteller, F., and McKneally, M. (1989). Randomized clinical trials in surgery. Int. J. Technology Assessment in Health Care 5: 317-332.

Meyer, L., Job-Spira, N., Bouyer, J., Bouvet, E., and Spira, A. (1991). Prevention of sexually transmitted diseases: A randomised community trial. J. Epidemiol. Community Health 45: 152-158.

Moertel, C.G., Fleming, T.R., Rubin, J. et al. (1982). A clinical trial of amygdalin (Laetrile) in the treatment of human cancer. New Engl. J. Med. 306: 201-206.

Murray, G.D. (1991). Statistical aspects of research methodology. Br. J. Surg. 78: 777-781.

Noseworthy, J.H., Ebers, G.C., Vandervoort, M.K., et al. (1994). The impact of blinding on the results of a randomized, placebo-controlled multiple sclerosis clinical trial. Neurology 44: 16-20.

NSABP (1992). NSABP Protocol P-1 (Breast Cancer Prevention Trial). Pittsburg, PA: NSABP Center Headquarters.

O'Bryan, T. and Walter, G. (1979). $Sankhy\bar{a}$ A, 41: 95-108.

Olkin, I. (1995). Meta analysis: Reconciling the results of independent studies. Statistics in Med. 14: 457-472.

O'Quigley, J. (1992). Estimating the probability of toxicity at the recommended dose following a phase I clinical trial in cancer. Biometrics 48: 853-862.

O'Quigley, J., Pepe, M., and Fisher, L. (1990). Continual reassessment method: A practical design for phase I clinical trials in cancer. Biometrics 46: 33-48.

O'Regan, B. and Hirshberg, C. (1993). Spontaneous Remission: An Annotated Bibliography. Sausalito, CA.: Institute of Noetic Sciences.

Osler, W. (1910). Man's Redemption of Man. London: Constable & Co.

Piantadosi, S. and Gail, M.H. (1995). Statistical Issues Arising in Thoracic Surgery Clinical Trials. Chapter 71 in F.G. Pearson, J. Deslauriers, R.J. Ginsberg, et al. (Eds.), Thoracic Surgery. New York: Churchill Livingstone.

Piantadosi, S. and Liu, G. (1996). Improved designs for phase I studies using pharmacokinetic measurements. Statistics in Med. 15: 1605-1618.

Ratain, M.J., Mick, R., Schilsky, R.L., and Siegler, M. (1993). Statistical and ethical issues in the design and conduct of phase I and II clinical trials of new anticancer agents. JNCI 85: 1637-1643.

Roberts, A.H., Kewman, D.G., Mercier, L., and Hovell, M. (1993). The power of nonspecific effects in healing: Implications for psychosocial and biological treatments. Clin. Psychol. Rev. 13: 375-391.

Ruberg, S.J. (1995a). Dose response studies. I. Some design considerations. J. Biopharmaceutical Statistics 5: 1-14.

Ruberg, S.J. (1995b). Dose response studies. II. Analysis and interpretation. J. Biopharmaceutical Statistics 5: 15-42.

Savage, L.J. (1954). The Foundations of Statistics. New York: John Wiley & Sons.

Simon, R., Wittes, R.E., and Ellenberg, S.S. (1985). Randomized phase II clinical trials. Cancer Treatment Reports 69: 1475-1381.

Simons, J.W., Jaffee, E.M., Weber, C. et al. (1997). Bioactivity of human GM-CSF gene transfer in autologous irradiated renal cell carcinoma vaccines. Cancer Research, in press.

Sommer, A. Tarwotjo, I., Djunaedi, E., West, K.P., Jr., and Loeden, A.A. (1986). Impact of vitamin A supplementation on childhood mortality: A randomized controlled community trial. Lancet, i, 1169-1173.

Sommer, A. and Zeger, S.L. (1991). On estimating efficacy from clinical trials. Statistics in Med. 10: 45-52.

Souhami, R.(1992). Large-Scale Studies. Chapter 13 in C.J. Williams (Ed.), Introducing New Treatments for Cancer: Practical Ethical and Legal Problems. Chichester: John Wiley & Sons.

Spiegelhalter, D.J., Freedman, L.S., and Parmar, M.K.B. (1994). Bayesian approaches to randomized trials. J. R. Statist. Soc. A 157: 357-416.

Stebbing, L.S. (1961). Philosophy and the Physicist. Middlesex, England: Penguin Books.

Storer, B.E. (1989). Design and analysis of phase I clinical trials. Biometrics 45: 925-937.

Walter, S.D. and Day, N.E. (1983). Estimation of the duration of a preclinical state using screening data. Am. J. Epidemiol. 118: 865-886.

Wetherill, G.B. (1963). Sequential estimation of quantal response curves (with discussion). JRSS B 25: 1-48.

Whitworth, J.A., Morgan, D., Maude, G.H., Luty, A.J., and Taylor, D.W. (1992). A community trial of ivermectin for onchocerciasis in Sierra Leone: Clinical and parasitological responses to four doses given at six-monthly intervals. Trans. R. Soc. Trop. Med. Hyg. 86: 277-280.

Wilde, D.J. (1964). Optimum Seeking Methods. Englewood Cliffs, N.J.: Prentice-Hall.

Wilson, E.O. (1992). The Diversity of Life. New York: W. W. Norton.

Winer, B.J. (1962). Statistical Principles in Experimental Design, 2nd Edition. New York: McGraw-Hill.

Wong, W.K. and Lachenbruch, P.A. (1996). Designing studies for dose response. Statistics in Med. 15: 343-359.

Yusuf, S., Collins, R., and Peto, R. (1984). Why do we need some large, simple, randomized trials? Statistics in Med. 3: 409-420.

CHAPTER 5

Bias and Random Error

5.1   Introduction

Error has two components, a purely random one and systematic one called bias. Understanding the differences between randomness and bias, and the sources of each, is the first step in being able to control them using experimental design. The terms "random error", "random variability", or just "variability" are often used to describe the play of chance, particularly when the effects of explanatory or predictive factors have already been taken into account. An operational definition of randomness might be *unexplainable fluctuations*, i.e., fluctuations that remain beyond our ability to attribute them to specific causes. New knowledge may show that some part of what was previously thought to be random is explainable.

"Bias" describes deviations that are not a consequence of chance alone. The exact consequences of bias may be difficult to see. However, it is usually simple to detect or understand factors that contribute to it. Sources of bias can often be understood well enough to be controlled. In real-world clinical trials, methodologists tend to focus as much on bias as a source of error as on random variation. This is because some biases, e.g., patient selection effects, appear to be strong compared with the size of many treatment effects.

Errors within experiments can be discussed in either a purely statistical context or in a larger clinical one. Although mathematical formalism is required to discuss the statistical context, ideas about the properties and behavior of random error and bias are basically the same in a clinical context. Most statistical discussions of random error (and bias) assume that a primary focus of the investigation is hypothesis testing. This framework is convenient and will be used here. However, adopting the usual perspective is not intended to be a general endorsement of hypothesis tests as the preferred method for making inferences. Furthermore, estimation is equally likely to be affected by random error and bias.

I begin by discussing general issues related to random error and bias and then focus on clinical and statistical contexts.

5.1.1 Random and systematic errors are distinct

Pure randomness has no preferred direction. This has two consequences. Statistically we expect its net or average effect to be zero. (Its expected value is zero.) Clinically, averaging over a large number of observations or a long enough period, we expect its relative effects to be inconsequentially small. This does not mean that chance hasn't affected a particular observation, but that it theoretically averages out to have no net effect in the long run. Maneuvers such as averaging after increasing the number of observations or repeating the experiment reduce the magnitude of random error. Because of sampling variability, subject-to-subject differences, measurement error, or other sources of noise, we can never completely eliminate random error. However, in most experiments, it can be controlled and reduced to acceptably low levels, by careful attention to the experimental design (e.g., sample size).

Bias, unlike random fluctuation, is a component of error that has a net direction and magnitude. In a statistical context, it cannot be eliminated by appealing to long run averages or expectation, although it can often be quantified. In a clinical context, bias can arise in numerous ways and can rarely be quantified precisely. But it can be large enough to invalidate the guesses of practitioners making unstructured treatment comparisons. Similarly, bias can invalidate poorly planned or conducted treatment comparisons. Bias yields a net effect in one direction or another and cannot be reduced by averaging after repetition or taking additional observations. The factors that produce bias may not be amenable to measurement, but can usually be removed or reduced by good design and conduct of the experiment.

The difference, and importance of distinguishing, between random variation and bias is analogous to sound or signal reproduction. In this analogy, the treatment effect is the sound level or signal strength, variation is like background noise, and bias is like distortion. Background noise (variation) may be important when the sound or signal level (treatment effect) is low. Reducing variation is like increasing the signal-to-noise ratio. In contrast, even when the noise is low, the sound produced may be distorted unless the system is designed and performing properly. *In contrast, even when the variation is low, the treatment effect may be biased unless the trial is designed and conducted properly.* Having a strong signal is not sufficient if there is too much distortion.

Example

Consider the behavior of two different estimators (or *methods of estimation*) of some parameter, Δ, which might be a treatment effect or treatment difference (Figure 5.1). Because of error, repeated use of either estimate would produce a distribution of values. One estimator, $\hat{\Delta}$, has random error but no bias, and the distribution of values we would obtain is centered around the true value, $\Delta = 1$. The second estimator, $\tilde{\Delta}$, has both random error and bias and its distribution is not centered around the true value. Many times, $\tilde{\Delta}$ yields answers similar to $\hat{\Delta}$ but, on average, $\tilde{\Delta}$ does not give the true value.

In practice, the investigator does not see a full distribution of values for any estimate, because the experiment is performed only once, or at most, a few times. Thus, the actual estimate obtained for Δ is a sample from a distribution. Because both $\hat{\Delta}$

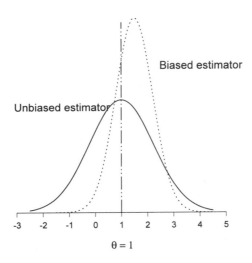

Figure 5.1 Hypothetical distributions of biased and unbiased estimators.

and $\widetilde{\Delta}$ in this example are subject to randomness, either can yield a value that is far enough away from the true value that we might conclude $\Delta \neq 1$ (e.g., after a hypothesis test). In this example, $\widetilde{\Delta}$ is closer, on average, to the true treatment effect than $\widehat{\Delta}$. Although not a general property, sometimes the overall performance (bias + random error) of a biased estimator can be better than that of an unbiased one.

5.2   Random Error

In this section, I assume that the estimators being employed are free of bias. I will return to examine the consequences of bias later in the chapter.

5.2.1   Hypothesis tests versus significance tests

Hypothesis testing has had a prominent role in developing modern ideas about the design and analysis of clinical trials and still provides a useful perspective on errors of inference. Following ideas put forth by Neyman and Pearson [e.g., 1933; Lehmann, 1986], hypothesis testing is an approach for choosing between two competing statistical hypotheses. Suppose the competing hypotheses are labeled H_0 and H_a and a summary of the data (or *statistic*), denoted by T, is selected. The hypothesis testing approach requires that we define a *critical region* in advance of taking data values, and then choosing H_0 or H_a, depending on whether or not T falls within the critical region.

Table 5.1 Random Errors from Hypothesis Tests and Other Types of Dichotomized Inferences

	Truth and Consequences	
Result of Test	H_0 True	H_0 False
Reject H_0	type I error	no error
Don't Reject H_0	no error	type II error

In practice, investigators seldom employ hypothesis testing in exactly this way. A different procedure, called *significance testing* [Cox and Hinkley, 1974] is used more commonly. A non-mathematical comparison of the two procedures is given by Salsburg [1990]. Assume that the probability distribution of the test statistic, T, is known or can be approximated when H_0 is true. The more extreme the actual value of T is, relative to this distribution, the less likely H_0 is to be true. The significance level is

$$p = \Pr\{T^* \geq T \mid H_o\}$$

where T is the value of the statistic based on the observed data. Thus, this "test" yields a significance level (or p-value) instead of a decision. The p-value is intended to help the investigator assess the strength of evidence for or against H_0. In reality, the p-value does not have this interpretation. The deficiencies of this approach will be discussed in Chapter 12.

The basic structures of hypothesis and significance tests are the same as are their properties with respect to random error. This is discussed in the next section.

5.2.2 Hypothesis tests are subject to two types of random error

The two types of random error that can result from a formal hypothesis test are shown in Table 5.1. The type I error is a "false positive" result and occurs if there is no treatment effect or difference but the investigator wrongly concludes that there is. The type II error is a "false negative" and occurs when investigators fail to detect a treatment effect or difference that is actually present. The *power* of the test is the chance of declaring a treatment effect or difference of a given size to be statistically significantly different from the null hypothesis value when the alternative hypothesis is true (i.e., the probability of *not* making a type II error).

These ideas are illustrated in Figure 5.2, which shows the distributions (assume they are normal) of a treatment effect estimator, $\hat{\Delta}$, under both the null hypothesis ($\Delta = 0$) and under an alternative hypothesis ($\Delta \neq 0$). The short vertical lines represent a "critical value" chosen from the type I error to reject the null hypothesis. For example, the critical value could be ± 1.96 standard deviations from the null hypothesis mean, which would yield a (two-sided) type I error of 5%. The following discussion will focus on only the upper critical value, although both have to be considered for a two-sided test.

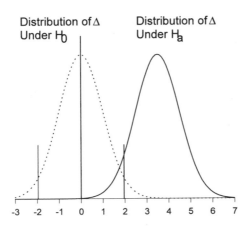

Distribution of Δ Under H_0 Distribution of Δ Under H_a

Figure 5.2 Distributions of a Treatment Effect under the Null and Alternative Hypotheses.

If the null hypothesis is true, $\widehat{\Delta}$ will come from the distribution of values centered at 0 ($\Delta = 0$). If $\widehat{\Delta}$ exceeds the critical value, the experimenter would find it unlikely that it came from the distribution centered at 0 and would reject the null hypothesis. This would constitute a type I error if the null hypothesis were true. If $\widehat{\Delta}$ does not exceed the critical value, the experimenter would not reject the null hypothesis.

If the alternative hypothesis is true, $\widehat{\Delta}$ comes from the distribution centered away from 0 ($\Delta \neq 0$). As before, the experimenter will reject the null hypothesis if $\widehat{\Delta}$ is greater than the critical value. However, if $\widehat{\Delta}$ is less than the critical value, the experimenter will not reject the null hypothesis, resulting in a type II error. When the alternative hypothesis is true, one would like to reject the null most of the time, i.e., have a test with high power.

The properties of the hypothesis test are determined by choosing the alternative hypothesis and the type I error level. If the alternative hypothesis is taken to be far away from the null, the test will have a high power. However, alternatives far away from the null may be unrealistic or uninteresting. The consequences of type I and type II errors are different. Aside from the fact that they are described and quantified under different assumptions about the true state of nature, maneuvers to control them need to be different. These are discussed in the following sections.

5.2.3 Type I errors are relatively easy to control

Usually there is only one factor that governs the chance of making a type I error, that is, the critical value. The experimentalist is free to choose the critical value to fix the chance of a type I error at any desired level. In other words, the chance of making a type I error is usually under the control of the investigator, even during the analysis of an experiment. In particular, the type I error rate does not depend on the size of the experiment. For example, in Figure 5.2, the type I error can be reduced by moving the critical value (short vertical line) to the right.

There are some circumstances in which the data analyst must consider more than just the critical value to control the type I error. Specifically, the type I error can become inflated when multiple tests are performed. This is likely to happen in two situations. The first is when investigators examine accumulating data and repeatedly perform statistical tests, as is done in sequential or group sequential monitoring of clinical trials. A second situation in which the type I error can become inflated occurs when many clinical outcomes or treatment groups are examined using multiple hypothesis tests. Although the type I error of each test can be controlled in the manner outlined above, the overall (experiment-wide) probability of an error can increase. In this second case, some corrections during analysis are possible. However, in both of these situations, the type I error should be carefully considered during the design of the trial. This point will be expanded in the discussion of sequential methods in Chapter 10.

5.2.4   The properties of confidence intervals are similar

In many circumstances, summarizing the observed data using point estimates and confidence intervals gives more information than using only hypothesis tests. Confidence intervals are always based (centered) on the observed or estimated effect and convey useful information regarding the precision of the estimate. This makes them more descriptive and useful than hypothesis tests or p-values, which are often inadequate for summarizing data (see Chapter 14). However, hypothesis tests and confidence intervals share some common properties. For example, we can usually reconstruct hypothesis tests from the confidence intervals. More specifically, a confidence interval is a collection of hypotheses that cannot be rejected at a specified α-level.

Suppose Δ is the true parameter value and investigators hypothesize that Δ_h is correct. A situation analogous to a type I error can occur if the confidence interval around the estimate of Δ excludes Δ_h (Figure 5.3A). The sample on which the confidence interval has been based was an atypical one, and we would wrongly conclude that the data were inconsistent with Δ_h, even though $\Delta_h \approx \Delta$. An error analogous to the type II error can occur when the confidence interval includes both Δ and Δ_h (Figure 5.3B). This can happen even when Δ_h is substantially different from Δ.

5.2.5   Using a one- or two-sided hypothesis test is not the right question

In comparative experiments, investigators frequently need to know if a one-sided hypothesis test is appropriate. When there is biological knowledge that the treatment difference can only go in one direction, a one-sided test may be appropriate. For example, when testing the effects of a non-toxic addition to a treatment, e.g., A versus

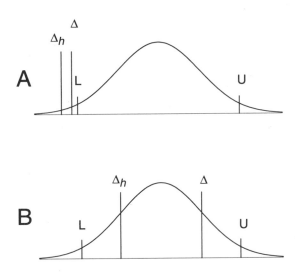

Figure 5.3 Confidence intervals. Δ_h **and** Δ **denote a hypothetical and true parameter value, respectively. U and L are the confidence bounds around the estimated parameter. (The true parameter value remains unknown.)**

A+B, where B can only augment the effect of A, a one-sided test may be sensible. It is not appropriate to employ a one-sided hypothesis test merely to reduce the required sample size, if the treatment difference could be in either direction.

Not all hypothesis tests are symmetric. If a new treatment is being compared with standard therapy, investigators will not be interested in demonstrating conclusively that the new treatment is *worse* than the standard. Learning that the new treatment is not superior to the standard is sufficient. This is essentially a one-sided question.

However, the directionality of the biological question in no way settles the appropriate probability of the type I error to use in a significance test. The critical value for the type I error rate is a standard of significance. Would investigators accept a lower standard of significance when the direction of a treatment difference is known than when it is not known? I think not, but this is precisely what would happen if a one-sided critical value were chosen for $\alpha = 0.05$ when otherwise a two-sided $\alpha = 0.05$ test would be used. In other words, preserving the type I error probability does not preserve the standard of evidence in favor of the treatment difference. A better procedure might be to employ a one-sided $\alpha = 0.025$ type I error, which would yield the same standard of significance as the conventional two-sided test. This would not reduce the sample size. Thus, the right question is the standard of evidence and not the direction of the hypothesis test. This discussion is not meant to define evidence in terms of the p-value.

5.2.6 *P*-values quantify the type I error

P-values are probability statements made under the null hypothesis (usually, the hypothesis of no clinical effect or difference). Suppose the null hypothesis is correct. Because of random variability, the estimated effect or difference will be different from zero. We could ask, "If the null hypothesis is correct, how likely were we to obtain the observed result, or one more extreme?" If the observed result is unlikely, we would take this as evidence that the null hypothesis is false. If we reject the null hypothesis in this situation, it is a type I error. The significance level, or *p*-value, is the probability of obtaining the observed result (or one further away from the null) when the null hypothesis is, in fact, true. If the observed result (or one more extreme) is relatively likely, we would not reject the null hypothesis.

If we could repeat our experiment many times, the estimates of clinical effect obtained would average out close to the true value (assuming no bias). Then, the probability distribution of the estimates would be evident and there would be little trouble in deciding if the assumption of no effect (or no difference) was correct. However, we usually perform only a single study, meaning that we cannot conclusively judge our hypothesis. Instead, we judge the estimate obtained, under an assumption of no effect. In this way of thinking, the probability distribution or uncertainty refers to the estimate obtained and not to the true treatment effect. Thus, the *p*-value is not a statement about the true treatment effect, but about estimates that might be obtained if the null hypothesis were true.

5.2.7 Type II errors depend on the clinical difference of interest

There are three factors that influence the chance of making a type II error. These are: the critical value for the rejection of the null hypothesis; the width of the distribution of the estimator under the alternative hypothesis; and the distance between the centers of the null and alternative distributions, i.e., the alternative treatment effect or difference (Figure 5.2). In principle, investigators have control over the rejection region (discussed above) and the width of the distribution. The width or variance of the distribution is a direct consequence of sample size.

The treatment effect or difference under the alternative hypothesis is not truly under investigator control. One can calculate power for different treatment effects that are *assumed*. If the treatment difference under the alternative hypothesis is increased, the type II error will appear to decrease. In other words, all trials have a high statistical power to detect treatment differences or effects of large enough size. Unfortunately, large treatment differences may not be plausible clinically, so the seemingly higher power to detect them is not helpful. To discuss power, investigators should keep in mind the smallest treatment effect that is of clinical importance. A small study can detect only large differences reliably, whereas a large study can detect small differences reliably.

These ideas can be made more clear by considering the accompanying power curve (Figure 5.4) for a hypothetical clinical trial comparing survival in two treatment groups. The power of the study is plotted against the assumed treatment difference

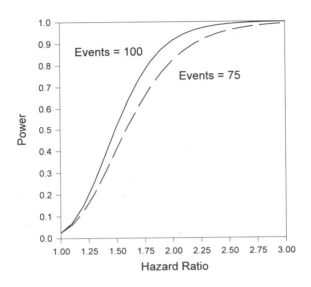

Figure 5.4 Power versus hazard ratio for the logrank test.

measured as a hazard ratio (ratio of median event times). A study with 100 events (solid line) has only 53% power to detect a hazard ratio of 1.5, but over 99% power to detect a threefold ratio. A smaller study of 75 events (dotted line), has lower power everywhere, but eventually reaches 90% power to detect a 2.1-fold hazard ratio. A more detailed discussion of power appears in Chapter 7.

5.2.8 *Post hoc* power calculations are not helpful

At the conclusion of a comparative clinical trial we usually know the estimated treatment effect and its variability. The power of the experiment is usually no longer a meaningful concern. The power characterizes a particular uncertainty before the trial is conducted, in particular the chance of rejecting the null if a certain alternative hypothesis is true. However, the experiment removes this uncertainty and provides more information about the treatment effect.

A possible exception to the futility of *post hoc* power calculations is the rare occasion when the study results are expressed only as a dichotomy, i.e., accept or reject the null hypothesis. If we don't know the magnitude of the treatment effect, the power of the trial against hypothetical effect sizes might be of some interest.

The power of a completed trial against the *observed* difference is likely to be low if the observed difference is smaller than the alternative hypothesis used to plan the study. However, the alternative treatment effect used to design the trial is no longer supported by the data. In other words, a *post hoc* power calculation will usually indicate only that the trial had lower power to detect effects smaller than that for which it was designed – an obvious state of affairs.

Example 7 *Suppose a trial is designed to detect a hazard ratio of 1.9 with 90% power between the treatment groups using a sample size of 100 events (Figure 5.4). Suppose also that, when the study is over, the estimated hazard ratio is 1.25. The power of the study to detect a hazard ratio of 1.25 as being statistically significant is only about 15% (Figure 5.4). Because $\Delta = 1.25$ is closer to the null hypothesis than $\Delta = 2.0$, it is clear that the power against the observed difference is lower than the power against the original alternative hypothesis. Knowing this does not help us to interpret the evidence provided by the trial. Also, calculating the power of the study against other alternative hypotheses that are not supported by the data will not be especially informative. When planning a new trial, we might need to determine the sample size that could detect a hazard ratio of 1.25 with some specified power.*

5.3 Clinical Biases

In this section, I consider estimates or clinical assessments that are subject to both bias and random error. When both are present, the total or average error is a sum of components attributable to each.

5.3.1 Relative size of random error and bias is important

When bias is present, its relative magnitude compared with random error is important. If the bias is small compared with random error, we would not expect it to be a large component of the total error. However, if bias is large compared with random error, it may be the principal component of the total error (Figure 5.5). A strong bias can yield an estimate very far from the true value, even with the wrong direction, i.e., a truly beneficial treatment might be seen as harmful or vice versa.

If we knew even the direction of a bias, we might be able to design informative studies or interpret results more clearly. For example, if we consistently overestimate the effect of treatment A, but a randomized trial shows it to be inferior to B, the study result will remain convincing. Unfortunately, investigators seldom know either the relative magnitude or direction of bias, so corrections are impossible. The only strategy is to prevent bias from occurring by using good design.

5.3.2 Bias arises from numerous sources

There are many potential sources and types of bias in medical studies. For a very detailed listing, see Sackett [1979]. Here I discuss only a few types that are commonly seen and can seriously affect inferences from clinical trials. I will refer to biases that are a consequence of inattention to study design and assessment criteria as structural biases. Some of these are listed in Table 5.2. Statistical biases are those

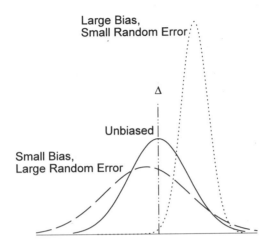

Figure 5.5 Relative size of bias and random error.

that arise from the selection of certain procedures, tests, or data manipulations, and are correctable by using alternative methods. Publication or reporting bias results from preferential selection of positive study results (i.e., those showing significant differences) over negative results (i.e., those failing to show a significant difference) when clinical trials are published (see Chapter 14).

Bias in the selection of the study cohort is a potentially limiting factor in the external validity of trial findings, especially SE studies. For randomized trials, this type of selection bias may not be as serious a problem, because it affects all groups equally and therefore does not influence the estimated treatment difference. In contrast, procedure selection (e.g., surgery versus medical treatment) can cause the treatment groups to be composed differently in a comparative trial and can therefore have an impact on the estimated treatment difference. More subtle selection biases can differentially affect treatment groups in a randomized trial.

Galen (c. 130–210 C.E.) created a system of medicine from the works of Hippocrates, Aristotle, and Plato, dominating Western and Islamic medicine for hundreds of years. His teachings were so highly respected that they were not disputed, despite credible observations contradicting some of them. Such authoritarianism can be a serious source of bias in clinical studies. This is illustrated by the following quote, attributed to Galen:

All who drink of this remedy recover in a short time, except those whom it does not help, who all die. Therefore, it is obvious that it fails only in incurable cases [Strauss, 1968].

Table 5.2 Some Types of Bias and Their Potential Effects on the Results of Clinical Trials

Selection bias:	May affect the external validity of the study.
Procedure selection:	Healthier patients may preferentially select or be selected for a particular treatment.
Post-entry exclusion:	Strong bias effects. Results no longer correspond to the target population.
Selective loss of data:	Variety of effects are possible.
Assessment bias:	Strength of effect can be either enhanced or diminished.
Retroactive definitions:	Strong anti-conservative bias is possible.

This reasoning is circular and defines prognosis in terms of outcome. The bias that results from retroactive definitions such as this can be very strong.

Inappropriate exclusion of eligible study subjects from the analysis is another way to create potentially strong biases. This can be a difficult source of bias to eliminate when there are seemingly excellent clinical reasons for making exclusions. However, whenever eligible patients are excluded from analysis, the experimental paradigm is broken, possibly leading to unwanted or unanticipated effects on estimation. This idea is developed further below and in Chapter 11, where handling of data imperfections is discussed.

Assessment bias is another familiar source of potential difficulty. Patients' self-assessments and clinicians' judgments lack objectivity when they have expectations about the treatment under study. Similar circumstances can arise from study groups, collaborators, or companies under external pressures such as time, money, or ego. Because trial designs that use subjective assessments are common, necessary, and important, controlling this bias is especially beneficial.

TM trials

Treatment mechanism trials generally employ objective methods of assessing the function, feasibility, or action of the treatment. Examples include pharmacologic outcomes, and physical or anatomic measurements. Because of this, properly performed TM studies can be subject to less bias than some later developmental trials. However, if subjective evaluation criteria are used or the investigator does not guard against his or her own assessment bias, the results of a TM trial can appear misleading. An example would be if the demonstration of a successful mechanism such as drug delivery or device function is equated with clinical efficacy.

DF trials

Dose-finding trials can be subject to biases that are not adequately appreciated. For example, dose escalations in oncology using traditional decision and stopping rules with pre-specified dose levels are essentially sequential trials. When they terminate because of toxicity, there is a tendency to underestimate the dose associated with the target level of toxicity. For example, if a dose escalation terminates because DLT is seen in 1 out of 3 patients, the true probability of toxicity is usually less than $1/3$. Operationally this is not a problem, but it can leave investigators with additional dose-finding necessary later in development. When properly implemented, the continual reassessment method of dose-finding is not as subject to this bias.

Recently, there have been suggestions that patients can select their own dose of a new drug in DF trials (within limits and after being properly informed about the risks and benefits). This strategy responds to ethical concerns that many patients on such trials receive ineffective doses and cannot benefit, because the drug levels are conservative early in the study. Using this strategy may confound dose with performance status or other important prognostic factors, causing investigators to mis-estimate the target dose or to overestimate efficacy. Whether or not such compromises are worthwhile will require a substantial amount of investigation.

SE trials

Safety and efficacy trials may be the most subject to bias of all types of trials, because: 1) they employ partly subjective or surrogate clinical endpoints, 2) they do not have internal controls, 3) they are relatively small with highly selected patient populations, and 4) some investigators tend to perform and emphasize subset and/or *post hoc* analyses. None of these characteristics necessarily induce bias, but they do nothing to discourage it. Patient selection effects can be strong in such trials, especially when they are performed within a single institution. Removal of patients from the analysis for reasons that are both outcomes and predictors, such as failing to complete therapy, can also bias the results.

CTE trials

Comparative treatment efficacy trials, particularly those with methodologic flaws, are also potentially subject to significant biases. Problems can result from using subjective endpoints, invalid surrogate endpoints, inappropriate comparison groups, and emphasizing analyses that are prone to error. However, well-designed and conducted CTE trials will minimize or eliminate such biases. Methods for doing so are sketched in the next section.

5.3.3   Controlling structural bias is conceptually simple

Relatively few methods are available, or needed, to eliminate or reduce structural bias. None of the methods and procedures discussed here is complicated, although each of them, at times, can conflict with other constraints imposed on a study. When large treatment effects are present, these methods of reducing bias may be unnecessary. However, when small to moderate treatment effects are present, these methods increase the strength of evidence from the trial.

Randomization

Randomization is the principal method available to the investigator designing a comparative study for reducing selection bias. It is effective because it guarantees that both observed and unobserved baseline differences between the treatment groups are attributable to chance, the effects of which can be quantified by the statistician. After accounting for chance, the remaining differences can be attributed to the treatment(s) reliably if other sources of bias have been eliminated. The benefits and necessity of randomization for reducing bias are not especially controversial. Inadequately performed randomization is associated with large treatment effects that are likely to be biased [Schulz, 1995]. Randomization is discussed in more detail in Chapter 9.

Masking

Masking (blinding) reduces assessment bias. Single masking means that the patients on the study are unaware of which treatment they receive. Masking can be accomplished by ensuring that both treatments look, feel, or taste the same and that the investigators do not know or reveal the treatment assignment to the patients. A masked placebo control is different from a no-treatment control. In the later case, the treatment difference will consist of the effects of the treatment plus the "placebo effect", which might be sizeable. For example, in studies comparing analgesics, patients who know they are receiving a new drug or procedure may have a bias in favor of its efficacy, causing them to overstate its effect. Thus, masking can improve the objectivity of partially subjective outcomes.

In many drug trials, masking can be accomplished effectively by using a placebo tablet or formulation that appears the same as the agent being tested. Double masking (double blind) implies that both patient and investigator responsible for assessing the outcome are unaware of which treatment is being administered. This type of masking further increases the usefulness of subjective endpoints, because investigators can also be influenced by their expectations. This is especially true if the investigator has been exposed to seemingly favorable pre-clinical data, believes strongly in the biological basis on which the therapy was developed, and/or has professional or financial interest in the success of the study. Effective treatment masking is essential in such cases.

Some trialists have made a case for triple masking, i.e., the situation where the Data Safety Monitoring Committee (DSMC) for a clinical trial is also unaware of the treatment assignment. This is intended to increase the objectivity of their decision to stop or continue a study. I believe the DSMC should not be masked. The DSMC is charged with making important decisions about the ongoing ethical and efficacy evidence from the study (Chapter 10). This role is difficult enough when treatment assignments are known to the DSMC members and may be impossible if they are masked. For example, suppose a major difference in non-life-threatening side effects is seen during a trial comparing standard therapy with a new treatment, but no difference in efficacy is evident. If standard therapy has a higher incidence of side effects, it might well be wise to allow the study to remain open to gather more knowledge about, and clinical experience with, the new treatment. Conversely, if the new treatment is the more toxic one, the trial could be stopped in favor of standard therapy. Masking of the DSMC in this situation would prevent them from doing an effective job.

Concurrent controls

A concurrent control group is a relatively resource intensive but effective method for reducing bias. It eliminates the confounding of treatment with calendar time and facilitates the use of randomization, which is the most reliable method for reducing bias due to treatment selection. There are many examples of strong trends in outcomes such as disease mortality over time [Silverman, 1985]. Such trends could render a historically controlled study uninterpretable, as discussed in Chapter 4. One does not need to examine a long interval of time to see time trends. For example, they are evident over short time intervals in areas such as supportive care of cancer and AIDS patients. Similar problems can affect inferences based on databases [Byar, 1980; 1991].

Objective assessments

In most situations, investigators have a choice about the methods that will be used to make clinical assessments of the major study endpoints. Whenever possible, the methods employed should be objective ones, to reduce assessment bias and increase the reproducibility of the findings. Objective assessments are those upon which independent reviewers would agree. Examples ranging from most objective to least objective are: quantitative laboratory measurements, vital status or survival time, time to disease progression or recurrence, outcomes based on predefined criteria such as toxicity or side effects, physician based judgments like functional indices, quality of life measurements, psychosocial assessments, and patient self-reports like pain intensity.

In a few circumstances, the most objective assessments may not be the best method of evaluating treatment. For example, when making assessments of pain intensity, the physician or nurse assessment may be poorly correlated with that from the patient [Grossman, Sheidler, Swedeen, et al., 1992]. Health professionals probably tend to underestimate pain and overestimate functional status. A better method for a clinical trial would be to use the patient's own assessment and employ masking to improve the reliability of the study.

Active follow-up and endpoint ascertainment

Even though endpoints such as disease recurrence and death are objective, the methods used to ascertain them may not be objective if investigators do not plan properly for conducting follow-up examinations. If a trial relies only on passive reporting of such events, the chance for bias is increased. For example, we cannot assume that patients who do not return to clinic for scheduled follow-up visits are alive and well. In contrast, if follow-up status is determined actively, e.g., with scheduled clinic visits or follow-up and phone contacts or home visits, the chance of ascertainment bias is reduced.

No post-hoc exclusions

After study entry, especially after treatment has begun, many study-related events that occur are likely to be correlated with one another. Some events will be causally related, while others are only weakly correlated, being connected through known or unknown third factors. In any case, one cannot realistically expect to select a subset of eligible study participants on the basis of one event and have them be comparable with regard to all other factors. For example, if we select a subset based on good treatment compliance, they are likely to differ from the subset of patients with poor compliance.

The consequence of this is that analyses of subsets of trial participants are subject to bias. One bias that can occur is a "selection bias", because patients predisposed to a particular outcome may be selected preferentially by the subset factor. The strength of this bias depends mostly on unobservable correlations between the selection factor and the outcome. Also, the results in small subsets may be heavily influenced by the outcomes in a few patients. Because little is typically known about the interplay of important factors defining and influencing the subset, it is better to prevent bias by avoiding these analyses.

In SE trials, these forces operate in addition to the selection effects of the eligibility criteria, which may be considerable. Thus, our usual inability to compare results, even informally, between institutions is worsened by subset analyses. In CTE randomized trials, the effect on treatment differences is not as great, unless the selection effect acts differently in the treatment groups. Despite the fact that subset analyses may not yield statistical tests with desirable properties, they may help explain the overall results of a trial or be useful for planning new studies.

5.4 Statistical Bias

Statisticians invariably try to avoid or reduce bias. However, there are circumstances in which it cannot be avoided, and even if it could be, a study might require too many resources to exclude all possible sources of bias. Unfortunately, even qualitative information about bias is difficult to obtain. In a few circumstances, investigators can quantify and correct a statistical bias.

5.4.1 Examples

Statistical bias can arise from some methods of analysis or estimation. Fortunately, such biases are usually not large and often are amenable to quantification and correction by other statistical means. One example of this is the effect of missing covariates in some non-linear regression models commonly used to analyze clinical trials. The relative treatment effects obtained from some models can be biased if necessary prognostic factors are omitted from the regression [Gail, Wieand, and Piantadosi, 1984; Gail, Tan, and Piantadosi, 1988]. This is in contrast to omitting terms from linear regressions where the remaining effects are estimated without bias (although with higher variances). Fortunately, the bias is not large in situations likely to be encountered commonly in clinical trials [Chastang, Byar, and Piantadosi, 1993].

Another situation that can produce a statistical bias occurs when a clinical trial is stopped early according to any of several guidelines commonly used for this purpose (discussed in Chapter 10). When a trial is terminated early because evidence favors rejecting the null hypothesis, the estimated treatment effect is biased in the direction of the alternative hypothesis. The earlier a trial is stopped, the larger is the potential for bias. Unfortunately, in this case, there is not a good correction for the bias, because its magnitude depends on the size of the true treatment effect, which is unknown. Thus, designs that permit early stopping might be unfavorable if investigators absolutely require an unbiased estimate of the treatment effect, even when an extreme alternative hypothesis is true.

5.4.2   Some statistical bias can be corrected

Perhaps the most commonly encountered statistical bias arises when estimating the variance of a random variable. Suppose s^2 is the estimate of a true population variance, σ^2, in which the sum of squared deviations (SSD) is customarily divided by $n - 1$:

$$s^2 = \frac{\sum_{i=1}^{n}(x_i - \overline{x})^2}{n - 1}.$$

Students often ask intuitively why the SSD is not divided by n, and are told that $n - 1$ is the "degrees of freedom". In fact,

$$v^2 = \frac{\sum_{i=1}^{n}(x_i - \overline{x})^2}{n}$$

is the maximum likelihood estimate (MLE) of σ^2, but is biased by the factor $(n - 1)/n$. Specifically, the expected value of v^2 is $\sigma^2(n - 1)/n$. Thus, it is not very biased, except in small samples. This bias can be corrected by multiplying v^2 by the factor $n/(n - 1)$, which yields s^2. It is a common feature of maximum likelihood estimates that they are biased in small samples. Their widespread use is a consequence of the fact that they are usually unbiased in large samples (e.g., consider the case just sketched), are efficient, and have asymptotic normal distributions.

Furthermore, when the sample comes from a normal distribution, the square root of the unbiased estimate of the variance is *not* an unbiased estimate of the standard deviation, i.e., s is not unbiased for the standard deviation, σ [Holtzman, 1950; Cureton, 1968]. This fact is often ignored. An unbiased estimator for σ is

$$\widehat{\sigma} = \sqrt{\frac{\sum_{i=1}^{n}(x_i - \overline{x})^2}{k}},$$

where

$$k = 2\left(\frac{\Gamma(\frac{n}{2})}{\Gamma(\frac{n-1}{2})}\right)^2.$$

5.4.3   Unbiasedness is not the only desirable attribute of an estimator

Although unbiasedness is a desirable characteristic of statistical estimators, there are other important and useful attributes, such as a small average overall error or mean squared error (MSE). (Consider the previous discussion regarding Figure 5.1.) Suppose η is an estimator of a parameter. The MSE is defined as

$$MSE = \int_{-\infty}^{\infty} (\eta - \theta)^2 f(\eta) \, d\eta \,, \tag{5.1}$$

where θ is the true value of the parameter and $f(\eta)$ is the probability density distribution of η. Because the MSE measures the average error, it could be smaller for a biased estimator compared with an unbiased one (Figure 5.5). Suppose $\overline{\eta}$ is the average or expected value of η. Equation 5.1 yields

$$MSE = \int_{-\infty}^{\infty} (\eta - \overline{\eta} + \overline{\eta} - \theta)^2 f(\eta) \, d\eta$$

$$= \int_{-\infty}^{\infty} \left((\eta - \overline{\eta})^2 + (\overline{\eta} - \theta)^2 + 2(\eta - \overline{\eta})(\overline{\eta} - \theta) \right) f(\eta) \, d\eta$$

$$= \int_{-\infty}^{\infty} (\eta - \overline{\eta})^2 f(\eta) \, d\eta + (\overline{\eta} - \theta)^2 + 0 \,.$$

The first term is the variance of η, the second term is b^2, the square of the bias of η for θ, and the third term is zero. Thus,

$$MSE = Var(\eta) + b^2.$$

This demonstrates that the relative sizes of bias and variance are important in determining the overall error, at least in a statistical sense. Unfortunately, these quantitative statistical relationships have no direct analogues in the domain of clinical bias where the magnitudes of possible systematic errors are usually unknown.

To follow the example in the previous section regarding the unbiased estimates of σ^2 and σ from the normal distribution, a minimum MSE estimate of the variance of a normal distribution [Stuart and Ord, 1987] is

$$\tilde{\sigma}^2 = \frac{\sum_{i=1}^{n}(x_i - \overline{x})^2}{n+1} \,.$$

Similarly, a minimum MSE estimate of σ is

$$\tilde{\sigma} = \sqrt{\frac{\sum_{i=1}^{n}(x_i - \overline{x})^2}{k}} \,,$$

where

$$k = 2 \left(\frac{\Gamma(\frac{n+1}{2})}{\Gamma(\frac{n}{2})} \right)^2 .$$

An example of where it is useful to consider (and minimize) MSE instead of bias arises in problems commonly encountered when estimating parameters in regression models with highly correlated predictor variables. In this circumstance, the ordinary maximum likelihood estimates are unstable and can yield values that have the wrong algebraic sign or incorrect significance levels. The problem can be corrected by using "ridge regression", in which a small amount of bias is permitted in the estimates, because it greatly reduces the total variability. Although the procedure has drawbacks, there are circumstances in which it is appropriate. See Draper and Smith [1981] for a discussion of this topic in the setting of linear models and Liu and Piantadosi [1997] for a discussion of ridge regression in some nonlinear models useful in clinical trial and prognostic factor analyses.

5.5   Summary

Random error and bias are qualitatively different types of errors that can affect inferences. Random error is a consequence only of chance and is most relevant to clinical trials in a statistical context. Bias is systematic error and is relevant primarily in a clinical context, although it can also arise in statistical estimation. A good experimental design will control both types of error.

When making inferences from hypothesis tests, there are two random errors possible. If the null hypothesis is true but the test rejects, this is a type I error. P-values quantify the type I error. If the alternative hypothesis is true (null hypothesis false) but the test fails to reject, this is a type II error. The power of a trial for a specific alternative is 1 minus the probability of a type II error.

Type I errors are relatively easy to control because they depend on the critical value chosen to reject the null hypothesis. The data analyst can choose this critical value. Type II errors are more difficult to control because they depend on the precision of the estimate or the sample size of the experiment. Therefore, the type II error can only be controlled by the design of the study rather than the analysis.

Like type II errors, bias can best be controlled by design methods rather than analyses. There are many sources of potential bias in clinical trials including patient selection, post-entry exclusion of subjects for reasons related to prognosis, selective loss of data, assessment bias, and improperly defined eligibility, response, or evaluability. Relatively simple methods can reduce or eliminate these and other biases. Bias reducing methods include randomization, treatment masking, objectively defined endpoints, active rather than passive ascertainment of outcomes, and not permitting *post hoc* exclusions.

Statistical biases, especially in estimation, occur frequently. They can usually be corrected mathematically or are of small magnitude, compared with errors in design and conduct of trials. In a few circumstances, biased estimation methods are deliberately utilized in an attempt to reduce the total (mean squared) error.

5.6   Questions for Discussion

1. Which provides stronger evidence against the null hypothesis: a small experiment with $p = 0.05$ or a large experiment with $p = 0.01$?

2. Discuss the difference between what is unknown and what is random in a statistical analysis. Are they the same? Are they modeled in the same way?

3. Type I and II error rates are often chosen entirely by convention. Discuss the most appropriate ways you can think of for setting the probabilities of type I and II error rates. Apply your reasoning to trials studying disease prevention compared with disease treatment.

4. When testing the equivalence of two treatments, what is the null hypothesis? In these so-called "equivalence trials", what happens to the type I and II errors? Should the test be one- or two-sided?

5. One can reconstruct a hypothesis test from confidence intervals. Do confidence intervals suffer from the same strengths and weaknesses as hypothesis tests? Discuss why or why not.

6. Suppose that the treatment difference estimated in a particular randomized trial is exactly equal to the true treatment difference, and that the p-value which results is $p = 0.025$. If the trial is repeated in the same way, what is the chance that the p-value from the new study will be less than 0.025?

7. SE trials frequently show promise of treatment benefit, even when informally compared with standard therapy. However, when the promising new treatments are studied in CTE trials, they often fail to show improvement over conventional therapy. Discuss reasons why this might happen.

Chapter References

Byar, D.P. (1980). Why data bases should not replace randomized clinical trials. Biometrics 36: 337-342.

Byar, D.P. (1991). Problems with using observational databases to compare treatments. Statistics in Med. 10: 663-666.

Chastang, C., Byar, D.P., and Piantadosi, S. (1988). A quantitative study of the bias in estimating the treatment effect caused by omitting a balanced covariate in survival models. Statistics in Med. 7(12): 1243-1255.

Cox, D.R. and Hinkley, D.V. (1974). Theoretical Statistics. London: Chapman and Hall.

Cureton, E.E. (1968). Unbiased estimation of the standard deviation. Am. Statistician. 22: 22.

Draper, N.R. and Smith, H. (1981). Applied Regression Analysis, Second Edition. New York: John Wiley & Sons.

Gail, M.H., Wieand, H.S., and Piantadosi, S. (1984). Biased estimates of treatment effect in randomized experiments with non-linear regressions and omitted covariates. Biometrika 71(3): 431-444.

Gail, M.H., Tan, W.-Y., and Piantadosi, S. (1988). Tests for no treatment effect in randomized clinical trials when needed covariates are omitted. Biometrika 75(1): 57-64.

Grossman, S.A., Sheidler, V.A., Swedeen, K., Mucenski, J., and Piantadosi, S. (1991). Correlation of patient and caregiver ratings of cancer pain. J. Pain Symptom Manage. 6(2): 53-57.

Holtzman, W.H. (1950). The unbiased estimate of the population variance and standard deviation. Am. J. Psychology 63: 615-617.

Lehmann, E.L. (1989). Testing Statistical Hypotheses, Second Edition. New York: John Wiley & Sons.

Liu, G. and Piantadosi, S. (1997). Ridge estimation in generalized linear models and proportional hazards regressions. Statistics in Medicine, submitted

Neyman, J. and Pearson, E.S. (1933). On the problem of the most efficient tests of statistical hypotheses. Phil. Trans. Roy. Soc. A. 231: 289-337.

Sackett, D.L. (1979). Bias in analytic research. J. Chron. Dis. 32: 51-63.

Salsburg, D. (1990). Hypothesis versus significance testing for controlled clinical trials: A dialogue. Statistics in Med. 9: 201-211.

Schulz, K.F. (1995). Subverting randomization in controlled trials. JAMA 274: 1456-1458.

Stuart, A. and Ord, J.K. (1987). Kendall's Advanced Theory of Statistics, Volume 1: Distribution Theory. Fifth Edition. New York: Oxford University Press.

Silverman, W.A. (1985). Human Experimentation. Oxford: Oxford University Press.

Strauss, M.B. (1968). Familiar Medical Quotations. Boston: Little, Brown.

CHAPTER 6

Objectives and Endpoints

6.1   Introduction

Clinical trials have both non-quantifiable purposes and quantitative objectives. The purpose of a trial might be to improve the treatment of a disease or condition. Successfully achieving this goal may depend on the qualitative outcome of the trial. For example, the management of a disease may not improve unless the new therapy under investigation is superior to conventional treatment. The objectives of a trial are the research questions phrased in concise quantitative terms. An example is to determine which therapy being investigated has superior efficacy or fewer side effects. Achieving objectives does not depend on the outcome of the trial, only on obtaining a valid result. Other examples of objectives include evaluating safety, pharmacology, or establishing equivalence.

Endpoints are the quantitative measurements implied or required by the objectives. An *endpoint* is determined in each study subject, whereas the *objectives* are met by the aggregate of endpoints. The best endpoints to use depend on specific clinical objectives stated in quantitative terms. For example, a clinical objective is to determine if a new surgical procedure "reduces peri-operative morbidity" compared with some standard method. However, the measurement of operative morbidity can be partly subjective, which may be an issue if more than one surgeon participates in the study. At least three aspects of morbidity might need to be defined. The first is a window of time, during which adverse events could be attributed plausibly to the operative procedure. The second is a list of diagnoses or complications to be included. The third is specification of procedures or tests required to establish each diagnosis definitively. Using these three criteria, a "morbid event" can be defined without much subjective interpretation and each patient can be classified as having or not having the endpoint.

A clinical objective may have more than one way of being quantified or may be described by more than one endpoint. For example, "improved survival" might mean prolonged median survival, higher five-year survival, or a lower death rate in the first year. These three definitions may require different methods of assessment and need not yield the same sample size or analysis plan. In the example above, peri-operative morbidity could be defined by any of several events or a composite. Knowing which endpoint and method of quantification to use in particular clinical circumstances is an essential task for the statistician.

Trials typically have a single primary objective or endpoint with additional secondary ones. It may not be feasible, or there may not be sufficient resources, to answer more than one primary question reliably. For example, we can only actively design control over the type II error for one objective. Secondary objectives have a statistical power that is determined passively by the sample size for the primary objective. Trials with many objectives require a multiplicity of statistical analyses, some of which may be based on subsets of the study cohort. This increases the possibility of error.

Each trial setting may be unique with respect to the efficiency and practicality of various endpoints. Investigators may also need to consider the cost-efficiency of various endpoints and choose a feasible one or allocate resources appropriately. A discussion from this perspective is given by Terrin [1990].

6.1.1   Prefer "hard" endpoints

"Hard" endpoints are clinical landmarks that are well defined in the study protocol, definitive with respect to the disease process, and require no subjectivity. Examples include death, disease relapse or progression, and many laboratory measurements. "Soft" endpoints are those that do not relate strongly to the disease process or require subjective assessments by the investigator or patient. Trying not to abuse terminology, we might say that hard endpoints are objectively measured, whereas soft endpoints are subjective. This distinction is not the same as that between definitive and "surrogate" endpoints, discussed below.

An example of why subjectivity is undesirable in clinical trial endpoints is the so-called *Hawthorne effect*, named after experiments at the Hawthorne Plant of the General Electric Company in the 1920s and 1930s [Homans, 1965]. These studies tested the effects of working conditions on productivity and demonstrated that even adverse changes could improve productivity. The research subjects were affected by the knowledge that they were being tested, illustrating that study participants can respond in unexpected ways to support the research hypothesis if they are aware of it. While such effects may be more likely when subjective endpoints are used, they can also influence hard outcomes that depend on changes in behavior.

Some useful and reliable endpoints fall between the extremes of "hard" and "soft". An example is pathologic classification, which is usually based on expert, experienced, and objective, judgment. Such endpoints are likely to be useful in clinical trials and prognostic factor studies, because they are valid and reliable. The underlying issue with endpoints is not their degree of hardness or subjectivity, but rather how error prone they are. The best endpoints are not prone to error and are repeatable. Even so, a good endpoint, such as vital status, can be made unreliable if investigators use poor methods of ascertainment.

In this chapter, I assume that a clinical trial is designed with quantitative objectives and that the endpoints are reliable. There may be perfectly valid designs that employ subjective or less reliable endpoints. Many such studies ask important clinical questions. An understanding of quantitative endpoints and measurements will carry over to more subjective ones.

6.2 Objectives

6.2.1 Estimation is the most common objective

Most clinical objectives translate into a need to *estimate* an important quantity. For example, the objective of the surgery study mentioned above might be to estimate the rate (risk or probability) of peri-operative morbidity. In oncology dose-finding (phase I) trials, the primary purpose is usually to estimate the maximum tolerated dose (MTD), defined as the dose associated with a specific probability of toxicity. More generally, one might view these trials as estimating the dose-toxicity function in a clinically relevant region (although conventional phase I designs are not very good at this). The objective of SE studies is usually to estimate response and toxicity probabilities using a fixed dose of drug or a specific treatment. CTE (or phase III) trials typically estimate treatment differences and ES (or phase IV) trials estimate rates of complications or side effects.

6.2.2 Selection can also be an objective

In some circumstances, trials are intended primarily to *select* a treatment that satisfies a set of important criteria, as opposed to simply estimating the magnitude of an effect. For example, the treatment with the highest response rate could be selected from among several alternatives in a multi-armed randomized SE trial. The size of such a study might not be sufficient to permit pairwise comparisons between the treatment groups with high power. In this situation, testing hypotheses about pairwise differences in the treatment effects may not be as important as simply ranking the estimated response rates.

Frequentist sequential trial designs (see Chapter 10) use significance tests to select the treatment that yields the most favorable outcome. When trials with these designs terminate early, the overall type I error is controlled, but the treatment effect or difference may be overestimated. These designs select the best treatment without providing an unbiased estimate of the difference. However, there are many situations where these designs are useful. For example, when choosing from among several developing treatments, it may be important to know which one is superior without being sure of the magnitude of difference.

6.2.3   Objectives require various scales of measurement

Clinical trial objectives require measurements that fall into one of four numeric categories. The first is *classification,* or determining into which of several categories an outcome fits. In these cases, the numerical character of the endpoint is nominal, i.e., it is used for convenience only. There is no meaning ascribed to differences or other mathematical operations between the numbers that describe outcomes. In fact, the outcomes need not be described numerically. An example of such a measurement is classifying a test result as normal, abnormal, or indeterminate. The results could be labeled 1, 2, or 3, but the numbers carry no intrinsic meaning.

A second type of objective requires *ordering* of outcomes that are measured on a degree, severity, or ordinal scale. An example of an ordinal measurement is severity of side effects or toxicity. In this case, we know that category 2 is worse (or better) than category 1, but not how much worse (or better) it is. Similarly, category 3 is more extreme, but the difference between 3 and 2 is not necessarily the same as the difference between 2 and 1. Thus, the rankings are important but the differences between values on the ordinal scale has no meaning.

Still other objectives are to *estimate differences* and lead to interval scales of measurement. On interval scales, ordering and differences between values is meaningful. However, there is an arbitrary zero point so that ratios or products of measures have no meaning. An example of an interval scale is temperature, which can be measured with an arbitrary zero point. A difference in temperature on a particular scale is meaningful, but the ratio of two temperatures is not.

Finally, the objectives of some studies are to *estimate ratios*. These lead to ratio scales on which sums, differences, ratios, and products are meaningful. Time from a clinical landmark such as diagnosis is an example of a ratio scale. Differences and ratios of time from diagnosis are meaningful. Examples of various scales of measurements for hypothetical data concerning age, sex, and treatment toxicity are shown in Table 6.1. Toxicity grade is an ordinal scale, age rank is an interval scale, age is a ratio scale, and sex code is nominal. The endpoints that are appropriate for each type of objective are discussed in the next section.

6.3   Endpoints

6.3.1   Endpoints can be quantitative or qualitative

Rigorously defined endpoints and prospective methods of assessing outcomes are among the characteristics that distinguish true experimental designs from other types of studies. Thus, the strength of evidence from a trial depends greatly on these aspects of design. The most important beneficial characteristics of the endpoint used in a study are: it must correspond to the scientific objective of the trial; and the method of endpoint assessment must be accurate and free of bias. These are important, not only for subjective endpoints like functional status or symptom severity, but also for more objective measures such as survival and recurrence times. These outcomes

Table 6.1 Examples of Different Data Types Frequently Used in Clinical Trials

ID Number	Age	Sex	Toxicity Grade	Age Rank	Sex Code
1	41	M	3	1	0
2	53	F	2	5	1
3	47	F	4	2	1
4	51	M	1	4	0
5	60	F	1	9	1
6	49	M	2	3	0
7	57	M	1	7	0
8	55	M	3	6	0
9	59	F	1	8	1
⋮	⋮	⋮	⋮	⋮	⋮
Scale:	ratio	category	ordinal	interval	nominal

usually become evident long after the treatment is begun, providing a chance that incomplete follow-up can affect the results.

There are several types of endpoints that are likely to be used in many types of trials. These include continuously varying measurements, dichotomous endpoints, event times, counts, ordered categories, unordered categories, and repeated measures. Measurements with established reliability and validity might be called *measures*. In the next section, each of these will be described with specific examples.

6.3.2 Measures are useful and efficient endpoints

Measurements that can theoretically vary continuously over some range are common and useful types of assessments in clinical trials. Examples include many laboratory values, blood or tissue levels, functional disability scores, or physical dimensions. In a study population, these measurements have a distribution, often characterized by a mean or other location parameter, and variance or other dispersion parameter. Consequently, these outcomes will be most useful when the primary effect of a treatment is to raise or lower the average measure in a population. Typical statistical tests that can detect differences such as these include the t-test or a non-parametric analog and analyses of variance (for more than two groups). To control the effect of confounders or prognostic factors on these outcomes, linear regression models might be used, as is often done in analyses of (co-)variance.

6.3.3 Some outcomes are summarized as counts

Count data also arise frequently in clinical trials. Count data are most common when the unit of observation is a geographic area or an interval of time. Geographic area is only infrequently a source of data in treatment trials, although we might encounter it in disease prevention studies. Counting events during time intervals is quite common in trials in chronic diseases, but the outcomes counted (e.g., survival) usually number 0 or 1. These special types of counts are discussed below.

Some assessments naturally yield data in the form of counts that can take on values higher than 0 or 1. For example, we might be interested in the cancer prevention effects of a non-steroidal anti-inflammatory agent on the production of colonic polyps. Between each of several examination periods, investigators might count the number of polyps seen during an endoscopic exam of the colon, and then remove them. During the study period, each patient would yield several correlated counts. In the study population, counts might be summarized as averages, or as an average intensity (or density) per unit of observation time.

6.3.4 Ordered categories are commonly used for severity or toxicity

Assessments of disease severity or the toxicity of treatments are most naturally summarized as ordered categories. For example, the functional severity of illness might be described as mild, moderate, or severe. The severity of a disease can sometimes be described as an anatomic extent, as in staging systems used widely in cancer. In the case of toxicities from cytotoxic anti-cancer drugs, five grades are generally acknowledged. Classifying individuals into a specific grade, however, depends upon the organ system affected. Cardiac toxicity, for example, ranges from normal rate and rhythm to atrial arrhythmias to ventricular tachycardia. Neurologic toxicity ranges from normal function, to somnolence, to coma. There is no overall scale of toxicity independent of organ system.

When used as a primary outcome or effect of treatment, ordered categories can capture much of the information in, but may be easier and more convenient to apply, than quantitative scores. For example, ordered categories might be useful in assessing outcomes for degree of impairment due to chronic arthritis, functional ability and muscular strength in multiple sclerosis, or functional ability in chronic heart disease. When measures are categorized for simplicity or convenience, investigators should retain the continuous measurements, whenever possible, to facilitate different analyses or definitions in the future.

Summarizing outcomes from ordered categories requires some special methods of analysis. One would not automatically look for linear trends across the categories, because the ordering itself may not be linear. For example, the difference between a Grade IV and Grade V side effect may not imply the same relative change as between Grade I and Grade II. Consequently, care must be exercised in the choice of analytic methods.

6.3.5 Unordered categories are sometimes used

Outcomes described as unordered categories are uncommon in clinical trials but are occasionally necessary. For example, following bone marrow transplantation for acute leukemia, some patients might develop acute graft versus host disease, others might develop chronic graft versus host disease, and others might remain free of either outcome. These outcomes are not graded versions of one another. In most circumstances unordered categorical outcomes can be reclassified into a series of dichotomies to simplify analyses.

6.3.6 Dichotomies are simple summaries

Some assessments have only two possible values, for example, present or absent. Examples include some imprecise measurements such as shrinkage of a tumor, which might be described as responding or not, and outcomes like infection which is either present or not. Inaccuracy or difficulty in accurate grading can make a measured value or ordinal assessment into a dichotomous one. In the study population, these outcomes can often be summarized as a proportion of "successes" or "failures". Comparing proportions leads to tests such as the chi-square or exact conditional tests. Another useful population summary for proportions is the odds, log-odds, or odds ratio for the outcome. The effect of one or more prognostic factors (or confounders) on this outcome can be modeled using logistic regression.

When summarizing proportions, one should be certain of the correct denominator to use. Problems can arise in two areas. First, there is a tendency to exclude patients from the denominator for clinical reasons, such as failure to complete an assigned course of treatment. The dangers of this are discussed in Chapter 11.

Second, the units of measurement of the denominator must be appropriate. For a proportion, the units of the denominator must be persons, as compared with person-years for a hazard. For example, if we compare the proportions of subjects with myocardial infarction in two cohorts, we might calculate r_1/n_1 and r_2/n_2, where r_1 and r_2 are the number of patients with the event. However, if the follow-up time in the two cohorts is very different, this summary could be misleading. It might be better to use the total follow-up time in each cohort as the denominator. This treats the outcome as a risk rate rather than a proportion.

6.3.7 Event times may be censored

Measurements of the time interval from treatment, diagnosis, or other baseline landmarks to important clinical events such as death (event times) are common and useful outcomes in chronic disease clinical trials. Survival time and time to disease progression are well-known examples of "definitive" event times, because the outcome is usually determined with minimal error. Many other intervals might be of clinical importance, such as time to hospital discharge or time spent on a ventilator. The distinguishing complication of event time measurements, like many longitudinal assessments, is the possibility of censoring. This means that some subjects being followed on the trial may not experience the event of interest by the end of the observation period.

The nature of patient accruals and event times in a clinical trial with staggered patient entry is shown in Figure 6.1. In this hypothetical study, patients are accrued until calendar time T. After T, there is a period of additional follow-up lasting to $T + \tau$. Some patients are observed to have events (denoted by x's) during the study period (e.g., #3 − #6). Others are lost to follow-up during the study, as denoted by the circles (e.g., #1), but may or may not have events after the study period. Still others

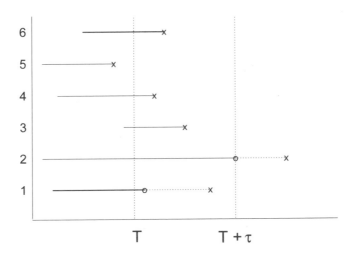

Figure 6.1 Accrual, follow-up, and censoring on an event time study.

remain event free at the end of the study, also denoted by circles (e.g., #2). Thus, subjects #1 and #2 are censored.

Censoring of event times most often occurs when an individual is followed for a period of time, but is not observed to have the event of interest. Thus, we know only that the event time was greater than some amount, but do not know its exact value. This is often called *right censoring*. Censoring can also occur if we observe the presence of a state or condition but do not know when it began. For example, suppose we are estimating the distribution of times from sero-positivity to clinical AIDS in patients at high risk of HIV. Some members of the cohort will already be sero-positive at the start of the observation period. The time to AIDS is censored for these observations, because we do not know the precise point of sero-conversion. This is often called *left censoring*. Event time data can also be *interval censored*, meaning that individuals can come in and out of observation. Most event time data are right censored only so that the term "censoring" most commonly means "right censoring".

The usual type of censoring in clinical trials is random (or type III) because the staggered entry and losses to follow-up produce unequal censoring times. Some laboratory experiments begin with all animals going on study at the same time and end after a fixed observation period. This produces type I censoring where all censored times are the same. Alternatively, if the investigator waits until a fixed proportion of the animals have had events, type II censoring is produced. Type I and II censoring are usually not seen in clinical trials.

Table 6.2 Example of Censored Event Time Data

ID Number	Exposure Time	Censoring Indicator
1	141	0
2	153	1
3	124	0
4	251	0
5	160	1
6	419	0
7	257	1
8	355	0
⋮	⋮	⋮

One does not discard censored or incomplete observations, but employs statistical methods to use the information about failure rates contained in the follow-up time. For example, if we followed a cohort of patients for 50 person-years of time, and observed no deaths, the event count would be zero, but we have learned something useful about the death *rate*. Using the information in censored observation times requires some special statistical procedures. Event time or "survival" distributions (e.g., life tables) might be used to summarize the data. Clinicians often use medians or proportions at a fixed time to summarize these outcomes. One of the most useful summaries is the hazard rate, which can be thought of as a proportion adjusted for follow-up time. The effect of prognostic factors or confounders on hazard rates can often be modeled using survival regression models.

Right censoring can occur administratively, as when the study observation period ends. However, it can also occur throughout a trial if study participants are lost to follow-up. The statistical methods for dealing with both of these situations are the same. All of the routine methods that account for right censoring assume that the censoring mechanism is independent of the outcome. This means that there is no information about the outcome in the fact that the event time is censored. If this is not true, a situation called *informative* censoring, then the usual methods of summarizing the data are likely to produce biased estimates. For example, suppose individuals are more likely to be censored just before they experience an event. Treating the censored observations as though they are independent of the event will cause one to under-estimate the event rate.

6.3.8   Event time data require two numerical values

To capture the information in event times, whether censored or not, it is necessary to record two data items for each individual. The first is the follow-up or exposure time. It is a measure such as number of days, weeks, months, or years of time. The second item needed is an indicator variable, which designates whether the event time records the interval to an event or to a censored point. Most often, the censoring indicator is given the value 1 for an event and 0 if the observation is censored. An example is shown in Table 6.2. If both left and right censoring are present, two indicator variables will be required.

The distribution of event times can be described in several ways. Often, it is summarized as the cumulative probability of remaining event-free over time. Because this method is used so commonly in survival applications, the resulting curves are often called "survival curves" even when the outcome is not death. The most commonly employed method for estimating survival curves is the product-limit method [Kaplan and Meier, 1958]. In many other situations, a more natural descriptive summary of the data is the overall hazard or event rate. Methods for describing such data are discussed in more detail in Chapter 12.

6.3.9   Composite outcomes instead of censoring

When studying treatments for a particular disease, investigators would prefer for the trial to count only events that relate specifically to that condition. There is often a clinical rationale for counting events unrelated to the target disease as censored observations. For example, in a large trial with a new treatment trying to prolong survival after cancer diagnosis, some patients will invariably die of non-cancer causes such as cardiovascular disease. It seems justified to censor these non-cancer events rather than count them as deaths. Unfortunately it is not.

When two or more failure processes affect a population (competing risks), investigators cannot expect to obtain unbiased estimates of risk for one cause by censoring all other events. If the failure processes are not independent of one another, as is usually the case, events attributable to one cause contain some information about events of other types. Not only is this true on a biological basis, but the reporting mechanisms may obscure connections. For example, a myocardial infarction listed as the primary cause of death may be secondary to an advanced state of the underlying disease. Therefore, the censored cardiovascular events are not independent of the cancer events, creating the potential for bias. Death due to accident may be partly a consequence of the patient's psychological state as a consequence of the underlying disease. Rather than making a doubtful assumption of independence, the study could be designed to count deaths from any cause as a composite outcome. This all-cause mortality is not subject to many biases and has a straightforward interpretation. Consequently, it is the preferred mortality endpoint for clinical trials.

6.3.10   Waiting for good events complicates censoring

In most event time studies, the interval of interest is measured from a hopeful clinical landmark, such as treatment, to a bad event, such as disease progression or death. Our perspective on censoring is that events such as disease progression or death could be seen with additional follow-up. In a few studies, however, investigators measure the waiting time to a good event. Short event times are better than long ones and censoring could be a more difficult problem than it is in survival studies.

For example, suppose patients undergoing bone marrow transplantation for hematologic malignancies are observed to see how long it takes the new bone marrow to "recover" or become functional. The restoration of bone marrow function is a good outcome but some patients may never recover fully or may die. Death from complications of not having a functioning bone marrow is more likely early rather than late in follow-up. In this circumstance, death censors time to recovery but the censoring paradigm is different than that discussed above. A short event time is good if it terminates with recovery but bad if it terminates with death (censoring). Long event times are not good but may be unlikely to end in death (censoring). This example illustrates the importance of understanding the relationship between the censoring process and the event process.

6.4   Surrogate Endpoints

A surrogate endpoint is one that is measured in place of the biologically definitive or clinically most meaningful endpoint. Typically, a definitive endpoint measures clinical benefit, whereas a surrogate endpoint is one that tracks the progress or extent of the disease. A good surrogate endpoint needs to be convincingly associated with a definitive clinical outcome so that it can be used as a reliable replacement. Investigators choose a surrogate when the definitive endpoint is inaccessible due to cost, time, or difficulty of measurement [Herson, 1989]. The difficulty in employing surrogate endpoints is more a question of their validity or strength of association with definitive outcomes than trouble designing, executing, or analyzing trials that use them.

Prentice [1994] offered a rigorous definition of a surrogate endpoint as

> a response variable for which a test of the null hypothesis of no relationship to the treatment groups under comparison is also a valid test of the corresponding null hypothesis based on the true endpoint.

An endpoint meeting this definition will be a good surrogate for the definitive outcome. A measurement that is merely correlated with outcome will not be a useful surrogate, unless it also reflects the effects of treatment on the definitive outcome. Surrogates may exist for efficacy, but there can be no convincing surrogates for safety.

Surrogate endpoints are sometimes called surrogate markers, intermediate, or replacement endpoints. The term "surrogate" may be the best overall descriptor and I will use it here. Some authors have distinguished auxiliary from surrogate endpoints [Fleming et al., 1994]. Auxiliary endpoints are those used to strengthen the analysis of a definitive endpoint data when the latter are weak because of a lack of events. Such endpoints can be used statistically to recover some of the information that is missing because of unobserved events. Auxiliary endpoints may be measurements such as biomarkers or other manifestations of the disease process. Also, intermediate endpoints can be distinguished from surrogate endpoints, particularly in the context of cancer prevention [Freedman and Schatzkin, 1992].

Table 6.3 Examples of Surrogate Endpoints Frequently Used in Clinical Trials

Disease	Definitive Endpoint	Surrogate Endpoint
HIV Infection	AIDS (or death)	CD4+ count
Cancer	mortality	tumor size reduction
Colon Cancer	disease progression	CEA level
Prostate Cancer	disease progression	PSA level
Cardiovascular Disease	hemorrhagic stroke	blood pressure
	myocardial infarction	cholesterol level
Glaucoma	vision loss	intraocular pressure

6.4.1 Surrogate endpoints are disease-specific

Surrogate endpoints are disease-specific because they depend on the mechanism of the condition under investigation. A universally valid surrogate probably cannot be found. Some examples of surrogate-definitive endpoint pairs are listed in Table 6.3. Trialists are interested in surrogate endpoints like these, because of their potential to shorten, simplify, and economize clinical studies. The potential gain is greatest in chronic diseases, where both the opportunity to observe surrogates and the benefit of doing so are high. However, surrogate endpoints are nearly always accompanied by questions about their validity. Trials with surrogate endpoints often require verification.

Some important characteristics of surrogate endpoints can be inferred from Table 6.3. First, a good surrogate can be measured relatively simply and without invasive procedures. Second, a surrogate that is strongly associated with a definitive outcome will likely be part of, or close to, the causal pathway for the true endpoint. In other words, the surrogate should be justified on biologically mechanistic grounds. Cholesterol level is an example of this, because it fits into the model of disease progression: high cholesterol $\Rightarrow$ atherosclerosis $\Rightarrow$ myocardial infarction $\Rightarrow$ death. This is in contrast to a surrogate like prostatic specific antigen (PSA), which is a reliable marker of tumor burden but is not in the chain of causation. We might say that cholesterol is a direct, and PSA is an indirect, surrogate. However, because of temporal effects, PSA rather than cholesterol may be more strongly associated with a definitive disease state.

Third, we would expect a good surrogate endpoint to yield the same inference as the definitive endpoint. This implies a strong statistical association, even though the definitive outcome may occur less frequently than the surrogate. Several authors have pointed out that this statistical association is not a sufficient criterion for a surrogate to be useful [e.g., Boissel et al., 1992]. Fourth, we would like the surrogate to have a short latency with respect to the natural history of the disease. Finally, a good surrogate should be responsive to the effects of treatment.

Cancer

In testing treatments for cancer prevention, surrogate endpoints are frequently proposed because of the long latency period for the disease. Also, we are most interested in applying preventive agents or measures to a population of patients without disease. Even populations at high risk may have only a small fraction of people developing cancer each year. These factors inhibit our ability to observe definitive events such as new cases of cancer or deaths attributed to cancer. This situation provides strong motivation for using surrogate endpoints like biomarkers, provided they are valid [Bogoch and Bogoch, 1994; Kelloff et al., 1994].

In studies of cancer therapy, investigators also find many reasons to be interested in surrogate endpoints [Ellenberg and Hamilton, 1989]. When the interval between treatment and a definitive endpoint is long, there is an opportunity for intercurrent events to confuse our assessment of the outcomes. Examples of these types of events are when the patient receives additional active treatments and deaths due to causes other than the disease under investigation.

Tumor size reduction (tumor response) is used as definitive endpoint and proposed as a surrogate endpoint in cancer clinical trials. In many SE trials, measurable tumor response is taken as evidence that the therapy is active against the disease. The degree of such activity often determines whether or not the treatment is recommended for continued testing in comparative trials. In CTE trials, tumor response is sometimes proposed as a surrogate for improved survival or longer disease free survival. However, the association between response and definitive event times is weak for most cancers. Consequently, tumor shrinkage (response) should not generally be used as the primary outcome variable in CTE trials. The rare exception might be for conditions in which reduction in tumor size provides a clinically important improvement in quality of life or reduced risk of complications.

"Cure" or "remission" are stronger types of tumor response that have been used as surrogate endpoints in some cancer trials. For example, permanent or long-term tumor shrinkage below the level of clinical detectability might be labeled a remission or cure as is commonly the case in studies of childhood hematologic malignancies. There are ample data to support the strong association between this type of endpoint and survival in these diseases. The connection is supported further by evidence that the failure rate diminishes to near zero or that the survival curve has a plateau in patients achieving remission, providing long-term survival for them. In other cancers, a disease free interval of, say, five years after disease disappearance, is often labeled as a "cure", but the failure (recurrence) rate may not be near zero. Thus, tumor response is not a uniformly good surrogate endpoint for all types of cancer.

Some cancer biomarkers have been considered reliable enough to serve as surrogate endpoints. Two well-known ones are prostatic specific antigen (PSA) and carcinoembryonic antigen (CEA), produced by some gastrointestinal malignancies. These markers are particularly useful for following disease status after treatment, when an elevation is strongly associated with recurrence. The usefulness of these and other biomarkers as surrogate endpoints remains to be established.

Cardiovascular diseases

Studies of cardiovascular diseases present opportunities to use potentially valid surrogate endpoints for definitive outcomes like mortality [Wittes, Lakatos, and Probstfield, 1989]. This is possible because we understand the mechanisms leading to many cardiovascular events fairly well and can measure entities in the causal path. For example, elevated blood pressure, serum cholesterol, left ventricular ejection fraction, and coronary artery patency are in the chain of events contributing to myocardial infarction and can be measured quantitatively. Sometimes these surrogates, or risk factors, are used as the primary endpoints in a trial, while in other cases they are secondary.

Because of the strong mechanistic connection between some cardiovascular surrogates and definitive outcomes, they may be used more effectively in trials in this setting than surrogates for cancer endpoints. However, interventions that modulate risk factors do not necessarily change definitive endpoints. If treatment modifies the risk factor through mechanisms unrelated to action on the definitive endpoint, we can be misled by a study using the factor as a surrogate endpoint.

HIV infection

In patients with HIV infection, CD4 positive lymphocyte count (CD4+) is a widely discussed candidate for a surrogate endpoint for clinical AIDS and death. Unfortunately, the available data suggest that CD4+ count is not reliable enough to serve as a valid surrogate endpoint. See Fleming [1994] for a review of this point. AIDS, by the Centers for Disease Control (CDC) clinical criteria, could be considered a surrogate for death because of the severely compromised immune system that it implies. Other clinically valid measures of immune function such as P-24 antigen levels and plasma HIV viral load have been suggested as possible surrogate endpoints but are unproven. Like SE cancer trials that use tumor response as an endpoint in spite of its poor utility as a definitive outcome, developmental trials in AIDS may be able to use measures of immune function to evaluate the potential benefit of new treatments.

Eye diseases

In trials studying diseases of the eye, Hillis and Seigel [1989] discuss some possible surrogate endpoints. On example is retinal vein occlusion, which can lead to loss of vision. Hypertensive vascular changes are a precursor to vein occlusion and can be observed non-invasively. However, in an eye affected by vein occlusion, the blood vessel changes may not be observable because of tissue damage. Observations in the opposite eye may be useful as a surrogate for the affected eye. Thus, the opposite eye is a surrogate for observing the state of the retinal vessels, which is a possible surrogate for vein occlusion. In this situation, the eye least affected by hypertensive vascular changes is likely to be used as a surrogate, leading to a biased underestimate of the relationship between the surrogate and the definitive endpoint.

A second example in eye diseases discussed by Hillis and Seigel [1989] is the use of intraocular pressure as a surrogate for long-term visual function in patients with glaucoma. The validity of this surrogate depends on certainty that the elevated pressure is a cause of optic nerve damage in glaucoma patients, that the pressure can be determined reliably with the type of measurements commonly used, and that lower intraocular pressure will result in better vision in the long term. Many recent trials of glaucoma therapy have followed this reasoning, correct or not, and used intraocular pressure as a surrogate endpoint.

6.4.2 Surrogate endpoints can make trials more efficient

Most clinical trials require an extended period of accrual and observation for each patient after treatment. This is especially true of comparative studies with event time as a primary outcome. Disease prevention studies, where event rates are low and event times are long because the study population is relatively healthy, are even more lengthy than most treatment trials. It can be impractical or very expensive to conduct studies that take such a long time to complete. Good surrogate endpoints can shorten such clinical trials, which explains why they are of particular interest in prevention trials. However, to be useful, a surrogate outcome needs to become manifest relatively early in the course of follow-up.

A simple example will illustrate the potential gain in efficiency using surrogate endpoints. Suppose we wish to test the benefit of a new anti-hypertensive agent against standard therapy in a randomized trial. Survival is a definitive endpoint and blood pressure is a surrogate. If it were practical and ethical to follow patients long enough to observe overall mortality, such a trial would need to be large. For example, using calculations discussed in detail in the next chapter, the difference between 95% and 90% overall mortality at five years requires 1162 subjects to detect as statistically significant with 90% power and a two-sided 0.05 α-level test. In contrast, if we use diastolic blood pressure as the endpoint, we could detect a reduction of as little as $1/2$ of a standard deviation using 170 patients with a trial duration of a few weeks or months. Larger reductions in blood pressure could be detected reliably using fewer patients. This hypothetical example is not meant to equate this benefit in mortality with this degree of blood pressure reduction. The benefit from such a small reduction is probably smaller. It does illustrate the potential difference in the scope of trials using surrogate endpoints.

In some instances, trials using surrogate outcomes may provide a clearer picture of the effects of treatment than those employing the "definitive" outcome. For example, suppose we are studying the effects of a treatment on the prevention of coronary occlusion in patients with high risk for this event. Clinicians react to these significant and morbid events when they occur by attempting to restore blood flow to the heart muscle using drugs, surgery, or other interventions and often make modifications in other aspects of the patient's treatment. Thus, coronary occlusion is an important clinical milestone and could be used as a basis for establishing the efficacy of treatments. A trial that used a "definitive" endpoint such as death could present a somewhat confusing picture of treatment efficacy. Some patients will live a long time after the first coronary occlusion, allowing non-cardiac complications to intervene. Also, the patient may change life-style or therapy after a coronary occlusion and there may be co-morbidities that influence the course of treatment. It may be difficult to describe or account for the effects of these changes on the natural history of the disease.

In other cases, the ethical acceptability of a trial can be enhanced by using surrogate endpoints. For example, suppose the definitive endpoint becomes apparent only after a long period of follow-up. A rigorous trial design comparing two therapies would likely require control of ancillary treatments administered during the follow-up period. However, restrictions on such treatments may be ethically problematic. In contrast, a valid surrogate endpoint that can be measured early in the post-treatment period allows the comparison of interest to proceed and permits physicians to respond with fewer constraints to changes in the patients' clinical status.

6.4.3   Surrogate endpoints have significant limitations

Although surrogate endpoints are used frequently for developmental trials and are occasionally helpful for comparative studies, they often have serious limitations. Sources of difficulty include the validity of the surrogate, coping with missing data, having the eligibility criteria depend on the surrogate measurement, and the fact that trials using these endpoints may be too small to reliably inform us about uncommon but important events. Of these, the validity of the surrogate endpoint is of most concern. For a recent review of surrogate endpoints and their limitations in various diseases, see Fleming and DeMets [1996].

Many surrogates are proposed because they appear to represent the biological state of disease, and observational data suggest that they are convincingly associated with the definitive outcome. The problem with trials using surrogates is that treatment effects on the definitive endpoints may not be predicted accurately by treatment effects on the surrogate. This problem can occur for two reasons. First is the imperfect association between the surrogate and the true outcome, which may not reflect the effects of treatment. Second is the possibility that treatment affects the true outcome through a mechanism that does not involve the surrogate.

A problem in the development cancer treatments arises when trying to evaluate cytostatic (rather than cytotoxic) drugs. The traditional endpoint for SE trials is response, which although a surrogate for benefit, is objective and widely understood. Some investigators have proposed new "clinical benefit" response criteria that could be useful for cytostatic drugs [Rothberg, et al., 1996]. (See Verweij, 1996 and Gelber, 1996 for discussions.) However, new endpoints will require validation with respect to disease status, treatment effects, and existing endpoints before being used to evaluate, and possibly discard, new drugs.

In cardiovascular diseases, there are sobering accounts of the recent use of surrogate endpoints in clinical trials. One example is the Cardiac Arrythmia Suppression Trial (CAST), which was a randomized, placebo controlled, double masked treatment trial with three drug arms [Cardiac Arrythmia Suppression Trial Investigators, 1989]. The drugs employed, encainide and flecainide, appeared to reduce arrhythmias, and therefore were promising treatments for reducing sudden death and total mortality. After a planned interim analyses, CAST was stopped early in two arms, because of a convincing *increase* in sudden deaths on the treatments. Control of arrhythmia, although seemingly justified biologically, is not a valid surrogate endpoint for mortality.

A randomized placebo controlled trial of milrinone, a phosphodiesterase inhibitor used as a positive inotropic agent in chronic heart failure, in 1088 patients also showed benefit on surrogate endpoints (measures of hemodynamic action) with increased long-term morbidity and mortality [Packer et al., 1991]. A similar failure of surrogate endpoints was seen in a randomized trial of the vasodilator flosequinan, compared with captopril in 209 patients with moderate to severe chronic heart failure [Cowley et al., 1994]. Flosequinan had similar long-term efficacy and mortality compared with captopril, but a higher incidence of adverse events.

Another example that does not speak well for the use of surrogate endpoints is the randomized study of fluoride treatment on fractures in 202 women with osteoporosis [Riggs et al., 1990]. Although bone mass was increased with fluoride therapy, the number of non-vertebral fractures was higher. Measures such as bone mass and bone mineral density are not valid surrogates for the definitive clinical outcomes.

A surrogate outcome in a specific disease may be useful for some purposes but not others. For example, surrogate outcomes in drug development may be appropriate for verifying the action of a drug under new manufacturing procedures or for a new formulation of an existing drug. Their use for a new drug in the same class as an existing drug may be questionable and their use for testing a new class of drugs may be inappropriate. For illnesses in which patients have a short life expectancy (e.g., advanced cancer and AIDS), it may be worthwhile to use treatments that improve surrogate outcomes, at least until efficacy can be verified definitively in earlier stages of disease.

6.5   Some Special Endpoints

6.5.1   Repeated measurements are not common in clinical trials

It is occasionally necessary in clinical trials to summarize endpoints repeatedly over some interval of time. An example is when comparing control of blood pressure on two or more experimental anti-hypertensive therapies. A trial could be designed using measurements before and after treatment to assess treatment differences. Because of the variability in blood pressure recordings, a better strategy might be to monitor blood pressure at frequent intervals, and/or with the patient in different positions, during the treatment period.

A major difficulty after implementing such a scheme is using all of the information collected for analysis. It can be difficult to implement statistical techniques that simultaneously use all of the longitudinal information collected, are robust to the inevitable missing data, and flexible enough to permit valid inferences concerning a variety of questions. Repeated measures analyses of variance and other methods of analyzing longitudinal data can be used. However, their complexity and higher cost and administrative needs for trial designs that require repeated assessments make these endpoints relatively uncommon.

6.5.2   Quality of life

Quality of life assessments are a special category of endpoints that are broadly used in clinical trials and other medical studies. These types of endpoints attempt to capture psychosocial features of the patient's condition, symptoms of the disease that may be distressing, and/or functional (physical) status and are important in chronic diseases like cancer. See Testa and Simonson [1996] for a recent review, and Chow and Ki [1994; 1996] for a discussion of statistical issues. It is easy to imagine situations in which the underlying disease is equally well controlled by either of two treatments, as measured by objective clinical criteria, but the quality of life might be superior with one treatment compared with the other. This could be a consequence of the severity and/or nature of the side effects, duration of treatment, or long-term consequences of the therapy.

Quality of life assessments are often made by summarizing items from a questionnaire (instrument) using a numerical score. Individual responses or assessments on the quality of life instrument might be summed, for example, for an overall score. Thus, quality of life assessment is a special case of a measured subjective endpoint. In other circumstances, quality of life assessments can be used as "utility coefficients" to weight or adjust other outcomes. This has been suggested in cancer investigations to create "quality-adjusted" survival times. Usually these quality-adjusted analyses require subjective judgments on the part of investigators in assigning utilities to various outcomes or conditions of the patient. For example, one could discount survival after chemotherapy for cancer by subtracting time with severe side effects from the overall survival time. This corresponds to a utility of zero for time spent in that condition. Because of the subjectivity required, quality-adjusted measurements often are not considered as reliable or rigorous as more objective measurements by many investigators.

6.6   Summary

The primary statistical objective of a clinical trial is usually to estimate some clinically important quantity, e.g., a treatment effect or difference. There may be numerous secondary objectives employing different endpoints, but the properties of the trial can usually only be controlled for one (primary) objective. Some trials are not designed to provide unbiased estimates of treatment effects, but instead select the "best" treatment from among several being tested.

Different scales of measurement may be required depending on the endpoint being used. Scales of measurement include nominal or categorical, ordered, interval (for estimating differences), and ratio. Aside from scales of measurements, endpoints can be classified as measures, categorical, counts, and event times. Event times are widely used endpoints for clinical trials, especially in chronic diseases like cancer, cardiovascular disease, and AIDS. Special statistical methods are required to cope with censored event times, which are frequently present in clinical trial data.

Trial methodologists continue to examine and debate the merits of surrogate endpoints, essentially on a study-by-study basis. Plausible surrogate endpoints have been proposed or used in cancer (e.g., tumor size), AIDS (e.g., CD4+ lymphocyte count), cardiovascular disease (e.g., blood pressure), and other disease trials. These types of endpoints can potentially shorten and increase the efficiency of trials. However, they may be imprecisely associated with definitive outcomes such as survival and can, therefore, yield misleading results.

6.7   Questions for Discussion

1.   Rank the different scales of measurement in order of their efficiency in using the available information. Discuss the pros and cons of each.
2.   Repeated measurements on the same study subjects increase precision. Because repeated measurements are correlated with one another, adding new study subjects may increase precision more. Discuss the merits and weaknesses of each approach.
3.   Surrogate or intermediate endpoints are frequently used in prevention trials. Discuss reasons why they may be more appropriate in studies of disease prevention than in studies of treatment.
4.   Read and comment on the study by the Chronic Granulomatous Disease Cooperative Study Group [N. Engl. J. Med. 324: 509-516, 1991].

Chapter References

Bogoch, S. and Bogoch, E.S. (1994). A checklist for suitability of biomarkers as surrogate endpoints in chemoprevention of breast cancer. J. Cellular Biochemistry, Supplement 19: 173-185.

Boissel, J.-P., Collet, J.-P., Moleur, P., and Haugh, M. (1992). Surrogate endpoints: A basis for a rational approach. Eur. J. Clin. Pharmacol. 43: 235-244.

CAST Investigators (1989). Preliminary report: Effect of encainide and flecainide on mortality in a randomized trial of arrythmia suppression after myocardial infarction. New Engl. J. Med 312: 406-412.

Chow, S.C. and Ki, F.Y.C. (1994). On statistical characteristics of quality of life assessment. J. Biopharmaceutical Statistics 1: 1-17.

Chow, S.C. and Ki, F.Y.C. (1996). Statistical issues in quality of life assessment. J. Biopharmaceutical Statistics 6: 37-48.

Cowley, A.J., McEntegart, D.J., Hampton, J.R., et al. (1994). Long-term evaluation of treatment for chronic heart failure: A 1 year comparative trial of flosequinan and captopril. Cardiovascular Drugs & Therapy 8(6): 829-836.

Ellenberg, S.S. and Hamilton, J.M. (1989). Surrogate endpoints in clinical trials: Cancer. Statistics in Med. 8: 405-413.

Fleming, T.R., Prentice, R.L., Pepe, M.S., and Glidden, D. (1994). Surrogate and auxiliary endpoints in clinical trials with potential applications in cancer and AIDS research. Statistics in Med. 13: 955-968.

Fleming, T.R. (1994). Surrogate markers in AIDS and cancer trials. Statistics in Med. 13: 1423-1435.

Fleming, T.R. and DeMets, D.L. (1996). Surrogate end points in clinical trials: Are we being misled? Ann. Intern. Med. 125: 605-613.

Freedman, L.S. and Schatzkin, A. (1992). Sample size for studying intermediate endpoints within intervention trials or observational studies. Am. J. Pub. Health 136: 1148-1159.

Gelber, R.D. (1996). Gemcitabine for pancreatic cancer: How hard to look for clinical benefit? An American perspective. Annals of Oncology 7: 335-337.

Herson, J. (1989). The use of surrogate endpoints in clinical trials (an introduction to a series of four papers). Statistics in Med. 8: 403-404.

Hillis, A. and Seigel, D. (1989). Surrogate endpoints in clinical trials: Ophthalmologic disorders. Statistics in Med. 8: 427-430.

Homans, G. (1965). Group factors in worker productivity. In H. Proshansky and B. Seidenberg (Eds.), Basic Studies in Social Psychology (pp. 592-604). New York: Holt, Rinehart, and Winston.

International Chronic Granulomatous Disease Cooperative Study Group (1991). A controlled trial of interferon gamma to prevent infection in chronic granulomatous disease. New Engl. J. Med 324: 509-516.

Kaplan, E.L. and Meier, P. (1958). Nonparametric estimation from incomplete observations. J. Am. Statist. Assoc. 53: 457-481.

Kelloff, G.J., Boone, C.W., Crowell, J.A., Steele, V.E., Lubet, R., and Doody, L.A. (1994). Surrogate endpoint biomarkers for phase II cancer chemoprevention trials. J. Cellular Biochemistry, Supplement 19: 1-9.

Packer, M., Carver, J.R., Rodeheffer, R.J., et al. (1991). Effect of oral milrinone on mortality in severe chronic heart failure. New Engl. J. Medicine 325: 1468-1475.

Patterson, B. and Piantadosi, S. (1989). Identification of endpoints: Selection and ascertainment. Chapter 19 in T. Moon, and M. Micozzi (Eds.), Nutrition and Cancer Prevention: The Role of Micronutrients. New York: Dekker.

Prentice, R.L. (1989). Surrogate endpoints in clinical trials: Definition and operational criteria. Statistics in Med. 8: 431-440.

Riggs, B.L., Hodgson, S.F., O'Fallon, W.M., et al. (1990). Effect of fluoride treatment on the fracture rate in postmenopausal women with osteoporosis.. New Engl. J. Med. 322: 802-809.

Rothenberg, M.L., Moore, M.J., Cripps, M.C. et al. (1996). A phase II trial of gemcitabine in patients with 5-FU-refractory pancreas cancer. Annals of Oncology 7: 347-353.

Terrin, M.L. (1990). Efficient use of endpoints in clinical trials: A clinical perspective. Statistics in Med. 9: 155-160.

Testa, M.A. and Simonson, D.C. (1996). Assessment of quality of life outcomes. New Engl. J. Med. 334: 835-840.

Verweij, J. (1996). The benefit of clinical benefit: A European perspective. Annals of Oncology 7: 333-334.

Wittes, J., Lakatos, E., and Probstfield, J. (1989). Surrogate endpoints in clinical trials: Cardiovascular diseases. Statistics in Medicine 8: 415-425.

CHAPTER 7

Sample Size and Power

7.1 Introduction

Questions regarding the quantitative properties of clinical trial designs, especially the correct power, best sample size, and optimal study duration, are among those most frequently posed by clinicians to statisticians. These questions are critical for most CTE trials and arise frequently in SE and ES studies. The size of a TM or DF investigation is not often an issue, because of the designs commonly used. I will discuss some approaches to these questions for all types of studies.

The underlying theme of sample size considerations in all clinical trials is *precision*. Precision of estimation is the characteristic of an experiment that is most directly a consequence of the size of the investigation. In contrast, validity, unbiasedness, and reliability do not necessarily relate to study size. The precision of an estimated parameter such as a mean, difference, proportion, rate, or ratio is a consequence of measurement error, person-to-person (and other) variability, number of replicates (e.g., sample size), experimental design, and methods of analysis. By specifying quantitatively the precision of measurement needed in an experiment, the investigator is implicitly outlining the sample size and, perhaps, other features of the study.

It is possible to specify precision directly for some studies. For example, we may need a sample size sufficient to estimate a mean diastolic blood pressure with a standard error of ± 2 mm Hg. In other circumstances, it may be preferable to specify the width of a confidence interval. For example, our sample size may need to be large enough for the 95% confidence interval around the mean diastolic blood pressure to be ± 4 mm Hg. In other studies, the size may be determined by the power of a hypothesis test. For example, we may need a sample size sufficient to yield 90% power to detect a 5-mm Hg difference as being statistically significant (using a specified type I error level). In all of these circumstances, a convenient specification of precision plus knowledge of variability will determine the sample size.

Table 7.1 Quantitative Design Parameters and Their Meanings Frequently Used in Clinical Trials

Power:	$1 - \beta$
β level:	type II error probability
α level:	type I error probability
Sample size:	number of experimental subjects
Number of events:	number of experimental subject who have a specific outcome
Study duration:	interval from beginning of trial to end of follow-up
Percent censoring:	percent of study participants left without an event by the end of follow-up
Allocation ratio:	ratio of sample sizes in the treatment groups
Accrual rate:	new subjects entered per unit of time
Loss to follow-up rate:	rate at which study participants are lost before outcomes can be observed
Follow-up period:	interval from end of accrual to end of study
Δ :	smallest treatment effect of interest based on clinical considerations

There are several approaches to specifying the precision that is needed in an experiment, including: 1) direct specification on the scale of measurement, 2) indirect specification through confidence limits, 3) the power of a statistical hypothesis test, 4) a guess based on ordinal scales of measuring effect sizes, and 5) *ad hoc* use of designs similar to those employed by other investigators. In this chapter, I will discuss primarily the second and third approaches.

CTE trials

For CTE studies, the discussion that follows emphasizes an approach based on a planned hypothesis test when the trial is completed. This is a convenient and frequently used perspective for planning the size of comparative trials and motivates the use of the term "power". The null hypothesis usually represents equivalence between the treatments. The alternative value for the hypothesis test is chosen to be the smallest difference of clinical importance between the treatments. Following this, the size of the study is planned to yield a high probability of rejecting the null hypothesis, if the alternative hypothesis is true. Therefore, the test statistic planned for the analysis dictates the exact form of the power equation. Even though the power equation depends on the test being employed, there is a similar or generic form for many different statistics.

Understanding the interrelationships between study design parameters in comparative trials (Table 7.1) can be challenging, even for familiar and commonly used endpoints. Because it is not possible to specify a universal approach to answering questions about power and sample size, I will discuss some basic ideas and examples on a case-by-case basis. Although some abbreviated sample size tables are presented below, it will be necessary to use the formulae for direct calculation of specific cases or to consult the original references for more extensive tabulations. For a more statistically oriented review of fixed sample size calculations, see Donner [1984] or Lachin [1981]. Tables and equations for specific purposes are presented in Machin and Campbell [1987], Shuster [1990], and Kraemer and Thiemann [1987]. Quantitative aspects of group sequential designs for comparative trials are discussed in Chapter 10.

The size and power of a comparative study can be expressed partly in terms of the intended type I and type II error rates. By convention, most power equations are written in terms of the normal quantiles for the type I and type II error rates (Z_α and Z_β), rather than the error probabilities themselves. The definitions of Z_α and Z_β follow from that for the cumulative normal distribution, which gives "lower" or "left" tail areas as:

$$\Phi(Z) = \int_{-\infty}^{Z} \frac{1}{\sqrt{2\pi}} e^{-\frac{x^2}{2}} \, dx. \qquad (7.1)$$

Then $1 - \alpha/2 = \Phi(Z_{1-\alpha/2})$ and $1 - \beta = \Phi(Z_{1-\beta})$. However, to simplify the notation slightly in the remainder of the chapter, I will define $Z_\alpha = \Phi^{-1}(1 - \alpha/2)$ and $Z_\beta = \Phi^{-1}(1 - \beta)$. For $\alpha = 0.05$, $Z_\alpha = 1.96$; and for $\beta = 0.10$, $Z_\beta = 1.282$.

7.1.1   Power calculations are approximations

There are two ways in which power and sample size calculations are approximations. First, the equations themselves are often based on approximations to the exact statistical distributions. For example, a useful and accurate equation for comparing means using the t-test can be based on a normal approximation with known variance (a so-called z-test). Second, the idea of predicting the number of patients or study subjects required in a study is itself an approximating process, because it depends on guesses about some of the parameters. For example, the accrual rate, censoring rate, or variance may be known only approximately.

One cannot take the estimated sample size or power that results from such approximations rigidly. We hope that our errors are small and the required sample size is accurate, generally within 5 or 10 percent of what is truly needed. However, we must be prepared to make the design more robust if some parameters are not known with sufficient precision. Usually this means increasing the sample size to compensate for overly optimistic assumptions. Furthermore, we should not allow small differences in sample size to dictate important scientific priorities, one way or the other. If it is essential clinically to achieve a certain degree of precision, then it is probably worthwhile to accrue 10% or 20% more participants to achieve it. Finally, some subjects are usually lost from the experiment, even in animal studies. We usually inflate the sample size to compensate for this, but the exact amount by which to do so is only an educated guess.

7.1.2 Power and sample size relationships are quadratic

Investigators are often surprised at how small changes in some design parameters yield large changes in the required sample size or study duration for experiments. At least for SE and CTE clinical trials, sample size tends to increase as the square, or inverse square of other design parameters. In general, the sample size increases as the square of the standard deviation of the treatment difference and the (sum of) normal quantiles for the type I and II error rates. Reducing the error rates increases Z_α and Z_β and increases the required sample size. Larger variability in the endpoint measurement increases the sample size. Also, the sample size increases as the inverse square of the treatment difference, i.e., detecting small treatment effects increases the required sample size greatly. These and other more quantitative ideas will be made more precise in the following sections.

7.2 Treatment Mechanism Studies

For many TM trials, sample size is not a statistical design concern. This is because convincing evidence of the reliability of treatment mechanism can often be obtained after studying only a few patients. Small sample size is not a rationale for conducting the entire TM study informally. For most types of treatments such as drugs and biologicals, a prospectively accrued study cohort is necessary. For treatments such as devices and surgery, where the technique may evolve from case to case, other designs may sometimes be used. DF studies, especially phase I trials, adapt to the accumulating results and therefore need a prospective design.

7.2.1 Sample size is an outcome of dose-finding studies

Usually it's not possible to specify the exact size of a phase I study in advance. Except in bioassay or other animal dose-response experiments, the size of the dose-finding trial depends on the outcomes observed. If the starting doses have been chosen conservatively, the trial will require more patients than if the early doses are near the MTD. Because the early doses are usually chosen conservatively, most phase I trials are less efficient (larger) than they could be if more were known about the MTD.

Regardless of the specific design used for a phase I trial, sample size, power, and the type I error rate are not the usual currency of concern regarding the properties of the study. Instead, such studies are dominated by clinical concerns relating to pharmacokinetic parameters, properties of the drug, and choosing a dose to use in later developmental trials. In the last few years, investigators have been paying more attention to the quantitative properties of phase I designs, particularly how well they inform us about the true dose-toxicity or dose-response function for the agent. Traditionally used dose escalation designs may not perform especially well in this regard, as discussed below.

Table 7.2 Simulated Phase I Study Using Modified Fibonacci Dose Escalation Scheme

Step	Dose Used	Patients Treated	Number of Responses
1	100	3	0
2	200	3	0
3	330	3	0
4	500	3	0
5	700	3	0
6	900	3	1
7	700	3	1
⋮	⋮	⋮	⋮

The MTD is operationally defined as the 700 unit dose.

7.2.2   Several classic DF designs have been described

A classic design for these studies is that of Dixon and Mood [1948], sometimes called the up-and-down method. In this design, equally spaced doses are chosen and the dose employed can go up or down after each patient is treated, depending on the response observed. After the data are collected, a probit model (cumulative normal distribution) can be fitted and the percentiles of the dose response function can be estimated. This design is most frequently used without the modeling step. The MTD is operationally defined to be the stopping dose.

Wetherill [1963] suggested using a grouped version of this design using groups of 2 or 3 patients. Another improvement is the use of a logit model which makes fitting easier without sacrificing flexibility. Again, the grouped design is often used without the modeling step. This is the basic design (three patients per group) most commonly used today in phase I studies (Table 7.2). Frequently, investigators treat additional patients at the final dose to have more clinical experience at the MTD.

Another design potentially useful for phase I studies is the stochastic approximation method [Robbins and Monro, 1951]. As with other approaches, a set of fixed dose levels is chosen and groups of patients can be used. If we denote the ith dose level by D_i and the ith response by Y_i, we then choose

$$D_{i+1} = D_i - a_i[Y_i - \theta] \, ,$$

where θ is the target probability of toxicity (or response) and a_i is a sequence of positive numbers converging to 0. For example, we might choose the a_i such that $a_i = c/i$, where c is the inverse of the slope of the dose-toxicity curve. It is clear that, when the response is close to θ, the dose level does not change (this is why the a_i are chosen to be decreasing in absolute value). The recommended dose (MTD) is the last design point. Although it has some desirable properties, this design is not used frequently.

7.2.3   There is no universal DF design

There is no standard or universally employed DF design for clinical trials. However, an approach similar to the following is often used in phase I cytotoxic drug trials (see also Storer [1989]). A conservative starting dose, based on animal or other preclinical data, is selected. For example, the starting dose might be taken to be 10% of the LD_{10} in rodents on a mg/kg basis. Then, a set of higher doses to be studied is specified in advance by the investigators. The range and dose increments are chosen according to a modified Fibonacci scheme, as discussed in Chapter 4. Three patients are treated at each dose. A dose limiting toxicity or side effect (DLT) is a serious or life-threatening, but reversible, side effect – except death, which is also dose limiting.

Escalations depend on how many patients out of groups of 3 experience DLT. If 0 out of three patients experience DLT, the next group receives the next higher dose. If 1 out of 3 patients have DLT, an additional 3 patients are accrued at the same dose. Of these, if 1 out of 6 experience DLT, the dose is then escalated. If 2 out of 6 have DLT, the escalations are stopped. If 2 or more out of 3 patients have DLT, the dose is reduced to the previous level. If this dose has already been studied in 6 patients, the trial is stopped. Otherwise, 3 more patients are entered at that dose to increase the clinical experience to 6 patients.

Although certain limitations of such a design are evident, it has some important advantages. The decision points and definitions are defined in advance and do not require elaborate statistical considerations. This is an important advantage in the clinic. The sample size, typically under 20 patients, is small, so that the study can be completed quickly. Finally, the design is familiar to many drug developers, allowing them to focus on clinical endpoints that are important when investigating new drugs.

7.2.4   Traditional DF designs can be improved

A potentially important improvement in phase I design, called the continual reassessment method (CRM), was suggested by O'Quigley, Pepe, and Fisher [1990] (see also O'Quigley and Chevret [1991]). Using this method, a starting dose is chosen and after the response is assessed, a one-parameter dose-toxicity model (e.g., logit curve with one free parameter) is fit to the data. This fitting process, or parameter estimation, is best accomplished using Bayesian methods. From the estimated dose-toxicity curve, we calculate the dose associated with the target probability of response. This estimated dose is the one used to treat the next patient. The process of treating, assessing response, model fitting, and dose estimation is repeated until it converges (no additional dose changes) or until a preset number of patients have been treated. Simulations show that the CRM is somewhat more efficient, i.e., reaches the actual MTD sooner, than the other designs discussed above.

The advantages of the CRM are that it requires only a starting dose as opposed to an entire set of doses specified in advance, the estimation method is unbiased, and it does not depend strongly on the starting dose. It has been claimed that the CRM has a tendency to treat a larger fraction of patients at higher doses, increasing the chances for serious toxicity from new drugs [Korn et al., 1994]. These deficiencies can be corrected by grouping patients (e.g., groups of three) and not allowing the escalation

SAMPLE SIZE AND POWER

154

to skip to high dose levels too quickly [Goodman, Zahurak, and Piantadosi, 1995].
Other modifications have been suggested by Faries [1994]. More recently, a likelihood, rather than a Bayesian, approach has been proposed for the CRM [O'Quigley
and Shen, 1996]. Despite the promise of this design, it has not yet been widely used
because many investigators are unfamiliar with it.

7.2.5 PK measurements can be used to improve CRM dose escalations

There is potential for further increasing the efficiency of the CRM using the information in pharmacokinetic (PK) measurements of the type that are routinely obtained
during phase I investigations [Piantadosi and Liu, 1997]. This method may be helpful when the PK measurements, usually derived by fitting compartmental models to
time-concentration data, carry information beyond that conveyed by dose because of
complexities in drug absorption, distribution, or elimination.

For example, suppose toxicity is believed to be a consequence of both the dose
of drug administered and the area under the time-concentration curve (AUC) for
blood. For relatively simple physiological distributions of drug, such as one- or two-
compartment models with first-order transfer rates, dose of drug and AUC are directly proportional, and therefore redundant in the information they carry. In such a
situation, we would not expect the addition of AUC to an escalation scheme based
on dose of drug to improve the efficiency of the dose-finding. However, if dose and
AUC become "uncoupled" because of complex pharmacokinetics, random variability, or other reasons, and AUC is a strong determinant of toxicity, then information
carried by AUC about toxicity may improve the efficiency of escalation schemes
based only on dose.

The CRM facilitates using ancillary information in the AUC or other PK measurements. Specifically, the basic CRM employs a parametric model of the probability
of toxicity as a function of dose. For example, if X_i is a random response variable
for the ith patient which takes the value 1 for a toxicity and 0 otherwise, a logistic
dose-toxicity function would specify

$$\Pr[X_i = 1] = \frac{1}{1 + e^{b_0 - b_1 \times D_i}},$$

where D_i is the dose of drug administered and b_0 and b_1 are population parameters which characterize the function. As dose increases, the probability of a toxic
response also increases.

Usually b_0 would be fixed at the start of the dose escalations and b_1 would be estimated from patient data during the escalations. After sufficient information becomes
available, both parameters can be estimated from the data. A Bayesian procedure can
be used, taking the parameter estimate to be the posterior mean of a distribution based
on the hypothesized prior distribution and the likelihood. For example,

$$\widehat{\beta}_1 = \frac{\int_0^\infty \beta_1 f(\beta_1)\mathcal{L}(\beta_1)\,d\beta_1}{\int_0^\infty f(\beta_1)\mathcal{L}(\beta_1)\,d\beta_1},$$

where $f(\beta_1)$ is the prior distribution for β_1 and $\mathcal{L}(\beta_1)$ is the likelihood function. These Bayesian estimates have desirable properties for the purposes at hand.

Using this formalism, the effect of AUC on toxicity could be incorporated as

$$\Pr[X_i = 1] = \frac{1}{1 + e^{b_0 - b_1 \times D_i - b_2 \times AUC_i}},$$

where b_2 is an additional population parameter. Thus, large AUCs increase the chance of toxicity and low AUCs decrease it in this model. Bayesian estimates for the parameters can be obtained using a joint prior distribution. An approach similar to this shows the possibility of increasing the efficiency of dose escalation trials based on statistical simulations [Piantadosi and Liu, 1996]. However, practical applications and experience with this method are currently lacking.

7.3   Safety and Efficacy Studies

7.3.1   Simple SE designs use fixed sample size

The goals of SE studies are typically to estimate a clinical endpoint with a specified precision. Examples of endpoints with clinical interest are average blood or tissue levels of a drug, the proportion of patients responding, with side effects, or meeting other pre-defined criteria, and population failure rates.

A useful measure of precision is the confidence interval around the estimated parameter. For example, narrow 95% confidence intervals indicate a higher degree of certainty about the location of a true effect than wide 95% confidence intervals do. Because confidence intervals depend on the number of subjects studied, precision specified in this way can be translated into requirements for sample size. For many phase II studies in oncology, the clinical outcome chosen is the proportion of patients showing objective evidence of treatment benefit. There are many methods for estimating confidence intervals for a proportion. See Vollset [1993] for a review. Here we consider only the conceptually easiest ways.

Consider as an example a trial in which patients with esophageal cancer are treated with chemotherapy prior to surgical resection. A complete response is defined as the absence of macroscopic and microscopic tumor at the time of surgery. We suspect that this might occur 35% of the time and would like the 95% confidence interval of our estimate to be $\pm 15\%$. Using the normal approximation to the binomial distribution, 95% confidence intervals for an estimated proportion, $\widehat{p}$, are

$$\widehat{p} \pm 1.96 \times \sqrt{\frac{p(1-p)}{n}}, \tag{7.2}$$

where n is the number of patients tested and 1.96 is the quantile from the normal distribution corresponding to a two-sided probability of 5% (equation 7.1). Because p is unknown, we usually substitute $\widehat{p}$ on the right-hand side of Equation 7.2. Then, this formula yields $0.15 = 1.96 \times \sqrt{0.35(1 - 0.35)/n}$ or $n = 39$ patients required to meet the stated requirements for precision. Because 35% is just an estimate of the proportion responding and some patients may not complete the study, the actual sample size to use might be increased slightly. Expected accrual rates can be used to estimate the duration of this study in a straightforward fashion.

A useful, but rough, guide for estimating sample sizes needed for proportions may be derived in the same way. Because $p(1-p)$ is maximal for $p = 0.5$, an approximate and conservative relationship between n, the sample size, and w, the width of the 95% confidence interval, is $n = 1/w^2$. To achieve a precision of $\pm 10\%$ (0.10) requires 100 patients, and a precision of $\pm 20\%$ (0.20) requires 25 patients. The quadratic nature of this relationship greatly increases the sample size needed to obtain high precision. This rule of thumb is not valid for proportions that deviate greatly from 0.5. For example, for proportions less than about 0.2 or greater than about 0.8, exact binomial methods should be used.

7.3.2   Exact binomial confidence limits are helpful

The method just sketched for SE studies uses 95% confidence intervals based on the normal approximation to the binomial distribution. This approximation may not be valid when p is extreme ($p < 0.2$ or $p > 0.8$), when the sample size is small, or when we require a high degree of confidence (e.g., 99% confidence intervals). Quantitative guidelines for deciding when to stop a phase II trial are often concerned with probabilities that fall into these ranges. For example, sometimes we might want to stop a trial if the incidence of serious side effects is greater than 10% or the success rate is less than 20%. In these circumstances, confidence limits based on the binomial distribution are more accurate than those based on a normal approximation. The ideas behind binomial confidence limits are as straightforward as those for continuous distributions and are based on tail areas.

The "tail areas" of the binomial distribution are obtained by summing probability terms. For example, suppose we observe r successes out of n trials. A $100(1 - \frac{\alpha}{2})\%$ lower confidence bound for the observed proportion r/n is the value of p that satisfies

$$\frac{\alpha}{2} = \sum_{k=0}^{r} \binom{n}{k} p^k (1-p)^{n-k} . \tag{7.3}$$

An upper $100(1 - \frac{\alpha}{2})\%$ confidence bound is the value of p that satisfies

$$\frac{\alpha}{2} = \sum_{k=r+1}^{n} \binom{n}{k} p^k (1-p)^{n-k} . \tag{7.4}$$

Note the resemblance of these formulae to equation 7.1. In general, these equations have to be solved numerically. Alternatively, some values can be found tabulated [Diem and Lentner, 1970]. Because this calculation is useful even when the normal approximation could be used, a flexible computer program for it is provided in Chapter 19.

Note that the confidence interval, like the binomial distribution, need not be symmetric around p even, when both tails contain the same fraction of the distribution.

It is customary to refer to confidence limits based on equations 7.3 and 7.4 as being "exact", because they use the correct probability distribution for $\hat{p}$, i.e., the binomial. In reality, they can still be approximate because of the discreteness of the distribution.

Example 8   *Suppose 3 of 19 patients respond to α-interferon treatment for multiple sclerosis. Exact 95% binomial confidence limits on the proportion responding are [0.03–0.40]. Approximate 95% confidence limits based on the normal approximation are [0.00–0.32]. (In this case, the normal approximation yielded a negative number for the lower 95% confidence bound.)*

An interesting special case arises when $r = 0$, that is, when no successes (or failures) out of n trials are seen. For $\alpha = 0.05$, the one-sided version of equation 7.4 is

$$0.95 = \sum_{k=1}^{n} \binom{n}{k} p^k (1-p)^{n-k} = 1 - \binom{n}{0} p^0 (1-p)^n$$

or

$$0.05 = (1-p)^n.$$

Thus, $\log(1-p) = \log(0.05)/n \approx -3/n$. This yields,

$$p \approx 1 - e^{-3/n} \approx \frac{3}{n}, \tag{7.5}$$

for $n \gg 3$. Actually, n does not need to be very large for the approximation to be useful. For example, for $r = 0$ and $n = 10$, the exact upper 95% confidence limit calculated from equation 7.4 is 0.26. The approximation based on equation 7.5 yields 0.30. When $n = 25$, the exact result is 0.11 and the approximation yields 0.12. So, as a general rule, to approximate the upper 95% confidence bound on an unknown proportion which yields 0 responses (or failures) out of n trials, use $3/n$. This estimate is sometimes helpful in drafting stopping guidelines for toxicity or impressing colleagues with your mental calculating ability.

Example 9   *The space shuttle flew successfully 24 times between April 12, 1981 and the January 28, 1986 Challenger disaster. What is the highest probability of failure consistent with such a series? In this case, we could calculate a one-sided 95% confidence interval. The exact solution to equation 7.4 yields $p = 0.117$. Equation 7.5 gives $p = 3/24 = 0.125$, close to the "exact" value. Although 24 is not a large denominator, the shuttle data did not rule out a high failure rate before the accident. Since 1981, there have been 50 additional successful space shuttle flights. If no improvements in launch procedures or equipment had been made (a highly doubtful assumption), an exact two-sided 95% binomial confidence interval on the probability of failure would be [0.0005–0.1065]. Thus, the current empirical evidence alone would not exclude a fairly high failure rate. (Some other interesting problems related to the Challenger can be found in Agresti [1996, p.135] and Dalal, Fowlkes, and Hoadley [1989].)*

Table 7.3 Exact Binomial Upper 95% Confidence Limits for r Responses Out of n Subjects

					r				
n	0*	1	2	3	4	5	6	7	8
5	.451	.716	.853	.947	.995				
6	.393	.641	.777	.882	.957	.996			
7	.348	.579	.710	.816	.901	.963	.996		
8	.312	.526	.651	.755	.843	.915	.968	.997	
9	.283	.482	.600	.701	.788	.863	.925	.972	.997
10	.259	.445	.556	.652	.738	.813	.878	.933	.975
11	.238	.413	.518	.610	.692	.766	.833	.891	.940
12	.221	.385	.484	.572	.651	.723	.789	.848	.901
13	.206	.360	.454	.538	.614	.684	.749	.808	.861
14	.193	.339	.428	.508	.581	.649	.711	.770	.823
15	.181	.320	.405	.481	.551	.616	.677	.734	.787

* One-sided confidence interval for $r = 0$, two-sided for all other cases.

7.3.3 Ineffective treatments can be discarded early

In diseases like cancer, SE studies assess the response rate of patients treated with new drugs or modalities. If the new treatment is ineffective (i.e., if the response rate is low) or there is too high an incidence of side effects, investigators would like to learn about it as early in the trial as possible and not place additional subjects on study. This has led to the widespread use of "early stopping rules" for these types of studies that permit accrual to be terminated before the planned fixed sample size end. Although a detailed look at this issue is given in Chapter 10, some designs are introduced here because they are widely used to determine the size of SE trials.

One simple quantitative approach to early stopping is the following: Suppose 0.20 is the lowest response rate that investigators consider acceptable for a new treatment (perhaps because standard therapy is as good or better than that). The exact binomial upper 95% confidence limit on 0 responses out of 12 tries is 0.20. Therefore, if none of the first 12 study participants respond, the treatment can be discarded because it most likely has a response rate less than 0.20. This type of rule was proposed by Gehan [1961] and is still used in phase II studies, because it is simple to employ and understand. It is easily modified using exact binomial confidence limits for target proportions other than 0.20 (Table 7.3). A more flexible approach to deal with this issue is to use two-stage designs, which are outlined in the next section.

7.3.4 Two-stage designs are efficient

Optimal two-stage designs for SE trials are discussed by Simon [1989]. The suggested design depends on two clinically important response rates p_0 and p_1 and type I and II error rates α and β. If the true probability of response is less than some clinically uninteresting level, p_0, the chance of accepting the treatment for further study is α. If the true response rate exceeds some interesting value, p_1, the chance of rejecting the treatment should be β. The study terminates at the end of the first stage only if the treatment appears ineffective. The design does not permit stopping early for efficacy.

The first stage (n_1 patients) is relatively small. If a small number ($\leq r_1$) of responses are seen at the end of the first stage, the treatment is abandoned. Otherwise, the trial proceeds to a second stage (n patients total). If the total number of responses after the second stage is large enough ($> r$), the treatment is accepted for further study. Otherwise, it is abandoned. The size of the stages and the decision rules can be chosen optimally to test differences between two response rates of clinical interest.

The designs can be specified quantitatively in the following way: Suppose the true probability of response using the new treatment is p. The trial will stop after the first stage if r_1 or fewer response are seen in n_1 patients. The chance of this happening is

$$B(r_1; p, n_1) = \sum_{k=0}^{r_1} \binom{n_1}{k} p^k (1-p)^{n_1-k},\tag{7.6}$$

which is the cumulative binomial mass function given above in equation 7.3. At the end of the second stage, the treatment will be rejected if r or fewer responses are seen. The chance of rejecting a treatment with true response probability p is the chance of stopping at the first stage plus the chance of rejecting at the second stage if the first stage is passed. We must be careful to count all of the ways of passing the first stage but not passing the second. The probability of rejecting the treatment is

$$Q = B(r_1; p, n_1) + \sum_{k=r_1+1}^{\min(n_1,r)} \binom{n_1}{k} p^k (1-p)^{n_1-k} B(r-k; p, n_2),\tag{7.7}$$

where $n_2 = n - n_1$.

When the design parameters, p_0, p_1, α, and β are specified, values of r_1, r_2, n_1, and n_2 can be chosen that satisfy the type I and type II error constraints. The design that yields the smallest *expected* sample size under the null hypothesis is defined as "optimal". Because a large number of designs could satisfy the error constraints, the search for optimal ones requires an exhaustive computer algorithm. Although many useful designs are provided in the original paper and some are tabulated here, a computer program for finding optimal designs is given in Chapter 19.

Trial designs derived in this way are shown in Tables 7.4 and 7.5. Multi-stage designs for SE studies can be constructed in a similar way. Three-stage designs have recently been proposed [Ensign et al., 1994]. However, two-stage designs are simpler and nearly as efficient as designs with more stages, or those that assess treatment efficacy after each patient. These designs are discussed in Chapter 10.

Table 7.4 Optimal Two-Stage Designs for SE (Phase II) Trials for $p_1 - p_0 = 0.20$ and $\alpha = 0.05$

p_0	p_1	β	r_1	n_1	r	n	$E\{n \mid p_0\}^*$
.05	.25	.2	0	9	2	17	12
		.1	0	9	3	30	17
.10	.30	.2	1	10	5	29	15
		.1	2	18	6	35	23
.20	.40	.2	3	13	12	43	21
		.1	4	19	15	54	30
.30	.50	.2	5	15	18	46	24
		.1	8	24	24	63	35
.40	.60	.2	7	16	23	46	25
		.1	11	25	32	66	36
.50	.70	.2	8	15	26	43	24
		.1	13	24	36	61	34
.60	.80	.2	7	11	30	43	21
		.1	12	19	37	53	30
.70	.90	.2	4	6	22	27	15
		.1	11	15	29	36	21

* Gives the expected sample size when the true response rate is p_0.

7.3.5   A Bayesian approach uses prior information

Consider the problem of planning a SE study when some information is already available about efficacy, e.g., the response rate for the new treatment. In the case of cytotoxic drug development, objective sources for this evidence may be animal tumor models, *in vitro* testing, phase I studies, or trials of pharmacologically related drugs. The evidence could be used to plan a SE trial to yield more precise information about the true response rate for the treatment. Thall and Simon [1994] discuss an approach for the quantitative design of such trials. Here I consider a rudimentary case using binomial responses to illustrate the components of a Bayesian approach. A useful tabulation of Bayesian confidence limits for a binomial proportion is given by Lindley and Scott [1995].

At the start of the trial, the Bayesian paradigm summarizes prior information about response probability in the form of a binomial probability distribution. Suppose the prior is taken to be equivalent to evidence that there have been r_1 responses out of n_1 patients on the treatment. This information about the true response rate, p, could be summarized as a binomial distribution

$$f(p) = \binom{n_1}{r_1} p^{r_1}(1-p)^{n_1-r_1}.$$

The current best estimate of the response rate is $\hat{p} = r_1/n_1$. The goal of the SE trial is to increase the precision of the estimate of $\hat{p}$ using additional observations.

Table 7.5 Optimal Two-Stage Designs for SE (Phase II) Trials for $p_1 - p_0 = 0.15$ and $\alpha = 0.05$

p_0	p_1	β	r_1	n_1	r	n	$E\{n \mid p_0\}^*$
.05	.20	.2	0	10	3	29	18
		.1	1	21	4	41	27
.10	.25	.2	2	18	7	43	25
		.1	2	21	10	66	37
.20	.35	.2	5	22	19	72	35
		.1	8	37	22	83	51
.30	.45	.2	9	27	30	81	42
		.1	13	40	40	110	61
.40	.55	.2	11	26	40	84	45
		.1	19	45	49	104	64
.50	.65	.2	15	28	48	83	44
		.1	22	42	60	105	62
.60	.75	.2	17	27	46	67	39
		.1	21	34	64	95	56
.70	.85	.2	14	19	46	59	30
		.1	18	25	61	79	43
.80	.95	.2	7	9	26	29	18
		.1	16	19	37	42	24

* Gives the expected sample size when the true response rate is p_0.

When the experiment is completed, the response rate can be estimated by $\widehat{p} = r/n$, where there are r responses out of n trials, and a confidence interval can be calculated (i.e., from equations 7.3 and 7.4). To assist with sample size determination, an alternate parameterization of equations 7.3 and 7.4 can be used,

$$0.025 = \sum_{k=0}^{r} \binom{n}{k} [\widehat{p} - w]^k [1 - (\widehat{p} - w)]^{n-k}, \tag{7.8}$$

and

$$0.025 = \sum_{k=r+1}^{n} \binom{n}{k} [\widehat{p} + w]^k [1 - (\widehat{p} + w)]^{n-k}, \tag{7.9}$$

where w is the width of the confidence interval. Specifying a value for w at the completion of the study and assuming a value for $\widehat{p}$, will allow investigators to calculate a total sample size by solving equations 7.8 and 7.9 for n. The additional observations to make will be $n - n_1$.

For example, suppose our prior information is equivalent to $n_1 = 15$ observations with $r_1 = 5$ responses and $\widehat{p} = 1/3$. Assume our final sample size should yield a 99% credible interval with width $w = 0.15$ and the true response rate is near $1/3$. Then, for the lower bound

$$0.005 = \sum_{k=0}^{r} \binom{n}{k} \left[\frac{1}{3} - 0.15\right]^{k} \left[1 - \left(\frac{1}{3} - 0.15\right)\right]^{n-k} , \qquad (7.10)$$

and for the upper bound

$$0.005 = \sum_{k=n+1}^{n} \binom{n}{k} \left[\frac{1}{3} + 0.15\right]^{k} \left[1 - \left(\frac{1}{3} + 0.15\right)\right]^{n-k} .$$

Equations 7.10 and **??** will be satisfied by $n = 57$ (with $r = 19$). This solution will also be approximately valid for $\hat{p}$ near $1/3$. Therefore, 42 additional observations in the SE study will satisfy the requirement for precision. An approximate solution can also be obtained from equation 7.2 with $Z_{\alpha} = 2.57$. Then,

$$n \approx 0.33 \times 0.66 \times (2.57/0.15)^2 = 64 ,$$

which compares favorably with the calculation based on exact confidence limits.

7.4   CTE Studies

7.4.1   How to choose type I and II error rates

Convention holds that most clinical trials should be designed with a two-sided α-level set at 0.05 and 80% or 90% power ($\beta = 0.2$ or 0.1, respectively). In practice, the type I and II error rates should be chosen to reflect the consequences of making the particular type of error. For example, suppose a standard therapy for a certain condition is effective and associated with few side effects. When testing a competing treatment, we would probably want the type I error rate to be small, especially if it is associated with serious side effects, to reduce the chance of a false positive. We might allow the type II error rate to be higher, indicating the lower seriousness of missing an effective therapy, because a good treatment already exists. Circumstances like this are commonly encountered when developing cytotoxic drugs for cancer treatment.

In contrast, suppose we are studying prevention of a common disease using safe agents such as diet or dietary supplements. There would be little harm in the widespread application of such treatments, so that the consequences of a type I error are not severe. In fact, some benefits might occur, even if the treatment was not preventing the target condition. In contrast, a type II error would be more serious because a safe, inexpensive, and possibly effective treatment would be missed. In such cases, there is a rationale for using a relaxed definition of "statistical significance", perhaps $\alpha = 0.10$, and a higher power, perhaps $\beta = 0.01$.

Special attention to the type I and II error rates may be needed when designing trials to demonstrate equivalence of two treatments. This topic is discussed below.

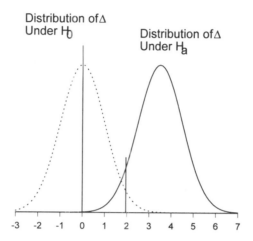
Distribution of Δ Under H_0

Distribution of Δ Under H_a

-3 -2 -1 0 1 2 3 4 5 6 7

Figure 7.1 Distributions of an estimator under the null and alternative hypotheses. Vertical lines are drawn at $\Delta = 0$ and $c = 1.96$ as explained in the text.

7.4.2 Comparisons using the *t*-test are a good learning example

Suppose the endpoint for a comparative clinical trial is a measurement so that the treatment comparison consists of testing the difference of the estimated means of the two groups. Assume the true means in the treatment groups are μ_1 and μ_2 and the standard deviation of the measurement in each patient is σ. Let the treatment difference be $\Delta = \mu_1 - \mu_2$. The null hypothesis is H_0: $\Delta = 0$. Investigators would reject the null hypothesis if $|\Delta|$ exceeds the critical value, c, where

$$c = Z_\alpha \times \sigma_\Delta$$

and σ_Δ is the standard deviation of Δ (Figure 7.1). In other words, if the estimated difference between the treatment means is too many standard deviations away from 0, we would disbelieve that the true difference is 0. Under the alternative hypothesis, the distribution of Δ is centered away from 0 (the right-hand curve in Figure 7.1).

The *power* of our statistical test is the area under the alternative distribution to the right of c, i.e., the probability of rejecting H_0 when the alternative hypothesis is true. This area can be calculated by standardizing c with respect to the alternative distribution

$$-Z_\beta = \frac{c - \Delta}{\sigma_\Delta} = \frac{Z_\alpha \times \sigma_\Delta - \Delta}{\sigma_\Delta},$$

i.e., by subtracting the mean of the alternative distribution and dividing by its standard deviation. The minus sign for Z_β comes from the fact that areas are tabulated from the left tail, whereas we are taking the area of the right tail of the distribution (equation 7.1). Thus,

$$-Z_\beta = \frac{Z_\alpha \times \sigma_\Delta - \Delta}{\sigma_\Delta} = Z_\alpha - \frac{\Delta}{\sigma_\Delta}$$

or

$$Z_\alpha + Z_\beta = \frac{\Delta}{\sigma_\Delta} . \tag{7.11}$$

Now

$$\sigma_\Delta = \sqrt{\frac{\sigma^2}{n_1} + \frac{\sigma^2}{n_2}} = \sigma\sqrt{\frac{1}{n_1} + \frac{1}{n_2}},$$

assuming the groups are independent and of sizes n_1 and n_2. Substituting into 7.11 and squaring both sides yields

$$\frac{1}{n_1} + \frac{1}{n_2} = \frac{\Delta^2}{(Z_\alpha + Z_\beta)^2\sigma^2}. \tag{7.12}$$

Now suppose $n_1 = rn_2$ (r is the *allocation ratio*) so that equation 7.12 becomes

$$\frac{1}{rn_2} + \frac{1}{n_2} = \frac{1}{n_2}\frac{r+1}{r} = \frac{\Delta^2}{(Z_\alpha + Z_\beta)^2\sigma^2}$$

or

$$n_2 = \frac{r+1}{r}\frac{(Z_\alpha + Z_\beta)^2\sigma^2}{\Delta^2} . \tag{7.13}$$

The denominator of the right-hand side of 7.13, expressed as $(\Delta/\sigma)^2$, is the square of the number of standard deviations between the null and alternative treatment means. All of the factors that affect the statistical power are evident from equation 7.13: the variance of an observation, the difference we are trying to detect, the allocation ratio, and the type I error level for the statistical comparison. Some convenient values that solve equation 7.13 are shown in Table 7.6.

Although this power equation has been derived assuming normal distributions (so called z-test), it yields values nearly correct for the t-test. One could increase accuracy by using quantiles from the t-distribution in place of Z_α and Z_β. However, when using the t-test, the power calculations are made more difficult by the need to evaluate the non-central t-distribution. Also, we have assumed that the variance is known. In some situations, the variance will be estimated from the observed data. This slightly increases the sample size required. However, the effect is small, amounting to an increase of only one or two subjects for sample sizes in the range of 20 [Snedecor and Cochran, 1980]. Consequently, the correction can be ignored for most clinical trials.

Although many important test statistics for clinical trials fit assumptions of normality, at least approximately, some important cases do not. For example, power and

Table 7.6 Approximate Total Sample Sizes for Comparisons Using the t-Test and Equal Group Sizes

	$\beta = 0.1$		$\beta = 0.2$	
Δ/σ	$\alpha = 0.05$	$\alpha = 0.10$	$\alpha = 0.05$	$\alpha = 0.10$
0.25	672	548	502	396
0.50	168	138	126	98
0.75	75	62	56	44
1.00	42	34	32	24
1.25	28	22	20	16
1.50	18	16	14	12

Δ is the difference in the treatment group means and σ is the standard deviation.

sample size equations for analyses of variance involve F-distributions which are computationally more cumbersome than Gaussian ones. Because these are uncommon designs for clinical trials, details are not given here. Approaches to this problem can be found in Winer [1971]. Some important non-normal cases more commonly encountered in clinical trials are discussed below.

7.4.3 Dichotomous responses are more complex

When the outcome is a dichotomous response, the results of a comparative trial can be summarized in a 2×2 table:

	Treatment	
Success	A	B
Yes	a	b
No	c	d

The analysis essentially consists of comparing the proportion of successes or failures in the groups, for example, $a/(a + c)$ versus $b/(b + d)$. The full scope of methods for determining power and sample size in this situation is large. A review of various approaches is given by Sahai and Khurshid [1996]. Here I discuss only the basics.

The usual analysis of such data would employ Fisher's exact test or the χ^2 test, with or without continuity correction. The exact test assumes that $a + b$, $c + d$, $a + c$ and $b + d$ are fixed by the design of the trial. However, in a trial, a and b are random variables, suggesting that the χ^2 test without continuity correction is appropriate. However, a fixed sample size with random treatment assignment leads to the exact test or χ^2 test with continuity correction. The sample size required for a particular trial can be different, depending on which perspective is taken [Pocock, 1982; Yates, 1984].

A derivation similar to the t-test above for comparing two proportions, π_1 and π_2, without continuity correction yields

$$n_2 = \frac{\left(Z_\alpha \sqrt{(r+1)\overline{\pi}(1-\overline{\pi})} + Z_\beta \sqrt{r\pi_1(1-\pi_1) + \pi_2(1-\pi_2)}\right)^2}{r\Delta^2}, \qquad (7.14)$$

where $\pi = (\pi_1 + r\pi_2)/(r+1)$ is the (weighted) average proportion and $\Delta = \pi_1 - \pi_2$. Convenient values that solve equation 7.14 for $r = 1$ are given in Tables 7.7 and 7.8. When $r = 1$, equation 7.14 can be approximated by

$$n_2 = \frac{(Z_\alpha + Z_\beta)^2 \left(\pi_1(1 - \pi_1) + \pi_2(1 - \pi_2)\right)}{\Delta^2}.$$

The calculated sample size must be modified when planning to use the χ^2 test with continuity correction. The new sample size must satisfy

$$n_2^* = \frac{n_2}{4} \left(1 + \sqrt{1 + \frac{2(r+1)}{rn_2\Delta}}\right)^2,$$

where n_2 is given by equation 7.14.

It is noteworthy that equation 7.14 could be solved algebraically for any single parameter in terms of the others. However, equation 7.14 cannot be solved simply for some parameters. For example, if we wish to determine the treatment difference that can be detected with 90% power, a sample size of 100 per group, equal treatment allocation, and a response proportion of 0.5 in the control group, equation 7.14 cannot be solved by elementary means. It can be solved using iterative calculations, i.e., starting with an initial guess for π_2 and using a standard method such as Newton's iterations to improve the estimate. This is a general feature of sample size equations: iterative methods are required to solve for some parameters. Consequently, good computer software is essential for performing such calculations which may have to be repeated many times before settling on the final design of a trial.

Equivalence

Some trials are designed to demonstrate the equivalence of two treatments. This may be necessary for new drugs when there is already a good standard therapy. To be useful, a new treatment could be as effective as standard therapy with fewer side effects, lower cost, greater convenience, or higher quality of life. In such cases, one might design a trial with the null hypothesis being "the treatments are different" and the alternative hypothesis being "the treatments are the same". This is a reversal of the usual situation where the null is the hypothesis of no difference. Furthermore, the test is one-sided because we don't wish to prove that the new treatment is significantly better or worse, only that it is equivalent. Thus, the roles of α and β are reversed and they must be selected with some thought.

The impact on sample size of choosing α and β in this way may not be great. It was shown above that the quantiles for type I and II error probabilities add together directly in many power formulae. However, the definition of "significant" may change depending on α and β, which could be consequential. In any case, a careful consideration of the consequences of type I and II errors will be useful before planning any trial. Approaches to power and sample size for equivalence trials are discussed by Roebruck and Kühn [1995] and Farrington and Manning [1990].

To demonstrate conclusively that two treatment effects are equivalent, a very large sample size is required. In equation 7.14, the sample size increases without bound as

Table 7.7 Approximate Sample Sizes for Comparisons Using the χ^2 Test without Continuity Correction with Equal Group Sizes

π_1	$\pi_2 - \pi_1$					
	.05	.10	.15	.20	.25	.30
.05	420	130	69	44	36	31
	570	175	93	59	42	37
.10	680	195	96	59	41	35
	910	260	130	79	54	40
.15	910	250	120	71	48	39
	1220	330	160	95	64	46
.20	1090	290	135	80	53	42
	1460	390	185	105	71	51
.25	1250	330	150	88	57	44
	1680	440	200	115	77	56
.30	1380	360	160	93	60	44
	1840	480	220	125	80	56
.35	1470	380	170	96	61	44
	1970	500	225	130	82	57
.40	1530	390	175	97	61	44
	2050	520	230	130	82	56
.45	1560	390	175	96	60	42
	2100	520	230	130	80	54
.50	1560	390	170	93	57	40
	2100	520	225	125	77	51

For each pair of π_1 and π_2, the upper number corresponds to $\alpha = 0.05$ and $\beta = 0.20$. The lower number corresponds to $\alpha = 0.05$ and $\beta = 0.10$.

$\pi_1 \rightarrow \pi_2$. However, the situation can be simplified if equivalence is defined to have a tolerance. For example, if we are willing to declare two proportions equivalent when $|\pi_1 - \pi_2| \leq \delta$, then equation 7.14 can be modified as

$$n_2 = \frac{(Z_\alpha + Z_\beta)^2 \left[\pi_1(1 - \pi_1) + \pi_2(1 - \pi_2)\right]}{[\delta - (\pi_1 - \pi_2)]^2} .$$

Most frequently, we would also assume $\pi_1 = \pi_2$. The sample size obtained from this calculation will be very sensitive to the definition of equivalence.

Example 10 *Suppose that the success rate for standard induction chemotherapy in adults with leukemia is 50% and that we would consider a new treatment equivalent to it if the success rate was between 40% and 60% ($\delta = 0.1$). The null hypothesis assumes that the treatments are unequal. Then, using an $\alpha = 0.10$ level test, we would have 90% power to reject non-equivalence with 428 patients assigned to each treatment group. In contrast, if equivalence is defined as $\delta = 0.15$, the required sample size decreases to 190 per group.*

Table 7.8 Approximate Sample Sizes for Comparisons Using the χ^2 Test without Continuity Correction with Equal Group Sizes

π_1	$\pi_2 - \pi_1$							
	.35	.40	.45	.50	.55	.60	.65	.70
.05	23	20	17	14	13	11	10	8
	31	24	21	18	16	13	12	11
.10	29	23	19	17	13	12	11	9
	36	29	24	20	17	16	13	11
.15	31	25	20	17	15	12	11	9
	40	31	26	22	18	16	13	11
.20	33	26	22	18	16	12	11	9
	43	33	28	23	18	16	13	11
.25	35	28	22	18	16	12	11	–
	45	36	29	23	18	16	12	–
.30	36	29	22	18	15	12	–	–
	46	36	29	23	18	16	–	–
.35	36	28	22	17	13	–	–	–
	46	36	28	22	17	–	–	–
.40	35	26	20	17	–	–	–	–
	45	32	26	20	–	–	–	–
.45	33	25	19	–	–	–	–	–
	43	32	24	–	–	–	–	–
.50	31	23	–	–	–	–	–	–
	40	29	–	–	–	–	–	–

For each pair of π_1 and π_2, the upper number corresponds to $\alpha = 0.05$ and $\beta = 0.20$. The lower number corresponds to $\alpha = 0.05$ and $\beta = 0.10$.

7.4.4   Hazard comparisons yield similar equations

Comparative clinical trials with event time endpoints require similar methods to estimate sample size and power. To test equality between treatment groups, it is common to compare the ratio of hazards (defined below) versus the null hypothesis value of 1.0. In trials with recurrence or survival time as the primary endpoint, the power of such a study depends on the number of events (e.g., recurrences or deaths). Usually there is a difference between the number of *patients* placed on study and the number of *events* required for the trial to have the intended statistical properties.

In the following sections, I give several similar appearing sample size equations for studies with event time outcomes. All will yield similar results. The sample size equations can be classified into those that use parametric forms for the event time distribution and those that do not (non-parametric). The equations use the ratio of hazards in the treatment groups, $\Delta = \lambda_1/\lambda_2$, where λ_1 and λ_2 are the individual hazards.

Exponential

If event times are exponentially distributed, some exact distributional results can be used. Suppose d observations are uncensored and $\widehat{\lambda}$ is the maximum likelihood estimate of the exponential parameter (see Chapter 12),

$$\widehat{\lambda} = \frac{d}{\sum t_i} ,$$

where the denominator is the sum of all follow-up times. Then $2d\lambda/\widehat{\lambda}$ has a chi-square distribution with $2d$ degrees of freedom [Epstein and Sobol, 1953; Halperin, 1952]. A ratio of chi-square random variables has an F distribution with $2d_1$ and $2d_2$ degrees of freedom [Cox, 1953]. This fact can be used to construct tests and confidence intervals for the hazard ratio. For example, a $100(1 - \alpha)\%$ confidence interval for $\Delta = \lambda_1/\lambda_2$ is

$$\widehat{\Delta} F_{2d_1,2d_2,1-\alpha/2} < \Delta < \widehat{\Delta} F_{2d_1,2d_2,\alpha/2} .$$

See Lee [1992] for some examples. Power calculations can be simplified somewhat using a log transformation, as discussed in the next section.

Other parametric

Under the null hypothesis, $\log(\Delta)$ is approximately normally distributed with mean 0 and variance 1.0 [George and Desu, 1974]. This leads to a power/sample size relationship similar to equation 7.13,

$$D = 4\frac{(Z_\alpha + Z_\beta)^2}{[\log(\Delta)]^2} , \tag{7.15}$$

where D is the total number of events required and Z_α and Z_β are the normal quantiles for the type I and II error rates. It is easy to verify that to have 90% power to detect a hazard ratio of 2.0 with a two-sided 0.05 α-level test, approximately 90 total events are required. It is useful to remember one or two such special cases because the formula may be difficult to recall.

A more general form for equation 7.15 is

$$\frac{1}{d_1} + \frac{1}{d_2} = \frac{[\log(\Delta)]^2}{(Z_\alpha + Z_\beta)^2} , \tag{7.16}$$

which is useful because it shows the number of events required in each group. Note the similarity to equation 7.7. Ideally, the patients should be allocated to yield equal number of events in the two groups. Usually this is impractical and not much different from allocating equal numbers of patients to the two groups. Equations 7.15 and 7.16 are approximately valid for non-exponential distributions as well, especially those with proportional hazards such as the Weibull.

Non-Parametric

To avoid parametric assumptions about the distribution of event times, a formula given by Freedman [1982] can be used. This approach is helpful when it is unreasonable to make assumptions about the form of the event time distribution. Under fairly flexible assumptions, the size of a study should satisfy

$$D = \frac{(Z_\alpha + Z_\beta)^2 (\Delta + 1)^2}{(\Delta - 1)^2}, \tag{7.17}$$

where D is the total number of events need on the study.

Example 11   *Using this formula, to detect a hazard rate of 1.75 as being statistically significantly different from 1.0 using a two-sided 0.05 α-level test with 90% power requires*

$$\frac{(1.96 + 1.282)^2 (1.75 + 1)^2}{(1.75 - 1)^2} = 141 \ events.$$

A sufficient number of patients must be placed on study to yield 141 events in an interval of time appropriate for the trial. Suppose that previous studies suggest that approximately 30% of subjects will remain event free at the end of the trial. The total number of study subjects would have to be

$$n = \frac{141}{1 - 0.3} = 202.$$

This number might be further inflated to account for study drop-outs.

7.4.5   Parametric and non-parametric equations are connected

Interestingly, equations 7.15 and 7.17 can be connected directly in the following way. For $\Delta > 0$, a convergent power series for the logarithmic function is

$$\log(\Delta) = \sum_{i=1}^{\infty} \frac{2}{2i - 1} \psi^{2i-1}, \tag{7.18}$$

where $\psi = (\Delta - 1)/(\Delta + 1)$. Using only the first term of equation 7.18 we have

$$\log(\Delta) \approx 2\psi.$$

Substituting this into equation 7.15, we get equation 7.17. The quantity $2(\Delta - 1)/(\Delta + 1)$ gives values closer to 1.0 than $log(\Delta)$ does, which causes equation 7.17 to yield higher sample sizes than equation 7.15.

The ratio of sample sizes given by the two equations, R, is

$$\sqrt{R} = \frac{\frac{1}{2} \log(\Delta)}{\psi} = \sum_{i=1}^{\infty} \frac{1}{2i - 1} \psi^{2i-2}.$$

Taking the first two terms of the sum,

$$\sqrt{R} \approx 1 + \frac{1}{3} \psi^2.$$

Table 7.9 Approximate Sample Sizes for Comparisons Using the Log Rank Test

Δ	$\beta = 0.1$		$\beta = 0.2$	
	$\alpha = 0.05$	$\alpha = 0.10$	$\alpha = 0.05$	$\alpha = 0.10$
1.25	844	688	630	496
	852	694	636	500
1.50	256	208	192	150
	262	214	196	154
1.75	134	110	100	80
	142	116	106	84
2.00	88	72	66	52
	94	78	70	56
2.25	64	52	48	38
	72	58	54	42
2.50	50	42	38	30
	58	48	42	34

Δ is the hazard ratio. The upper row is for the exponential parametric assumption (equation 10) and the lower row is a non-parametric assumption (equation 7.16).

For $\Delta = 2$, $\psi = \frac{1}{3}$, and

$$\sqrt{R} = 1 + \frac{1}{27}$$

or $R \approx 1.08$. Thus, equation 7.17 should yield sample sizes roughly 8% larger than equation 7.15, for hazard ratios near 2.0. This is in accord with Table 7.9.

7.4.6 Formulae accommodate unbalanced treatment assignments

In some circumstances, it is useful to allocate unequally sized treatment groups. This might be necessary if one treatment is very expensive, in which case the overall cost of the study could be reduced by unequal allocation. In other cases, we might be interested in a subset of patients on one treatment group. If d_1 and d_2 are the treatment group sizes, define $r = d_2/d_1$ to be the allocation ratio. Then equation 7.16 becomes

$$d_1 = \frac{r+1}{r} \frac{(Z_\alpha + Z_\beta)^2}{[\log(\Delta)]^2} . \qquad (7.19)$$

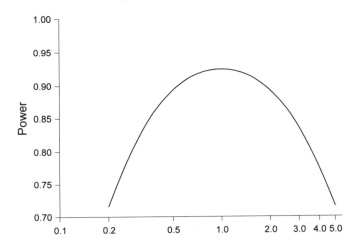

Figure 7.2 Power vs. allocation ratio for event time comparisons.

The effect of unequal allocations can be studied from this equation. Suppose the total sample size is held constant, i.e.,

$$D = d_1 + d_2 = d_1 + rd_1 = d_1(r+1)$$

or $d_1 = D/(r+1)$. Then equation 7.19 becomes

$$D = \frac{(r+1)^2}{r} \frac{(Z_\alpha + Z_\beta)^2}{[\log(\Delta)]^2} . \qquad (7.20)$$

From this we have

$$power = \Phi\left(\frac{\sqrt{Dr}}{r+1}\log(\Delta) - Z_\alpha\right).$$

A plot of power versus r using this equation is shown in Figure 7.2.

As the allocation ratio deviates from 1.0, the power declines. However, this effect is not very pronounced for $0.5 \leq r \leq 2$. Thus, moderate imbalances in the treatment group sizes can be used without great concern about loss of power or the need to increase total sample size.

7.4.7 A simple accrual model can also be incorporated

Often, it is important to estimate the length of time required to complete a clinical trial with event time endpoints. This is true in studies of many chronic diseases like cancer and AIDS. Consider a trial that accrues patients over an interval of time from 0 to T. After time T, the study does not terminate, but continues without new accru-

Table 7.10 Accrual Times That Satisfy Equation 7.22 with Equal Group Sizes

Event Rates		Accrual Rate						
λ_1	λ_2	20	30	40	50	75	100	200
.1	.15	20.4	15.6	13.0	11.3	8.9	7.5	5.1
	.20	9.9	7.8	6.6	5.8	4.6	3.9	2.7
	.25	6.9	5.5	4.7	4.1	3.3	2.8	2.0
.15	.20	31.2	22.7	18.3	15.6	11.8	9.8	6.4
	.25	12.9	9.9	8.2	7.2	5.6	4.8	3.2
	.30	8.5	6.6	5.5	4.9	3.9	3.3	2.2
.20	.30	16.9	12.5	10.2	8.8	6.8	5.7	3.8
	.35	10.4	7.9	6.6	5.7	4.5	3.8	2.5
	.40	7.7	5.9	4.9	4.3	3.4	2.9	2.0

$\alpha = 0.05$, $\beta = 0.10$, and $\tau = 0$.

als while those patients already on study are followed for events (Figure 7.1). This scheme is advantageous because individuals accrued close to the end of the study ordinarily would not be followed long enough to observe many events. Using a period of additional follow-up permits subjects accrued near T to contribute information to the study.

Under the assumptions of Poisson accrual rates and exponentially distributed failure times, the study parameters in this case should satisfy

$$\sum_{i=1}^{2} \frac{2 (\lambda_i^*)^2}{n \lambda_i} \frac{1}{\lambda_i^* T - e^{-\lambda_i^* \tau}(1 - e^{-\lambda_i^* T})} = \frac{[\log(\Delta)]^2}{(Z_\alpha + Z_\beta)^2}, \qquad (7.21)$$

where the subscript indicates group 1 or 2, λ is the event rate, $\lambda_i^* = \lambda_i + \mu$, which is the event rate plus μ, a common loss to follow-up rate, T is the accrual period, τ is the period of additional follow-up, and the other parameters are as above [Rubinstein, Gail, and Santner 1981]. This equation must be used thoughtfully to be certain that the time scales for the event rates and accrual periods are the same (e.g., years, or months, etc.). Numerical methods are required to solve it for the event rates, accrual time, and follow-up time parameters. The other parameters can be found algebraically. Values of accrual time that satisfy equation 7.21 for various other parameter values are shown in Table 7.10.

Example 12 *A randomized clinical trial is planned to detect a 2-fold reduction in the risk of death following surgery for non-small cell lung cancer using adjuvant chemotherapy versus placebo. In this population of patients, the failure rate is approximately 0.1 per person-year of follow-up on surgery alone. Investigators expect to randomize 60 eligible patients per year. Assuming no losses to follow-up and type I and II error rates of 5% and 10%, respectively, equation 7.21 is satisfied with $T = 2.75$ and $\tau = 0$. This is the shortest possible study because accrual continues to*

the end of the trial, i.e., is maximized. The total accrual required is $60 \times 2.75 = 165$
subjects. However, those individuals accrued near the end of the study may con-
tribute little information to the treatment comparison because they have relatively
little time at risk and are less likely to have events than those accrued earlier. As
an alternative design, investigators consider adding a 2-year period of follow-up on
the end of the accrual period, so that individuals accrued late can be followed long
enough to observe events. This type of design can be satisfied by $T = 1.66$ *and*
$\tau = 2$, *i.e., these parameters will yield the same number of events as those above.*
Here the total accrual is $60 \times 1.66 = 100$ *patients and the total trial duration is* 3.66
years. Thus, this design option allows trading follow-up time for up-front accruals.
This strategy is often possible in event time studies. Follow-up time and accruals
can be exchanged to yield a favorable balance while still producing the necessary
number of events in the study cohort.

In its original form, equation 7.21 is somewhat difficult to use and the sample size
tables often do not have the needed entries. If the exponential terms in equation 7.21
are replaced by first-order Taylor series approximations, $e^{\lambda x} \approx 1 - \lambda x$, we obtain

$$n \approx \tilde{\lambda} \frac{(Z_\alpha + Z_\beta)^2}{T\tau[\log(\Delta)]^2} ,$$

where $\tilde{\lambda}$ is the harmonic mean of λ_1 and λ_2. This approximation yields accrual rates
which are slightly conservative. Nevertheless, it is useful in situations where the
first-order approximation is valid, for example, when the event rates are low. This
might be the case in disease prevention trials where the population under study is
high risk but the event rate is expected to be relatively low.

7.5   ES Trials

ES (phase IV) studies are large safety trials, typified by post-marketing surveillance,
and are intended to uncover and accurately estimate the frequency of uncommon side
effects that may have been undetected in earlier studies. The size of such studies
depends on how low the event rate of interest is in the cohort under study and how
powerful the study needs to be.

7.5.1   Model rare events with the Poisson distribution

Assume that the study population is large and that the probability of an event is small.
Also, assume that all subjects are followed for approximately the same length of time.
The number of events, D, in such a cohort would follow the Poisson distribution. The
probability of observing exactly r events is

$$\Pr[D = r] = \frac{(\lambda m)^r e^{-\lambda m}}{r!} ,$$

where λ is the event rate, and m is the size of the cohort. The chance of observing r or fewer events is the tail area of this distribution or

$$\Pr[D \leq r] = \sum_{k=0}^{r} \frac{(\lambda m)^k e^{-\lambda m}}{k!} .$$

The study should be large enough to have a high chance of seeing at least one event when the event rate is λ.

Example 13 *The chance of seeing at least one event in the Poisson distribution is*

$$\beta = 1 - \Pr[X = 0] = 1 - e^{-\lambda m},$$

or $m = -log(1 - \beta)/\lambda$. *If* $\lambda = .001$ *and* $\beta = 0.99$, *then* $m = 4605$. *In other words, if we studied 4605 patients and observed no events, we would have a high degree of certainty that the event rate was lower than 0.1%.*

Confidence intervals on λ can be calculated in a fashion similar to those for the binomial distribution above. In some cases, comparative trials are designed with discrete outcomes having a Poisson distribution. Power computations in these cases are discussed by Gail [1974].

7.6   Other Considerations

7.6.1   Increase the sample size for non-adherence

Frequently, patients on randomized clinical trials do not comply with the treatment to which they were assigned. Here we consider a particular type of non-adherence, called drop-in, where patients intentionally take the other (or both) treatment(s). This might happen in an AIDS trial, for example, where study participants want to receive all treatments on the chance that one of them would have a large benefit. A more general discussion of the consequences of non-adherence is given by Schechtman and Gordon [1994]. Non-adherence, especially treatment cross-over, always raises questions about how best to analyze the data. Such questions are discussed in Chapter 11.

Drop-ins diminishes the difference between the treatment groups, requiring a larger sample size than one would need to detect the same therapeutic effect in perfectly complying subjects. Investigators frequently inflate the sample size planned for a trial on an *ad hoc* basis to correct for this problem. For example, if 15% of subjects are expected to fail to comply, one could increase the sample size by 15% as though the analysis would be based on compliant patients only. This strategy is helpful, because it increases the power of the trial, but is based on the incorrect assumption that non-compliers can be removed from the analysis.

Sometimes it is possible to determine quantitatively the consequence of non-adherence on the power of a comparative clinical trial. As an example, suppose that the trial endpoint is survival and that a fixed proportion of study participants in each group cross over to the opposite treatment. For simplicity, we assume that the compliant proportion is p, and is the same in both groups, and that patients only drop-in to the other treatment. Denote the hazard ratio in compliant subjects by Δ and in partially compliant subjects by Δ'. Then, for the same type I and II error rates, the required number of events are D and D', respectively. Considering equation 7.19, the sample size inflation factor, R, that corrects for different hazard ratios satisfies

$$R = \frac{D'}{D} = \frac{(\Delta - 1)^2 (\Delta' + 1)^2}{(\Delta + 1)^2 (\Delta' - 1)^2} .$$

Expressing Δ' in terms of Δ will put this equation in a usable form.

To accomplish this, assume that $\Delta' = \lambda'_1 / \lambda'_2$, where λ'_1 and λ'_2 are the composite hazards in the two treatment groups after non-compliant patients are taken into account. In the first treatment group, p subjects have hazard λ_1 and $1 - p$ have hazard λ_2. Assume that the "average" hazard in this group is the weighted harmonic mean,

$$\lambda'_1 = \frac{2}{\frac{p}{\lambda_1} + \frac{1-p}{\lambda_2}} .$$

Similarly, in the second treatment group,

$$\lambda'_2 = \frac{2}{\frac{1-p}{\lambda_1} + \frac{p}{\lambda_2}} .$$

Therefore,

$$\Delta' = \frac{1 + p(\Delta - 1)}{\Delta + p(\Delta - 1)} .$$

From this, it is straightforward to show that

$$\frac{\Delta' + 1}{\Delta' - 1} = \frac{\Delta + 1}{\Delta - 1} \frac{1}{2p - 1} .$$

Substituting into the equation defining R,

$$R = \frac{D'}{D} = \frac{(\Delta - 1)^2 (\Delta' + 1)^2}{(\Delta + 1)^2 (\Delta' - 1)^2} = \frac{1}{(2p - 1)^2} ,$$

which gives the inflation factor as a function of the adherence rate.

When all patients comply, $p = 1$ and $R = 1$. If 95% of patients in each group comply (5% "drop-in" to the opposite group), $R = 1/(1.9 - 1)^2 = 1.23$. In other words, to account for 5% non-adherence of this type, the number of events has to be inflated by 23%. If the non-adherence is 10%, the sample size inflation factor is 56%, illustrating the severe attenuation of the treatment difference that this type of problem can cause. Similar equations can be derived for drop-outs or when the drop-in rates are different in the two groups.

Table 7.11 Simulated Lifetable to Estimate Study Size and Duration Assuming Exponential Event Times

Time Interval	Number Accrued	Number on Study	Events in Interval	Number Event Free	Cumulative Events
1	30	30	4	26	4
2	30	56	8	48	12
3	30	78	11	67	23
4	30	97	14	83	37
5	30	113	16	97	53
6	30	127	18	109	71
7	30	139	19	120	90
⋮	⋮	⋮	⋮	⋮	⋮

7.6.2 Simulated lifetables can be a simple design tool

Sometimes one does not have a software package, computer, or programmed calculator available, but still wishes to have a rough idea of how long a trial might take to complete. Assuming we can calculate the number of events needed from an equation like 7.15 or 7.17, a basic lifetable can be constructed to show how long such a study might take. The only additional piece of information required is the accrual rate.

The procedure is fairly simple. For each interval of time, calculate 1) the number of patients accrued, 2) the total number at risk, 3) the number of events in the interval produced by the overall event rate, and 4) the cumulative number of events. When the cumulative number of events reaches its target, the trial will stop. As an example, suppose we wish to know how long a trial will take that requires 90 events and has event rates of 0.1 and 0.2 per person-year in the two treatment groups. Accrual is estimated to be 30 patients per year. Table 7.11 shows the calculations. Here I have assumed the overall event rate is

$$\bar{\lambda} = 2/(\frac{1}{\lambda_1} + \frac{1}{\lambda_2}) = \frac{2}{10 + 5} = 0.14 \,,$$

i.e., the harmonic mean of the two event rates. In the seventh year of the lifetable, the cumulative number of events reaches 90. Thus, this study would require approximately seven years to complete. In the event that accrual was stopped after five years, a similar calculation shows that the trial would take nine years to yield 90 events.

This method is approximate because it assumes that all patients accrued are at risk for the entire time interval, there are no losses from the study, and both the event rate and accrual rate are constant. Also, not all accruals are always accounted for at the end of the table because of round-off error. These problems could be corrected with a more complex calculation, but this one is useful because it is so simple.

7.6.3   Computer programs simplify calculations

The discussion in this chapter demonstrates the need for flexible and fast, user-friendly, computer software to alleviate hand calculations. Most statisticians who routinely perform such calculations have their own programs, commercial software, tables, or other labor-saving methods. Good software packages can greatly simplify these calculations, saving time, increasing flexibility, and allowing the trialist to focus on the conceptual aspects of design. Most commercial programs are periodically updated. It is important to weigh ease of use and cost. Often, the easier a program is to use, the more costly it is. A few programs are described below.

First is the *Clinical Trials Design Program*, which includes many of the formulae described here as well as some other useful ones [Piantadosi, 1990]. This program permits solving for any design parameter in terms of the others and uses algebraic or numerical methods as needed. All of the parameters are entered in a simple format on a single form and the calculation of the unknown parameter is done by pressing a single key. Multiple calculations are automatically tabulated for later printing. This program is relatively expensive, costing over $200 in 1995.

A different computer program, *Power and Sample Size* (PASS) is sold by NCSS Software. It also performs most of the calculations outlined here and permits simple power curves to be graphed. The price of this program is approximately $150. It is a useful learning device and the price may be discounted for students. Recently, a *Windows* version has become available [Hintze, 1996].

A newer program for power and sample size is *nQuery Advisor* by Statistical Solutions [Elashoff, 1995]. It is *Windows* based and easy to use. This program performs many sample size calculations, but permits solving only for power, sample size, or effect size. Other parameters are assumed to be fixed. This program can also graph power versus sample size and costs about $475.

Other computer programs are available for 1) general power calculations (see Goldstein [1989] for a review) and 2) specialized purposes (e.g., group sequential designs). These latter programs will be discussed in Chapter 19. Some complexities such as time varying drop-out and event rates can be handled [Wu, Fisher, and DeMets, 1980].

7.6.4   Simulation is a powerful and flexible design alternative

It is not uncommon to encounter circumstances in which one of the numerous sample size equations is inadequate or based on assumptions known to be incorrect. In these situations, it is often possible to study the behavior of a particular trial design by simulating the data that might result and then analyzing it. If this process is repeated many times with data generated from the appropriate model with a random component, the distribution of various trial outcomes can be seen. The process of simulating data, sometimes called the "Monte Carlo method", is widely used in statistics to study analytically intractable problems.

An example of a situation in which the usual assumptions might be inaccurate occurs in prevention clinical trials studying the effects of treatments such as diet or life-style changes on the time to development of cancer. In this circumstance, it is likely that the effect of the treatment gradually phases in over time. Thus, the risk (hazard) ratio between the two treatment groups is not constant over time. However, a constant hazard ratio is an assumption of all of the power and sample size methods presented above for event time endpoints. It is also difficult to deal analytically with time-varying hazard ratios. Additionally, the loss rates or drop-in rates in the treatment groups are not likely to be constant over time. An appropriate way to study the power of such a trial might be to use simulation.

Simulations can facilitate studies in other situations. Examples include studying dose escalation algorithms in DF trials, the behavior of flexible grouped designs, and making decisions about early stopping. Reasonable quantitative estimates of trial behavior can be obtained with 1000–10,000 replications. Provided the sample size is not too great, these can usually be performed in a reasonable length of time on a microcomputer.

7.6.5 Power curves are sigmoid shaped

I emphasized earlier the need to specify the alternative hypothesis when discussing the power of a comparative trial. It is often helpful to examine the power of a trial for a variety of alternative hypotheses (Δ) when the sample size is fixed. Alternatively, the power for a variety of sample sizes for a specific Δ is also informative. These are "power curves" and generally have a sigmoidal shape with increasing power as sample size or Δ increases. It is important to know if a particular trial design is a point on the plateau of such a curve, or lies more near the shoulder. In the former case, changes in sample size or Δ will have little effect on the power of the trial. In the latter case, small changes can seriously affect the power.

As an example, consider the family of power curves shown in Figure 7.3. These represent the power of a clinical trial using the log rank statistic to detect differences in hazard ratios as a function of Δ. Each curve is for a different number of total events and all were calculated from equation 7.17 as

$$1 - \beta = \Phi(Z_\beta) = \Phi\left(\sqrt{d}\frac{\Delta - 1}{\Delta + 1} - Z_\alpha\right) .$$

For any sample size, the power increases as Δ increases. In other words, even a small study has a high power against a sufficiently large alternative hypothesis. However, only large trials have a high power to detect smaller (and clinically realistic) alternative hypotheses, and retain power, even if some sample size is lost.

7.7 Summary

Sample size and power are quantitative specifications of the statistical design properties of clinical trials, especially comparative studies. These quantifications, although approximate, are useful and necessary for designing trials and planning for resource utilization. A frequentist perspective is commonly adopted for performing sample

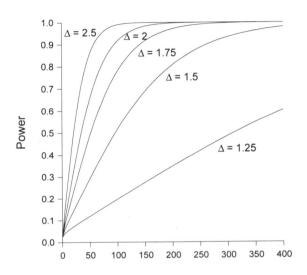

Figure 7.3 Power versus number of events for the logrank test.

size and related calculations. Other design parameters that may be important to spec-ify quantitatively besides sample size and power include the intended type I error rate, the number of events in an event-time study, accrual rate and duration, losses to follow-up, allocation ratio, total study duration, and the smallest treatment differ-ence of clinical importance. The actual importance of each of these depends on the type of trial and its specific design.

The sample size needed for a phase I trial is usually an outcome of the study, although it is frequently less than 20–25 patients. The exact sample size cannot usu-ally be specified in advance, because the study stops only after pre-specified clinical criteria are met. For dose-finding, fairly simple and familiar study designs usually suffice, although some newer methods such as the continual reassessment method can perform better. Designs that explicitly incorporate pharmacokinetic information into the dose escalation may make these studies more efficient.

Developmental studies, like SE trials, which look for evidence of treatment ef-ficacy, can employ a fixed sample size. The sample size can be determined as a consequence of the precision required to estimate the response, success rate, or fail-ure rate of the treatment. These trials usually require 25–50 subjects. When faced with evidence of low efficacy, investigators wish to stop a SE trial as early as possi-ble. This motivates the use of quantitative early stopping rules, sequential, or staged designs that minimize the number of patients given an unpromising treatment. When evidence about efficacy is available from previous studies, a Bayesian SE design may be useful.

Sample size and power relationships for CTE trials depend on the particular test statistic used to compare the treatment groups. Sample size increases as the type I and type II error rates decrease. Sample size decreases as the treatment difference (alternative hypothesis) increases or as the variance of the treatment difference decreases. For event-time studies, the currency of design is the number of events required to detect a particular hazard ratio. The actual sample size needed to yield the required number of events depends on the degree of censoring and the duration of the trial and its follow-up. Non-adherence with assigned treatment may increase the required number of study participants dramatically.

Besides analytic power and sample size equations, statistical simulation may be a useful way to study the quantitative properties of some trial designs. These could be as simple as a single hypothetical life table constructed under the assumptions of the trial, accrual, and treatment alternatives. More complex simulations could help quantify the effects of non-adherence or other analytically intractable problems in trials. Specialized, flexible computer programs are necessary for performing the required calculations efficiently. Depending on the shape of the power curve, small changes in design parameters can have large or small effects on the power of the study against a fixed alternative.

7.8 Questions for Discussion

1. How large a study is required to estimate a proportion with a precision of ± 0.1 (95% confidence limits)? How large a study is required to estimate a mean value with precision ± 0.1 standard deviation (95% confidence limits)?

2. What is the largest proportion consistent with 0 successes out of 5 binomial trials? Define what you mean by "consistent with". What about 0 out of 10, 12, 15, and 20 trials?

3. Using the normal approximation, confidence limits for a proportion are symmetric around the point estimate. Exact binomial confidence limits can also be constructed to be symmetric around the point estimate. Give some numerical examples for $p \neq 0.05$ and discuss the advantages and disadvantages of this approach.

4. Suppose a series of binomial trials is stopped when the first "success" occurs. What distribution should be used for confidence intervals on the probability of success? Give some numerical examples.

5. A SE trial is planned with a fixed sample size of 25 patients, expecting 5 (20%) of them to "respond". Investigators will stop the study if 0 of the first 15 patients respond. What is the chance that a treatment with a true response rate of 20% will be discarded by such an approach? What about a treatment with a true response rate of 5%? Discuss the pros and cons of this simple rule for early stopping.

6. Standard treatment produces successes in 30% of patients. A new treatment will be pursued only if it seems to increase the success rate by 15%. Write a

formal statistical methods section for a protocol using an appropriate design for this situation.

7. A staged SE trial design uses the following stopping rules: 0/5, 1/10, 2/15 and 5/5, 9/10, 13/15. These correspond approximately to lower and upper 95% confidence bounds on $p = 0.5$. If the study stops early, the estimated proportion of successes will be biased. For example, when the true $p = 0.5$ and the 5/5 upper boundary is hit, the apparent p is 0.75. When the lower 2/15 boundary is hit, the apparent p is 0.13. Discuss ways to systematically investigate this bias.

8. A CTE randomized trial is investigating the reduction in mortality attributable to reduced dietary fat. Investigators choose $\alpha = 0.05$ (two-sided) and $\beta = 0.10$ for the trial design. Discuss the appropriateness of these choices.

9. Suppose the trial in Question 8 is studying the use of a synthetic fat substitute instead of dietary modification. Does your opinion of $\alpha = 0.05$ and $\beta = 0.10$ change? Why or why not?

10. A CTE randomized trial will compare the means of the two equally sized treatment groups using a t-test. How many patients are required to detect a difference of 0.5 standard deviations using $\alpha = 0.05$ (two sided) and $\beta = 0.20$? How does the sample size change if twice as many patients are assigned to one treatment as the other?

11. Suppose investigators wish to detect the difference between the proportion of successes of $p_1 = 0.4$ and $p_2 = 0.55$, using equal treatment groups with $\alpha = 0.05$ (two-sided) and $\beta = 0.10$. How large must the trial be? Suppose the allocation ratio is 1.5:1 instead of 1:1?

12. Investigators will compare survival on two treatments using the logrank statistic. What sample size is required to detect a hazard ratio of 1.5, assuming no censoring?

13. Five-year survival on standard treatment is 40%. If a new treatment can improve this figure to 60%, what size trial would be required to demonstrate it using $\alpha = 0.05$ (two-sided) and $\beta = 0.10$? How does this estimated sample size compare with one obtained using equation 7.15 for the difference of proportions? Discuss.

14. Compare the sample sizes obtained from equation 7.18 with those obtained by recasting the problem as a difference in proportions and using equation 7.15. Discuss.

15. Considering equation 7.17, what is the "optimal" allocation of subjects in a trial with a survival endpoint?

16. One could employ a Bayesian or frequentist approach to specifying the size of a SE clinical trial. Discuss the strengths and weaknesses of each and when they might be used.

Chapter References

Agresti, A. (1996). An Introduction to Categorical Data Analysis. New York: John Wiley & Sons.

Cox, D.R. (1953). Some simple tests for Poisson variates. Biometrika 40: 354-360.

Dalal, S.R., Fowlkes, E.B., and Hoadley, B. (1989). Risk analysis of the space shuttle: Pre-Challenger prediction of failure. J. Am. Statist. Assoc. 84: 945-957.

Diem, K. and Lentner, C. (Eds.) (1970). Scientific Tables, 7th Edition. Basel/ CIBA-Geigy.

Dixon, W.J. and Mood, A.M. (1948). A method for obtaining and analyzing sensitivity data. J. Am. Statist. Assoc. 43: 109-126.

Donner, A. (1984). Approaches to sample size estimation in the design of clinical trials – A review. Statistics in Med. 3: 199-214.

Elashoff, J.D. (1995). nQuery Advisor User's Manual. Los Angeles: Dixon Associates.

Ensign, L.G., Gehan, E.A., Kamen, D.S., and Thall, P.F. (1994). An optimal three-stage design for phase II clinical trials. Statistics in Med. 13: 1727-1736.

Epstein, B. and Sobel, M. (1953). Life testing. J. Am. Statist. Assoc. 48: 486-502.

Faries, D. (1994). Practical modifications of the continual reassessment method for phase I cancer clinical trials. J. Biopharmaceutical Statistics 4: 147-164.

Farrington, C.P. and Manning, G. (1990). Test statistics and sample size formulae for comparative binomial trials with null hypothesis of non-zero risk difference or non-unity relative risk. Statistics in Med. 9: 1447-1454.

Freedman, L.S. (1982). Tables of the number of patients required in clinical trials using the logrank test. Statistics in Med. 1, 121-9.

Gail, M. (1974). Power computations for designing comparative Poisson trials. Biometrics 30(2): 231-237.

Gehan, E.A. (1961). The determination of the number of patients required in a preliminary and follow-up trial of a new chemotherapeutic agent. J. Chron. Dis. 13: 346-353.

George, S.L. and Desu, M.M. (1974). Planning the size and duration of a clinical trial studying the time to some critical event. J. Chron. Dis. 27: 15-24.

Goldstein, R. (1989). Power and sample size via MS/PC-DOS computers. Am. Statistician 43: 253-260.

Goodman, S.N., Zahurak, M.L., and Piantadosi, S. (1995). Some practical improvements in the continual reassessment method for phase I studies. Statistics in Med. 14: 1149-1161.

Halperin, M. (1952). Maximum likelihood estimation in truncated samples. Ann. Math. Stat. 23: 226-238.

Hintze, J.L. (1996). PASS User's Guide: Power Analysis and Sample Size for Windows. Kaysville, UT: NCSS.

Korn, E.L., Midthune, D., Chen, T.T., Rubinstein, L.V., Christian, M.C., and Simon, R.M. (1994). A comparison of two phase I trial designs. Statistics in Med. 13: 1799-1806.

Kraemer, H.C. and Thiemann, S. (1987). How Many Subjects? Newbury Park, CA: Sage Publications.

Lachin, J.M. (1981). Introduction to sample size determination and power analysis for clinical trials. Controlled Clin. Trials 2: 93-113.

Lee, E.T. (1992). Statistical Methods for Surival Data Analysis, Second Edition. New York: John Wiley & Sons.

Lindley, D.V. and Scott, W.F. (1995). New Cambridge Statistical Tables, Second Edition. Cambridge: Cambridge University Press.

Machin, D. and Campbell, M.J. (1987). Statistical Tables for the Design of Clinical Trials. Oxford: Blackwell.

O'Quigley, J., and Chevret, S. (1991). Methods for dose finding studies in cancer clinical trials: A review and results of a Monte Carlo study. Statistics in Med. 10: 1647-1664.

O'Quigley, J., Pepe, M., and Fisher, L. (1990). Continual reassessment method: A practical design for phase I clinical trials in cancer. Biometrics 46: 33-48.

O'Quigley, J. and Shen, L.Z. (1996). Continual reassessment method: A likelihood approach. Biometrics 52: 673-684.

Piantadosi, S. and Liu, G. (1996). Improved dose escalation designs for phase I studies using pharmacokinetic measurements. Statistics in Medicine 15: 1605-1618.

Piantadosi, S. (1990). Clinical Trials Design Program. Cambridge, UK: BIOSOFT.

Robbins, H. and Monro, S. (1951). A stochastic approximation method. Annals Math. Stat. 22: 400-407.

Roebruck, P. and Kühn, A. (1995). Comparison of tests and sample size formulae for proving therapeutic equivalence based on the difference of binomial probabilities. Statistics in Med. 14: 1583-1594.

Rubinstein, L.V., Gail, M.H., and Santner, T.J. (1981). Planning the duration of a comparative clinical trial with loss to follow-up and a period of continued observation. J. Chron. Dis. 34: 469-479.

Sahai, H. and Khurshid, A. (1996). Formulae and tables for the determination of sample sizes and power in clinical trials for testing differences in proportions for the two-sample design: A review. Statistics in Med. 15: 1-21.

Schechtman, K.B. and Gordon, M.O. (1994). The effect of poor compliance and treatment side effects on sample size requirements in randomized clinical trials. J. Biopharmaceutical Statistics 4: 223-232.

Shuster, J.J. (1990). Handbook of Sample Size Guidelines for Clinical Trials. Boca Raton, FL: CRC Press.

Simon, R. (1989). Optimal two-stage designs for phase II clinical trials. Controlled Clinical Trials 10: 1-10.

Snedecor, G.W. and Cochran, W.G. (1980). Statistical Methods. Seventh Edition. Ames, IA: Iowa State University Press.

Storer, B.E. (1989). Design and analysis of phase I clinical trials. Biometrics 45: 925-937.

Thall, P.F. and Simon, R. (1994). A Bayesian approach to establishing sample size and monitoring criteria for phase II clinical trials. Controlled Clin. Trials 15: 463-481.

Vollset, S.E. (1993). Confidence intervals for a binomial proportion. Statistics in Med. 12: 809-824.

Wetherill, G.B. (1963). Sequential estimation of quantal response curves (with discussion). JRSS B 25: 1-48.

Winer, B.J. (1971). Statistical Principles in Experimental Design, Second Edition. New York: McGraw-Hill.

Wu, M., Fisher, M., and DeMets, D. (1980). Sample sizes for long-term medical trial with time-dependent dropout and event rates. Controlled Clinical Trials 1: 109-121.

Yates, F. (1984). Tests of significance for 2×2 contingency tables (with discussion). JRSS A 147: 426-463.

CHAPTER 8

The Study Cohort

8.1 Introduction

There is a well-known report by Moertel et al. [1974] describing response rates to 5-fluorouracil treatment for colon cancer in phase II trials. The authors show that essentially the same treatment for the same extent of disease as tested by 21 different investigators varied between 8% and 85%. Many of the response rates were estimated in studies with patient populations over 40 subjects, suggesting that random variation in the response rate is not the only reason for the observed differences. (See also Moertel and Reitemeier [1969], Moertel and Thynne [1982], and Leventhal and Wittes [1988].) How can rigorously performed studies of the same treatment yield such large differences in outcome?

Differences in outcome like these can be a consequence of many factors. However, given the same eligibility criteria for the various studies, only a few factors are likely to yield effects on outcome as strong as those seen: patient selection (or, equivalently, uncontrolled prognostic factors); different definitions of response; and differences in analysis such as post-treatment exclusion of some patients. Of these, patient selection factors may be the most difficult for investigators to control. I will use the term "eligibility criteria" to denote formal (written) specifications of inclusion/exclusion factors for a study, and "selection factors" to describe uncontrolled inclusion/exclusion factors.

Even when study eligibility criteria are carefully drafted and seemingly followed precisely by different investigators, they usually permit enough heterogeneity in the treatment groups at different institutions so that the results can vary considerably [e.g., Toronto Leukemia Study Group, 1986]. Although each patient individually meets the eligibility criteria, other prognostic or selection factors may be influential and systematically different at different institutions, contributing to variability in outcomes. As in the studies cited above, the differences in "outcomes" that are really differences in selection can be large enough to affect clinical inferences.

Apart from defining prognosis and encouraging homogeneity, another practical effect of eligibility criteria is to define the accrual base (i.e., accrual rate) for the trial. Every criterion tends to restrict the composition of the study cohort and prolong accrual. Because of this, the eligibility criteria can have important consequences for the resources that a trial will require. Also, the utility of a homogeneous study cohort produced by detailed eligibility criteria must be balanced against enhanced external validity resulting from looser criteria and a more heterogeneous population.

8.2   Defining the Study Cohort

The consequences of eligibility or selection effects may be most important for developmental studies. In fact, the utility of case reports, case series, and database analyses depends, in part, on the difficult task of comparing selection effects that determine how individuals were included in the collection of observations. In TM trials, preliminary evidence of efficacy can be influenced strongly by patient selection, although the primary goals of such studies are often unaffected. For DF (phase I) trials, selection issues arise because side effects, toxicity, or other determinants of dose can be a consequence of previous treatment and/or the underlying disease. For example, patients with advanced cancer may have been previously treated and have minimal reserve organ function. The maximum tolerated dose estimated in these patients is likely to be lower than in untreated patients or healthy study subjects.

It may be more difficult to isolate a biological effect of treatment if the study cohort consists of patients with a variety of disease types than if the study is performed in a homogeneous population. A narrowly defined cohort may have some external validity for others with the same disease, especially if the treatment appears to be beneficial. Investigators may have difficulty interpreting the results from a heterogeneous cohort, especially if the treatment does not appear to be beneficial.

In SE trials, the consequences of selection and eligibility factors may be even greater. These studies estimate the tolerability of a new therapy and are often performed in a single institution. It is natural to make direct, but statistically informal, comparisons between SE study results for different treatments. Unfortunately, this often confounds treatment effects with institutional selection effects, many of which can be as large as, or larger than, the treatment difference.

8.2.1   The trial may select patients with better or worse prognosis

Epidemiologists have defined the "healthy worker effect", a name for the observation that the general health of individuals who are employed is better than average. In other words, employed individuals may be unsuitable controls for case-control studies when case ascertainment is based on hospitalized patients. There are similar circumstances where patients who participate in a clinical trial have more favorable outcomes than those who refuse, even if the treatment is not effective [Tygstrup, Lachin, and Juhl, 1982]. This selection effect, which could be called the "trial participant effect", can be quite strong. It is of concern in situations where one treatment requires better baseline health and organ system function than alternative therapies. For example, this is common for surgical treatments where, on average, patients must be healthier to undergo an operative procedure than to receive medical therapy. However, even within surgical treatment, selection effects can be pronounced [Davis et al., 1985].

For example, currently there is interest in surgical lung volume reduction (LVR) for patients with chronic obstructive pulmonary disease (COPD), especially emphysema. Case series suggest that surgical removal of portions of the lung appears to improve pulmonary function and exercise tolerance in some patients. However, there are strong selection effects favoring those patients able to tolerate LVR. In a hypothetical randomized comparison of medical versus surgical management of COPD, surgical eligibility would be a prerequisite, making it likely that even study participants on medical therapy will have a better than average outcome. Similar circumstances surround "ventricular remodeling", a proposed surgical treatment for end-stage congestive heart failure, in which a portion of heart muscle is removed to improve cardiac function.

The impact of the trial participant effect is, to a certain degree, unavoidable in non-comparative designs. In randomized comparative trials, it is less of a problem, provided the selection effects do not help form the treatment groups differentially. Treatment *differences* are unlikely to be affected by selection effects that operate prior to randomization. However, if selection effects operate differentially in the treatment groups, because of either poor design or patient exclusions after treatment, problems with bias and study interpretation can occur, even in randomized trials.

An analytic example

The quantitative impact of selection effects can be seen in a theoretical example. Suppose we are interested in the average chance that individuals will respond to a particular treatment (response rate), and that this response probability, p, has a statistical distribution from person to person in the population. In other words, not everyone has exactly the same probability of responding to the treatment. For simplicity, assume that the differences from person to person are due only to chance and that the distribution of response probabilities in the population, denoted by $f(p)$, follows a standard beta distribution [Johnson and Kotz, 1970],

$$f(p) = \frac{1}{B(r, s)} p^{r-1} (1 - p)^{s-1},$$

for $0 \le p \le 1$, where $B(r, s) = \Gamma(r)\Gamma(s)/\Gamma(r + s)$ is the beta function. The reason for choosing this functional form for the distribution of response probabilities, aside from the fact that p ranges between 0 and 1, is purely convenience.

If all individuals in the population have an equal chance of being included in the study cohort (i.e., the trial cohort is selected randomly from the population), the expected value of the observed response rate will be the expected value of p in the population, which is

$$E(p) = \int_0^1 p \frac{1}{B(r,s)} p^{r-1} (1-p)^{s-1} dp = \frac{B(r+1,s)}{B(r,s)} = \frac{r}{r+s}.$$

This is what we would expect intuitively. For example, when $r = s$, the beta distribution is symmetric and the mean equals 0.5.

In contrast, suppose that there is a selection effect operating and individuals with a specific or narrow range of response probabilities are preferentially chosen for the trial. Such a selection effect could arise from non-random sampling of the population or could be constructed intentionally to choose those with a higher (or lower) response probability. Again for convenience, assume that this "weighting" of the study sample can also be summarized as a beta distribution,

$$w(p) = \frac{1}{B(a,b)} p^{a-1}(1-p)^{b-1}.$$

In other words, those with a response probability equal to $a/(a+b)$ are most likely to be chosen for the study cohort. However, individuals with *any* response probability *could* be included, because the beta distribution is continuous and covers the entire interval $(0,1)$. Note that $\int_0^1 w(p)dp = 1$. Using a sample subject to this type of selection, the expected response rate in the study cohort will be the average in the population *weighted* by the selection distribution,

$$
\begin{aligned}
E^*(p) &= \int_0^1 p\, w(p) \frac{1}{B(r,s)} p^{r-1}(1-p)^{s-1} dp \\
&= \frac{1}{B(a,b)} \frac{1}{B(r,s)} \int_0^1 p^{a+r-1}(1-p)^{b+s-2} dp \\
&= \frac{B(a+r,b+s-1)}{B(a,b) \cdot B(r,s)}.
\end{aligned}
$$

In general, this expected response rate in the study cohort is not equal to $r/(r+s)$, the mean value in the population, illustrating the potential for bias due to the selection effects. Only when all individuals in the population have an equal chance of being selected for the study (a uniform distribution or $a = b = 1$), or when there is no population variability, will the population and study cohort response probabilities be the same.

To illustrate this numerically, if $r = s = 5$, $a = 3$, and $b = 2$ (Figure 8.1), the true average probability of response in the population will be 0.5. However, in the study cohort,

$$\frac{B(3+5, 2+5-1)}{B(3,2) \cdot B(5,5)} = \frac{105}{143} = .734,$$

demonstrating the strong bias that is possible from nonrandom selection. Selection criteria that define a cohort narrowly in terms of response probability can produce a larger bias than broad selection. It is possible for non-uniform selection to yield no bias. For example, consider the previous case with $a = b = 5$. A randomized

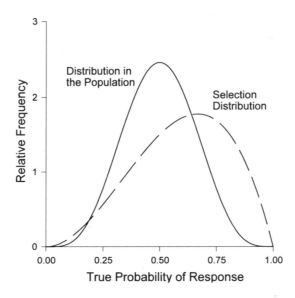

Figure 8.1 Distribution of true response probabilities in a population and selection probabilities for a study cohort.

comparative design will yield an unbiased estimate of the treatment *difference* in this situation, unless the treatment effect depends on the true response probability (e.g., treatment–covariate interaction). This illustrates again the benefit of a randomized concurrent control group.

8.2.2   Define the study population using eligibility and exclusion criteria

Because of the possible effects of prognostic and selection factors on differences in outcome, the eligibility criteria for the study cohort need to be defined thoughtfully. At least two philosophies have been proposed [Yusuf et al., 1990]. One approach is to define eligibility criteria with considerable restricting detail, increasing the homogeneity of the study cohort, reducing the variability in the estimated treatment effect, and possibly minimizing the size of the study. Studies designed in this way can yield clear and convincing evidence of biological effects, but may have less external validity than some other strategies. An alternative approach is to simplify and expand the eligibility criteria, permitting heterogeneity in the study cohort, and cope with the increased variability by increasing the sample size. This approach is suggested by advocates of large-scale trials (LST), CTE studies that appear to increase external validity because of their large and diverse study cohort (Chapter 4).

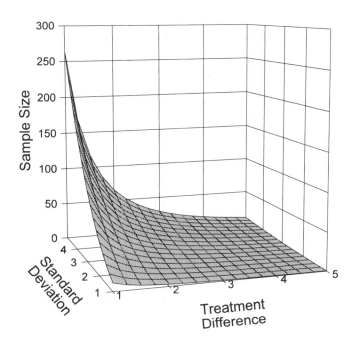

Figure 8.2 Sample size as a function of standard deviation and treatment difference.

Both of these approaches are useful in some situations and both have serious shortcomings in others. For example, LS trials are inappropriate for developmental studies, where it is usually more important to demonstrate a biological effect convincingly than prove its general validity. In either case, both the internal and external validity of a trial can depend strongly on the study cohort. In turn, the cohort is defined, at least operationally, by the eligibility criteria *and their interpretation* by the investigators. In many circumstances, the eligibility criteria are interpreted by less experienced investigators or study administrators, who may not be familiar with subtle intentions. The somewhat subjective nature of eligibility criteria needs to be considered when planning the study.

An example of the relationship between the required sample size of a comparative study, the standard deviation of the outcome measure, and the treatment difference of clinical importance is shown in Figure 8.2. This figure was plotted using points obtained from equation 7.13. Small changes in the standard deviation (actually the standard deviation divided by the treatment difference) do not strongly affect the sample size. However, the relationship between these two factors is an inverse square, so that larger differences substantially affect the sample size required. This motivates using a homogeneous cohort to minimize the size of the trial.

In many instances, endpoints may be evaluated more easily if certain complicating factors are prevented by patient exclusions. For example, if patients with recent non-pulmonary malignancies are excluded from a lung cancer trial, evaluation of tumor recurrences and second primaries might be made simpler. If and when disease progresses or recurs, investigators would be more certain that it was a consequence of the index cancer, rather than a pre-existing condition.

Ethical considerations also suggest that patients who are unlikely to benefit from the treatment (e.g., because of organ system dysfunction) not be allowed to participate in the trial. Presumably, the risk/benefit ratio will not be favorable for these individuals if the treatment carries much risk, as it often does in cancer trials. Whenever possible, quantitative parameters such as laboratory values should be used to make inclusionary and exclusionary definitions rather than qualitative clinical assessments. For example, some studies in patients with advanced cancer might call for a "life expectancy of at least 6 months". A more useful and reproducible criteria would be Karnofsky performance status greater than, say, 70.

8.2.3 Quantitative selection criteria should be used

The potential vagaries of interpretation can be reduced by stating inclusion and exclusion criteria quantitatively. In many clinical trials, especially those using drugs or cytotoxic therapy, the trial eligibility criteria require demonstrating good major organ system reserve, such as "normal" renal and hepatic function. The eligibility criteria might be specified in terms of normal values for key blood tests. However, "normal" lab values may differ from hospital to hospital and some sense of institutional norms is probably needed when specifying the criteria. For surgical treatment trials, the principle of using quantitative selection criteria is the same, but may extend to other organ systems such as pulmonary function.

One quantitative measure that should not routinely be used as an exclusionary criterion is age. Although advanced age is a good surrogate for declining functional reserve in many organ systems, one should not automatically exclude older persons from the study unless specific physiologic, anatomic, or other criteria require it. In studies of fatal illnesses such as AIDS, cancer, and some heart diseases, some studies attempt to exclude patients who have a very poor prognosis. Given the difficulties of prognosticating, criteria should be based on objective functional scores.

8.2.4 Comparative trials are not as sensitive to selection

In a sense, investigators can never precisely define the study cohort. Instead, they define the target population using selection and exclusion criteria and accept the fact that the study sample actually accrued will likely be different. The difference between the target population and those on the study may adversely affect external validity, as discussed above. For example, suppose a pharmacologic trial of a cytotoxic drug for cancer accrues patients who have been treated with other regimens but have had progressive disease. The organ system function of these individuals may appear normal when, in fact, their reserve has been lowered by prior therapy. Consequently, toxicities may occur at lower doses than they would in untreated patients.

This could yield an MTD that is too low, making the drug appear to have a response rate too low to be used as front-line therapy.

In randomized trials, this problem may not be as much of a concern. Although selection factors may render the trial cohort somewhat different from the general disease population, the relative treatment effect is more likely to be externally valid than in developmental trials. The only way that the relative treatment effect (or treatment difference) would be estimated incorrectly in an RCT is if the treatment effect is, to a large degree, a function of the characteristics of the cohort. In other words, if there is a treatment–covariate interaction, the relative treatment effect may be sensitive to selection factors. Because these types of interactions are uncommon, the actual composition of the cohort in an RCT is not as important for external validity as it is in developmental trials.

8.3   Assessing Accrual

Often in clinical trials, we think of measuring or anticipating accrual and determining other trial parameters, such as study duration, from it. In some circumstances, accrual may be under the control of the investigators. This can happen, for example, in multicenter trials, where additional institutions can be added to increase accrual.

One unfortunate and preventable mishap in conducting clinical trials is to plan and initiate a study, only to have it terminate early because of low accrual. This is a waste of resources and time for all those involved in the study. This situation can be avoided with some advanced planning and assumptions about the trial. First, investigators should know the accrual rate that is required to complete the study in a certain fixed period of time. Most researchers would like to see comparative treatment trials completed within five years and pilot or feasibility studies finished within a year or two. Disease prevention trials may take longer. In any case, the accrual rate required to complete a study within the time allowed can usually be estimated easily from the total sample size required.

Second, investigators need to obtain *realistic* estimates of the accrual rate. The number of patients with a specific diagnosis can often be determined from hospital or clinic records, but it is a large overestimate of potential study accrual. It must be reduced by the proportion of subjects likely to meet the eligibility criteria, and again by the proportion of those willing to participate in the trial (e.g., consenting to randomization). This latter proportion is usually less than half. Study duration can then be projected based on this potential accrual rate, which might be $1/4$ to $1/2$ of the patient population.

Third, investigators can project trial duration based on a worst-case accrual. The study may still be feasible under such contingencies. If not, plans for terminating the trial because of low accrual may be needed so as not to waste resources. Accrual estimates from participating institutions other than the investigator's own are often overly optimistic. How long will the study take as a single-institution trial?

8.3.1   Use a run-in period

Occasionally, accrual of eligible patients is not a concern, but the trial and its interpretation are likely to be complicated by the failure of many patients to adhere to the
treatment. When there is a potential for this to occur, a run-in period could be used
to increase the fraction of individuals on the study who comply with the treatment.
During the run-in period, eligible patients are monitored for treatment compliance,
using a placebo, for example. This monitoring can be complicated to implement.
Methods suggested for compliance monitoring include simple assessments like self-
reports, pill or medication counts, or more complex assessments, such as those based
on blood or urine samples. In any case, patients who are found to have poor compliance with the treatment can then be dropped from the study before the treatment
period begins.

It is possible that such a run-in period could decrease the external validity of the
trial. In the real world, patients regularly fail to comply with recommended treatments. A trial done under different circumstances with highly compliant patients
may overestimate the effectiveness of the treatment. This criticism is potentially
valid. However, it may be more important to establish the efficacy of the treatment
before deciding if it can be applied broadly.

8.3.2   Estimate accrual quantitatively

To estimate potential accrual more accurately, a formal survey of potential participants can be done before the trial begins. As patients are seen in clinic over a period
of time, investigators can keep a record to see if potential participants match the eligibility criteria. To estimate the proportion of eligible patients willing to give consent,
one could briefly explain the proposed study and ask if they would (hypothetically)
be willing to participate. These accrual surveys are most useful in multi-center collaborative groups that have a track record for performing studies. Often, databases
exist in these groups, which can be used effectively to help estimate accrual.

The expected number of events on the study can be modeled

Modeling the cumulative number of events in the study cohort is helpful for predicting the required duration of a trial with time to event endpoints. It can also be used to
predict cost and paper flow [Piantadosi and Patterson, 1987]. Suppose that subjects
are accrued over an interval of time $[0, T]$, at the end of which accrual is terminated.
Denote the accrual rate, survival function, and hazard function by $a(t)$, $S(t)$, and
$\lambda(t)$ respectively. The number of events observed at an arbitrary time t depends on
individuals accrued at all earlier times. To be counted as an event at t, an individual
must have been accrued at $u < t$, survived $t - u$ units of time, and had an event at t.
If $n(t)$ represents the number of events at t,

$$n(t) = \int_0^\tau a(u)\, S(t-u)\, \lambda(t-u)\, du, \qquad (8.1)$$

where $\tau = \min(t, T)$, i.e., the upper limit of integration extends only to the minimum
of t and T. We now make the simplifying assumptions of constant accrual $a(t) = a_0$,

and exponential survival so that equation 8.1 becomes

$$n(t) = a_0 \lambda \int_0^T e^{-\lambda \cdot (t-u)} \, du.$$

Then,

$$n(t) = \begin{cases} a_0 \left(1 - e^{-\lambda t}\right) & , \text{ if } t \leq T \\ a_0 \left(e^{-\lambda(t-T)} - e^{-\lambda t}\right) & , \text{ if } t > T \end{cases} . \tag{8.2}$$

The cumulative number of events observed before t is

$$D(t) = \int_0^t n(u) \, du.$$

Using the simplifying assumptions above and equation 8.2, we have

$$D(t) = \begin{cases} \frac{a_0}{\lambda} \left(\lambda t + e^{-\lambda \cdot t} - 1\right) & , \text{ if } t \leq T \\ \frac{a_0}{\lambda} \left(\lambda T + e^{-\lambda \cdot t} - e^{-\lambda \cdot (t-T)}\right) & , \text{ if } t > T \end{cases} . \tag{8.3}$$

Note that

$$\lim_{t \to 0} D(t) = 0$$

and

$$\lim_{t \to \infty} D(t) = a_0 T,$$

where $a_0 T$ is simply the total accrual.

Similar arguments apply to non-constant accrual and non-exponential survival distributions. However, obtaining practical results analogous to equations 8.2 and 8.3 is difficult or impossible for complicated functions.

Example 14 *Suppose a clinical trial requires 180 events to achieve its planned power. If accrual proceeds at a constant rate of 80 subjects per year for 4 years and the event rate is 0.13 per person-year of follow-up, how many events will have taken place after 4 years? We assume exponential survival. Substituting into equation 8.3 yields*

$$D(3) = \frac{80}{0.13} \times (0.13 \times 4 + e^{-0.13 \cdot 4} - 1) = 70 \; events.$$

The study will be only 40% finished, with respect to events, after 4 years. However, additional events will accumulate more quickly after 4 years due to the size of the study cohort. The number of subjects remaining on-study at 4 years is $320 - 70 = 250$ and the length of time required to observe 180 events is just under 7 years.

8.4   Other Considerations for the Study Cohort

8.4.1   Barriers can hinder trial participation

Among adult cancer patients in the U.S., less than 3% participate in clinical trials [Gotay, 1991]. Similar levels of participation in research studies would probably be found for many diseases. Exceptions might include AIDS and some uncommon pediatric conditions. Although the reasons for lack of participation are complex, they fall into three general categories: physician, patient, and administrative.

The reasons that physicians give for failing to enter eligible patients onto clinical trials include the perception that trials interfere with the physician–patient relationship and difficulties with informed consent [Taylor, Margolese, and Soskolne, 1984]. In some cases, participation in a trial may threaten the supposed expertise and authority of the physician. This is likely to be less of a problem in the future as patients become more active in choosing from among treatment options. The increasing use of second opinions instituted by patients and insurers and, patients' assertive participation in multiple AIDS treatments are examples.

Informed consent procedures can be cumbersome, intimidating, and time consuming. Often patients who give consent do not retain the detailed knowledge about the treatments or the study that investigators would like them to. This suggests difficulties with the consent process that may discourage patients and their families from completing it. Many consent forms are not written at an appropriate reading level. The process tends to overstate risks and understate benefits from participating in research studies as a way of minimizing the liability of investigators and their institutions. An accurate portrayal of these details would require excessively long and technical consent documents.

Some investigators are implicitly or explicitly formulating the idea that patients have a *right* to participate in research studies [Elks, 1993]. This new right is seen to arise as an extension of the principle of autonomy. I believe this notion is incorrect because it presupposes benefits from participation that may not exist. This is true on the individual participant level and also on a group or societal level. This point will be expanded below. Furthermore, this right cannot be exercised universally, even if it exists because the number of clinical trials is too small.

Many patients are mistrustful of the medical establishment, even though they trust their individual physicians. Recent public reactions to proposed changes in health care, such as managed, care indicate this. Even stronger reactions are often evident among racial and ethnic minority groups regarding participation in clinical trials. Of the small amount of research that has been done in this area, results related to cancer suggest three points: 1) patients are not well informed about trials, 2) they believe that trials will be of personal benefit, and 3) patients are mistrustful [Roberson, 1994]. Such factors help explain the low minority participation on many research studies.

Table 8.1 General Characteristics and Orientation of Efficacy and Effectiveness Trials

Characteristic	Efficacy Trial	Effectiveness Trial
Purpose	Test a biological question	Assess effectiveness
Number of participants	Less than 1000	Tens of thousands
Cost	Moderate	Large
Orientation	Treatment	Prevention
Cohort	Homogeneous	Heterogeneous
Data	Complex and detailed	Simple
Focus of inference	Internal validity	External validity
Eligibility	Strict	Relaxed

8.4.2 Efficacy versus effectiveness trials

There are two views of the role of clinical trials in evaluating medical therapies today. They overlap considerably with regard to the methodology that is required, but can generate differences of opinion about the appropriate study sample to enroll, coping with data imperfections (Chapter 11), and the best settings for applying clinical trials. The first view is that trials are primarily developmental tools used to make inferences about biological questions. These types of studies tend to be smaller than their counterparts (discussed below) and employ study cohorts that are relatively homogeneous. Studies with these characteristics are sometimes called "efficacy" trials, a term and distinction incorrectly attributed to Cochrane [1972]. With this perspective, investigators tend to emphasize the internal validity of the study and generalize to other settings based primarily on biological knowledge.

A second perspective on trials is that they are evaluation tools used to test the worth of interventions that should be applied on a large scale. They are motivated by the fact that a biologically sound therapy may not be effective when applied outside the controlled setting of a developmental trial. These trials are large, applied in heterogeneous populations, and use simple methods of assessment and data capture. In Chapter 4, I referred to these studies as large-scale (LS) trials. They have also been called "effectiveness trials", "large simple", and "public health" trials. Investigators conducting these trials tend to emphasize the external validity of the studies and expect that their findings will have immediate impact on medical practice.

A concise summary of the difference between these types of studies is shown in Table 8.1. These characterizations are approximations and simplifications. It is easy to find studies that fit neither category well or have elements of both. As we have already seen, some treatments become widely accepted and validated without using any structured methods of evaluation. Other treatments are developed using both types of studies at different times. Viewed in this way, we can see that the proper emphasis of clinical trials is not an "either-or" question about effectiveness or efficacy. Both pathways and types of studies have useful roles in developing and disseminating medical therapies.

The importance of these distinctions for the study cohort primarily relates to the breadth of the eligibility criteria. For any particular trial, these criteria should be broad enough to permit inclusion of enough patients to answer the research question quickly. However, the criteria should not permit more heterogeneity than is clinically useful. For example, the bioavailability of a compound may be in question and could be established using a small number of study subjects who meet fairly narrow eligibility criteria. Questions about the bioavailability in different individuals are important, but could be answered by combining the study result with other biological knowledge. It may not be efficient to try to determine this empirically.

8.4.3   Representation

In recent years, the clinical trials community has focused a great deal of attention on the composition of study cohorts, particularly with regard to their gender and minority make-up. A perception developed early that women and minorities were "under represented" in clinical studies of all types and that this was a problem for scientific inference [e.g., Roberson, 1994; Schmucker and Vesell, 1993; Sechzer et al., 1994].

The legislative solution for this problem was contained in the NIH Revitalization Act of 1993 [Public Law103-43, 1993]:

> The Director of NIH shall ensure that the trial is designed and carried out in a manner sufficient to provide for a valid analysis of whether the variables being studied in the trial affect women or members of minority groups, as the case may be, differently than other subjects in the trial.

Some exceptions to this requirement are permitted, although the law explicitly excludes cost as a reason for noncompliance. There are many scientific reasons why one would test for treatment–sex (or race) interactions in specific circumstances. However, to require *always* testing for them while ignoring the consequences of known effect modifiers such as major organ function, and to increase the cost of performing trials to do so, requires something other than a scientific perspective.

As for the under-representation belief, in the case of women, reliable and convincing data to support or refute such a claim are simply not available [Mastroianni, Faden, and Federman, 1994]. Data from published studies suggest that female:male participation of individuals in clinical trials is about 2:3. Published female-only trials tend to be larger than male-only studies, and there were probably as many female-only trials as male-only trials before the law was passed [Gilpin and Meinert, 1994]. For ethnic subsets, few data are available.

NIH and FDA Guidelines

The response of scientists at NIH to the requirements of the law is evident in the guidelines published to implement them [DHHS, 1994]. The guidelines essentially restrict the applicability of the law to phase III trials and require an assessment of existing evidence from animal studies, clinical observations, natural history, epidemiology, and other sources to determine the likelihood of "significant differences of clinical or public health importance in intervention effect". When such differences are expected, the design of the trial must permit answering the primary question in each subset. When differences in treatment effects are not expected, are known not to exist, or are unimportant for making therapeutic decisions, the composition of the study group is unimportant. In cases where the evidence neither supports nor refutes the possibility of different treatment effects, representation is required, although "the trial will not be required to provide high statistical power for each subgroup".

In view of the wording of the law, the NIH guidelines are helpful because they intend to restore a scientific perspective on the design of phase III trials. When no conclusive information about treatment–covariate interactions is available, a "valid analysis" is implicitly defined as being unbiased, because trials with low statistical power are permitted. Presumably, very large interactions would be evident from such designs. However, if "valid analysis" means "unbiased" as opposed to "high statistical power", then some clinically important interactions could remain undetected. This seems to be contrary to the intent of the law. Thus, there does not appear to be a reasonable scientific perspective that can be superimposed on the law and the "fix-up" is inescapably empirical.

The FDA guidelines concerning women of childbearing potential [DHHS, 1993] also attempt to impose scientific thinking on an empirical law. They deal with the issues in a more mechanistic fashion, emphasizing the role of pharmacokinetic analyses in detecting possible gender differences. Also, the exclusion of women of child-bearing potential from early trials has been eliminated. Additionally, the FDA states

> . . . representatives of both genders should be included in clinical trials in numbers adequate to allow detection of clinically significant gender-related differences in drug response [DHHS, 1993].

Although questions of "validity" and "power" are not addressed, this statement seems to be at odds with the NIH guidelines. Nowhere in the guidelines does it say explicitly that FDA will refuse drug approval on the basis of failure to study patients adequately representative of those with the disease. One can easily imagine circumstances in which this would be reasonable, and other situations in which it would not be.

An interesting example arose recently when the FDA approved the use of Tamoxifen for treatment of male breast cancer, virtually exclusively on the basis of biological similarity of the disease to female breast cancer, rather than on the results of well-performed clinical trials in men. Furthermore, during advisory committee review of the issue, there was little, if any, discussion of male-female differences in response to Tamoxifen. Outcomes such as this are consistent with a biology-based approach to the issues, but are at odds with the current law and written policy.

Treatment–covariate interactions

One reason for requiring a cohort with a particular composition (e.g., age, sex, or ethnic background) on a clinical trial is to be able to study interactions between the treatment and the covariate. For example, if males and females are likely to have clinically significantly different treatment effects, the trial should probably be designed to permit studying the difference. To accomplish this efficiently, equal numbers of

males and females should be accrued rather than proportions representative of those
with the disease.

The cost of testing treatment–covariate interactions can be high, even for balanced covariates. For example, the variance of the difference of two means, analogous to a main effect, is $2\sigma^2/n$, where the variance of an observation is σ^2 and n
observations contribute to each mean. The variance of the difference of differences,
analogous to a treatment–covariate interaction, is $4\sigma^2/n$. Thus, twice as many subjects are required for a test of treatment–covariate interaction to yield the same precision as an overall test of treatment effect. Covariate imbalances will decrease the
precision. Ordinarily, we would not design trials to detect such effects with high
precision, unless it was very important to learn about them.

8.5   Summary

A clinical trial cohort is defined by the eligibility and exclusion criteria. The criteria are chosen with a target population in mind, but often the study cohort will not
closely resemble the intended population. This selection effect is a consequence of
interpretations by the investigators and chance and limits the comparability of different single-arm studies, even though they have the same selection criteria. In randomized comparative trials, the selection effects are the same in all treatment groups,
validating the comparisons.

Realistic quantitative assessments of accrual are necessary when planning a clinical trial. Simple mathematical models can help predict the expected duration of a
study and the number of events that will be observed over time.

In the last few years, there has been a great deal of interest in the gender and ethnic
composition of trial participants. This interest arises, in part, from concerns about the
generalizeability of trial results. Large heterogeneous study populations offer some
advantages for generalizing results empirically, but may not be optimal for proving
biological principles. Removing barriers to trial participation and employing representative cohorts is essential for the health of medical studies. However, required
representation in clinical trials could be a hindrance to acquiring new knowledge if
it consumes too many resources.

8.6   Questions for Discussion

1. Suppose the population consists of only two types of individuals. Half of all
    patients have a response probability of 0.25 and the other half have a response
    probability of 0.40. If both types of patients are equally likely to be accrued
    on a trial, what response probability can we expect to observe? How will
    this change if the eligibility criteria select 2:1 in favor of those with a higher
    response probability?

2. Suppose the accrual rate onto a trial is constant and the event times (survival)
    are exponentially distributed with hazard λ. After the accrual period, there is

a fixed-length follow-up period. Derive expressions for the number of events and cumulative number of events as functions of time and these parameters. Illustrate how follow-up time (or total study duration) can be substituted for new accruals.

3. Response data from a clinical trial will be analyzed using a linear model. For the ith patient,

$$Y_i = \beta_0 + \beta_1 T_i + \beta_2 X_i + \gamma T_i X_i,$$

where T and X are binary indicator variables for treatment group and covariate, respectively, Y is the response, and the other parameters are to be estimated from the data. γ models the interaction between treatment and covariate. Using ordinary least squares (or maximum likelihood), what is the relative magnitude of $Var\{\beta_1\}$, $Var\{\beta_2\}$, and $Var\{\gamma\}$? Discuss.

4. One way to generalize the results from clinical trials is empirical. This perspective suggests that, if females are not in the study population, the results do not pertain to them. Another way to generalize is biological. This perspective suggests that learning about males informs us about females insofar as biological similarities will allow. Discuss the merits and deficiencies of each point of view.

Chapter References

Cochrane, A.L. (1972). Effectiveness and Efficiency. London: Nuffield Provincial Hospital Trust.

Davis, S., Wright, P.W., Schulman, S.F. et al. (1985). Participants in prospective, randomized clinical trials for resected non-small cell lung cancer have improved survival compared with nonparticipants in such trials. Cancer 56: 1710-1718.

Department of Health and Human Services (DHHS) (1994). NIH Guidelines on the Inclusion of Women and Minorities as Subjects in Clinical Research. Federal Register 59: 14508-14513.

Department of Health and Human Services (DHHS) (1993). NIH Guideline for the Study and Evaluation of Gender Differences in the Clinical Evaluation of Drugs; Notice. Federal Register 58, 39406-39416.

Elks, M.L. (1993). The right to participate in research studies. J. Lab. Clin. Med. 122: 130-136.

Gilpin, A.K. and Meinert, C.L. (1994). Gender bias in clinical trials? Proceedings of the Society for Clinical Trials, Houston, Texas.

Gotay, C.C. (1991). Accrual to cancer clinical trials: Directions from the research literature. Soc. Sci. Med. 33: 569-577.

Johnson, N.L. and Kotz, S. (1970). Continuous Univariate Distributions. Boston: Houghton Mifflin.

Leventhal, B.G. and Wittes, R.E. (1988). Research Methods in Clinical Oncology. New York: Raven Press.

Mastroianni, A.C., Faden R., and Federman, D. (Eds.) (1994). Women and Health Research: Ethical and Legal Issues of Including Women in Clinical Studies. Washington, DC: National Academy Press.

Moertel, C.G. and Reitemeier, R.J. (1969). Advanced Gastrointestinal Cancer. Clinical Management and Chemotherapy. New York: Harper and Row.

Moertel, C.G., Schutt, A.J., Hahn, R.G., and Reitemeier, R.S. (1974). Effects of patient selection on results on phase II chemotherapy trials in gastrointestinal cancer. Cancer Chemother. Rep. 58: 257-260.

Moertel, C.G. and Thynne, G.S. (1982). Large Bowel. In J.F. Holland and E. Frei III (Eds.), Cancer Medicine (pp.1830-1859). 2nd edition. Philadelphia: Lea and Febiger.

Piantadosi, S., and Patterson, B. (1987). A method for predicting accrual, cost, and paper flow in clinical trials. Controlled Clin. Trials 8: 202-215.

Public Law 103-43 (1993). Clinical Research Equity Regarding Women and Minorities. Public Law 103-43, Subtitle B, Sec. 131.

Roberson, N.L. (1994). Clinical trial participation. Cancer 74: 2687-2691.

Schmucker, D.L. and Vesell, E.S. (1993). Underrepresentation of women in clinical drug trials. Clin. Pharmacol. Ther. 54: 11-15.

Sechzer, J.A., Rabinowitz, V.C., Denmark, F.L., McGinn, M.F., Weeks, B.M., and Wilkens, C.L. (1994). Sex and gender bias in animal research and in clinical studies of cancer, cardiovascular disease, and depression. Ann. N.Y. Acad. Sci. 736: 21-.

Taylor, K.M., Margolese, R.G., and Soskolne, C.L. (1984). Physicians' reasons for not entering eligible patients in a randomized clinical trial of surgery for breast cancer. New Engl. J. Med. 310: 1363-1367.

Toronto Leukemia Study Group (1986). Results of chemotherapy for unselected patients with acute myeloblastic leukaemia: Effect of exclusions on interpretation of results. Lancet 1: 786-788.

Tygstrup, N., Lachin, J.M., and Juhl, E. (Eds.) (1982). The Randomized Clinical Trial and Therapeutic Decisions. New York: Marcel Dekker.

Yusuf, S., Held, P., Teo, K.K., and Toretsky, E.R. (1990). Selection of patients for randomized controlled trials: Implications of wide or narrow eligibility criteria. Statistics in Med. 9: 73-86.

CHAPTER 9

Treatment Allocation

9.1 Introduction

There are several different ways in which physicians can recommend treatments for patients. The most common is the way in which the physician in clinical practice ordinarily uses the diagnosis, characteristics of the individual patient, medical knowledge, opinion, patient preference, and constraints produced by the circumstances to recommend a treatment. Treatment choice made in this way does not facilitate investigating questions of efficacy, unless differences in outcome are very large. Therefore, this type of treatment selection is not a consideration in clinical trials.

A second type of treatment assignment occurs when physicians use a single therapy exclusively. This could be a consequence of following a non-comparative study protocol. More commonly, it happens because teaching suggests that there is a single best therapy for a particular condition. However, exclusive use of one treatment can result from opinion, tradition, dogma, or individual or institutional preferences. In any case, physicians using a single therapy do not control treatment allocation, selection bias, or confounders. These shortcomings are evident when comparing case series from different times, institutions, or clinics. Treatment assignments made in this way are haphazard with respect to assessing treatment *differences*, and are not a consideration in comparative clinical trials, except to differentiate the allocation method from that used in true experimental designs.

The third way of making treatment choices is based on active control of the alternatives and allocation process by the investigator, with the purpose of avoiding biases and correlations. This method of treatment allocation can be performed deterministically, randomly, or by a mixture of the two, usually called constrained randomization. Treatment assignments made in this way are directly relevant to true experimental designs. Although non-random but unbiased treatment assignment schemes (e.g., alternating assignments) can serve the purpose of eliminating bias, they are subject to *discovery* by investigators and would reveal information about future assignments. This, in turn, could permit a systematic difference in the treatment groups (bias) if patients with a particular characteristic are sequenced according to knowledge of the assignment scheme. In contrast, properly constructed and used random schemes are not subject to discovery (unless too tightly constrained) and, therefore, are more convincing ways of eliminating biased assignments.

9.1.1   Allocation is concerned with practical issues

When choosing an allocation scheme for a clinical trial, there are three technical considerations: reducing bias, producing a balanced comparison, and quantifying errors attributable to chance. The allocation scheme should convincingly satisfy these objectives or the outcome of the trial may be questioned. Bias in treatment assignment can be reduced or eliminated when prognostic factors do not differentially affect the composition of comparison groups. Operationally, this means that control over individual assignments is removed from the investigator. Credibility requires the assignment process to be non-discoverable. Although a non-discoverable deterministic assignment scheme can remove bias and balance prognostic factors, it is usually easier and more convincing to employ a random assignment scheme.

Issues surrounding the methods and administration of randomized treatment allocation appear as though they should be straightforward. There are few circumstances where simple methods of treatment assignment in clinical trials are inappropriate. Problems with simple allocation schemes tend to be small in magnitude and arise only infrequently. However, there are several different methods of treatment allocation commonly used for "randomized" studies [Kalish and Begg, 1985]. We refer to them collectively as randomization, although each may have different properties and advantages. Also, we tend to equate *impartial* assignment with *balanced* assignment. Although this is not necessarily correct, when treatment groups do not meet our expectation of being balanced (with respect to both group size and risk factor composition), we tend to view the trial results with more suspicion and concern than when the comparison groups are well balanced. Therefore, balance is a practical component of credibility.

There are three potential problems that motivate the use of randomized treatment assignments in comparative clinical trials. The first is the wide variation in clinical outcomes relative to the magnitude of effects or differences that treatments are likely to produce. Good study design, including randomization, helps control and quantify this variability. The second motive arises because of selection bias, or as Miettinen [1983] described it, "confounding by indication". This means that individuals with certain characteristics are more likely to receive particular treatments, confounding the effects of the therapy with prognostic factors. Without randomization, selection of patients for particular treatments could yield differences of a clinically important size but due only to bias.

Third, researchers are usually unable to characterize why individuals receive a particular treatment or define homogeneous risk strata for non-randomized comparisons. If we could characterize quantitatively the relationship between risk factors and treatment choice outside a trial, the effect of selection could be undone, yielding an unbiased treatment comparison. Alternatively, if we knew all prognostic factors, we could define homogeneous risk strata and make treatment comparisons within each. The treatment differences could then be pooled across strata to yield a valid overall estimate. The most practical and convincing way to avoid these problems is to use random treatment assignment.

9.2   Randomization

In some cultures, chance phenomena were a means of communicating with the gods or were associated with chaos and darkness. In some, unpredictability was associated with danger. In other cultures, randomness has been a time-honored method to apportion blame and remove human bias. As Barrow [1991] says in his brief but interesting discussion of this topic in a cosmological context,

> ... dabbling with random devices was serious theological business, not something to be trifled with or merely studied for the fun of it.

In contemporary Western society, we use randomization more for demonstrating a convincing lack of bias than for superstitious reasons, e.g., coin flips before sporting contests and choosing straws for unpleasant tasks. In clinical trials, researchers use randomization for its objectivity in removing bias.

In Western science, randomization was suggested formally by R. A. Fisher in the 1920s [Box, 1980] and used in medical studies by Bradford Hill and Richard Doll in Great Britain in the 1940s. In the United States, randomization was advocated by early trialists such as Tom Chalmers and Paul Meier. It continues to be widely used for preventing bias in allocating treatments in comparative clinical trials and is popular because of its simplicity and reliability.

In an early single-masked tuberculosis treatment clinical trial in the United States, randomization was used slightly differently than it is today. The investigators stated

> The 24 patients were then divided into two approximately comparable groups of 12 each. The cases were individually matched, one with another, in making this division. ... Then, by a flip of the coin, one group became identified as group I (sanocrysin-treated) and the other as group II (control) [Amberson et al., 1931].

Today, investigators seldom have treatment groups already composed and ready for randomization as a whole. Instead, each individual patient is usually randomized independently, although both procedures are logically equivalent. Even when the experimental unit is a group rather than an individual, we may not be able to randomize all clusters at once. Current practice and theory associated with randomization is discussed by Lachin, Matts, and Wei [1988] and Lachin [1988a; 1988b]. For a discussion of the timing of randomization, see Durrleman and Simon [1991].

9.2.1 Randomization prevents influence of unknown factors

Randomization is an effective means for reducing bias in treatment selection, because it guarantees that treatment assignment will not be based on patients' prognostic factors. This prevents the investigators from consciously or unconsciously assigning better prognosis patients to a treatment that they hope will be superior. Because selection bias can influence outcomes as strongly as many treatment effects, preventing it is an important benefit of randomization.

Selection bias is not the only one which plagues clinical studies. Treatment administration, outcomes assessment, and counting endpoints can all be biased, in spite of random treatment assignment.

Example 15 *Consider an unblinded trial with randomization between treatment and no treatment. The placebo effect will contribute to the apparent efficacy of the treatment. In other words, it may bias the estimated treatment effect. In contrast, if the same trial employs a placebo control, the estimated treatment difference should not be biased.*

Thus, randomization does not guarantee complete objectivity in a trial and must be combined with other design strategies to reduce bias.

A second, and more far-reaching, benefit of randomization is that it prevents confounding, even if the investigator is unaware that the effects exist and/or has not measured them. One argument against randomization is that it is unnecessary because confounders can be controlled in the analysis by using statistical adjustment procedures. However, prevention is better than control. Furthermore, the extent to which confounding can be controlled reliably depends on two additional assumptions: 1) the investigators are aware of, and have measured, all the important confounders in the experimental subjects, and 2) the assumptions underlying the statistical models or other adjustment procedures are known to be correct. Randomization obviates these problems. Critics sometimes overlook this last point, which provides randomized studies with their high degree of inferential directness and credibility.

Thus, randomization corrects many of the important limitations of studies with non-randomized controls. It prevents effects from unknown prognostic factors and eliminates differential treatment selection effects, whether due to patient choice or physician judgment. Randomization facilitates defining start of treatment and controls time trends in the disease, patient population, diagnostic methods, and ancillary care. Interesting examples where investigators did not make the mistake of claiming definitive treatment differences in a non-randomized comparison for reasons similar to those just outlined are given by Green and Byar [1984]. One example is based on the report by Byar et al. [1979].

Although the benefits of randomization are considerable, there are methodologic problems and biases that it cannot eliminate. One example is limitation of the external validity of a trial. Eligibility restrictions that reduce variability in trials limit the spectrum of patients studied and consequently can reduce the external validity of findings. A second problem is the limited treatment algorithm that most clinical trials study. The experimental structure simplifies and restricts interventions to control them. This may not reflect how the treatments are used in actual practice. A third problem that randomization alone cannot eliminate is bias in the ascertainment of outcomes. Treatment masking and other design features are needed to eliminate this bias.

9.2.2   Haphazard assignments are not random

In many nonexperimental study designs, the methods by which patients came to receive the treatments they actually got are unknown. Presumably, the treating physicians used information at hand in the usual way to select treatments which they felt were best. At the worst, the physicians were ineffective at this and the treatments were assigned in a haphazard fashion. Even in such a case, treatment comparisons based on these data lack credibility and reliability compared with those from a randomized trial. Haphazard assignments are not random and cannot be relied upon to reduce bias. When reviewing the results of a comparative trial, we want to be convinced that accidents or selection and other biases are not responsible for differences observed.

If one could be certain that patients presented themselves for study entry in a purely random fashion and that investigators would use no prognostic information whatsoever to assign treatments, then virtually any allocation pattern would be effectively random. For example, a trial might employ alternating treatment assignments, under the assumption that the patients available are a temporally random sample of those with the disease under study. While this might be credible, it relies on the additional assumption of random arrival in the clinic. Investigators would prefer to control randomization convincingly instead of leaving it to chance!

9.2.3   Simple randomization can yield imbalances

Simple randomization makes each new treatment assignment without regard to those already made. In other words, a simply randomized sequence has no memory of its past history. While this has important advantages, it can also produce certain unwanted effects in a clinical trial. The most common adverse consequence is an imbalance in the number of subjects assigned to one of the treatments. For example, suppose we are studying two treatments, A and B, and we randomize a total of N subjects with probability $p = 0.5$ to each treatment group. When the trial is over, the size of the two treatment groups will not, in general, be equal. In fact, the chance that $N_A = N_B = N/2$ is only

$$\Pr[X = N/2] = \binom{N}{\frac{N}{2}} \left(\frac{1}{2}\right)^N ,$$

which can be quite small. For example, when $N = 100$, the chance of the randomization yielding exactly 50 subjects per group is only about 8%.

It is informative to consider the probability of imbalances greater than or equal to some specified size. Using properties of the binomial distribution, the expected number of assignments to each of two groups is

$$E\{N_A\} = E\{N_B\} = Np \,,$$

and the variance of the number of assignments is

$$Var\{N_A\} = Var\{N_B\} = Np(1-p).$$

When $N = 100$ and $p = 1/2$, the variance of N_A is 25. An approximate 95% confidence bound on the number of assignments to treatment A is $N_A \pm 1.96 \times \sqrt{25} \approx N_A \pm 10$. Thus, we would expect more than a 60/40 imbalance in favor of A (or B) 5% of the time using simple randomization.

This problem of imbalance becomes more noticeable when we must account for influential prognostic factors. Even if the number of treatment assignments is balanced, the distribution of prognostic factors may not be. For example, suppose there are k independent dichotomous prognostic factors, each with probability 0.5 of being "positive". We compare two treatment groups with respect to the proportion of subjects with a positive prognostic factor. Using a type I error of 5% for the comparison, the chance of balance on any one variable is 0.95. The chance of balance on all k factors is 0.95^k (assuming independence). Thus, the chance of finding at least one factor unbalanced is $1 - 0.95^k$. When $k = 5$, the chance of at least one statistically significant imbalance is 0.23, explaining the frequency with which this problem is noticed.

From a practical point of view, large imbalances in the number of treatment assignments or the distribution of covariates can lessen the credibility of trial results. Even though statistical methods can account for the effects, if any, of imbalances that occur by chance, we are usually left feeling uneasy by large or significant differences in baseline characteristics between the treatment groups. For large, expensive, and unique trials to be as credible as possible, the best strategy is to prevent the imbalances from occurring in the first place. One way to control the magnitude of imbalances in these studies is to use constrained, rather than simple, randomization. There are two general methods of constrained randomization – blocked randomization and minimization. These will be discussed in the next sections.

9.3 Constrained Randomization

9.3.1 Blocking improves balance

Randomization in blocks is a simple constraint that improves balance in the number of treatment assignments in each group [Matts and Lachin, 1988]. A "block" contains a pre-specified number and proportion of treatment assignments. The size of each block must be an exact integer multiple of the number of treatment groups. A sequence of blocks makes up the randomization list. Within each block, the order of the treatments is randomly permuted, but they are exactly balanced at the end of

Table 9.1 All Possible Permutations of Two Treatments in Blocks of Size 4

Within-Block	Permutation Number					
Assignment Number	1	2	3	4	5	6
1	A	A	A	B	B	B
2	A	B	B	B	A	A
3	B	A	B	A	B	A
4	B	B	A	A	A	B

each block. After making all the assignments in each block, the treatment groups are exactly balanced as intended.

To see that this scheme is constrained randomization, consider two treatment groups, A and B, and blocks of size $N_A + N_B$. During the randomization, the current number of assignments in a block made to treatment A is n_A and likewise for B. At the start of each new block, we reset $n_A = n_B = 0$. Then, the blocking constraint can be produced by setting the probability of assignment to treatment A to

$$\Pr[A] = \frac{N_A - n_A}{N_A + N_B - n_A - n_B} \tag{9.1}$$

for each assignment. When N_A assignments have been made in a block, $n_A = N_A$ and the probability of getting A is 0. When N_B assignments have been made, the probability of getting A is 1. This is a useful way to generate blocked assignments by computer. To make each new assignment, we compare a random number, u, uniformly distributed on the interval $(0,1)$ to $\Pr[A]$. If $u \le \Pr[A]$, the assignment is made to A. Otherwise, it is made to B.

Suppose there are two treatments, A and B, and blocks of size 4 are used. There are six possible permutations of two treatments in blocks of size 4 (Table 9.1). The assignment scheme consists of a string of blocks chosen randomly (with replacement) from the set of possible permutations. If we are unlucky enough to stop the trial halfway through a block in which the first two assignments are A's, the imbalance will be only 2 extra in favor of treatment A. This illustrates that the maximum imbalance is one-half of the block size.

The number of orderings of the treatments within small blocks is not very large. Usually it makes sense to use relatively small block sizes to balance the assignments at frequent intervals. Suppose there are 2 treatments and the block size is $2b$. Then, there are $\binom{2b}{b}$ different permutations of the assignments within blocks. If the trial ends exactly halfway through a block, the excess number of assignments in one group will be no greater than b and is likely to be less. Blocking in a similar fashion can be applied to unbalanced allocations or for more than two treatments. For more than two treatments, the number of permutations can be calculated from multinomial coefficients and the assignments can be generated from formulae similar to equation 9.1.

In an actual randomization, all blocks do not have to be the same size. Varying the length of each block (perhaps randomly) makes the sequence of assignments appear more random and can help prevent discovery. These sequences are not much more difficult to generate or implement than fixed block sizes. In practice, one could choose a small set of block sizes from which to select. For example, for two treatments, we could randomly choose from among blocks of length 2, 4, 6, or any multiple of 2. For three treatments, the block sizes would be multiples of 3.

9.3.2 Blocking and stratifying balances prognostic factors

To balance several clinically important prognostic factors, the randomization can be blocked and stratified. Every prognostic factor combination can be made an individual stratum, with blocking in each. Then, the treatment assignments will be balanced in each stratum, yielding balanced risk factors in each treatment group. This balance can improve the power of trials [Palta, 1985].

An example using blocks of size 4 should help make this clear (Table 9.2). Suppose there are two prognostic factors, age (young versus old) and sex. To balance both, we would form four strata: young-female, young-male, old-female, and old-male. Blocked assignments are generated for each stratum. Each patient receives the next treatment assignment from the stratum into which he or she fits and the strata do not necessarily all fill at the same rate.

In a blocked stratified trial such as this, we could stop the trial when all strata are half filled, all with an excess of assignments on A (or B). For example, the sequence of assignments depicted in Table 9.2 could end halfway through all current blocks and with the last two assignments being AA (or BB). Block #2 in the old-female stratum is of this type. This situation creates the largest imbalance that could occur.

For a trial with b assignments of each treatment in every block (block size $= 2b$) and k strata, the size of the maximum imbalance using blocked strata is $b \times k$. In other words, each stratum could yield an excess of b assignments for the same treatment. The same is true if b is the *largest* number of assignments possible to one treatment in a block in each of k strata when a variable block size is used. If b_j represents the largest excess number of assignments possible in a block in the jth stratum (not necessarily the same for all strata), the largest imbalance (total excess number of assignments on one group) possible is $b_1 + b_2 + \ldots + b_k$.

Admittedly, we would have to be very unlucky for the actual imbalance to be at the maximum when the study ends. For example, suppose there are b assignments of each type in every block and the trial ends randomly and uniformly within a block. In other words, there is no increased likelihood of stopping on either a particular treatment assignment or position within a block. Assume that all blocks are the same size. The chance of stopping in every stratum exactly halfway through a block is

$$u = \left(\frac{1}{2b}\right)^k,$$

and the chance that the first half of all k blocks has the same treatment assignment is

Table 9.2 Example of Blocked Stratified Treatment Assignments with Equal Allocation in Two Groups

Block Number	Strata			
	Males		Females	
	Young	Old	Young	Old
1	A	B	B	A
1	B	B	A	B
1	B	A	B	A
1	A	A	A	B
2	A	B	A	B
2	A	A	B	B
2	B	B	A	A
2	B	A	B	A
⋮	⋮	⋮	⋮	⋮

$$v = \binom{2b}{b}^{-k}.$$

Then uv is the chance of ending on the worst imbalance. For 2 treatments and 4 strata with all blocks of size 4 ($b = 2$), as in the example above, the maximum imbalance is $2 \times 4 = 8$. The chance of stopping with an imbalance of 8 in favor of one treatment or the other is only

$$uv = 2 \times \left(\frac{1}{4}\right)^4 \times \binom{4}{2}^{-4} = 6.03 \times 10^{-6}.$$

The chance of a lesser imbalance is greater.

Stratified randomization *without* blocking will not improve balance beyond that attainable by simple randomization. In other words, simple randomization in each of several strata is equivalent to simple randomization overall. Because a simple random process has no memory of previous assignments, stratification serves no purpose, unless the assignments are constrained within strata. Another type of constraint that produces balance using adaptive randomization is discussed below.

9.3.3 Other considerations regarding blocking

One can inadvertently counteract the balancing effects of blocking by having too many strata. For example, if each patient winds up in his or her own stratum uniquely specified by a set of prognostic factors, the result is equivalent to having used simple randomization. Plans for randomization must take this possible problem into account and use only a few strata, relative to the size of the trial. In other words, most blocks should be filled because unfilled blocks permit imbalances.

If block sizes are too large, it can also counteract the balancing effects of blocking. Treatment assignments from a very large block are essentially equivalent to simple randomization, except toward the end of the block. For example, consider equation 9.1 for $Pr[A]$ when N_A and N_B are very large. Then, $Pr[A] \approx \frac{1}{2}$ for all the early assignments in a block.

Because at least the last assignment in each block (and possibly up to half of some blocks) is not random (i.e., determined from the previous assignments), the block size should not be revealed to the clinical investigators. If the investigators know the block size, then some assignments are potentially discoverable. Sometimes random block sizes can be used, provided all possible sizes are small, to reduce or eliminate the chance that an investigator will acquire knowledge about future treatment assignments. For example, in a two-group trial, choosing randomly from among block sizes of 2, 4, and 6 yields assignments that would look almost purely random if revealed, except that they are fairly closely balanced.

Blocking can also be used with unequal treatment allocation. For example, suppose we wish to have a 2:1 allocation in favor of treatment A. Block sizes that are multiples of three could be used with two-thirds of the assignments allocated to treatment A. At the end of each block, the treatment allocation will be exactly 2:1 in favor of treatment A.

One advantage of blocked assignments, with or without strata, is that they can be generated on paper in advance of the trial and placed in notebooks accessible to the staff responsible for administering the treatment allocation process. An excess number of assignments can be generated and used sequentially as accrual proceeds. The resulting stream of assignments will have the intended properties and will be easy to prepare and use. Excess assignments not used at the end of the study can be ignored.

9.4 Adaptive Randomization

Adaptive randomization is a process in which the probability of assignment to the treatments in a clinical trial does not remain constant, but is determined by the current balance and/or composition of the groups. In a sense, this same characteristic holds true for blocked randomization. However, adaptive randomization is a more general idea and can be used to adjust the treatment assignment probabilities in response to numerical balance, prognostic factor, or risk composition of the groups, or outcomes. General discussions of this method can be found in Hoel, Sobel, and Weiss [1975], Efron [1971], and Pocock and Simon [1975]. Urn designs (biased coin randomization) and minimization are two types of adaptive treatment allocation.

9.4.1 Urn designs also improve balance

An alternative to blocking to prevent large imbalances in the numbers of assignments made to treatment groups is a technique based on urn models [Wei and Lachin, 1988]. Urn models are ubiquitous devices in probability and statistics, which are helpful in illustrating important concepts. Imagine an urn containing one red and one white ball. To make a treatment assignment, a ball is selected at random. If the ball is red, the assignment is to treatment A. A white ball yields treatment B. After use, the ball is replaced in the urn. This procedure is equivalent to simple randomization with probability of $1/2$ of receiving either treatment.

To discourage imbalances, however, a slightly different procedure might be used. Suppose we begin with one ball of each color in the urn and the first ball picked is red. Then the original ball plus an additional *white* ball might be placed in the urn. With the next choice, there is one red ball and two white balls in the urn, yielding a higher probability of balancing the first treatment assignment. With each draw, the chosen ball and one of the opposite color are placed in the urn. Suppose n_A and n_B represent the current number of red and white balls, respectively, in the urn. Then, for each assignment,

$$\Pr[A] = \frac{n_B}{n_A + n_B} \ .$$

When the number of draws is small, there tends to be tighter balance. As the number of draws increases, the addition of a single ball is less important and the process begins to behave like 1:1 simple randomization. At any point, when equal numbers of assignments have been made for each group, the probability of getting a red or white ball on the next draw is $1/2$. This process could also be used for stratified assignments.

This urn procedure might be useful in trials where the final sample size is going to be small and tight balance is needed. These assignments can also be generated in advance and stratified, if necessary, to balance a prognostic factor. For example, Table 9.3 shows the first few treatment assignments from a two-group, two-stratum sequence. Any sequence is possible, but balanced ones are much more likely.

9.4.2   Minimization yields tight balance

Other schemes to restrict randomization to yield more balance in treatment groups are based on minimization as suggested by Pocock and Simon [1975] and Begg and Iglewicz [1980]. To implement minimization, a measure of imbalance based on the current number of treatment assignments (or the prognostic factor composition of the treatment groups) is used. Before the next treatment assignment is made, the imbalance that will result is calculated in two ways: 1) assuming the assignment is made to A, and 2) assuming it is made to B. The treatment assignment that yields the smallest imbalance is chosen. If the imbalance would be the same either way, the choice is made randomly.

The strengths of this scheme are that it can produce a tighter balance than blocked strata. However, it has the drawback that one must keep track of the current measure of imbalance. This is not a problem for computer-based randomization schemes, which are frequently used today. Also, when minimization is employed, *none* of the assignments (except perhaps the first) is necessarily made randomly. This would seem to prevent the use of randomization theory in analysis. However, treating the data as though they arose from a completely randomized design is commonly done and probably results in few errors of inference. At least in oncology, many multi-institutional "randomized" studies actually employ treatment allocation based on minimization.

Table 9.3 Example of Stratified Treatment Assignments Using an Urn Model

Stratum 1				Stratum 2			
n_a	n_b	Pr[A]	Treatment	n_a	n_b	Pr[A]	Treatment
1	0	0.500	A	1	0	0.500	A
1	1	0.333	B	1	1	0.333	B
2	1	0.500	A	1	2	0.500	B
3	1	0.400	A	1	3	0.600	B
4	1	0.333	A	1	4	0.667	B
4	2	0.286	B	2	4	0.714	A
5	2	0.375	A	3	4	0.625	A
5	3	0.333	B	4	4	0.556	A
5	4	0.400	B	4	5	0.500	B
6	4	0.455	A	5	5	0.545	A
7	4	0.417	A	5	6	0.500	B
8	4	0.385	A	6	6	0.538	A
8	5	0.357	B	6	7	0.500	B
8	6	0.400	B	7	7	0.533	A
8	7	0.438	B	7	8	0.500	B
9	7	0.471	A	7	9	0.529	B
10	7	0.444	A	7	10	0.556	B
10	8	0.421	B	8	10	0.579	A
11	8	0.450	A	8	11	0.550	B
11	9	0.429	B	9	11	0.571	A
⋮	⋮	⋮	⋮	⋮	⋮	⋮	⋮

$Pr[A]$ is the probability of assignment to treatment A calculated prior to the assignment.

9.4.3 Play the winner

Other methods for making treatment allocations in clinical trials have been suggested to meet certain important constraints. For example, Zelen [1969] and Wei and Durham [1978] suggested making treatment assignments according to a "play the winner" rule, to minimize the number of patients who receive an inferior treatment in a comparative trial. One way of implementing this scheme is as follows: Suppose that randomization to one of two groups is made by the logical equivalent of drawing balls labeled A or B from an urn, with replacement. For the first patient, the urn contains one ball of each type (or an equal number of each). The first patient is assigned on the basis of a random draw. If the assigned treatment "fails", a ball of the other type is added to the urn. The next patient therefore has a higher probability of receiving the other treatment. If the first treatment "succeeds", a ball of the same type is added to the urn. Thus, the next patient has a higher probability of receiving the same therapy.

This method has the advantage of preferentially using what appears to be the best treatment for each assignment after the first. However, implementing it in the manner

Table 9.4 Results from an ECMO Clinical Trial using Play the Winner Randomization

Patient Number	Treatment Assignment	Outcome
1	ECMO	Success
2	Control	Failure
3	ECMO	Success
⋮	⋮	⋮
10	ECMO	Success

described requires being able to assess the final outcome in each study subject before placing the next patient on the trial. This may not always be feasible. A more flexible approach is to use a multi-stage design with adjustment of the allocation ratio, to favor the treatment arm that appears to be doing the best at each stage. This approach can also be used with outcomes that are not dichotomous. Some investigators believe that trials designed in this way may be viewed more favorably than conventional designs by patients and Institutional Review Boards.

A design of this type was used in a clinical trial of extracorporeal membrane oxygenation (ECMO) versus standard therapy for newborn infants with persistent pulmonary hypertension [Bartlett et al., 1985]. Based on developmental studies over ten years, ECMO appeared to be a potentially promising treatment for this fatal condition when it was tested in a clinical trial in 1985. Using the Wei and Durham method of urn randomization, the trial was to be stopped when the urn contained 10 balls favoring one treatment. This stopping rule was chosen to yield a 95% chance of selecting the best treatment when $p_1 \geq 0.8$ and $p_1 - p_2 > 0.4$, where p_1 and p_2 are the survival probabilities on the best and worst treatments, respectively.

Some of the data arising from the trial (in the stratum of infants weighing more than 2 kilograms) are shown in Table 9.4. The first patient was assigned to ECMO and survived. The second patient received conventional treatment and died. All subsequent patients were randomly assigned to ECMO. The trial was terminated after 10 patients received ECMO, but 2 additional patients were non-randomly assigned to ECMO. Because of the small sample size, one could consider testing the data for statistical significance using Fisher's exact test, which conditions on the row and column totals of the 2×2 table. However, the analysis should not condition on the row and column totals because, in an adaptive design such as this, they contain information about the outcomes.

This trial was unusual from a number of perspectives: the investigators felt fairly strongly that ECMO was more effective than conventional therapy before the study was started; an adaptive design was used; consent was sought only for patients assigned to experimental therapy (see below); and the stopping criterion was based on selection or ranking of results. Ware and Epstein [1985] discussed this trial, stating that, from the familiar hypothesis testing perspective, the type I error rate for a trial with this design is 50%.

The ECMO trial is also unusual because of the subsequent controversies that it sparked. Not all of the discussions stem from the design of the trial; much is a consequence of the clinical uncertainties. However, alternative designs may have helped resolve the clinical questions more clearly. For example, a design with an unequal treatment allocation (discussed below) might have reduced some of the uncertainty. For a clinical review of the ECMO story, see the paper by O'Rourke [1991]. Ethical issues were discussed by Royall [1991].

9.5   Other Issues Regarding Randomization

9.5.1   Administration of the randomization

The beneficial effects of randomization for reducing bias can be undone if future treatment assignments are discoverable by investigators. Potentially, this information could be available if all treatment assignments are listed in advance of the study in a notebook or folder and dispensed as each patient goes on study, as is commonly done. This problem could arise if clinical investigators responsible for placing patients on study and selecting treatment are involved with, or have access to, the randomization process. To convincingly demonstrate that this has not occurred, the administration of the randomization process should be physically separated from the clinical investigators.

In multi-center trials, this is commonly accomplished by designating one of the institutions, or an off-site location, to serve as a trial coordinating center. Treatment assignments are then made by telephone or secure computer access. The concern about access to treatment assignments may be more relevant in single-institution studies, where the clinical investigators often administratively manage their own trials. It is sometimes necessary for the investigators to manage treatment assignment for reasons of accessibility or convenience. When this is required, extra care should be taken to keep the assignments secure.

Example 16 *Investigators conducted a multi-center randomized trial of low tidal volume versus standard ventilation in patients with adult respiratory distress syndrome. Because the patients were all ventilator-dependent and hospitalized in intensive care units (ICU), it was necessary to have the capability to randomize treatment assignments 24 hours each day. This could not be accomplished easily using an independent study coordinator. Instead, it was more efficient to designate one of the participating ICUs as the randomization center and have the nursing staff always available there perform an occasional randomization. This ICU environment is potentially "hostile" to performing such tasks rigorously. Nevertheless, a suitably written computer program helped the randomization proceed routinely. The program contained password protection for each randomization and safeguards to prevent tampering with either the program itself or the sequence of treatment assignments. Initially, stratified randomized assignments from the computer program were made with a block size of 8. Interestingly, after 3 of the first 4 assignments in one* *stratum were made to the same treatment group, the ICU nurses became convinced that the program was not functioning "randomly". This illustrates the scrutiny that the sequence of assignments is likely to get. Reassuring investigators that the program was operating correctly was a strong suggestion about the (fixed) block size. Consequently, the randomization program was modified to use a variable block size.*

This example illustrates that, under special circumstances, treatment assignments can be protected from tampering, while still permitting flexibility and convenience. Of course, no safeguards are totally effective against a determined unscrupulous investigator. For example, one might be able to defeat seemingly secure randomization programs by running two copies. The second copy would permit experimentation that could help to determine the next treatment assignment. The most secure randomization for 24-hour-per-day availability is provided by centralized, automated, dial-in computer applications kept at a location remote from the clinic.

The use of sealed envelopes managed by clinical investigators is sometimes proposed as a method of randomization. Although expedient, it should be discouraged as a method of treatment allocation, because it is potentially discoverable, error prone, and will not provide as convincing evidence of lack of bias as treatment allocation methods that are independent of the clinicians. Even so, sometimes sealed envelopes are the only practical allocation method. This may be the case when trials are conducted in settings with limited resources or research infrastructure, such as some developing countries or in some clinical settings where 24-hour-per-day treatment assignment is needed. Assignments using sealed envelopes should be periodically audited against a master list maintained centrally.

9.5.2   Computers generate pseudorandom numbers

I am always fascinated that some investigators seem reluctant to employ truly random methods of generating numbers in preference to computer-based (pseudorandom) methods. Consider the familiar Plexiglas apparatus filled with numbered ping pong balls, which is often used to select winning numbers for lottery drawings. This is a reliable and convincingly random method for selecting numbers and could well be used for treatment assignments in clinical trials, except that it is slow and inconvenient.

Computers, in contrast, generate pseudorandom numbers quickly. The numbers are generated by a mathematical formula that yields a completely predictable sequence if one knows the constants in the generating equation and the starting seed. The resulting stream of numbers will pass most important tests for randomness, in spite of its being deterministic, provided the seed and constants are chosen wisely. Excellent discussions of this topic are given by Knuth [1981] and Press et al. [1992].

The most commonly used algorithm for generating a sequence of pseudorandom numbers, $\{N_i\}$, is the linear congruential method. This method uses a recurrence formula to generate N_{i+1} from N_i which is

$$N_{i+1} = aN_i + c \pmod{k},$$

where a is the *multiplier*, c is the *increment*, and k is the *modulus*. Modular arithmetic takes the remainder when N is divided by k. This method can produce numbers that appear random and distributed uniformly over the interval $(0,1)$.

There are some important limitations to this method of generating pseudorandom numbers. The stream of numbers can be serially correlated and it will eventually repeat after no more than k numbers. The sequence will have a short period if a, c, and k are not carefully chosen, so that one must be cautious about using untested random number generators built-in to computer systems. Also, the formula and number stream are sensitive to the hardware of the particular computer system. These are important points for statistical simulation, but, perhaps, not so critical for clinical trial treatment assignments, because the operative benefit of randomization is that the assignments are made impartially.

In any case, the reader should realize that 1) computers generate *pseudo*-random numbers, 2) the method of generation is subject to mistakes that could lead to pseudo-random number streams with very undesirable properties, and 3) extra care is needed to have good pseudorandom number generators or ones that yield identical results on all computer systems. It seems we have come full circle now in terms of treatment allocation. The "randomization" of computer-based methods is actually a non-discoverable- seemingly random, deterministic allocation scheme. Used with care, it is perfectly appropriate for "randomized" assignments in clinical trials.

9.5.3   Randomization justifies type I errors

In addition to eliminating bias in treatment assignments, a second benefit of randomization is that it guarantees the correctness of certain statistical procedures and control of type I errors in hypothesis tests. For example, the important class of statistical tests known as permutation (or randomization) tests of the null hypothesis are validated by the random assignment of patients to treatments. To understand this, we must discuss some aspects of analysis now, even though it is jumping ahead in the scheme of our study of clinical trials. An in-depth discussion of permutation tests is given by Good [1994].

The validity of randomization tests is motivated by the exchangeability of treatment assignments in a clinical trial. Under a population model, two samples from the same population are exchangeable. This might be the view of a randomized clinical trial where, under the null hypothesis, the sample observations from the two treatments are exchangeable. Alternatively, we could motivate such tests by a randomization model as suggested by R. A. Fisher. Under this model, the outcomes from the experiment are viewed as fixed numbers and the null hypothesis states that treatment has no effect on these numbers. Then the group assignments are exchangeable under this null hypothesis.

Suppose there are two treatments, A and B, N patient assignments in total, $N/2$ patients in each treatment group, and treatment assignments have been made by simple randomization. Let Y_i be the response for the ith patient, $\overline{Y}_A$ and $\overline{Y}_B$ be the average responses in the two treatment groups, and $\Delta = \overline{Y}_A - \overline{Y}_B$. The null hypothesis states that there is no difference between the treatment groups, i.e., $H_0 : \Delta = 0$. Stated another way, the treatment assignments and the responses are independent of one another and exchangeable under the null hypothesis. If so, any ordering of the treatment assignments is equally likely under randomization and all should yield a "similar" Δ.

Following this idea, the null hypothesis can be tested by forming all permutations of treatment assignments independently of the Y_i's, calculating the distribution of the Δ's that results, and comparing the observed Δ to the permutation distribution. If the observed Δ is atypical (i.e., if it lies far enough in the tail of the permutation distribution), we would conclude that the distribution arising from the null hypothesis is an unlikely origin for it. In other words, we would reject the null hypothesis. This procedure is "exact", in the sense that the distribution generated is the only one that we need to consider and can be completely enumerated by the permutation method.

Number of permutations

The number of permutations for even modest sized studies is very large. For example, the number of permutations for two treatment groups, A and B, using simple random allocation with N_A and N_B assignments in each group, is

$$M = \binom{N_A + N_B}{N_A} = \binom{N_A + N_B}{N_B} = \frac{(N_A + N_B)!}{N_A! N_B!},$$

which is the binomial coefficient for N objects (treatment assignments) taken N_A (or N_B) at a time. The formula is valid when $N_A \neq N_B$. This number grows very rapidly with $N_A + N_B$. For more than two treatments, the number of permutations is given by the multinomial coefficient

$$M = \binom{N}{N_A, N_B, \cdots} = \frac{N!}{N_A! N_B! \cdots},$$

where $N = N_A + N_B + \ldots$ is the total number of assignments. This number also grows very rapidly with N.

When blocking is used, the number of permutations is smaller, but still becomes quite large with increasing sample size. For two treatments with b assignments in each fixed block and all blocks filled, the number is

$$M = \binom{2b}{b}^k,$$

where the number of blocks is k. A more general formula for blocks of variable size is

$$M = \prod_{i=1}^{r} \binom{N_{A_i} + N_{B_i}}{N_{A_i}}^{k_i},$$

where there are r different sized blocks and k_i of each one. Here also, the formula is valid when $N_{A_i} \neq N_{B_i}$. This last formula can also be adapted to cases where the last block is not filled. Examples of the number of permutations arising from two-treatment group studies of various sizes are shown in Table 9.5.

Implementation

Because the number of permutations from even modest size studies is so large, it is impractical to use exact permutation tests routinely in the analysis of clinical trials, despite the desirable characteristics of the procedure. A more economical approach, which relies on the same theory, is to sample randomly (with replacement) from the set of possible permutations. If the sample is large enough, although considerably smaller than the total number of possible permutations, the resulting distribution will accurately represent the exact permutation distribution and will be suitable for making inferences. For example, one might take 1000 or 10,000 samples from the permutation distribution. Such a procedure is called a "randomization test", although this term could be applied to permutation tests as well. The terminology is not important, as long as one realizes that the exact permutation distribution can be accurately approximated by a sufficiently large sample.

An example of a permutation test is shown in Table 9.6. Here there were 5 assignments in each of two groups, yielding a total of 252 possible permutations, conditional on the number in each group being equal. For each possible permutation, let $\Delta = \overline{X}_B - \overline{X}_A$. The 5 responses on A and B were $\mathbf{X} = \{1.1, 1.3, 1.2, 1.4, 1.2, 1.5, 2.0, 1.3, 1.7, 1.9\}$. From these, the Δ's that would be obtained for each permutation of treatment assignments are shown in Table 9.6, ordered by the size of Δ. Only the upper half of the permutations are listed – the mirror-image half (i.e., A and B switching places) has Δ's that are the negative of those in the table. Figure 9.1 shows the permutation distribution. Suppose the observed Δ was 2.2, the sequence of assignments actually being $BABBBAABAA$, (from permutation number 2), which lies above the 0.012 percentile of the distribution. Thus, we would reject the null hypothesis of no treatment difference. The validity of this procedure relies on nothing, except the use of randomization in allocating treatment assignments: no assumptions about statistical distributions or models have been made. Similar procedures can be applied to event data from clinical trials [Freedman, Sylvester, and Byar, 1989; Ohashi, 1990].

Permutation and randomization tests are appealing because they can be applied to virtually any test, they do not depend on the sample size, and they require few assumptions beyond the use of randomization. They have not been as widely applied as many other tests, probably because of the amount of computing resources required. However, recent improvements in computing performance on all platforms make randomization tests very attractive.

9.6   Unequal Treatment Allocation

Usually comparative trials employ an equal allocation of subjects to each of the treatments under study. To maximize the efficiency (power) of the primary comparison, this is often the best approach. However, the trial may be designed intentionally to employ unequal group sizes to meet important secondary objectives. Then, unbalanced designs can be more efficient than equal allocation for meeting all study objectives. Examples where this can be useful include important subset analyses, large

Table 9.5 Number of Possible Permutations of Two Treatment Assignments for Different Block and Sample Sizes

Total Sample Size	Block Size			
	2	4	8	∞
4	4	6	6	6
8	16	36	70	70
16	256	1296	4900	12870
24	4096	46656	343000	2.7×10^6
56	2.68×10^8	7.84×10^{10}	8.24×10^{12}	7.65×10^{15}
104	4.50×10^{15}	1.71×10^{20}	9.69×10^{23}	1.58×10^{30}

The calculation assumes all blocks are filled. An infinite block size corresponds to simple randomization.

differences in the cost of treatments, and when the responses have unequal variances. For a review of unequal allocation, see Sposto and Krailo [1987].

Some investigators feel that unbalanced random assignment reflects a preference for the more frequently employed treatment. This view is not correct (at least with any sensible allocation ratio). Randomization is employed in the presence of equipoise to eliminate selection bias. This same rationale applies to unequal allocation. Furthemore, one cannot correct a lack of equipoise by appealing to a collective ethic that does less harm on average. It is either appropriate to randomize or not. The need to use an unbalanced allocation should be separated from the decision to randomize, and is more properly based on other study objectives as outlined below.

9.6.1   Subsets may be of interest

It may be important to acquire as much experience with a new treatment as possible, while also comparing it with standard therapy. In this case, an unequal allocation of subjects, e.g., 2:1 in favor of the new treatment, may allow important additional experience with the new treatment without substantially decreasing the efficiency (power) of the comparison. Similarly, subsets of patients who receive the new treatment (e.g., older patients) may be of interest and unequal allocation may increase their number. The sensitivity of power to the allocation ratio was discussed in Chapter 7.

9.6.2   Treatments may differ greatly in cost

When one treatment is much more expensive than the other in a two-group clinical trial, the total cost of the study will be minimized by an unequal allocation of subjects. Fewer patients would be allocated to the more expensive treatment. Obviously, the lowest total cost is incurred when no patients are placed on the most expensive therapy. However, this tendency must be offset by the need to meet the statistical objectives of the comparison. Thus, the cost function and the "power" or "precision" function of the trial can be optimized together.

Table 9.6 Lower Half of the Permutation Distribution for Ten Balanced Treatment Assignments in Two Groups

Permutation	Δ	Permutation	Δ	Permutation	Δ
AAABABBABB	2.4	AAABBBBABA	1.0	ABBAAABBBA	0.4
ABAAABBABB	2.2	BAAAABBBAB	1.0	BAABAABBBA	0.4
AAAAABBBBB	2.2	AABBAABBAB	1.0	BBAAABAABB	0.4
ABABAABABB	2.0	AAABBABBAB	1.0	BBBAAABAAB	0.4
AAAABBBABB	2.0	BBABAABAAB	0.8	ABABBAAABB	0.4
AABAABBABB	2.0	ABABAABBBA	0.8	ABBBAAAABB	0.4
AAABAABBBB	2.0	AAAABBBBBA	0.8	BAAAABABBB	0.4
ABAAAABBBB	1.8	AABAABBBBA	0.8	BAAABBBABA	0.4
BAAAABBABB	1.8	ABAAABABBB	0.8	BABAABBABA	0.4
AAABBABABB	1.8	ABAABABBAB	0.8	BBAABABAAB	0.4
AABBAABABB	1.8	ABAABBBABA	0.8	AABABBAABB	0.4
ABAABABABB	1.6	ABBAABBABA	0.8	AABBAAABBB	0.4
ABABABBAAB	1.6	BAABABBABA	0.8	AAABBAABBB	0.4
ABBAAABABB	1.6	AABBABAABB	0.8	BAAABABBAB	0.4
BAABAABABB	1.6	BAAABBBAAB	0.8	BABAAABBAB	0.4
AAAABABBBB	1.6	BABAABBAAB	0.8	ABABBBBAAA	0.2
AABAAABBBB	1.6	AAABBBAABB	0.8	ABBBABBAAA	0.2
AAABABBBAB	1.6	AABBBABAAB	0.8	ABAABAABBB	0.2
BAAAAABBBB	1.4	ABBAAABBAB	0.8	ABBABABABA	0.2
ABAAABBAB	1.4	BAABAABBAB	0.8	BAABBABABA	0.2
BBAAAABABB	1.4	AABABBBABA	0.6	BBAAAABBBA	0.2
AAABBBBAAB	1.4	BBAAABBABA	0.6	AABBBAAABB	0.2
AABABABABB	1.4	ABAABBAABB	0.6	ABABABABAB	0.2
AABBABBAAB	1.4	ABABBABABA	0.6	BABABABAAB	0.2
ABABABBABA	1.2	ABBBAABABA	0.6	BBABAAAABB	0.2
AAAABBBBAB	1.2	AAAABBABBB	0.6	ABBAAAABBB	0.2
AABAABBBAB	1.2	AAABBABBBA	0.6	BAAABBAABB	0.2
ABAABBBAAB	1.2	AABAABABBB	0.6	BAABAAABBB	0.2
ABBAABBAAB	1.2	ABBABABAAB	0.6	BABAABAABB	0.2
BAAABABABB	1.2	BAAAABBBBA	0.6	BABBAABABA	0.2
BAABABBAAB	1.2	BAABBABAAB	0.6	AABABABBBA	0.2
BABAAABABB	1.2	BABBAABAAB	0.6	AAABBBBBAA	0.2
ABABAABBAB	1.2	BBAAAABBAB	0.6	AABBABBBAA	0.2
AAABABBBBA	1.2	AABBAABBBA	0.6	AAABBBABAB	0.0
ABAAABBBBA	1.0	ABABAAABBB	0.6	AABABAABBB	0.0
ABABBABAAB	1.0	ABBAABAABB	0.6	ABAABBBBAA	0.0
ABBBAABAAB	1.0	BAABABAABB	0.6	ABBAABBBAA	0.0
ABABABAABB	1.0	AABABABBAB	0.6	BAAABABBBA	0.0
BBAAABBAAB	1.0	BBABAABABA	0.4	BAABABBBAA	0.0
AAABABABBB	1.0	AABBBABABA	0.4	BABAAABBBA	0.0
AABABBBAAB	1.0	ABAABABBBA	0.4	BBAAAAABBB	0.0
AABBABBABA	1.0	ABABABBBAA	0.4	BBAABABABA	0.0

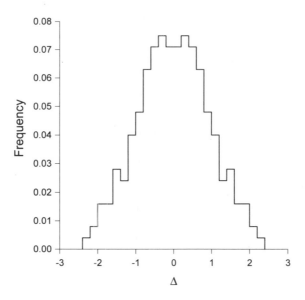

Figure 9.1 Example permutation distribution from ten treatment assignments.

For example, suppose the total cost of a trial, C, is given by

$$C = c_1 n_1 + c_2 n_2 = c_1 n_2 r + c_2 n_2 = n_2(c_1 r + c_2) , \qquad (9.2)$$

where n_1 and n_2 are the group sizes, c_1 and c_2 are fixed costs per subject on the two treatments, and r is the allocation ratio ($n_2 = r n_1$). Also if the sample size satisfies

$$n_2 = \frac{r+1}{r} \frac{(Z_\alpha + Z_\beta)^2 \sigma^2}{\Delta^2} = \frac{r+1}{r} N \qquad (9.3)$$

(equation 7.14), then the total cost can be found by combining equations 9.2 and 9.3,

$$C = \left(c_2 + c_1 r + \frac{c_2}{r} + c_1 \right) N. \qquad (9.4)$$

The best allocation ratio might be the one that minimizes the total cost as a function of sample size. The allocation ratio that minimizes total cost in equation 9.4 can be found by equating the derivative with respect to r to zero. Therefore, r will satisfy,

$$0 = \frac{dC}{dr} = \left(c_1 - \frac{c_2}{r^2} \right) N$$

or

$$r = \sqrt{\frac{c_2}{c_1}}.$$

In other words, the optimum allocation ratio for this simple case is the square root of the inverse of the costs per treatment. It is not a function of any design parameters except the treatment costs. If $c_2/c_1 = 10$, for example, the cost-minimizing allocation ratio will be approximately 3:1 in favor of the less expensive treatment.

9.6.3 Variances may be different

Suppose the means, μ_1 and μ_2, of two treatment groups are being compared using a test, for which the statistic is

$$t = \frac{\mu_1 - \mu_2}{\sqrt{\frac{\sigma_1^2}{n_1} + \frac{\sigma_2^2}{n_2}}} ,$$

where the variances, σ_1^2 and σ_2^2, are not necessarily equal. Because of this, one may wish to change the allocation ratio (i.e., n_1 and n_2) to make the test as efficient as possible. For fixed μ_1 and μ_2, the test statistic is maximized when the denominator is minimized, or when $\sigma_1^2/n_1 + \sigma_2^2/n_2$ is minimized. For $N = n_1 + n_2$, the minimum satisfies

$$0 = \frac{\partial}{\partial n_1} \left(\frac{\sigma_1^2}{n_1} + \frac{\sigma_2^2}{N - n_1} \right)$$

or

$$\frac{\sigma_2^2}{\sigma_1^2} = \left(\frac{N - n_1}{n_1} \right)^2 ,$$

from which the optimal fraction in group 1 is found to be

$$\frac{n_1}{N} = \frac{\sigma_1}{\sigma_1 + \sigma_2} .$$

Therefore, the optimal allocation ratio is

$$r = \frac{n_1}{n_2} = \frac{\sigma_1}{\sigma_2} .$$

In other words, more subjects should be placed in the group where the measured response is less precise.

9.7 Randomization Before Consent

Partly in response to the difficulties of getting patients to accept randomization, Zelen [1979; 1990] suggested a "pre-randomized" scheme, which works in the following way. Suppose a new therapy is being compared with standard treatment. Eligible patients are randomized before being approached to participate in the trial. If the treatment assignment is standard therapy, the patient is offered the standard as a matter of routine and randomization and consent need not be discussed. If the randomized assignment is the new therapy, the patient is approached for consent. If the patient refuses, he or she is offered standard therapy. The final comparison is between the groups based on randomized assignment. A double randomized consent has also been suggested, in which those initially assigned to standard therapy are also asked if they will accept the treatment. A review of these designs is given by Parmar [1992].

The randomization before consent strategy can increase the number of trial participants. However, it creates some difficulties that limit its use. For example, in the analysis by treatment assigned, the patients who refuse their assignment dilute the treatment difference. If the trial is analyzed by treatment received, there is potential for bias. Most importantly, the design has difficulty passing ethical review, because patients assigned to standard therapy are part of a research study without being properly informed (highlighting a double standard for consent on research studies). For example, the patients on standard therapy are not given the chance to obtain the new treatment. Some may not wish to participate in the study for reasons not directly related to treatment.

This design was used in the ECMO trial discussed above although only a single patient was assigned to conventional therapy. A second trial of ECMO was conducted using this consent procedure [O'Rourke et al., 1989]. This pre-randomization was thought to be necessary, because of the lack of equipoise on the part of the investigators. This trial, like the one before it and non-randomized studies, supported the efficacy of ECMO compared with conventional therapy. This second ECMO study also raises a number of important issues about trial conduct discussed by Meinert [1989] and Chalmers [1989]. A few other trials have used randomization before consent, including some collaborative studies in the U.S. and Europe [Parmar, 1992].

Because of its practical and ethical difficulties, pre-randomization should probably not be routinely used for treatment assignments in clinical trials. Although there may be special circumstances that warrant its use and it can increase accrual, traditional randomized designs seem to be better suited to the objectives of comparative trials and the limits of ethical standards.

9.8   Summary

Treatment allocation in clinical trials and other true experimental designs is characterized by active control of the treatments and the process used to make assignments. The practical concerns in choosing an allocation scheme for comparative studies are reducing bias, quantifying random errors, and increasing the credibility of results. Simple or constrained randomization satisfies the practical concerns and offers important theoretical advantages over other methods of allocation. Randomization reduces or eliminates biases in treatment assignment, guarantees the expectation that unobserved confounders will be controlled, validates control over type I error, and motivates an important class of analyses.

Despite its appeal, the actual realization of a simple randomization scheme can result in chance imbalances in influential prognostic factors or the size of treatment groups. This can be prevented using constrained randomization. Constraints frequently used include blocking and stratifying, adaptive randomization, and minimization. These methods, while theoretically unnecessary, encourage covariate balance in the treatment groups, which tends to enhance the credibility of trial results. Unequal group sizes might be used when it minimizes the cost of a trial or facilitates secondary objectives.

Administering treatment assignments may be as important as using an unbiased allocation method. The assignments should be supervised and conducted by individuals who have no vested interest in the results of the trial. The method employed should be convincingly tamper-proof and distinct from the clinic site. The beneficial effects of randomization in reducing bias can be undone if investigators can discover future treatment assignments.

9.9   Questions for Discussion

1. Simple randomization is used in a two-group CTE trial with 100 participants. The probability of being assigned to treatment A is $p = 0.5$. What is the chance that treatment A will end up having between 48 and 52 assignments? Using a 0.05 α-level test, what is the chance that the groups will be so unbalanced that investigators would conclude that $p \neq 0.5$?

2. Simple randomization is used in a two-group CTE trial. The probability of being assigned to either treatment is 0.5. How many independent binary covariates would one need to test to be 50% certain of finding at least one "significantly" unbalanced in the treatment groups? How about being 95% certain?

3. A clinical trial with four groups uses treatment assignments in blocks of size 4 in each of 8 strata. What is the maximum imbalance in the number of treatment assignments that can occur? What is the chance of this happening? What is the chance that the trial will end exactly balanced?

4. Investigators have written a computer program to generate random integers between 0 and 32767. The output is tested repeatedly and found to satisfy a uniform distribution across the interval. Even integers result in assignment to group A and odd ones to group B. When the actual assignments are made, group B appears to have twice as many assignments as group A. How can this happen? Can this generator be used in any way? Why or why not?

5. A new random number generator is tested and found to satisfy a uniform distribution. Values below the midpoint are assigned to treatment A. When the actual assignments are made, there are very few "runs" of either treatment (i.e., $AA, AAA, \ldots, BB, BBB, \ldots$). How would you describe and quantify this problem? Can this generator be used after any modifications? If so, how?

6. A trial with 72 subjects in each of two groups uses randomized blocks of size 8. The data will be analyzed using a permutation test. You find a fast computer that can calculate 10 permutation results each second and start the program. How long before you have the results? Can you suggest an alternative?

7. In a randomized clinical trial with a survival endpoint, one treatment costs twice as much as another. What allocation ratio minimizes the total cost of the trial?

Chapter References

Amberson, J.B., Jr., McMahon, B.T., and Pinner, M. (1931). A clinical trial of sanocrysin in pulmonary tuberculosis. Am. Rev. Tuberc. 24: 401-404

Barrow, J.D. (1991). Theories of Everything. Oxford: Clarendon Press.

Bartlett, R.H., Roloff, D.W. Cornell, R.G., Andrews, A.F., Dillon, P.W., and Zwischenberger, J.B. (1985). Extracorporeal circulation in neonatal respiratory failure: A prospective randomized study. Pediatrics 76: 479-487.

Begg, C.D. and Iglewicz, B.A. (1980). A treatment allocation procedure for sequential clinical trials. Biometrics 36: 81-90.

Box, J.F. (1980). R. A. Fisher and the design of experiments, 1922-1926. Am. Statistician 34: 1-7.

Byar, D.P., Green, S.B., Dor, P., Williams, E.D., Colon, J., van Gilse, H.A., Mayer, M., Sylvester, R.J., and Van Glabbeke, M. (1979). A prognostic index for thyroid carcinoma. A study of the EORTC Thyroid Cancer Cooperative Group. European J. Cancer 15: 1033-1041.

Chalmers, T.C. (1989). A belated randomized control trial. Pediatrics 85: 366-368.

Durrleman, S. and Simon, R. (1991). When to randomize? J. Clin. Oncol. 9: 116-122.

Efron, B. (1971). Forcing a sequential experiment to be balanced. Biometrika 58: 403-417.

Freedman, L., Sylvester, R., and Byar, D.P. (1989). Using permutation tests and bootstrap confidence limits to analyze repeated events data from clinical trials. Controlled Clinical Trials 10: 129-141.

Good, P. (1994). Permutation Tests. New York: Springer -Verlag.

Hoel, D.G., Sobel, M. and Weiss, G.H. (1975). A survey of adaptive sampling for clinical trials. In: R.M. Elashoff (Ed.), Perspectives in Biometrics. New York: Academic Press.

Green, S.B. and Byar, D.P. (1984). Using observational data from registries to compare treatments: The fallacy of omnimetrics. Statistics in Med. 3: 361-370.

Kalish, L.A., and Begg, C.B. (1985). Treatment allocation methods in clinical trials: A review. Statistics in Med. 4: 129-144.

Knuth, D. (1981). Seminumerical Algorithms, 2nd Edition, Vol. 2 of The Art of Computer Programming. Reading, MA: Addison-Wesley.

Lachin, J.M. (1988a). Properties of simple randomization in clinical trials. Controlled Clin. Trials 9: 312-326.

Lachin, J.M. (1988b). Statistical properties of randomization in clinical trials. Controlled Clin. Trials 9: 289- 311.

Lachin, J.M., Matts, J.P., and Wei, L.J. (1988). Randomization in clinical trials: Conclusions and recommendations. Controlled Clin. Trials 9: 365-374.

Matts, J.P., and Lachin, J.M. (1988). Properties of permuted-block randomization in clinical trials. Controlled Clin. Trials 9: 327-344.

Meinert, C.L. (1989). Extracorporeal membrane oxygenation trials (commentary). Pediatrics 85: 365-366.

Miettinen, O. (1983). The need for randomization in the study of intended effects. Statistics in Med. 2: 267-271.

Ohashi, Y. (1990). Randomization in cancer clinical trials: Permutation test and development of computer program. Environmental Health Perspectives 87: 13-17.

O'Rourke, P.P. (1991). ECMO: Where have we been? Where are we going? Respiratory Care 36: 683-694.

O'Rourke, P.P., Crone, R.K., Vacanti, J.P., Ware, J.H., Lillehei, C.W., Parad, R.B., and Epstein, M.F. (1989). Extracorporeal membrane oxygenation and conventional medical therapy in neonates with persistent pulmonary hypertension of the newborn: A prospective randomized study. Pediatrics 84: 957-963.

Palta, M. (1985). Investigating maximum power losses in survival studies with nonstratified randomization. Biometrics 41: 497-504.

Parmar, M.K.B. (1992). Randomization Before Consent. Ch. 14 in C.J. Williams (Ed..). Introducing New Treatments for Cancer: Practical, Ethical, and Legal Problems. Chichester: John Wiley & Sons.

Pocock, S. and Simon, R. (1975). Sequential treatment assignment with balancing for prognostic factors in the controlled clinical trial. Biometrics 31: 103-115.

Press, W.H., Teukolsky, S.A., Vetterling, W.T., and Flannery, B.P. (1992). Numerical Recipes in C: The Art of Scientific Computing. Second Edition. Cambridge: Cambridge University Press.

Royall, R.M. (1991). Ethics and statistics in randomized clinical trials. Statistical Science 6: 52-88.

Sposto, R., and Krailo, M.D. (1987). Use of unequal allocation in survival trials. Statistics in Medecine 6: 119-25.

Ware, J.H. and Epstein, M.F. (1985). Extracorporeal circulation in neonatal respiratory failure: A prospective randomized study (commentary). Pediatrics 76: 849-851.

Wei, L.J. and Durham, S. (1978). The randomized play-the-winner rule in medical trials. J. Am. Stat. Assoc. 73: 840-843.

Wei, L.J. and Lachin, J.M. (1988). Properties of the urn randomization in clinical trials. Controlled Clin. Trials 9: 345-364.

Zelen, M. (1969). Play the winner rule and the controlled clinical trial. J. Am. Stat. Assoc. 64: 131-146.

Zelen, M. (1979). A new design for randomized clinical trials. N. Engl. J. Med. 300: 1242-1245.

Zelen, M. (1990). Randomized consent designs for clinical trials: An update. Statistics in Med. 9: 645-656.

CHAPTER 10

Data-Dependent Stopping

10.1 Introduction

Continuing a clinical trial should be an active affirmation by the investigators that the scientific and ethical milieu requires and permits it, rather than a passive activity based only on the fact that the study was begun. As the trial proceeds, investigators must consider ongoing aspects of ethics, the precision of scientific results, data quality, and resource availability in deciding whether or not to continue the study. The most appropriate source of information on which to base this decision is the accumulating data, although sometimes information from outside the study may be relevant. This explains the idea of "data-dependent stopping" from which decisions about continuing the trial are based on the evidence currently available.

The problem of correctly gathering and interpreting information accumulating during a clinical trial is often referred to as "interim analysis" or "early stopping". Strictly speaking, an interim analysis need not address the question of study termination for reasons of efficacy. It might be done for administrative or quality control reasons. However, the most interesting and difficult questions are those surrounding early termination, so that will be the focus of my discussion. In any case, pre-planned and structured information gathering during a trial is probably the most reliable way to proceed for all purposes.

In this chapter, I discuss ways of minimizing errors that can result from interim looks at accumulating trial data and ways of improving decision making. This discussion pertains only to two-group trials and a single major endpoint. Methods for data-dependent stopping fall into four general categories: likelihood, Bayesian, frequentist, and others. There is a large literature base related to this topic. A good current source of information is an issue of *Statistics in Medicine* containing papers from a workshop on early stopping rules in cancer clinical trials [Souhami and Whitehead, 1994]. For older but useful reviews, see Gail [1982; 1984], Rubinstein and Gail [1982], Freedman and Spiegelhalter [1989], Fleming and DeMets [1993], Berry [1985], Pocock [1993], or Fleming, Green, and Harrington [1984]. There

Table 10.1 Some Reasons Why a Clinical Trial Might Be Stopped Early

- Treatments are found to be convincingly different by impartial knowledgeable experts.
- Treatments are found to be convincingly not different by impartial knowledgeable experts.
- Side effects or toxicity are too severe to continue treatment in light of potential benefits.
- The data are of poor quality.
- Accrual is too slow to complete the study in a timely fashion.
- Definitive information becomes available from outside the study, making the trial unnecessary or unethical.
- The scientific questions are no longer important because of other developments.
- Adherence to the treatment is unacceptably poor, preventing an answer to the basic question.
- Resources to perform the study are lost or no longer available.
- The study integrity has been undermined by fraud or misconduct.

is little in the clinical trials literature on the monitoring and stopping of trials with more than two treatment groups. Exceptions are the papers by Hughes [1993] and Proschan, Follmann, and Geller [1994]. In addition to statistical guidelines for interim analyses, I discuss some computer programs that can assist with the necessary computations.

10.1.1 Trials can be stopped for a variety of reasons

Some practical reasons for terminating a trial early are shown in Table 10.1. My use of the term "data-dependent stopping" to describe *all* of these aspects of trial monitoring is broader than usual, because the term is applied often only to the statistical aspects of planning for study termination. Because one cannot easily separate the statistical aspects of trial monitoring from the administrative ones, I will use the term to refer to both.

The simplest approach to formalizing the decision to stop a clinical trial is to use a fixed sample size. Fixed sample size designs are easy to plan, carry out, stop, and analyze, and the estimated treatment effects will be unbiased if the trial is performed and analyzed properly. Often, however, investigators have important reasons to examine and review the accumulating data while a study is ongoing. If convincing evidence becomes available during the trial about either treatment differences, safety, or the quality of the data, there may be an imperative to terminate accrual and/or stop the study before the final fixed sample size has been reached. Assessment of study progress from an administrative perspective, updating collaborators, and monitoring treatment compliance also require that the data be reviewed during the study.

There are two decision landmarks when monitoring a study: when to terminate accrual and when to publish results. Some investigators view these as one and the same, but it is often useful to separate them in studies with prolonged follow-up (e.g., survival studies). As sketched in Chapter 7, one can advantageously trade accrual rate, accrual time, or follow-up time for events in these types of trials.

It is routine to view the stopping decision as symmetric with respect to the outcome of the trial. For example, whether A is superior to B or B is superior to A, the quantitative aspects of the stopping guidelines are often taken to be the same or similar. The clinical circumstances are usually not symmetric, however. If A is standard and B is a new treatment, we would likely wish to stop a CTE trial: 1) when B cannot be superior to A rather than when it is convincingly worse, or 2) when B is convincingly better than A. Thus, stopping guidelines for efficacy should be drafted considering the asymmetric consequences of the differences implied, and supplemented with expert opinion.

10.1.2 There is tension in the decision to stop

Reviewing, interpreting, and making decisions about clinical trials based on interim data is necessary, but error prone. Before the data are complete and verified, one will get an imprecise view of most aspects of the study. If preliminary information is disseminated to study investigators, it may inappropriately affect their objectivity about the treatments. If statistical tests are performed repeatedly on the accumulating data, the chance of making a type I error is increased. In spite of these potential problems, investigators are vitally interested in the ongoing status of a trial and need summaries of the data in a useful format and with an appropriate level of detail to stay informed without corrupting the study.

There are pressures to terminate a trial at the earliest possible moment. These include the need to minimize the size of the trial and the number of patients treated on the inferior arm. Also, investigators are concerned about cost and other economic issues surrounding the study, and timeliness in disseminating results. These pressures to shorten a trial are opposed by reasons to continue the study as long as possible. Benefits of longer, larger trials include increasing precision and reducing errors of inference, obtaining sufficient power to account for the effects of prognostic factors, the ability to examine clinically important subgroups, and gathering information on secondary endpoints, which may be obtained only in the context of an ongoing trial. Thus, there is a natural tension between the needs to stop a study and those tending to continue it.

Example 17 *This tension can be illustrated by the second clinical trial of extra-corporeal membrane oxygenation (ECMO) versus standard treatment for newborn infants with persistent pulmonary hypertension [O'Rourke et al., 1989]. (This study, and the first trial of ECMO, were briefly discussed in Chapter 9.) Thirty-nine new-born infants were enrolled in a trial comparing ECMO with conventional medical therapy. In this study, randomization was terminated on the basis of 4 deaths in 10*

infants treated with standard therapy compared with 0 of 9 on ECMO (p = 0.054).
Regardless of how one evaluates the data, the evidence from such a small trial is not
an ideal basis on which to base changes in clinical practice. If ECMO is a truly ef-
fective treatment, the failure to adopt it broadly because of weak evidence favoring
it is also an ethical problem.

Example 18   *The Second International Study of Infarct Survival (ISIS-2) is an ex-*
ample of a trial that continued past the point at which many practitioners would have
been convinced by the data. In this study, the streptokinase versus placebo compar-
ison was based on 17,187 patients with myocardial infarction [ISIS-2, 1988]. After
five weeks, the death rate in the placebo group was 12.0% and in the streptokinase
group was 9.2% (p = 10^{-8}). With regard to this outcome, convincing evidence in
favor of streptokinase was available earlier in the trial. However, the impact of this
study on practice is largely related to its precision, which would have been dimin-
ished by early stopping. An earlier overview of 22 smaller trials had little effect on
practice, even though the estimate it produced in favor of streptokinase was similar.

10.1.3 There are several statistical approaches for evaluating incomplete evidence

To facilitate decision making about statistical evidence while a trial is still ongoing,
several quantitative methods have been developed. These include frequentist approaches (e.g., fixed sample size, fully sequential, and group sequential methods),
Bayesian methods, decision-theoretic approaches, and likelihood based methods.
Evaluating incomplete evidence from a comparative trial is one area of statistical
theory and practice that tends to highlight differences between all of these, but particularly Bayesian and frequentist approaches. No method of study monitoring is
completely satisfactory in all circumstances, although certain aspects of the problem
are better managed by one method or another. Frequentist methods appear to be the
most widely applied in practical situations. For a general discussion of monitoring
alternatives, see Gail [1984]. Some practical issues are discussed in DeMets [1990].

Statistical guidelines for early stopping can be classified further in two ways:
those based only on the current evidence at the time of an interim analysis and those
that attempt to predict the outcome after additional observations have been taken
(such as those that would be obtained if the trial continued to its fixed sample size
conclusion). Frequentist procedures that use only the current evidence include sequential and group sequential methods, alpha spending functions, and repeated confidence intervals. Stochastic curtailment is a frequentist method that uses predictions
based on continuation of the trial. Corresponding Bayesian methods are based on the
posterior distribution or a predictive distribution.

Regardless of the method used to help quantify evidence, investigators must separate the statistical guidelines and criteria used for stopping boundaries from the
qualitative and equally important aspects of monitoring a clinical trial. Although the
statistical criteria are useful tools for addressing important aspects of the problem,
they suffer from several shortcomings. They tend to oversimplify the information

relevant to the decision and the process by which it is made. The philosophy behind, and the results of, the various statistical approaches are not universally agreed upon and they are sometimes inconsistent with one another. These problems set the stage for formal ways of introducing expert opinion into the monitoring process, discussed below.

Similarities

These different statistical methods to facilitate early termination of trials do have several things in common. First, all methods require the investigators to state the questions clearly and in advance of the study. This demands a priority for the various questions that a trial will address. Second, all methods for early stopping presuppose that the basic study is properly designed to answer the research questions. Third, all approaches to early stopping require the investigator to provide some structure to the problem beyond the data being observed. For example, fixed sample size methods essentially assume that the interim data will be inconclusive. The frequentist perspective appeals to the hypothetical repetition of a series of identical experiments and the importance of controlling type I errors. Bayesian approaches require specifying prior beliefs about treatment effects, and decision methods require constructing quantitative loss functions. Any one of these approaches may be useful in specific circumstances or for coping with specific problems.

Fourth, except for using a fixed sample size, the various approaches to early stopping tend to yield quantitative guidelines with similar practical performance on the same data. Perhaps this is not surprising because they are all ways of reformulating evidence from the same data. In any specific study, investigators tend to disagree more about the non-statistical aspects of study termination, making differences between quantitative stopping guidelines relatively unimportant.

Fifth, investigators pay a price for terminating trials early. This is true whether explicit designs are used to formalize decision making or *ad hoc* procedures are used. Unless investigators use designs that formalize the decision to stop, it is likely that the chance for error will be increased or the credibility of the study will suffer. Studies that permit or require formal data-dependent stopping methods as part of their design are more complicated to plan and carry out and, when such trials are stopped early, the estimates of treatment differences can be biased. Also, accurate data may not be available as quickly as they are needed. Good formal methods are not available to deal with multiple endpoints such as event times, safety, and quality of life or to deal effectively with new information from outside the trial itself. Finally, there is a difficult to quantify but very important question of how convincing the evidence will be if the study is terminated early.

No method is a substitute for judgment. Investigators should keep in mind that the sequential boundaries are *guidelines* for stopping. The decision to stop is considerably more complex than capturing information in a single number for a single endpoint would suggest. Although objective review and consensus regarding the available evidence is needed when a stopping boundary is crossed, the decision cannot be made on the basis of the statistic alone. Mechanisms for making such decisions are discussed later in this chapter.

Differences and criticisms

There are substantial differences between the various approaches to study monitoring and stopping, at least from a philosophical perspective. For example, the frequentist approach measures the evidence against the null hypothesis using the α-level of the hypothesis test. However, hypotheses with the same α-level may have different amounts of evidence against them and Bayesian methods reject this approach [Anscombe, 1963; Cornfield, 1966a 1966b]. For monitoring, frequentist methods have three additional problems. First, they lack the philosophical strength and consistency of Bayesian methods. Second, they are difficult to use if the monitoring plan is not followed. Finally, the estimated treatment effects at the end of the trial are biased if the study is terminated early according to one of these plans. This is discussed below.

Bayesian approaches rely on choosing a prior distribution for the treatment difference, which summarizes prior evidence and/or belief. This can be a weakness of the method because a prior probability distribution may be difficult to specify, especially for clinicians. Apart from this, a statistical distribution may be a poor representation of one's knowledge (or ignorance). Even if we ignore these problems, different investigators are likely to specify a different prior distribution. Its exact form is somewhat arbitrary.

Decision theoretic approaches require specifying a loss function that attempts to capture the consequences of incorrect conclusions. This usually requires an over-simplification of losses and the consequences of incorrect conclusions. These approaches use the idea of a "patient horizon", which represents those who are likely to be affected by the trial. The magnitude of the patient horizon has a quantitative effect on the stopping boundary.

10.2   Likelihood Methods

Likelihood methods for monitoring trials are based principally or entirely on the likelihood function constructed from an assumed probability model. The likelihood function is frequently used for testing hypotheses, but it also provides a means for summarizing evidence from the data without a formal hypothesis test. Here we consider a likelihood method originally developed for testing, but use it as a pure likelihood-based assessment of the data.

10.2.1   Fully sequential designs test after each observation

One could assess the treatment difference after each experimental subject is accrued, treated, and evaluated. Although this approach would allow investigators to learn about treatment differences as early as possible, it can be impractical for studies that require a long period of observation after treatment before evaluating the outcome. (An alternative perspective on this view is offered below.) This approach is definitely useful in situations where responses are evident soon after the beginning of

236   DATA-DEPENDENT STOPPING

treatment. It is broadly useful to see how quantitative guidelines for this approach
can be constructed.

The first designs that used this approach were developed by Wald [1947] to improve reliability testing and are called sequential probability (or likelihood) ratio tests
(SPRT). As such, they were developed for testing specific hypotheses using the likelihood ratio test, and could be classified as frequentist procedures. More generally
as suggested above, the likelihood function is a summary of all the evidence in the
data and the likelihood ratio does not have to be given a hypothesis testing interpretation. Therefore, I have classified the SPRT as a likelihood method, in spite of it
being a "test". Frequentist methods are discussed below.

SPRT boundaries for binary outcomes

Consider a binary response from each study subject that becomes known soon after receiving treatment. We are interested in knowing if the estimated probability
of response favors p_1 or p_2, values of clinical importance chosen to facilitate decisions about early stopping. We will test the evidence in favor of p_1 or p_2, using the
likelihood ratio test [Stuart and Ord, 1991], a commonly used statistical procedure.
Because the response is a Bernoulli random variable for each subject, the likelihood
function is binomial,

$$\mathcal{L}(p, \mathbf{X}) = \prod_{i=1}^{N} p^K (1 - p)^{N-K},$$

where $\mathbf{X} = \{r_1, r_2, r_3, \ldots r_N\}$ is the data vector, r_i is 1 or 0 depending on whether
the ith subject responded or not, K is the total number of responses, and N is the
number of subjects tested. The likelihood is a function of both the data, $\mathbf{X}$, and the
unknown probability of success, p. To assess the strength of evidence in favor of p_1
or p_2 quantitatively, we calculate the likelihood ratio assuming each one is the correct
value given the data,

$$R = \frac{\mathcal{L}(p_1, \mathbf{X})}{\mathcal{L}(p_2, \mathbf{X})} = \left(\frac{p_1}{p_2}\right)^K \left(\frac{1 - p_1}{1 - p_2}\right)^{N-K}.$$

If R is large, the evidence favors p_1 and if R is small, it favors p_2. When $R = 1$,
there is no evidence either way. Thus, we can define two critical values for R: R_U
causes us to favor p_1 and R_L favors p_2. The likelihood ratio summarizes the data
and could be used as easily at the end of the trial after all data are available.

When analyzing interim data, we can calculate the likelihood ratio and stop the
study only if the evidence in favor of p_1 or p_2 is the same as it would have been for
the final (fixed) sample size. Thus, the stopping criteria, expressed as the likelihood
ratio, are constant throughout the study. This means that to stop early, we must satisfy
either

$$\left(\frac{p_1}{p_2}\right)^k \left(\frac{1 - p_1}{1 - p_2}\right)^{n-k} \geq R_U \qquad (10.1)$$

or

$$\left(\frac{p_1}{p_2}\right)^k \left(\frac{1-p_1}{1-p_2}\right)^{n-k} \leq R_L, \qquad (10.2)$$

where we *currently* have k responses out of n subjects tested. It is more convenient to express the stopping criteria either in terms of k versus n or $\pi = k/n$ versus n, where π is the observed proportion of responders. Values of π (and, therefore, k and n) which satisfy equations 10.1 and 10.2 are "boundary values".

Equation 10.1 or 10.2 can be solved for k as

$$\log(R) = k \log\left(\frac{p_1}{p_2}\right) + (n-k)\log\left(\frac{1-p_1}{1-p_2}\right),$$

where $R = R_U$ or $R = R_L$. Thus,

$$k = \frac{\log(R) - n\log(\frac{1-p_1}{1-p_2})}{\log(\Theta)}, \qquad (10.3)$$

where Θ is the odds ratio, and

$$\pi = \frac{k}{n} = \frac{\frac{\log(R)}{n} - \log(\frac{1-p_1}{1-p_2})}{\log(\Theta)}. \qquad (10.4)$$

A similar derivation has been given by Wald [1947] and Duan-Zheng [1990].

Equation 10.3 is helpful because it shows that the boundary values of k and n are linearly related. We will obtain an upper or lower boundary, depending on whether we substitute R_U or R_L into equations 10.3 or 10.4. Choosing R_U and R_L is somewhat arbitrary, but for "strong" evidence, we might take

$$R_U = R_L = 32.0.$$

A weaker standard of evidence might use

$$R_U = R_L = 8.0.$$

To make a tighter analogy with frequentist testing procedures, choices which attempt to satisfy controlling the type I and type II error level of the comparison [Wald, 1947] might be

$$R_L = \frac{1-\alpha}{\beta}$$

and

$$R_U = \frac{\alpha}{1-\beta},$$

where $\alpha = 0.05$ and $\beta = 0.20$, for example. Plots of π versus n for several values of R_U and R_L are shown in Figure 10.1. Early in the trial, only extreme values of π (or k) will provide convincing evidence to stop the study.

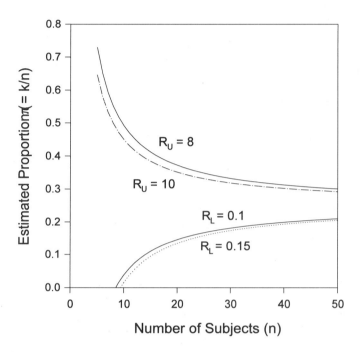

Figure 10.1 SPRT boundaries for a binomial outcome calculated from equation 10.4. $p_1 = .17, p_2 = .35.$

SPRT boundaries for event rates

Similar equations can be used to derive the boundaries for a sequential likelihood ratio test for deciding if evidence favors either of two event rates, λ_1 and λ_2. Again, the hypothesis testing perspective is convenient but unnecessary. For event times with a Weibull distribution with shape parameter v and possible right censoring, the likelihood ratio test for H_0: $\lambda_1 = \lambda_2$ is

$$R = \frac{\prod_{i=1}^{N} e^{-\lambda_1 t_i^v} \lambda_1^{z_i} (vt_i^{v-1})^{z_i}}{\prod_{i=1}^{N} e^{-\lambda_2 t_i^v} \lambda_2^{z_i} (vt_i^{v-1})^{z_i}} = \frac{e^{-\lambda_1 \sum_{i=1}^{N} t_i^v} \lambda_1^d}{e^{-\lambda_2 \sum_{i=1}^{N} t_i^v} \lambda_2^d}, \tag{10.5}$$

where N is the total number of subjects under study, and z_i is a binary indicator variable for each subject such that $z_i = 1$ if the ith subject has failed and $z_i = 0$ if the ith subject is censored. The exponential distribution is a special case of the Weibull with $v = 1$. Note that $d = \sum z_i$ is the total number of failures. Equation 10.5 can be written

$$R = e^{-(\lambda_1 - \lambda_2)T} \Delta^d, \tag{10.6}$$

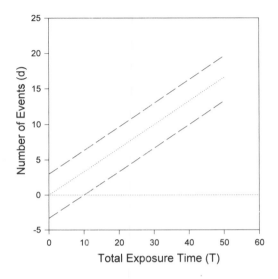

Figure 10.2 SPRT stopping boundaries for event rate comparisons. Note that the vertical axis is number of events and not the failure rate.

where $\Delta = \lambda_1/\lambda_2$ and $T = \sum_{i=1}^{N} t_i^v$ is the total "effective" exposure time for all study subjects. Taking logarithms and solving equation 10.6 for d yields

$$d = \frac{\log(R) + (\lambda_1 - \lambda_2)\,T}{\log(\Delta)}\;,\tag{10.7}$$

which shows the linear relationship between d and T. A plot of number of events versus total exposure time using this equation with $\nu = 1$ is shown in Figure 10.2. If λ had been plotted instead of d, the graph would resemble Figure 10.1.

Alternatively, solving for the boundary value $\frac{d}{T} = \lambda$ yields

$$\lambda = \frac{d}{T} = \frac{\frac{\log(R)}{T} + \lambda_1 - \lambda_2}{\log(\Delta)}\;.\tag{10.8}$$

These equations express the stopping boundary value, d or λ, in terms of T, the current "total" exposure time in the trial cohort. T is an ordinary total exposure time when $v = 1$. For $v \neq 1$, it is similar to a "weighted" total. For the upper boundary, one would choose $R = R_U$ and λ_1 and λ_2 would be given values that reflect clinically relevant high and low failure rates. For the lower boundary, $R = R_L$. After observing T units of total follow-up time in the cohort, the observed failure rate can be compared with the corresponding boundary point to help decide whether or not to stop the trial.

Using SPRT boundaries

The SPRT is an appealing method for constructing stopping guidelines for a number of reasons. First, it is based on the likelihood function, an efficient summary of the data and one of the few points of agreement for all of the data-dependent stopping methods commonly used. Second it is conceptually and mathematically relatively simple to employ. Third, it permits continuous monitoring of study outcomes, which is a natural and flexible use for most clinicians. Finally, it is simple to interpret, both when designing the guidelines and in the event that a boundary is reached. These points assume that the statistical model is correct.

These types of designs, although optimal from certain perspectives, have been criticized as impractical for clinical trials, because the outcome or response must be known quickly, and because the boundary is "open", i.e., there is a chance that the interim estimate of the event rate will never touch a boundary and the trial will not terminate. The first criticism is not as problematic as it might seem at first because, if the outcome is not evident immediately for each subject in the trial, one can use instead the subjects who have been followed long enough to be assessed.

For binary outcomes that require a prolonged period of observation, it is as though study subjects are in a "pipeline" with a delay, during which a response cannot occur. Only when they emerge from the other end of the pipeline can they be evaluated for response. The longer the delay, the less ability there is to stop the trial immediately because patients remain in the pipeline. Even so, the basic methodology of the fully sequential design remains applicable. For event rates, every increment in follow-up time contributes to the estimate of the failure rate. Therefore, all patients accrued contribute continuously to the information needed to monitor the study. In fact, even after accrual stops, the follow-up time is increasing and could lead to having the ratio reach a boundary.

The problem of never encountering a stopping boundary in an SPRT trial is harder to deal with. The accumulating evidence from a trial may never favor either para-meter within a reasonable period of time. In this case, the study must be interpreted as yielding evidence, which does not distinguish between p_1 and p_2. This may be a perfectly appropriate assessment of the evidence, so that this characteristic is not necessarily a drawback. Also we may be interested in more than p_1 and p_2.

At least three possible solutions to the "problem" exist. After a fixed number of patients have been accrued (or a fixed total follow-up time), the trial could be de-clared finished with the evidence favoring neither alternative. This is probably the most correct representation of the evidence. Alternatively, the inconclusive circum-stance could be taken conservatively as evidence in favor of the null hypothesis. This would increase the type II error from the frequentist point of view. Finally, the design could be replaced by one which is guaranteed to terminate at a stopping boundary at some point. Such designs are termed "closed" and are discussed in the section on frequentist methods (below).

10.3 Bayesian Methods

Bayesian methods for statistical monitoring of trials seem to have much appeal to clinicians and have a strong philosophical foundation, but have not been widely used. Bayesian methods for trials in general are discussed by Berry [1985] and Freedman and Spiegelhalter [1989]. A concise review of Bayesian methods for monitoring clinical trials is given by Freedman, Spiegelhalter, and Parmar [1994]. Robust Bayesian methods are discussed by Carlin and Sargent [1996]. Additional Bayesian methods for single-arm trials are discussed by Thall, Simon, and Estey [1995; 1996].

Problems of inference can arise when the assessment of evidence about the treatments depends on the plans for analyses in the future, as it does in frequentist methods. This problem is acute when considering, for example, a trial "result" with a statistical significance level of 0.03. If this is the final analysis of a fixed sample size study, we might conclude that the findings are significant and be willing to stand by them. However, if we learn that the result is only the first of several planned interim analyses (especially one using a very conservative early stopping boundary), the frequentist will be unwilling to embrace the same evidence as being convincing. A similar situation might arise if different investigators are monitoring the same study using different frequentist stopping boundaries. Problems increase if a trial is extended beyond its final sample size. The strict frequentist, having "spent" all of the type I error during the planned part of the trial, cannot find any result significant if the study is extended indefinitely.

Bayesian monitoring methods avoid these problems, because the assessment of evidence does not depend on the plan for future analyses. Instead, the interim data from the trial are used to estimate the treatment effect or difference and Bayes rule is used to combine the prior distribution and the experimental evidence, in the form of a likelihood, into a posterior distribution. The posterior distribution is the basis for recommendations regarding the status of the trial. If the posterior distribution is shifted far in one direction, the probability that the treatment effect lies in one region will be high and the inference will favor that particular treatment. If the posterior distribution is more centrally located, neither treatment will be convincingly superior. Thus, these posterior probabilities can be used to make decisions about stopping the trial or gathering additional evidence.

10.3.1 Bayesian example

To illustrate the Bayesian monitoring method, consider a randomized controlled trial with survival as the main endpoint. We suppose that investigators planned to detect a hazard ratio of 2.0 with 90% power using a fixed sample size of 90 events. Suppose also that investigators plan one interim analysis approximately halfway through the trial and a final analysis. The logarithm of the hazard ratio is approximately normally distributed, making it simpler to work on that scale. The variance of the log-hazard distribution is approximately $1/d_1 + 1/d_2$, where d_1 and d_2 are the numbers of events in the treatment groups. Under the null hypothesis of no treatment difference, the log hazard ratio is 0 and for a hazard ratio of 2.0, the logarithm is 0.693.

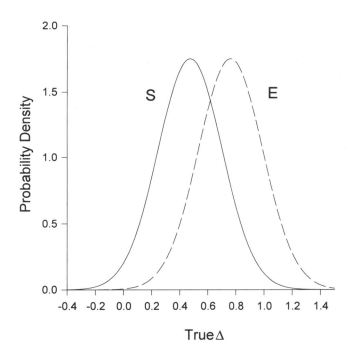

Figure 10.3 Bayesian posterior distributions for monitoring a trial with event rate outcomes based on a skeptical (S) or enthusiastic prior (E).

Skeptical prior

For a prior distribution, investigators summarize the evidence as being equivalent to a distribution with zero mean and a standard deviation of 0.35. If correct, random samples from this distribution would exceed 0.693 only 2.5% of the time. This corresponds to having observed approximately 32 events on the treatments with an estimated risk ratio of 1.0. This particular prior distribution, if based only on strength of belief, expresses some skepticism about the treatment benefit.

At the time of the interim analysis, there are 31 events in one group and 14 in the other, with the hazard ratio estimated to be 2.25. We can summarize this evidence as a normal distribution centered at $\log(2.25) = 0.811$ with a standard deviation of $\sqrt{1/31 + 1/14} = 0.32$. Then, the mean of the posterior distribution is

$$\mu_p = \frac{(0 \times 32 + 0.811 \times 45)}{(32 + 45)} = 0.474$$

and the standard deviation of the posterior distribution is

$$\sigma_p \approx \sqrt{\frac{4}{32 + 45}} = 0.228.$$

These quantities can be used to calculate probabilities about the current estimate of the treatment effect (hazard ratio). For example, the probability that the true hazard ratio exceeds 2.0 is

$$\Pr\{\Delta > 2.0\} = 1 - \Phi\left(\frac{\log(2.0) - 0.474}{0.228}\right) = 1 - \Phi(0.961) = 0.168,$$

where $\Phi(\cdot)$ is the cumulative normal distribution function and Δ is the true hazard ratio. In other words, there is not convincing evidence to terminate the trial, using this skeptical prior distribution.

Enthusiastic prior

For comparison, consider what happens when investigators are subjectively enthusiastic about the new treatment. They quantify their opinion in the form of a different prior distribution, centered at the alternative hypothesis, but with the same variance as the skeptical prior. If true, random samples from this distribution would yield hazard ratios in excess of 2.0 50% of the time. Following the calculations now, the posterior mean is

$$\mu_p' = \frac{(0.693 \times 32 + 0.811 \times 45)}{(32 + 45)} = 0.762 \,,$$

with the same standard deviation as that obtained above. Investigators would then estimate the chance that the true hazard ratio exceeds 2.0 as

$$\Pr\{\Delta > 2.0\} = 1 - \Phi\left(\frac{\log(2.0) - 0.762}{0.228}\right) = 1 - \Phi(-0.302) = 0.682.$$

Furthermore, the chance that the true hazard ratio exceeds 1.75 is 81%, which might lead some investigators to want the trial terminated because of efficacy.

This example illustrates both the Bayesian method and its dependence on the choice of a prior distribution for the treatment effect. In many actual cases, one would not choose either of these distributions as a prior for monitoring purposes, preferring instead to let the evidence from the trial stand more on its own by employing a "less informative" density function. An example of this might be a normal distribution, which is made to be very flat by virtue of having a large variance. This would correspond to having few prior observations. Such a distribution might be chosen by investigators who prefer not to influence monitoring decisions greatly with information from outside the trial.

10.4 Decision-Theoretic Methods

One can approach the problem of stopping or continuing a clinical trial at the time of an interim analysis as a decision-theory question. Given a prior distribution for the treatment difference and a utility function, it is possible to construct optimal group sequential tests for terminating the trial. Similarly, any particular group sequential test is optimal under some assumed prior and utility, which can be determined using this approach. Like the likelihood and Bayesian methods, decision-theoretic approaches do not control the type I error properties of the stopping procedure. Fixing the probability of a type I error in advance does not lead to stopping guidelines with optimal decision-theoretic properties.

Many of the designs that have been developed using this approach have been impractical and have not been applied to actual clinical trials. A principal difficulty is that the exact designs are sensitive to the "patient horizon", which is the number of patients who stand to benefit from the selected therapy. It is usually difficult or impossible to specify this number. Despite this shortcoming, it is useful to examine the general properties of this approach. With it, subjective judgments are isolated and formalized as utility functions and prior distributions. The utility function quantifies the benefit from various outcomes and the prior distribution is a convenient way to summarize knowledge and uncertainty about the treatment difference before the experiment is conducted. Using these tools, the behavior of decision rules can be quantified and ranked according to their performance.

Standard group sequential stopping rules (discussed below) have been studied from a decision-theoretic view and found to be lacking [Heitjan, Houts, and Harvey, 1992]. When the utility functions and prior distributions are symmetric, the group sequential methods commonly employed are optimal. However, when a trial is judged by how well it improves the treatment of future patients, symmetric utilities may not be applicable, and standard group sequential stopping rules perform poorly.

Lewis and Berry [1994] discussed trial designs based on Bayesian decision theory, but evaluated them as classical group sequential procedures. They show that the clinical trial designs based on decision theory have smaller average costs than the classical designs. Moreover, under reasonable conditions, the mean sample sizes of these designs are smaller than those expected from the classical designs.

10.5 Frequentist Methods

Sequential and group sequential clinical trial designs have been developed from the perspective of hypothesis testing, which permits trial termination when a test of the null hypothesis of no difference between the treatments rejects. As interim assessments of the evidence (e.g., tests of the null hypothesis) are carried out, the test statistic is compared with a pre-specified set of values called the "stopping boundary". If the test statistic exceeds or crosses the boundary, the statistical evidence favors stopping the trial.

By repeatedly testing accumulating data in this fashion, the type I error level can be increased. Constructing boundaries that preserve the type I error level of the trial, but still permit early termination after multiple tests, is part of the mechanics of frequentist sequential trial design. A simplified example will illustrate the effect.

Example 19 *Suppose we take the data in n non-overlapping batches (independent of one another) and test treatment differences in each one using $\alpha = 0.05$. If the null hypothesis is true, the chance of not rejecting each batch is $1 - 0.05 = 0.95$. Because of independence, the chance of not rejecting all batches is 0.95^n. Thus, the chance of rejecting one or more batches (i.e., the overall type I error) is $1 - 0.95^n$. The overall type I error, α^*, would be*

$$\alpha^* = 1 - (1 - \alpha)^n,$$

where α is the level of each test.

This example is only slightly deficient. In an actual trial, the test is performed on overlapping groups as the data accumulate so that the tests are not independent of one another. Therefore, the type I error may not increase in the same way as it would for independent tests, but it does increase nonetheless. One way to correct this problem is for each test to be performed using a smaller α to keep α^* at the desired level.

10.5.1 Triangular designs are "closed"

A complete discussion of the theory of sequential trial designs is beyond the scope of this book. This theory is extensively discussed by Whitehead [1992] and encompasses fixed sample size designs, SPRT designs, and triangular designs. A more concise summary is given by Whitehead [1994]. Computer methods for analysis are discussed by Duan-Zheng [1990]. Here I sketch sequential designs for censored survival data while trying to avoid some of the complexities of the theory. For a recent clinical application of the triangular design, see Moss, Hall, Cannom, et al. [1996].

As in the case of fixed sample size equations, assume that the measure of difference between treatment groups is $\Delta = \log(\lambda_1/\lambda_2)$, the logarithm of the hazard ratio. At the time of the ith failure, we have observed d_{i1} and d_{i2} failures in the treatment groups from n_{i1} and n_{i2} subjects who remain at risk. Consider the logrank statistic, which measures the excess number of events on the control treatment over that expected

$$Z = \sum_{i=1}^{N} \frac{n_{i1}d_{i2} - n_{i2}d_{i1}}{n_i},$$

where $n_i = n_{i1} + n_{i2}$. The variance of this quantity is

$$V = \sum_{i=1}^{N} \frac{d_i(n_i - d_i)n_{i1}n_{i2}}{(n_i - 1)n_i^2},$$

where $d_i = d_{i1} + d_{i2}$. V is a measure of the amount of information in the data. For equal sized treatment groups and a small proportion of events, $V \approx D/4$ where D is the total number of events.

To monitor the trial, Z_j and V_j will be calculated at the jth monitoring point. It is necessary to assume that V_j does not depend on $Z_1, \ldots Z_{j-1}$ so that the stopping rules cannot be manipulated. This can be accomplished by using a fixed schedule of interim analysis times. At the jth interim analysis, if Z_j is more extreme than a specified boundary point, the trial will be stopped. The boundaries depend on $V_1, \ldots V_j$. It is customary to draw them on a plot of Z versus V. Figure 10.4 shows an example for the triangular test. For discrete rather than continuous monitoring, the boundaries must be modified slightly, yielding a "Christmas tree" shape.

The mathematical form of the boundaries can be derived from two considerations. The first is the usual power requirement which states that the probability of rejecting the null hypothesis when the hazard ratio is Δ_a should be $1 - \beta$. The second consideration relates the upper boundary, Z_u and the lower boundary Z_ℓ, to V as

$$
\begin{aligned}
Z_u &= a + cV \\
Z_\ell &= -a + 3cV.
\end{aligned}
$$

In the very special case when $\beta = \alpha/2$, we have

$$
a = \frac{-2\log(\alpha)}{\Delta_a}
$$

and

$$
c = \frac{\Delta_a}{4} \; .
$$

However, the restriction on α and β that produces this simplification is not generally applicable and one must resort to numerical solutions for other cases.

10.5.2 Group sequential designs may be easier to construct and apply

In many circumstances, investigators do not need to assess treatment differences after every patient is accrued. When monitoring large (multi-center) trials, it is more common for data about efficacy to be available only at discrete times, perhaps once or twice each year. When assessments are made at discrete intervals but frequently enough, the trial can terminate nearly as early as if it were monitored continually. This is the idea of group sequential methods. Typically, only a handful of interim looks need to be performed.

The statistical approach to group sequential boundaries is to define a critical value for significance at each interim analysis so that the overall type I error criterion will be satisfied. Suppose there are a maximum of R interim analyses planned. If the values of the test statistics from the interim analyses are denoted by $Z_1, Z_2, \ldots, Z_R$, the boundary values for early stopping can be denoted by the points $B_1, B_2, \ldots, B_R$. At the jth analysis, the trial stops with rejection of the null hypothesis if

$$
Z_j \geq B_j, \quad for \; 1 \leq j \leq R.
$$

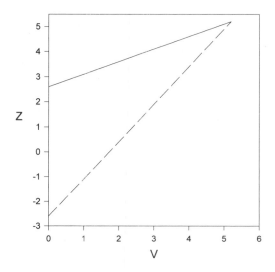

Figure 10.4 Triangular test stopping boundaries.

Many commonly used test statistics have "independent increments" so that the interim test statistic can be written

$$Z_j = \frac{\sum_{i=1}^{j} Z_i^*}{\sqrt{j}} \ ,$$

where Z_i^* is the test statistic based on the ith group's data. This greatly simplifies the calculation of the necessary interim significance levels. Although the boundaries are constructed in a way that preserves the overall type I error of the trial, one may construct boundaries of many different shapes, which satisfy the overall error criterion. However, there are a few boundary shapes that are commonly used. These are shown in Figure 10.5 and the numerical values are given in Table 10.2.

Specific group sequential boundaries

The Pocock boundary uses the same test criterion for all tests performed, $Z_i = Z_c$ for $1 \leq i \leq R$, where Z_c is calculated to yield the desired overall type I error rate. Using this boundary, it is relatively easy to terminate a trial early. However, the procedure suffers from the undesirable feature that the final test of significance is made with a larger critical value (smaller p-value) than that conventionally used for a fixed sample size trial. In theory, the final significance level after three analyses could be between, say, 0.05 and 0.0221 (Table 10.2). If one had not used a group sequential procedure, the trial would show a significant difference. However, because the sequential procedure was used, the result is not "significant". This is an uncomfortable position for investigators.

Table 10.2 Some Frequently Used Group Sequential Stopping Boundaries with Z Scores and Significance Levels for Different Numbers of Interim Analyses.

Interim Analysis Number	O'Brien – Fleming		Haybittle – Peto		Pocock	
	Z	p	Z	p	Z	p
			$R = 2$			
1	2.782	.0054	2.576	.0100	2.178	.0294
2	1.967	.0492	1.960	.0500	2.178	.0294
			$R = 3$			
1	3.438	.0006	2.576	.0100	2.289	.0221
2	2.431	.0151	2.576	.0100	2.289	.0221
3	1.985	.0471	1.960	.0500	2.289	.0221
			$R = 4$			
1	4.084	5×10^{-5}	3.291	.0010	2.361	.0158
2	2.888	.0039	3.291	.0010	2.361	.0158
3	2.358	.0184	3.291	.0010	2.361	.0158
4	2.042	.0412	1.960	.0500	2.361	.0158
			$R = 5$			
1	4.555	5×10^{-6}	3.291	.0010	2.413	.0158
2	3.221	.0013	3.291	.0010	2.413	.0158
3	2.630	.0085	3.291	.0010	2.413	.0158
4	2.277	.0228	3.291	.0010	2.413	.0158
5	2.037	.0417	1.960	.0500	2.413	.0158

The Haybittle-Peto boundary corrects this problem, because the final significance level is very close to that conventionally employed, e.g., it is near 0.05. It is harder to terminate the trial early, but the final analysis resembles the hypothesis test that would have been used in a fixed sample size design. Similarly, the O'Brien-Fleming design uses boundaries that yield nearly conventional levels of significance for the final analysis but make it hard to terminate the trial early. For these, $Z_j = Z_c / \sqrt{R/j}$, where again, Z_c is calculated to control the overall type I error rate [O'Brien and Fleming, 1979]. One needs very strong evidence to stop early when using this boundary.

10.5.3 Alpha spending designs permit more flexibility

One of the principal difficulties with the strict application of group sequential stopping boundaries is the need to specify the number and location of points for interim analysis in advance of the study. As the evidence accumulates during a trial, this lack of flexibility may become a problem. It may be more useful to be able to adjust the timing of interim analyses and, for the frequentist, to use varying fractions of the

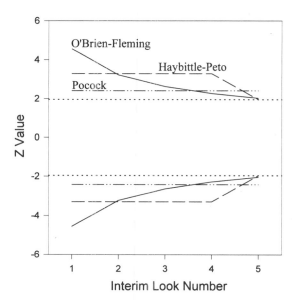

Figure 10.5 Group sequential stopping boundaries from Table 10.2.

overall type I error for the trial. Such an approach was developed and called the "alpha spending function" [DeMets and Lan, 1994; Lan and DeMets, 1983]. See also Hwang and Shih [1990].

Suppose there are R interim analyses planned for a clinical trial. The amount of information available during the trial is called the information fraction and will be denoted by τ. For grouped interim analyses, let i_j be the information available at the jth analysis, $j = 1, 2, \ldots, R$, and let $\tau_j = i_j/I$ be the information fraction, where I is the total information. For studies comparing mean values based on a final sample size of N, $\tau = n/N$, where n is the interim accrual. For studies with time-to-event endpoints, $\tau \approx d/D$, where d is the interim number of events and D is the planned final number. The alpha spending function, $\alpha(t)$, is a smooth function on the information fraction such that $\alpha(0) = 0$ and $\alpha(1) = \alpha$, the final type I error rate desired. The alpha spending function must be monotonically increasing.

If the values of the test statistics from the interim analyses are denoted by Z_1, Z_2, $\ldots$, Z_j, the boundary values for early stopping are the points B_1, B_2, $\ldots$, B_j, such that

$$\Pr\{|Z_1| \geq B_1, \text{ or } |Z_2| \geq B_2, \cdots, \text{ or } |Z_j| \geq B_j\} = \alpha(\tau_j).$$

Using this definition, the O'Brien-Fleming boundary discussed above is

$$\alpha_{OF}(\tau) = 2 \left[1 - \Phi \left(\frac{Z_\alpha}{\sqrt{\tau}} \right) \right],$$

where $\Phi(x)$ is the cumulative standard normal distribution function. The Pocock boundary discussed above is

$$\alpha_P(\tau) = \alpha \log(1 + \tau(e - 1)).$$

Many other spending functions have been constructed [Hwang and Shih, 1990].

10.5.4 Early stopping may yield biased estimates of treatment effect

One drawback of sequential and group sequential methods is that, when a trial terminates early, the estimates of treatment effect will be biased. This can be undestood intuitively. If the same study could be repeated a large number of times, chance fluctuations in the estimated treatment effect in the direction of the boundary would be more likely to result in early termination than fluctuations away from the boundary. Therefore, when the boundary is touched, these variations would not average out equally, biasing the estimated treatment effect. The sooner a boundary is hit, the larger the bias in the estimated treatment effect. This effect can create problems with the analysis and interpretation of a trial that is terminated early [e.g., Emerson and Banks, 1994].

For example, consider a randomized comparative group sequential trial with 4 analyses using an O'Brien-Fleming stopping boundary. If the true treatment effect is 0.0, there is a small chance that the stopping boundary will be crossed at the third analysis. This would be a type I error. This probability is 0.008 for the third analysis, upper boundary. Among trials crossing the upper boundary there, the average Z-score for the treatment effect is approximately 2.68. When the true treatment effect is 1.0, 50% of the trials will cross the upper boundary. Among those crossing at the third interim analysis, the average Z-score is 2.82. When the true treatment effect is 2.0, 98% of trials will terminate on the upper boundary. Among those crossing at the third interim analysis, the average Z-score is 3.19. These results, each determined by statistical simulation of 10,000 trials, illustrate the bias in estimated treatment effects when a boundary is crossed.

One could consider correcting for this bias using a Bayesian procedure that modifies the observed treatment effect by averaging over all possible "prior" values of the true treatment effect. However, such a procedure will be strongly affected by the properties of the assumed prior distribution and therefore may not be a good solution to the problem of bias. In other words, the true prior distrubution of treatment effects is unknown, making it impossible to reliably correct for the bias.

Because of this bias, the trialist must view these sequential designs as "selection designs" that terminate when a treatment satisfies the stopping criteria. In contrast, fixed sample size trials might be termed "estimation designs", because they will generally provide unbiased estimates of the treatment effect or difference. One should probably not employ a selection design when it is critical to obtain unbiased estimates of the treatment effect. A fixed sample size design would be more appropriate in such a situation. Similarly, when early stopping is required for efficient use of study resources or ethical concerns, a selection design should be used in place of the fixed sample size alternative.

10.6 Other Monitoring Tools

10.6.1 Conditional power

The early stopping methods discussed above have assumed that the trial should be terminated only when the treatments are significantly different. Alternatively, we might wish to stop a clinical trial when the interim result is unlikely to change after accruing more subjects. The accumulated evidence might convincingly demonstrate that the treatments are equivalent, for example. Investigators would want to terminate a study if it is virtually certain to end without a rejection of the null hypothesis, even if carried to the planned fixed sample size. It is possible to quantify the power of the study to yield an answer different from that seen at an interim analysis and base a monitoring plan on this approach. This is called *conditional power* [Lan, DeMets, and Halperin,1984; Lan, Simon, and Halperin, 1982]. Some additional practical aspects are discussed by Andersen [1987].

Example 20 *Suppose we are testing a questionable coin to see if it yields heads 50% of the time when flipped. If π is the true probability of heads, we have $H_0 : \pi = \Pr[heads] = 0.5$ or $H_a : \pi = \Pr[heads] > 0.5$. Our fixed sample size plan might be to flip the coin 500 times and reject H_0 if*

$$Z = \frac{N_H - 250}{\sqrt{500 \times .5 \times .5}} \geq 1.96 ,$$

where N_H is the number of heads obtained and $\alpha = 0.025$. Stated another way, we reject H_0 if $N_H \geq 272$. Suppose we flip the coin 400 times and observe 272 heads. There would be little point in performing the remaining 128 trials because we are sure to reject the null hypothesis.

Partial sums

To illustrate how conditional power works in a one-sample case, suppose that we have a sample of size N from a $N(\mu, 1)$ distribution and we wish to test $H_0 : \mu = 0$ vs. $H_a : \mu > 0$. Furthermore, assume that we have a test statistic, $Z_{(N)}$, which is based on the mean of a sample from a Gaussian distribution,

$$Z_{(N)} = \frac{\sum_{i=1}^{N} x_i}{\sqrt{N}} ,$$

where we reject H_0 if $Z_{(N)} > 1.96$. Using a standard fixed sample size approach (equation 7.12), we solve $\theta = \sqrt{N}\mu = (Z_\alpha + Z_\beta)$ for N to obtain the sample size.

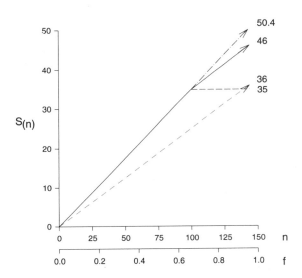

Figure 10.6 Projected partial sums during a trial.

Part way through the trial when n subjects have been accrued, the test statistic is

$$Z_{(n)} = \frac{\sum_{i=1}^{n} x_i}{\sqrt{n}} = \frac{S_n}{\sqrt{n}},$$

where $1 \leq n \leq N$, and S_n is the partial sum. It is easy to show that $E\{S_n\} = n\mu$ and $Var\{S_n\} = n$. More importantly, using S_n, the increments are independent, i.e., $E\{S_N \mid S_n\} = S_n + E\{S_{N-n}\}$ and $Var\{S_N \mid S_n\} = N - n$. The expected value of S_n increases linearly throughout the trial. Therefore, we can easily calculate the probability of various outcomes conditional on observing certain interim results. This is represented by Figure 10.6 showing a plot of S_n versus n and the following example.

Example 21 *Suppose $\mu = 0.25$ and $\sqrt{N}\mu = (1.96 + 1.04) = 3$, so that $N = 144$. After $n = 100$ patients, suppose $S_{100} = 35$ ($Z_{100} = 35/\sqrt{100} = 3.5$). There are at least three scenarios under which we would like to project the end of the trial given the interim results: C1) the current trend continues to the end, C2) the original alternative hypothesis continues to the end of the trial, and C3) the original null hypothesis continues to the end of the trial. Other scenarios may be important to consider also. The method of calculation is shown in Table 10.3. For C1,*

$$\Pr\{Z_{(144)} \geq 1.96 \mid Z_{(100)} = 3.5, \ \mu = 0.25\}$$
$$= \quad \Pr\{S_{144} \geq 23.52 \mid S_{100} = 35, \ \mu = 0.25\}$$

Table 10.3 Projected Partial Sums During a Trial under Three Assumptions about the Trend

Case	μ	$E\{S_{144}\vert S_{100}\}$	$\text{Var}\{S_{144}\vert S_{100}\}$
C1	0.25	$35 + (144 - 100) \times 0.25 = 46.0$	$144 - 100 = 44$
C2	0.35	$35 + (144 - 100) \times 0.35 = 50.4$	44
C3	0.00	$35 + (144 - 100) \times 0.00 = 35.0$	44

$$= \quad \Pr\left\{\frac{S_{144} - 46.0}{\sqrt{44}} \geq \frac{23.52 - 46.0}{\sqrt{44}} \;\Big|\; S_{100} = 35,\ \mu = 0.25\right\}$$

$$= \quad \Pr\{\Phi(x) \geq -3.39\}$$

$$= \quad 0.99965$$

Similarly, for C2,

$$\Pr\{Z_{(144)} \geq 1.96 \mid Z_{(100)} = 3.5,\ \mu = 0.35\}$$

$$= \quad \Pr\left\{\frac{S_{144} - 50.4}{\sqrt{44}} \geq \frac{23.52 - 50.4}{\sqrt{44}} \;\Big|\; S_{100} = 35,\ \mu = 0.35\right\}$$

$$= \quad \Pr\{\Phi(x) \geq -4.05\}$$

$$= \quad 0.99997,$$

and for C3,

$$\Pr\{Z_{(144)} \geq 1.96 \mid Z_{(100)} = 3.5,\ \mu = 0.0\}$$

$$= \quad \Pr\left\{\frac{S_{144} - 35.0}{\sqrt{44}} \geq \frac{23.52 - 35.0}{\sqrt{44}} \;\Big|\; S_{100} = 35,\ \mu = 0.35\right\}$$

$$= \quad \Pr\{\Phi(x) \geq -1.73\}$$

$$= \quad 0.95818.$$

Because of the high chance of rejecting the null hypothesis regardless of assumptions about the trend, investigators would probably terminate this study early.

B -values

The method of conditional power can be improved by making it independent of the actual sample size [Lan and Wittes, 1988]. To do so, we define the *information fraction* of the trial as $f = n/N$. Then we define

$$Z_f = Z_{(n)} = \frac{\sum_{i=1}^{n} x_i}{\sqrt{n}} = \frac{S_n}{\sqrt{n}},$$

and

$$B_f = \frac{\sum_{i=1}^{n} x_i}{\sqrt{N}} = \frac{S_n}{\sqrt{n}}\sqrt{\frac{n}{N}} = Z_f\sqrt{f}.$$

Note that $B_1 = Z_1 = Z_{(N)}$ and that B_f and $(B_1 - B_f)$ are independent. Also, the conditional mean of B_1 is $B_f + (1-f)\theta$ and the conditional variance of B_1 is $1-f$. The example above can be reworked in terms of B-values.

Example 22 $\mu = 0.25$ and $\theta = \sqrt{N}\mu = (1.96 + 1.04) = 3$, so that $N = 144$. After $n = 100$ patients, $f = 100/144 = .69444$ and $B_{.694} = 3.5\sqrt{.69444} = 2.9167$. The three scenarios under which we would like to project the end of the trial given the interim results are C1) $\theta = 3$, C2) $\theta = 2.9167/.69444 = 4.2001$, and C3) $\theta = 0$. For C1,

$$
\begin{aligned}
&\Pr\{Z_{(144)} \geq 1.96 \mid Z_{(100)} = 3.5,\ \mu = 0.25\} \\
=\ &\Pr\{S_{144} \geq 23.52 \mid S_{100} = 35,\ \mu = 0.25\} \\
=\ &\Pr\left\{ \frac{S_{144} - 46.0}{\sqrt{44}} \geq \frac{23.52 - 46.0}{\sqrt{44}} \ \middle|\ S_{100} = 35,\ \mu = 0.25 \right\} \\
=\ &\Pr\{\Phi(x) \geq -3.39\} \\
=\ &0.99965.
\end{aligned}
$$

Similarly, for C2,

$$
\begin{aligned}
&\Pr\{Z_{(144)} \geq 1.96 \mid Z_{(100)} = 3.5,\ \mu = 0.35\} \\
=\ &\Pr\left\{ \frac{S_{144} - 50.4}{\sqrt{44}} \geq \frac{23.52 - 50.4}{\sqrt{44}} \ \middle|\ S_{100} = 35,\ \mu = 0.35 \right\} \\
=\ &\Pr\{\Phi(x) \geq -4.05\} \\
=\ &0.99997,
\end{aligned}
$$

and for C3,

$$
\begin{aligned}
&\Pr\{Z_{(144)} \geq 1.96 \mid Z_{(100)} = 3.5,\ \mu = 0.0\} \\
=\ &\Pr\left\{ \frac{S_{144} - 35.0}{\sqrt{44}} \geq \frac{23.52 - 35.0}{\sqrt{44}} \ \middle|\ S_{100} = 35,\ \mu = 0.35 \right\} \\
=\ &\Pr\{\Phi(x) \geq -1.73\} \\
=\ &0.95818.
\end{aligned}
$$

Here again, the study will almost certainly yield a significant result so that it would be logical to terminate it at this point.

10.7 Some Software

A recurring problem in implementing new or difficult methods of design and analysis is the availability of reliable, flexible, and reasonably priced computer software to facilitate the computations. For the Bayesian and likelihood based methods discussed above, the calculations are simple enough to be performed by hand. To my knowledge, there is no commercially available software to accomplish those calculations.

For calculating group sequential boundaries, the program *EaSt* [Cytel Software, 1993] is available for IBM-compatible microcomputers. Although the user interface is somewhat awkward, the program is accurate and reasonably priced. It also permits including stopping boundaries for both the null hypothesis and the alternative hypothesis. For fully sequential frequentist designs, illustrated above by the triangular design, there is *PEST* [Whitehead, Brunier, and Facey, 1992], a commercially available program also for IBM PCs. It requires a fairly high level of expertise from the user and is very expensive. Because of these features, it is a workable solution only for the investigator who needs to perform such calculations frequently.

Conditional power calculations using B-values can be performed using the program cpower.exe provided on the disk that accompanies this book. See Chapter 19 for additional details.

10.8   Monitoring and Interim Reporting

In addition to formally specifying statistical criteria for study termination, investigators use interim analyses to assess other important aspects of an ongoing trial. Deficiencies in any of several areas could be reason to stop the trial. These include accrual, data quality, safety, and other items listed in Table 10.1. Thus, the statistical stopping guidelines discussed above become part of a broader trial monitoring activity. A number of authors have discussed this broad issue and offer useful perspectives for the clinician and trialist alike [Geller, 1987; Green, Fleming, and O'Fallon, 1987; O'Fallon, 1985]. An interesting discussion in the context of cardiovascular disease is given by the Task Force of the Working Group on Arrhythmias of the European Society of Cardiology [1994].

Aside from terminating a study early because of outcomes or data quality, there are other reasons why investigators may want a view of trial data as they accumulate. Problems with patient accrual or recruitment may become evident and require changes in the study protocol or investigator interactions with prospective participants. In some cases, incentives or recruitment programs may need to be initiated. Additionally, monitoring and judicious interim reporting can help maintain investigator interest in, and enthusiasm for, the study. It is natural for highly motivated investigators to wonder about study progress and be curious about results. Not all such curiosity can or should be satisfied by interim reports, but they can serve to maintain active interest. Finally, it may be necessary to make other adjustments in the trial design, such as sample size, on the basis of information from the early part of the study [Herson and Wittes, 1992].

10.8.1 Monitoring of single-center studies relies on periodic investigator reporting

The practical issues in trial monitoring may be somewhat different for multi-center clinical trials than for single-institution studies. The funding and infrastructure for multi-center trials usually permits a separate monitoring mechanism for each study or group of related studies. For single academic institutions conducting a variety of trials, such as cancer centers, the same oversight mechanism may be required to deal with many varied clinical studies. In such settings, the responsibility for study conduct and management may reside more with the individual investigator than it does in collaborative clinical trial groups.

A typical mechanism to assist single institutions in monitoring clinical trials sponsored by their faculty is an annual report. It is the responsibility of the study principal investigator to prepare the report and submit it to the oversight committee, which may be the Institutional Review Board or a similar body. This report should contain objective and convincing evidence that the study is safe and appropriate to continue. As a minimum, the renewal report should address the following concerns.

- *Compliance with governmental and institutional oversight.* The investigator should document that all of the necessary regulations have been satisfied.
- *Review of eligibility.* Document that there is a low frequency of ineligible patients being placed on study.
- *Treatment review.* Most or all patients should have adhered to the intended treatment. Frequent non-adherence may be a sign of problems with the study design, eligibility, or conduct.
- *Summary of response.* For diseases like cancer where response to treatment is a well defined and widely used measure of efficacy, investigators should summarize responses and the criteria used to judge them.
- *Summary of survival.* For most serious chronic diseases, the survival (or disease-free survival) experience of the study cohort is important. In any case, events possibly related to adverse consequences of the treatment need to be summarized.
- *Adverse events.* Convincing evidence of safety depends on accurate, complete, and timely reporting of all adverse events related to the treatment. Investigators sometimes attribute adverse events to causes other than the investigational treatment, such as to the underlying disease. This aspect of the annual report merits careful review.
- *Safety monitoring rules.* Many study protocols have formal guidelines or statistical criteria for early termination. The data must be summarized appropriately and compared with these guides.
- *Audit and other quality assurance reviews.* Data audits examine some of the issues outlined above and other aspects of study performance. The results of such audits and other process quality review should be available for consideration by the oversight committee.

10.8.2 Decisions about early termination are aided by a DSMC

It is common practice when conducting clinical trials to have data and questions reviewed periodically by a Data and Safety Monitoring Committee or Board (DSMC or DSMB) to assist investigators with the decision to stop a trial or make other modifications of the study based on unexpected findings in the data. In recent years, the role of DSMCs has become vital for monitoring multi-center studies and its conceptual functions have become fairly well standardized. Other names for the DSMC are "data monitoring committee" or just "monitoring committee".

There are several reasons why DSMCs have become widely used. First, they provide a workable mechanism for coping with the problem of protecting the interests and safety of study participants, while preserving the scientific integrity of the trial. The DSMC is intellectually and financially independent of the study investigators. This gives investigators and observers confidence that decisions will be made independently of academic and economic pressures. Finally, many sponsors of trials (e.g., NIH) support or require such a mechanism. For example, the National Heart Lung and Blood Institute (NHLBI) has explicit guidelines for data quality assurance that emphasize the DSMC mechanism [NHLBI, 1994a; 1994b]. Similar policies have recently been adopted by the National Cancer Institute [National Cancer Institute, 1996]. Although the DSMC mechanism has strengths, it also has some weaknesses (discussed below).

Composition of DSMCs

DSMCs are usually composed of a combination of clinical, statistical, epidemiological, laboratory, data management, and ethical experts. All members of the DSMC should be knowledgeable about the circumstances surrounding the trial and should not have any vested interest in the outcome. Of course, the committee members will have a scientific interest in the outcome, but only to the extent that they would like to see a valid and well-performed trial. Individuals with any financial or other conflicts of interest should not be members of the DSMC.

Monitoring committees often consist of 3 to 10 members, depending on the size of the trial and complexity of the issues. It is good practice to include some experienced members on every DSMC. A new committee should not be constructed entirely from inexperienced members, even if they are all experts. Multidisciplinary and/or multi-national membership may be helpful, because some issues may require these varying perspectives. Individuals who would make good DSMC members are usually known to the trial investigators. There is no formal source for such expertise except for personal contacts. Experienced trial methodologists, clinical experts, ethicists, and investigators who have conducted similar studies are good sources for DSMC members.

Investigators and trialists do not agree universally on whether or not the DSMC should include an investigator from the trial. To the extent that the role of the DSMC is to protect the interests of the patients, a clinical investigator can be a member. To the extent that the DSMC should preserve the scientific integrity of the trial, a clinical investigator may be unnecessary or inappropriate. This question need not be very difficult to resolve. For example, a clinical investigator could participate in safety and data quality related aspects of the DSMC deliberations but be excluded from discussions regarding efficacy and possible early termination of the trial because of convincing treatment differences. An investigator or other individual with particular expertise can be a non-voting member of the Committee.

In institutions that conduct many clinical trials simultaneously, such as large comprehensive cancer centers, a single DSMC may review multiple studies or may even monitor all ongoing trials. The role or emphasis of this committee may be broader than simply safety and efficacy monitoring. For example, such a committee may help investigators with protocol development and review, setting institutional priorities for potentially competing studies, monitoring adverse events, and renewing protocols and other administrative matters. These functions are distinct from those usually performed by the Institutional Review Board.

There are other questions that an impartial view of the data can help answer beside evaluating treatment or side effects. For example, the need for ancillary studies, secondary questions, or requests for the data might be evaluated by the DSMC. The committee will meet once or twice each year (more often if the study progress or issues require it) and review formal reports of study outcomes. Because of the potential for this interim information to affect the clinicians' interactions with patients, the DSMC's meetings and the data presented to it are kept confidential. Reports typically address a number of issues vital to decision making about the trial and are not disseminated.

Masking

The DSMC should not be masked as to treatment assignment. Doing so can inhibit interpretation of important details. For example, if clinically significant differences in safety or efficacy between treatment groups are evident, the DSMC could wrongly attribute them to one treatment or another. Thus, unexpected results can be missed until the end of the trial. Masking of the DSMC can facilitate some aspects of the scientific integrity of the trial. However, masking probably cannot improve patient safety and should be discouraged. Because the DSMC will be aware of treatment assignment and must make important decisions based on limited data, the members should be selected thoughtfully.

Meeting format and reporting responsibilities

The DSMC will meet usually at the same time that trial investigators review the progress of their studies. This often occurs semi-annually, for example. The frequency of meetings depends on how quickly information in the trial accumulates. The deliberations of the DSMC are confidential and there should be no discussion or dissemination of any results outside the Committee meetings. A fairly standard but flexible format for meetings has evolved in many trial settings. It includes a graded degree of confidentiality, depending on the aspect of the study being discussed. Topics from non-confidential to most confidential are: 1) relevant information from outside the trial, 2) accrual and study progress, 3) safety data, 4) efficacy differences, 5) DSMC speculations.

For example, the general progress of the study (e.g., accrual) can be discussed in an open forum. Additionally, scientific information from outside the study can be brought to the attention of the Committee and investigators. This might include results or progress on related trials. Attendance at this portion of the meeting can include the sponsor, study chair (PI) or other investigators, and statistical center personnel in addition to the DSMC members.

A more restricted portion of the meeting follows this. Discussions and summary data concerning safety should probably be restricted to the sponsor, study chair, study statistician, and the DSMC. Discussions and data presented by treatment group should be closed to investigators, except for the trial statistician or designee who presents quantitative findings to the DSMC. During this portion of the meeting, outcome data on safety and efficacy by treatment group are presented and discussed. No formal decisions are made by the DSMC during this part of the meeting.

Following the presentation of safety and efficacy data by treatment group, the DSMC meets alone in executive session. During these deliberations, decisions or recommendations regarding changes in the study are made. These decisions can then be transmitted to the appropriate group representative. In some clinical trials, the DSMC reports to the sponsor. This is the case, for example, in many NIH-sponsored trials. Other times, the Committee reports to the principal investigator or study chair. In the AIDS Clinical Trial Group, the DSMC reports to the Executive Committee of the group. There are many workable models, provided the recommendations of the DSMC are considered seriously by those ultimately responsible for the conduct of the study. In rare cases, the investigators may choose not to follow the course of action suggested by the DSMC. This can lead to a great deal of friction between the investigators and the DSMC, sometimes resulting in resignations from the monitoring committee.

10.8.3 The DSMC assesses baseline comparability

Before recommending termination of a clinical trial because of treatment or side effects, the DSMC will establish that any observed differences between the treatment groups are not due to imbalances in patient characteristics at baseline. When such differences are present and thought to be of consequence for the outcome, the treatment effect typically would be "adjusted" for the imbalance, perhaps using methods discussed in Chapter 13. Without the exploratory adjusted analyses, the trial might continue under the assumption that the differences are, in fact, a consequence only of baseline imbalances. This is likely to be a risky assumption. Familiar statistical methods will usually suffice to assess baseline balance and determine its impact on the observed outcome.

Baseline imbalances by themselves are not likely to be a cause for much concern. For example, in a well-conducted randomized trial, they must be due to chance. However, because imbalances can undermine the appearance or credibility of a trial, some interventions might be proposed to correct them. These could include modifications of blocking or other methods employed to create balance.

10.8.4 The DSMC reviews accrual and timeliness of study completion

Design assumptions

Another consideration for the DSMC that reflects on the decision to continue is the rate of accrual onto the trial and the projected duration of the study based on the current trends. Often, the accrual rate at the beginning of a trial is slower than that projected when the study was designed or slower than that required to finish the trial in a timely fashion. In many studies, the accrual rate later increases and stabilizes. In any case, after accrual has been open at all centers for several months, investigators can get a reliable estimate of how long it will take to complete the study under the original design assumptions and the observed accrual and event rates.

At this early point in the trial, it may be evident that design assumptions other than the projected accrual rate are inaccurate. For example, the drop-out rate may be higher than expected, the event rate may be lower than planned (because trial participants are often at lower risk than the general population with the same disease), or the intervention may not be applied in a manner sufficient to produce its full effect (e.g., some dietary interventions). Each of these circumstances could significantly prolong the length of time necessary to complete the study. Unless remedial actions are taken, e.g., increasing accrual by adding study centers, the trial may be impossible to complete. The DSMC may recommend that these studies terminate prematurely.

Resource availability

It may also happen that some of the limited resources available to conduct the clinical trial are being consumed more rapidly than planned. Money is likely to be at the top of this list, but one would have to consider shrinking human resources as well. Difficulties obtaining rare drugs are another example. Occasionally, irreplaceable expertise is lost, for example, because of the death of an investigator. Any of these factors may substantially impede the timely completion of a study.

10.8.5 Data quality is a major focus of the DSMC

Even when the design assumptions and observed accrual rate of an ongoing clinical trial suggest that the study can be completed within the planned time, problems with data quality may cause the DSMC to recommend stopping. Evidence of problems with the data may become available after audits or as a result of more passive observations. An audit can be a useful device for the DSMC to assure them that data errors do not contribute to any treatment differences that are observed.

Routinely, the DSMC will review patient eligibility. Minor deviations from the protocol eligibility criteria are common and are not likely to have any consequence for the internal or external validity of the trial. These minor errors are study dependent, but might include things such as errors of small magnitude in the timing of registration or randomization or baseline laboratory values which are out of bounds. More serious eligibility violations undermine the internal validity of the trial and might include things such as randomizing patients who have been misdiagnosed or those with disease status that prevents them from benefiting from the treatment. Usually in multi-center trials, eligibility violations occur in less than 10% of those accrued. If the rate is much higher than this, it may be a sign of internal quality control problems.

The DSMC cannot perform its duties without up-to-date data and the database cannot be updated without a timely and complete submission of data forms. Monitoring this activity is relatively easy for the coordinating center and can be a reliable way of spotting errors or sloppy work. While there are numerous reasons why forms might be submitted behind schedule, there are not so many why they would be chronically delayed or extremely late. The percentage of forms submitted to the coordinating center within a few weeks or months of their due date should be high, e.g., over 90%.

In nearly all trials, there is a set of laboratory or other tests that needs to be completed either as a part of eligibility determination or to assess the baseline condition of the patient. Investigators should expect that the number of such tests would be kept to the minimum required to address the study question and that 100% of them are performed on time. One must not assume that missing data are "normal". Failure of study centers or investigators to carry out and properly record the results of these tests may be a sign of serious shortcomings that demand an audit or closing accrual at the clinic. The DSMC will be interested in the completion rate of these required tests.

Treatment compliance or adherence is another measure of considerable importance in the evaluation of data quality. Viewing trials from the intention-to-treat (ITT) perspective (see Chapter 11), the only way to ensure that the ITT analysis yields an estimate of treatment effect that is also the effect of actually receiving the treatment is to maintain a high rate of treatment adherence. When adherence breaks down it might be a sign of one or more of the following: 1) serious side effects, 2) patients too sick to tolerate the therapy or therapies, 3) poor quality control by the investigators, or 4) pressures from outside the study (e.g., other treatments). In any case, poor adherence threatens the validity of the study findings and may be cause for the DSMC to stop the trial.

10.8.6 The DSMC reviews safety and toxicity data

Safety and toxicity concerns are among those most carefully considered by the DSMC. There are three characteristics of side effects that are relevant: the frequency of side effects; their intensity or seriousness; and whether or not they are reversible. Frequent side effects of low intensity which are reversible by dose reduction or other treatment modifications are not likely to be of much consequence to the patients or concern to the investigators. In contrast, even a rarely occurring toxicity of irreversible or fatal degree could be intolerable in studies where patients are basically healthy or have a long life expectancy.

In diseases like cancer or AIDS, serious but reversible toxicities are likely to be common side effects of treatment and are frequently accepted by patients because of the life-threatening nature of their illness. In fact, in the cytotoxic drug treatment of many cancers, the therapeutic benefit of the treatment may depend on, or be coincident with, serious but reversible toxicity. This idea is especially important when considering the design of phase I trials in oncology. Here experienced investigators may realize that the implications of serious toxicity are not as far-reaching as they would be in many other diseases.

10.8.7 Efficacy differences are assessed by the DSMC

Efficacy, or the lack of it, is the most familiar question to evaluate when considering the progress of a trial. The importance of learning about efficacy as early as possible has ethical and resource utilization motivations. Before attributing any observed differences in the groups to the effects of treatment, the DSMC will be certain that the data being reviewed are of high quality and that baseline differences in the treatment groups cannot explain the findings. Statistical stopping rules like the ones outlined earlier in this chapter may be of considerable help in structuring and interpreting efficacy comparisons.

It is possible that efficacy and toxicity findings during a trial will be discordant, making the question of whether or not to stop the study more difficult. For example, suppose that a treatment is found to offer a small but convincing benefit in addition to a small but clinically important increase in the frequency and severity of side effects. On balance, these findings may not be persuasive for terminating the trial. In this situation, it may be important to continue the study to gather more precise information or data about secondary endpoints.

10.8.8 The DSMC should address a few practical questions specifically

From a practical perspective, the DSMC needs to answer only a few questions to provide investigators with the information required to complete the experiment.

Should the trial continue?

The most fundamental question, and the one most statistical monitoring guidelines are designed to help answer, is "should the study be stopped?". When the efficacy and toxicity information is convincing, the DSMC will likely recommend stopping. However, there is room for differences of opinion about what is, to a large degree, a subjective assessment.

Clinical trials yield much more information than just a straightforward assessment of treatment and side effect differences. There are many secondary questions that are often important motivations for conducting the trial. Also, the database from the study is a valuable resource that can be studied later to address ancillary questions and generate new hypotheses. Much of this secondary gain from a completed clinical trial can be lost when the study is stopped early. If the window of opportunity for performing comparative studies closes, as it might if the DSMC terminates the trial, some important questions will remain unanswered. Therefore, the DSMC should weigh the decision to stop carefully and in the light of the consequences of losing ancillary information.

Should the study protocol be modified?

If the trial is to continue, the DSMC may ask if the study protocols should be modified on the basis of the interim findings. A variety of modifications may be prudent, depending on the clinical circumstances. For example, side effects may be worrisome enough to adjust the frequency or timing of diagnostic tests, but not serious (or different) enough to stop the trial. If more than one treatment comparison is permitted by the study design (e.g., in a factorial trial), convincing stopping points may be reached for some treatment differences but not for others. Thus, the structure of part of the trial could be changed, while still allowing the remaining treatment comparisons to be made.

Numerous other types of modifications may be needed after an interim look at the data. These include changes in the consent documents or process, improvements in quality control of data collection, enhancing accrual resources, changes in treatment to reduce drop-outs or non-adherence, or changes in the eligibility criteria or their interpretation. In some cases, one or more treatments or treatment schedules will have to be modified, hopefully in ways that preserve the integrity of the biological question being asked.

Does the DSMC require other views of the data?

Another practical question for the DSMC is whether or not the data have been presented in sufficient detail and proper format to examine the monitoring questions. Remaining questions could be answered by additional views of the data, analysis of certain subsets, or presentation of supporting details. These could be important considerations for two reasons. First, preparation of additional analyses and supporting documentation may not be a trivial task for the statistical office. It could require extra quality control effort and verification of interim data. Second, continuation of the trial may strongly depend on subtle findings or those in a small percentage of the study participants. In such cases, it is likely that some ways of viewing the results will not display the influential findings. An unfortunate encounter with fraudulent or fabricated data would illustrate this.

Should the DSMC meet more/less frequently?

Interesting trends in the data might prompt the DSMC to meet more often than originally planned. Such a decision could create problems for some statistical monitoring plans, which is a reason to use as flexible an approach as possible. In the same way, slower accrual or a lower event rate than originally projected could prolong the interval between DSMC meetings. In terms of "information time" for the trial, the meeting may occur at the recommended intervals. However, in terms of calendar time, the frequency could change.

Are there other recommendations by the DSMC?

Finally, there are other recommendations that may result from the DSMC review. An example would be changes in the Committee itself, perhaps adding expertise in specific areas. If recruitment goals are not being met, the DSMC might recommend initiating efforts to improve it, such as interactions with target populations through community leaders or organizations. Sometimes for multi-center trials, a meeting of the investigators may increase enthusiasm and clear up minor problems with accrual. In any case, the DSMC should be viewed and should act as objective experts who have in mind the best interests of all parties associated with the study. As such, the Committee will feel free to recommend any course of action that enhances the safety and quality of the clinical trial.

10.8.9 The DSMC mechanism has potential weaknesses

Although DSMCs can satisfy the need for informed impartial decision making in clinical trials, the mechanism has potential shortcomings. Trial investigators are often not permitted to be part of the DSMC so that this important perspective may be under-represented during deliberations. Although clinical investigators are in a state of equipoise when a trial begins, experience, knowledge, or opinion gained during the study can eliminate it. However, the DSMC may artificially preserve the state of equipoise either because members do not have the clinical experiences of working with the treatments and patients or because they employ somewhat artificial statistically based termination criteria (discussed above). Also, these stopping guidelines typically consider only a single outcome whereas the decision to stop a trial may depend on several factors.

The relationship between the DSMC and trial sponsor can sometimes be an issue. In some trials sponsored by NIH, the DSMC reports to the sponsoring institute only, and not to the study investigators or local IRBs. The sponsor has no written obligation to inform the investigators about DSMC recommendations. For example, the sponsor may not agree with DSMC concerns and may not convey recommendations to the study investigators. However, the investigators are the ones who carry ethical obligations to the patients. Thus, a policy that does not require DSMC recommendations to be transmitted to study investigators does not honor all ethical obligations.

Because of their composition and function, DSMCs can emphasize impartiality over expertise. Overzealous adherence to statistical stopping criteria could be a manifestation of this. Some DSMCs remain masked to treatment assignments to increase impartial assessments of differences that may become evident. It is hard to see how a DSMC can adequately assure patient safety while masked. Finally, there are occasional suggestions from trialists that studies employing DSMCs tend to stop too soon leaving important secondary questions unanswered.

10.9 Summary

It is appropriate, if not ethically imperative, for investigators to examine the accumulating results from a clinical trial in progress. Information from the trial may convince investigators to close the study early for reasons of patient safety. Reasons why a trial might be stopped earlier than initially planned include: the treatments are convincingly different (or equivalent); side effects are too severe or adherence is too low; the data are of poor quality; or needed resources are lost or are insufficient. The tendency to stop a study for these or other reasons is balanced by an imperative to gather complete and convincing evidence about the objectives.

Making inferences about treatments based on incomplete data can be error prone. Investigators must place additional structure on the interim analyses beyond the usual end-of-study plans to minimize errors. There are several approaches to accomplishing this, including frequentist methods that control the type I error, likelihood-based methods, Bayesian approaches, and decision theory. The product of each of these approaches to early stopping is a set of quantitative guidelines that help investigators evaluate the strength of the available evidence and decide if the trial should be terminated. All methods require timely and accurate interim reporting of data.

Frequentist methods for constructing early stopping guidelines (boundaries) have gained widespread acceptance. They control the overall type I error of the trial and are relatively simple and flexible to implement and interpret. However, they have the drawback that the same data can yield different inferences depending on the monitoring plans of the investigators. Likelihood methods base the decision to stop a trial early on achieving the same strength of evidence (measured by likelihood ratios) as one would obtain for the final analysis. Bayesian methods have similar characteristics but allow subjective notions of strength of evidence to play a part in the decision to stop.

In the commonly used group sequential boundaries, the decision to stop or not is taken at a small number of discrete points during the trial, typically once or twice each year. Additional flexibility in the timing and type I error control can be gained by using an alpha spending function approach. Fully sequential frequentist methods, likelihood methods such as the SPRT, and most Bayesian monitoring methods permit assessment of interim data continuously. Besides stopping when the "null hypothesis" appears to be false, trials may be terminated early if, after some point, there is little chance of finding a difference. Conditional power calculations are one means to facilitate this.

Statistical guidelines for the primary endpoint are not the only consideration when assessing the interim evidence from a clinical trial. Side effects, unanticipated events, data quality, secondary objectives, and evidence from outside the trial may all reflect on the decision to continue. Also, the sponsor or investigators may have other obligations or interests that can conflict with objective evaluation of trial data. Because monitoring can be complicated, many clinical trials use a formal Data Safety Monitoring Committee (DSMC) to assist with the task and insure patient safety. After reviewing interim data, the DSMC could recommend a variety of actions including stopping the trial, modifying the study protocol, examining additional data, or making a new assessment of the evidence sooner than originally planned.

10.10 Questions for Discussion

1. Investigators plan a SE clinical trial to study the efficacy and side effects of a new genetically engineered treatment vaccine against prostate cancer. The toxicity is likely to be low and the potential treatment effect, based on animal studies, could be high. The clinicians are anxious to finish the trial as quickly as possible because of cost and scientific priorities. Sketch and defend a trial design that you believe would be appropriate under these circumstances.

2. The probability of success on standard therapy for a disease is 50%. A new treatment is being tested and investigators would like to end the trial if evidence supports a success rate of 75%. Construct, graph, and explain what you believe to be appropriate statistical monitoring guidelines for this trial.

3. In a clinical trial comparing treatments to improve survival following AIDS, investigators plan to adopt a new treatment if the evidence suggests a hazard ratio of 1.75 (new treatment is superior). Investigators prefer a Bayesian approach to monitoring and analysis. Prior to the trial, some data are available indicating a hazard ratio of 1.6 based on 50 events. During the trial, a hazard ratio of 2.0 is observed with 60 and 30 events in the treatment groups. What is your quantitative assessment of the evidence and would you favor continuing the trial?

4. Two statisticians are helping to conduct, monitor, and analyze a trial with a single planned interim analysis and a final analysis. At the interim, the statisticians perform some calculations independently and agree that the study should be continued. (Because they agree to recommend continuing the trial, the statisticians do not discuss details of their interim analyses.) At the final analysis, the p-value turns out to be 0.035. To their consternation, the statisticians discover that they have used different boundaries for the analyses and one can declare the final result "significant" while the other cannot. Discuss how you can help them out of this problem.

5. A trial is planned to accrue a maximum sample size of 80 patients. After 60 have been accrued, $Z = 25/\sqrt{60} = 3.23$. Should the trial be continued? Justify your recommendation.

6. For the previous problem, calculate the information fraction, f, and the B-value, B_f.

Chapter References

Andersen, P.K. (1987). Conditional power calculations as an aid in the decision whether to continue a clinical trial. Controlled Clinical Trials 8: 67-74.

Anscombe, F.J. (1963). Sequential medical trials. J. Am. Stat. Assoc. 58: 365-383.

Berry, D.A. (1985). Interim analyses in clinical trials: Classical vs. Bayesian approaches. Statistics in Med. 4: 521-526.

Carlin, B.P. and Sargent, D.J. (1996). Robust Bayesian approaches for clinical trial monitoring. Statistics in Med. 15: 1093-1106.

Cornfield, J. (1966a). Sequential trials, sequential analysis, and the likelihood principle. Am. Statistician 20: 18-23.

Cornfield, J. (1966b). A Bayesian test of some classical hypotheses with applications to sequential clinical trials. J. Am. Stat. Assoc. 61: 577-594.

Cytel Software Corporation (1992). EaSt. A Software Package for the Design and Interim Monitoring of Group Sequential Clinical Trials. Cambridge, MA.: Cytel Software.

DeMets, D.L. (1990). Data monitoring and sequential monitoring – An academic perspective. Journal of Acquired Immune Deficiency Syndrome 3(suppl. 2): S124-S133.

DeMets, D.L. and Lan, K.K.G. (1994). Interim analysis: The alpha spending function approach. Statistics in Med. 13: 1341-1352.

Duan-Zheng, X. (1990). Computer Analysis of Sequential Medical Trials. New York: Ellis Horwood.

Emerson, S.S. and Banks, P.L.C. (1994). Interpretation of a Leukemia Trial Stopped Early, Chapter 14 in Nicholas Lange et al. (Eds.), Case Studies in Biometry, New York: John Wiley & Sons.

Fleming T.R., Green S.J., and Harrington D.P. (1984). Considerations for monitoring and evaluating treatment effects in clinical trials. Controlled Clin. Trials 5: 55-66.

Fleming, T.R. and DeMets, D.L. (1993). Monitoring of clinical trials: Issues and recommendations. Conrolled Clin. Trials 14: 183-197.

Freedman, L.S., Spiegelhalter, D.J., and Parmar, M.K.B.? (1989). Comparison of Bayesian with group sequential methods for monitoring clinical trials. Controlled Clinical Trials 10: 357- 367.

Gail, M.H. (1982). Monitoring and Stopping Clinical Trials. Chapter 15 in Valerie Mike and Kenneth Stanley (Eds.), Statistics in Medical Research, New York: John Wiley & Sons.

Gail, M. (1984). Nonparametric frequentist proposals for monitoring comparative survival studies. Handbook of Statistics 4: 791-811.

Geller, N.L. (1987). Planned interim analysis and its role in cancer clinical trials. J. Clinical Onc. 5: 1485-1490.

Green, S.J., Fleming, T.R., and O'Fallon, J.R. (1987). Policies for study monitoring and interim reporting of results. J. Clinical Onc. 5: 1477-1484.

Heitjan, D.F., Houts, P.S., and Harvey, H.A. (1992). A decision-theoretic evaluation of early stopping rules. Statistics in Medicine 11: 673-683.

Herson, J., and Wittes, J. (1993). The use of interim analysis for sample size adjustment. Drug Info. J. 27: 753-760.

Hughes, M.D. (1993). Stopping guidelines for clinical trials with multiple treatments. Statistics in Med. 12: 901-915.

Hwang, I.K. and Shih, W.J. (1990). Group sequential designs using a family of type I error probability spending functions. Statistics in Medicine 9: 1439-1445.

ISIS-2 Collaborative Group (1988). Randomized trial of intravenous streptokinase, oral aspirin, both, or neither among 17,187 cases of suspected acute myocardial infarction. Lancet, ii, 349-360.

Lan, K.K.G. and DeMets, D.L. (1983). Discrete sequential boundaries for clinical trials. Biometrika 70: 659-663.

Lan, K.K., DeMets, D.L., and Halperin, M. (1984). More flexible sequential and non-sequential designs in long-term clinical terms. Commun Statist-Theor. Meth. 13: 2339-2353.

Lan, K.K.G., Simon, R., and Halperin, M. (1982). Stochastically curtailed tests in long-term clinical trials. Commun. Stat.-Sequential Analysis 1: 207-219.

Lan, K.K.G. and Wittes, J. (1988). The B-value: A tool for monitoring data. Biometrics 44: 579-585.

Lewis, R.J. and Berry, D.A. (1994). Group sequential clinical trials: A classical evaluation of Bayesian decision-theoretic designs. J. Am. Statist. Assoc. 89: 1528-1534.

Moss, A.J., Hall, W.J., Cannom, D.S, et al. (1996). Improved survival with an implanted defibrillator in patients with coronary disease at high risk for ventricular arrhythmia. New Engl. J. Med. 335: 1933-1940.

National Cancer Institute (1996). NCI Cooperative Group Data Monitoring Committee Policy (unpublished).

NHLBI (1994a). NHLBI Guidelines for Data Quality Assurance in Clinical Trials and Large Epidemiologic Studies (unpublished).

NHLBI (1994b). NHLBI Guide for Data and Safety Monitoring Boards (unpublished).

O'Brien, P.C., and Fleming, T.R. (1979). A multiple testing procedure for clinical trials. Biometrics 35: 549-556.

O'Fallon, J.R. (1985). Policies for interim analysis and interim reporting of results. Cancer Treat. Rep. 69 (10): 1101-1106.

O'Rourke, P.P., Crone, R.K., Vacanti, J.P., Ware, J.H., Lillehei, C.W., Parad, R.B., and Epstein, M.F. (1989). Extracorporeal membrane oxygenation and conventional medical therapy in neonates with persistent pulmonary hypertension of the newborn: A prospective randomized study. Pediatrics 84: 957-963.

Pocock, S. (1993). Statistical and ethical issues in monitoring clinical trials. Statistics in Med. 12: 1459-1469. (See also the discussion which follows.)

Proschan, M.A., Follmann, D.A., and Geller, N.L. (1994). Monitoring multi-armed trials. Statistics in Med. 13: 1441-1452.

Rubinstein, L.V., and Gail, M.H. (1982). Monitoring rules for stopping accrual in comparative survival studies. Controlled Clinical Trials 3: 325-343.

Souhami, R.L. and Whitehead, J. (Eds.) (1994). Workshop on Early Stopping Rules in Cancer Clinical Trials, Robinson College, Cambridge, U.K., 13-15 April, 1993. Statistics in Med. 13: 1289-1500.

Task Force of the Working Group on Arrhythmias of the European Society of Cardiology (1994). The early termination of clinical trials: Causes, consequences, and control – with special reference to trials in the field of arrhythmias and sudden death. Circulation 89: 2892-2907.

Thall, P.F., Simon, R., and Estey, E.H. (1995). Bayesian sequential monitoring designs for single-arm clinical trials with multiple outcomes. Statistics in Med. 14: 357-379.

Thall, P.F., Simon, R., and Estey, E.H. (1996). A new statistical strategy for monitoring safety and efficacy in single-arm clinical trials. J. Clin. Oncology 14: 296-303.

Wald, A. (1947). Sequential Analysis. New York: John Wiley & Sons.

Whitehead, J. (1992). The Design and Analysis of Sequential Clinical Trials, Second Edition. New York: Ellis Horwood.

Whitehead, J. (1994). Sequential methods based on the boundaries approach for the clinical comparison of survival times. Statistics in Med. 13: 1357-1368.

Whitehead, J., Brunier, H., and Facey, K. (1992) PEST: Planning and Evaluation of Sequential Trials, User's Manual.

CHAPTER 11

Counting Patients and Events

11.1 Introduction

The findings from a clinical trial can be sensitive to how investigators resolve imperfections in the data. Imperfections arise mainly when experimental subjects do not adhere precisely with some aspect of the protocol. Non-adherence is usually not an extensive problem in experiments other than clinical trials. For example, when it occurs in laboratory and animal studies, lack of adherence to the study plan tends to be minimal so that it has relatively little impact on the analysis and interpretation of the experiment. In contrast, clinical trials are characterized, even dominated on occasion, by imperfect data arising from non-adherence with the protocol. Patients fail to follow the experimental protocol precisely because of their independence and autonomy and because of unforeseen clinical circumstances. The consequences of imperfect data depend on where the problem occurs in the experimental design and how the investigators resolve them.

Problems with data can be classified as *protocol non-adherence, missing or incomplete observations*, or *methodologic errors*. This categorization is similar to commonly used terms such as missing and incomplete observations, treatment dropouts, treatment cross-overs, eligibility errors, uncounted events, and lack of adherence to planned schedules [Gail, 1985]. Data imperfections are either correctable or permanent. Correctable mistakes are those derived through faulty definitions from source data that are free of error. Permanent, or uncorrectable, imperfections occur when the source data are lost or are in error. Both correctable and permanent errors can occur at any point in the experimental paradigm.

The difficulty with imperfections is how best to reconcile them with the experimental structure upon which reliable inference depends. This problem has been approached from two perspectives. One view has been called "explanatory"; the other "pragmatic", terms coined 30 years ago [Schwartz and Lellouch, 1967; Schwartz, Flamant, and Lellouch, 1980]. Other terms used to describe the same distinction are "efficacy" versus "effectiveness" (Chapter 8) and "explanatory" versus "management" [Sackett, 1983]. The explanatory perspective emphasizes acquiring information, while the pragmatic perspective focuses on making decisions. These perspectives have practical implications for how the analyst deals with trial design issues, as well as data imperfections. This chapter emphasizes the pragmatic perspective.

11.1.1 Explanatory and pragmatic approaches compete

Suppose investigators are studying the effect of pre-operative chemotherapy on disease recurrence and survival in patients with early stage non-small cell lung cancer. They plan a randomized trial with the treatment groups consisting of surgery (S) versus chemotherapy (C) plus surgery. A biologist might view the question like a laboratory experiment, and could isolate the effect of chemotherapy by scheduling surgery at the same time following randomization in both treatment groups. Thus, patients in the S group would wait a period of time before having surgery. The waiting time in the S group corresponds to the chemotherapy period in the $C + S$ group. This design attempts to estimate the effect of chemotherapy.

In contrast, a clinician might view this design as unrealistic, noting that physicians and patients will be unwilling to wait for surgery. In practice, patients receiving surgery alone would have their operations immediately after diagnosis. This leads to a (different) practical design, where surgery is scheduled at once in the S group but after chemotherapy in the $C + S$ group. Although this design cannot isolate the effect of chemotherapy strictly, it is pragmatic and attempts to select the superior treatment as used in actual practice.

The two trial designs are superficially the same, but demonstrate an important conceptual difference. The explanatory trial attempts to estimate what has been called "method-effectiveness" [Meier, 1991; Sheiner and Rubin, 1995], while the pragmatic one addresses "use-effectiveness". One cannot say which is the superior or correct approach, only that both questions are relevant and important and that both types of queries cannot always be answered by the same trial. Similarly, when resolving data imperfections arising from non-adherence with the study protocol, explanatory and pragmatic views may each suggest methods based on relevant and important questions. However, like the design problem just outlined suggests, there is no guarantee that the questions can be answered from the existing data. The final resolution depends on the specific circumstances.

Distinguishing between explanatory and pragmatic approaches is a useful device to investigate different philosophies about coping with protocol non-adherence and other data imperfections, as well as some design issues. However, it is not possible to label all approaches to such problems in this way. Moreover, it is not possible to say exactly what methods the explanatory or pragmatic views will emphasize in every circumstance. In any case, I will continue to use the labels in this chapter as a descriptive device.

11.2 Nature and Consequences of Specific Data Imperfections

Not all imperfections produce missing data. Imperfections could result from inappropriately "correcting" data that are properly missing. These and other types of data imperfections are avoidable. For example, patients who are too ill to comply with a demanding course of treatment should not be included in the study population, because they are not likely to adhere to the treatment. Unavoidable imperfections are those due to human error, patients lost to follow-up, and some types of missing observations such as when patients refuse to undergo tests or clinic visits, because they feel ill. Data imperfections can also be a consequence of poor study methodology, chance, or lack of protocol adherence. These topics are discussed below.

11.2.1 Prevent methodologic errors

Protocols sometimes contain improper plans that can create, or exacerbate, imperfections in the data. A common example of this is **evaluability criteria** which attempt to define what it means to receive treatment. (Already there is a potential problem because the definition of "receiving treatment" would not be important unless exclusions based on it were planned.) Investigators define "evaluable" patients as those who receive all planned courses of therapy. A biological rationale permits removing inevaluable patients from the analysis, because the treatment did not have an opportunity to work. This may be particularly relevant in SE trials.

For example, suppose patients are accrued to a SE trial. N_E are evaluable, of whom R_E have a favorable outcome. N_I are inevaluable, of whom R_I have a favorable outcome (usually $R_I = 0$). The estimate of benefit among all patients is $P = (R_E + R_I)/(N_E + N_I)$, and that for evaluable patients is $P_E = R_E/N_E$. It appears that the estimate from evaluable patients has a firmer biological basis. This approach seems persuasive, because the plans are described in advance and acknowledge the biological fact that treatment can't work unless a patient receives it. Attempts to isolate and estimate biological effects of treatment are explanatory, as compared with pragmatic analyses for which evaluability is immaterial. Evaluability criteria can create missing data, although the explanatory perspective sees them as irrelevant.

There are fundamental problems with this approach. Evaluability criteria define inclusion retroactively, that is, on the basis of treatment adherence, which is an outcome. In other words, patients are partly selected on the basis of an outcome. Although treatment adherence is also a predictor of subsequent events, exclusions based on it implicitly assume that adherence is a baseline factor, which it is not. These problems create a potential for bias. Other **retroactive definitions** are also likely to create bias. For example, suppose comparison groups are defined using outcome or future events such as tumor response in cancer studies. Patients who respond must have lived long enough to do so, whereas patients who did not respond may have survived a shorter time. Therefore, survival or other event time comparisons can be biased. This problem is discussed by Anderson et al. [1985].

The pragmatic perspective is a better one for coping with this issue. The pragmatist recognizes that the trial does not guarantee an assessment of biological effect. In fact, the concept of biological effect degenerates if patients cannot adhere to the treatment. The trial does assure an unbiased estimate of treatment benefit if all eligible patients are included in the analysis. The way to assure that the pragmatic estimate of benefit is close to the explanatory estimate of biological effect is to select treatments and design and conduct the trial so that there is a high degree of adherence. For CTE studies that attempt to show equivalence, this is particularly important, because $P_E > P$.

Avoiding the pitfalls of evaluability analyses is not always easy. A way to assess the potential for trouble is to imagine applying the evaluation definition to a new patient at the required clinical landmark. If information from the patient's future is required, the definition is probably inappropriate. Any analysis plan that eliminates eligible patients from the study is likely to create a bias.

11.2.2 Statistical methods can cope with some types of missing data

In most circumstances, **unrecorded data** imply that a methodologic error has occurred. This may not be the case if measurements were omitted during follow-up, because investigators did not know that the information was important. When this occurs frequently, especially in baseline or other clinically important assessments, it may be evidence of a fundamental problem with study design or conduct. Sometimes data may be missing for reasons associated with other patient characteristics or outcomes. Other times, it is essentially random occurrence, for example, because of human error during data entry.

The explanatory way of coping with uncounted events, because they are seemingly unrelated to the outcome of interest (e.g., non-cardiac deaths in a cohort with time to myocardial infarction as the primary study outcome), might be to censor such observations. If events seemingly unrelated to the outcome of interest are, in fact, independent of the outcome, the explanatory approach might be appropriate. In other words, not counting or censoring the seemingly unrelated events would address a useful question about the *cause specific* event rate and would not be subject to bias.

In clinical trials with longitudinal components such as time-to-event studies, some patients are likely to be **lost to follow-up**. In other words, the follow-up period may not be long enough for investigators to observe events in all patients. This can happen when a study participant is no longer accessible to the investigators because the patient does not return for clinic visits or has moved away. It can also happen when the follow-up period is shortened due to limited resources or error. Follow-up information is also lost when the earliest event time is the patient's death, which prevents observing all later event times such as disease progression or recurrence. In this case, the competing risks of death and disease progression result in lost data. This can be a problem in studies of chronic disease, especially in older populations.

If losses to follow-up occur for reasons not associated with outcome, they have little consequence for affecting the study result, except to reduce precision. If investigators know that losses to follow-up are independent of outcome, the explanatory and pragmatic views of the problem are equivalent. In a trial with survival time as the main outcome, patients might stop coming to clinic for scheduled follow-up visits, because they are too ill or have, in fact, died. In this case, being lost to follow-up is not a random event but carries information about the outcome. Such problems could affect the treatment groups of a randomized trial differently, producing a bias. In any case, studies designed with active follow-up and active ascertainment of endpoints in the participants will be less subject to this problem than those that rely on passive methods of assessing individual outcomes.

When losses occur frequently, even if they are not associated with the outcome, the external validity of the trial might be open to question. In studies using survival or disease recurrence/progression time as the major outcome, these losses to follow-up should occur in less than five percent of the trial participants when the study is conducted by experienced researchers. Often these types of missing data are not correctable but are preventable by designs and infrastructure that use active follow-up and ascertainment of events.

Investigators cannot reliably assume that losses are random events and conduct analyses that ignore them, particularly if they occur often. Every effort should be made to recover lost information rather than assuming that the inferences will be correct "as though all patients were followed completely". Survival status can sometimes be updated through the *National Death Index* or local sources. Active efforts to obtain missing information from friends or family members are also frequently successful.

There are clinical rationalizations why investigators permit **uncounted events** in the study cohort. Suppose a drug trial is being conducted in patients at high risk of death due to myocardial infarction. Because these patients are likely to be older than low risk individuals, some study participants might die from other diseases before the end of the trial. Some investigators might prefer not to count these events, because they do not seem to carry information about the effect of treatment on the target cause of death. Failure to count all such events can bias estimates of treatment effect. Sackett and Gent [1979] have some sensible advice on this point.

On the other hand, it is likely that different causes of failure compete with one another and that failure of one type carries some information about other types of failure. Being lost to follow-up may be associated with a higher chance of disease progression, recurrence, or death, for example. Death from suicide, infection, or cardiovascular causes may be associated with recurrence or progression of chronic disease such as cancer or AIDS. In cases such as these, one cannot expect to estimate a cause specific event rate without bias by censoring the seemingly unrelated events. Instead, the pragmatist would rely on a composite and well-defined endpoint such as time to disease recurrence or death from any cause (disease free survival). Alternatively, time to death from any cause (overall survival) might be used. Censoring seemingly unrelated event times is usually a correctable error.

11.2.3 Protocol non-adherence is common

Ineligible patients are a form of missing data with respect to the external validity of the trial. We don't usually think about eligibility in these terms, but it is precisely the concern raised regarding inclusiveness or representation in the study cohort. Potentially, this problem can be ameliorated by using a large heterogeneous study cohort. However, this may not always be possible because of resource limitations. This problem is interesting but peripheral to the focus of this chapter.

In most clinical trials, it is common to find errors that result in ineligible patients being placed on study. These **eligibility errors** are a relatively common type of protocol non-adherence. If the eligibility criteria are defined objectively and are based only on information available before study entry or randomization, the consequences of such errors will be minimal. In contrast, if the criteria are partly subjective, or are defined improperly using outcome information, errors and the methods of resolving them carry greater consequences.

Objective eligibility criteria are less prone to error than subjective ones. Objective criteria include quantitative measurements such as age, the results of laboratory tests, and some categorical factors such as sex. Partly subjective criteria include some measures like extent of disease, histologic type, and the patient's functional capacity. These criteria are clinically well defined, but require some element of expert opinion to specify them. This subjectivity can sometimes produce an error. Subjective criteria are those based on patient self-report or solely on physician judgment. These may not be appropriate eligibility criteria, although they may be the gold standard for some assessments such as quality of life and pain.

Patients can fail to comply with nearly any aspect of treatment specification. Common **treatment non-adherence** problems are reduced or missed doses and improper scheduling. All treatment modalities are subject to such errors including drugs, biologicals, radiotherapy, surgery, life-style changes, diet, and psychosocial interventions. Failure to comply with, or complete, the intended treatment can create a strong, but incorrect, rationale to remove patients from the final analysis. Evaluability criteria, mentioned above, are a type of non-adherence. Removing eligible but non-compliant patients from the analysis can create serious problems. In general, criteria that permit such removals are a methodologic error. Approaches to the analysis in the presence of treatment non-adherence are discussed in the section regarding intention-to-treat (below).

Ineligible patients who were mistakenly placed on study can be analyzed in two ways: included with the eligible patients from the trial cohort (pragmatic approach), or removed from the analysis (explanatory approach). In a randomized comparative trial, if the eligibility criteria are objective and determined from pre-study criteria, neither of these approaches will create a bias. However, excluding patients from any study can diminish the external validity of the results.

If there is any potential for the eligibility determination to be applied retroactively, because of subjective interpretation of the criteria or methodologic error in the protocol design, the pragmatic and explanatory approaches have quite different properties. In particular, excluding patients in this situation can affect the treatment groups in a randomized comparison differently and produce a bias. The principal difficulty is that patient exclusions produce the possibility that eligibility will be confounded with outcome.

For example, suppose a randomized trial compares medical versus surgical therapy for the same condition. Patients randomized to surgery may need evaluations and criteria beyond those required for patients to receive medical therapy. Simple examples are normal EKGs and good pulmonary function. If retroactive exclusions are based on such tests, they can differentially affect the treatment groups, yielding patients with a better prognosis in the surgical arm. This problem could be avoided by requiring all trial participants to pass the same (pre-surgical) criteria. However, such a policy would exclude many patients eligible for medical therapy, reducing the generalizations that can be made from the trial. Thus, it is not necessarily the best course of action.

Treatment non-adherence is a special type of protocol non-adherence that has received a great deal of attention in the clinical trials literature, because it is a common problem and there are different ways to cope with it when analyzing most trials. These are discussed in detail in the next section.

11.3   Treatment Non-Adherence

There has been considerable investigation into the problems surrounding treatment non-adherence. Most work has focused on ways of measuring or preventing non-adherence and proposed ways of improving statistical estimates of treatment effects when adherence is a problem. There is a chronic debate about the advantages and problems of analyses based on treatment assigned compared with those based on treatment received in comparative trials. See Newell [1992] or Lewis and Machin [1993] for concise reviews. This section will highlight some of the issues surrounding this "intention-to-treat" debate.

11.3.1   Intention-to-treat is a policy of inclusion

Intention-to-treat (ITT) is the idea, often stated as a principle, that patients on a randomized clinical trial should be analyzed as part of the treatment group to which they were assigned, even if they did not actually receive the intended treatment. The term "intention-to-treat" appears to have been originated by Hill [1961]. It can be defined generally as the analysis that

> includes all randomised patients in the groups to which they were randomly assigned, regardless of their adherence with the entry criteria, regardless of the treatment they actually received, and regardless of subsequent withdrawal from treatment or deviation from the protocol [Fisher et al., 1990].

Thus, ITT is an approach to several types of protocol non-adherence. "Treatment received" (TR) is the idea that patients should be analyzed according to the treatment actually given, even if the randomization called for something else. I can think of no other issue which perpetually generates so much disagreement between clinicians, some of whom prefer treatment received analyses, and statisticians, who usually prefer intention-to-treat approaches.

Actually, there is a third type of analysis that often competes in this situation, termed "adherers only". This approach discards all those patients who did not comply with their treatment assignment. Most investigators would instinctively avoid analyses that discard information. I will not discuss "adherers only" analyses for this reason and also because doing so will not help illuminate the basic issues.

Suppose a trial calls for randomization between two treatments, A and B. During the study, some patients randomized to A actually receive B. I will denote this group of patients by B_A. Similarly, patients randomized to B who actually receive A will be designated A_B. ITT calls for the analysis groups to be $A + B_A$ compared with $B + A_B$, consistent with the initial randomization. TR calls for the analysis groups to be $A + A_B$ compared with $B + B_A$, consistent with the treatment actually received. Differences in philosophy underlying the approaches and the results of actually performing both analyses in real clinical trials fuel debate as to the correct approach in general.

With some careful thought and review of empirical evidence, this debate can be decided mostly in favor of the statisticians and ITT, at least as an initial approach to the analysis. In part, this is because one of the most useful perspectives of an RCT is as a test of the null hypothesis of no treatment difference, a circumstance in which the ITT analysis yields the best properties. However, it is a mistake to adhere rigidly to either perspective. It is easy to imagine circumstances where following one principle or the other too strictly is unhelpful or inappropriate. The potential utility of TR analyses should probably be established on a study-by-study basis as part of the trial design (analysis plan). Then, differences between TR and ITT results will not influence one's choice.

11.3.2 Coronary Drug Project results illustrate the pitfalls of exclusions based on non-adherence

The potential differences between ITT and TR analyses have received attention in the clinical trials literature since the early work by the Coronary Drug Project Research Group (CDP) [Coronary Drug Project Research Group, 1980]. The CDP trial was a randomized, double-blind, placebo-controlled, multi-center clinical trial, testing the efficacy of the cholesterol lowering drug clofibrate on mortality. In the CDP, there was speculation that patients who adhered to the clofibrate regimen received a demonstrable benefit, while those who did not comply would have a death rate similar to the placebo group. This type of analysis is shown in Table 11.1, where adherence is defined as those patients taking more than 80% of their medication. The event rates in Table 11.1 have been adjusted for age, sex, and several other prognostic factors. The results appear to support the biological hypothesis that clofibrate is effective and that treatment adherence is necessary to achieve the benefit of the drug.

However, an identical analysis of patients receiving placebo demonstrates why results based on adherence can be misleading (Table 11.2). Patients who adhered to placebo show an even larger "treatment" benefit than those adhering to clofibrate.

Table 11.1 Comparison of Death Rates for Clofibrate Compliers and Non-Compliers in the Coronary Drug Project

| | Clofibrate | |
Status	Compliers	Non-Compliers
Alive	269	602
Dead	88	106

The odds ratio is 0.54 (0.39–0.75). The difference between compliers and non-compliers is statistically significant ($p = 0.0001$).

Thus, we cannot attribute the reduced mortality in the adhering patients to the drug. Instead, it must be a consequence of factors associated with patients adhering to medication. These could be other treatments, disease status, life-style, or unknown factors. In any case, comparison of groups based on adherence is potentially misleading.

11.3.3 Statistical studies support the ITT approach

Several authors have studied ITT and alternative approaches using analyses of existing data or simulation [Lee et al., 1991; Peduzzi et al., 1991; Peduzzi et al., 1993]. There is a consensus supporting ITT analyses. Lee et al. [1991] studied several types of analyses in a trial of phenobarbital in children with febrile seizures. They concluded that the ITT analysis was preferred and that analyses based on treatment received may confuse rather than help the interpretation of results.

Peduzzi et al. [1991] analyzed data from the Veterans Administration coronary bypass surgery study using TR and four other approaches. The ITT analysis yielded a non-significant treatment difference ($p > 0.99$), whereas the TR approach showed a survival advantage for the surgical therapy group ($p < 0.001$). Based on these findings and simulations, the authors conclude that ITT analyses should be the standard for randomized clinical trials. Similar conclusions were obtained in a second study [Peduzzi et al., 1993].

Lagakos, Lim, and Robins [1990] discuss the similar problem of early treatment termination in clinical trials. They conclude that ITT analyses are best for making inferences about the unconditional distribution of time to failure. The size of ITT analysis tests is not distorted by early treatment termination. However, a loss of power can occur. They propose modifications to ordinary logrank tests that would restore some of the lost power without affecting the size of the test.

11.3.4 Trials can be viewed as tests of treatment policy

It is unfortunate that investigators conducting clinical trials cannot guarantee that the patients who participate will definitely complete (or even receive) the treatment assigned. This is, in part, a consequence of the ethical principle of respect for individual autonomy. Many factors contribute to patients' failure to complete the intended therapy, including severe side effects, disease progression, patient or physi-

Table 11.2 Comparison of Death Rates for Placebo Compliers and Non-Compliers in the Coronary Drug Project

| | Placebo | |
Status	Compliers	Non-Compliers
Alive	633	1539
Dead	249	274

The odds ratio is 0.45 (0.37–0.55). The difference between compliers and non-compliers is statistically significant ($p \ll 0.0001$).

cian strong preference for a different treatment, and a change of mind. In nearly all circumstances, failure to complete the assigned therapy is partially an outcome of the study and, therefore, may produce a bias if used to subset patients for analysis. From this perspective, a clinical trial is a test of treatment policy, not a test of treatment received. ITT analyses avoid bias by testing policy or programmatic effectiveness.

From a clinical perspective, post-entry exclusion of eligible patients is analogous to using information from the future. For example, when selecting a therapy for a new patient, the clinician is primarily interested in the probability that the treatment will benefit the new patient. Because the clinician has no knowledge of whether or not the patient will complete the treatment intended, he or she has little use for inferences that depend on events in the patient's future. By the time treatment adherence is known, the clinical outcomes may also be known. Consequently, at the outset, the investigator will be most interested in clinical trial results that do not depend on adherence or other events in the patient's future. If the physician wishes to revise the prognosis when new information becomes available, then an analysis that depends on some intermediate success might be relevant.

11.3.5 ITT analyses can't always be applied

The limitations of the ITT approach have been discussed by Feinstein [1991] and Sheiner and Rubin [1995]. A breakdown in the experimental paradigm can render an analysis plan based on ITT irrelevant for answering the biological question. This does not mean that TR analyses would be the best solution because they are subject to errors of their own. There may be no entirely satisfactory analysis when the usual or ideal procedures are inapplicable because of unanticipated complications in study design or conduct. On the other hand, when the conduct of the trial follows the experimental paradigm fairly closely, as is often the case, analyses such as those based on ITT are frequently the most appropriate.

Example 23 *Busulfan is a preparative regimen for the treatment of hematological malignancies with bone marrow transplantation. In a small proportion of patients, the drug is associated with veno-occlusive disease (VOD) of the liver, a fatal complication. Clinical observations suggested that the incidence of VOD might be eliminated with appropriate dose reduction to decrease the area under the time-concentration curve (AUC) of the drug, observable after patients are given a test* *dose. Furthermore, the efficacy of the drug might be improved by increasing the dose in patients whose AUC is too low. These considerations led to a randomized trial design in which patients were assigned to two treatments consisting of the same drug but used in different ways. Group A received a standard fixed dose, while group B received a dose adjustment, up or down, to achieve a target AUC, based on the findings of a test dose. Partway through the trial, the data were examined to see if dose adjustment was reducing the incidence of VOD. Interestingly, none of the patients assigned to B actually required a dose adjustment because, by chance, their AUCs were all within the targeted range. On treatment A, some patients had high AUCs and a few experienced VOD. The intention-to-treat analysis would compare all those randomized to B, none of whom were dose adjusted, with those on A. Thus, the ITT analysis could not carry much information about the efficacy of dose adjustment. On the other hand, when the trial data were examined in conjunction with pre-existing data, the clinical investigators felt ethically compelled to use dose adjustment and the trial was stopped.*

In special circumstances, TR analyses can yield estimated treatment effects that are closer to the true value than those obtained from the ITT analyses. However, this improved performance of the TR approach depends upon also adjusting for the covariates responsible for cross-over. Investigators would have to know factors responsible for patients failing to get their assigned treatment, and incorporate those factors in correct statistical models describing the treatment effect. This is usually not feasible, because investigators do not know the reasons why, or the covariates associated with, patients failing to complete their assigned treatment. Even if the factors that influence non-adherence are known, their effect is likely to be more complex than simple statistical models can capture. Thus, the improved performance of TR methods in this circumstance is largely illusory.

Sommer and Zeger [1991] present an alternative to TR analyses that permits estimating efficacy in the presence of non-adherence. This method employs an estimator of biological efficacy that avoids the selection bias that confounds the comparison of compliant subgroups. This method can be applied to randomized trials with a dichotomous outcome measure, regardless of whether a placebo is given to the control group. The method compares the compliers in the treatment group to an inferred subgroup of controls, chosen to avoid selection bias.

Efron and Feldman [1991] discuss a statistical model that uses adherence as an explanatory factor and apply their method to data from a randomized placebo controlled trial of cholestyramine for cholesterol reduction. Their method provides a way to reconstruct dose response curves from adherence data in the trial. This and similar approaches based on models are likely to be useful supplements to the usual conservative ITT analyses and can recover valid estimates of method effectiveness when non-adherence is present [Sheiner and Rubin, 1995].

Treatment effects in the presence of imperfect adherence can be bounded using models of causal inference that do not rely on parametric assumptions. Examples of this is the work by Robins [1989], Manski [1990], and Balke and Pearl [1994]. These methods permit estimating the extent to which treatment effect estimates based on

ITT can differ from the true treatment effect. These methods show promise, but have not been widely applied in clinical trials.

11.3.6 Trial inferences depend on the experimental design

The best way to reconcile the legitimate clinical need for a good biological estimate of treatment efficacy and the statistical need for unbiased estimation and correct error levels is to be certain that patients entered on the trial are very likely to complete the assigned therapy. In other words, the eligibility criteria should exclude patients with characteristics that might prevent them from completing the therapy. This is different from excluding patients solely to improve homogeneity. For example, if the therapy is lengthy, perhaps only patients with good performance status should be eligible. If the treatment is toxic or associated with potentially intolerable side effects, only patients with normal function in major organ systems would be likely to complete the therapy.

It is a fact that the potential inferences from a clinical trial and the potential correctness of those inferences are a consequence of both the experimental design and the methods of analysis. One should not employ a design with particular strengths and then undo that design during the data analysis. For example, if we are certain that factors associated with treatment decisions are known, there might be very little reason to randomize. One could potentially obtain correct inferences from a simple database. However, if there are influential prognostic factors (known), then a randomized comparative trial offers considerable advantages. These advantages should not be weakened by ignoring the randomization in the analysis. Finally, there may be legitimate biological questions that one cannot answer effectively using rigorous designs. In these circumstances, it is not wise to insist on an ITT analysis. Instead, an approximate answer to a well-posed biological question will be more useful than the exact answer to the wrong question.

11.4 Summary

Clinical trials are characterized by imperfect data as a consequence of protocol non-adherence, methodologic error, and incomplete observations. Inferences from a trial can depend on how the investigators resolve data imperfections. Two approaches to such questions have been called "explanatory" and "pragmatic". The pragmatic approach tends to follow the statistical design of an experiment more closely. The explanatory approach may make some assumptions to try to answer biological questions.

Data imperfections that have the most potential for influencing the results of a trial arise from patients who do not adhere with assigned treatment or other criteria. Non-adherence encourages some investigators to remove patients from the analysis. If the reasons for exclusion are associated with prognosis or can affect the treatment groups differently, as is often the case, the trial results based on exclusions may not be valid.

Intention-to-treat is the principle that includes all patients for analysis in the groups to which they were assigned, regardless of protocol adherence. This approach is sometimes at odds with explanatory views of the trial, but usually provides a valid test of the null hypothesis. Approaches based on analyzing patients according to the treatment they actually received may be useful for exploring some clinical questions, but should not be the primary analysis of a randomized clinical trial. Investigators should avoid any method that removes eligible patients from the analysis.

11.5 Questions for Discussion

1. In some retrospective cohort studies, patients who have not been followed for a while in clinic could be assumed to be alive and well. Discuss how such an assumption could create bias.
2. Generalizing the idea of intention-to-treat to developmental trials, one might require that all patients who meet the eligibility criteria should be analyzed as part of the treatment group. Discuss the pros and cons of this approach.
3. Discuss specific circumstances in a CTE trial that might make it difficult to apply the intention-to-treat approach.
4. Read the paper by Stansfield et al., [1993] and discuss the inclusion/exclusion properties of the analysis.
5. Apply the method of Sommer and Zeger [1991] to the data from the Coronary Drug Project assuming the placebo compliance data were not available. How does the method compare to the actual estimated relative risk? Discuss.

Chapter References

Anderson, J.R., Cain, K.C., Gelber, R.D., and Gelman, R.S. (1985). Analysis and interpretation of the comparison of survival by treatment outcome variables in cancer clinical trials. Cancer Treat. Rep. 69: 1139-1144.

Balke, A.A. and Pearl, J. (1994). Universal formulas for treatment effects from noncompliance data. Technical Report R-199-A, Cognitive Systems Laboratory, UCLA.

Coronary Drug Project Research Group (1980). Influence of adherence to treatment and response of cholesterol on mortality in the Coronary Drug Project. New Engl. J. Med. 303: 1038-1041.

Efron, B. and Feldman, D. (1991). Compliance as an explanatory variable in clinical trials. J. Am. Stat. Assoc. 86: 9-17.

Feinstein, A.R. (1991). Intention-to-treat policy for analyzing randomized trials: Statistical distortions and neglected clinical challenges. Chapter 28 in J.A. Cramer and B. Spilker (Eds.), Patient Compliance in Medical Practice and Clinical Trials, New York: Raven Press.

Fisher, L.D., Dixon, D.O., Herson, J., Frankowski, R.K., Hearron, M.S., and Peace, K.E. (1990). Intention-to-treat in clinical trials, in K.E. Peace (Ed.), Statistical Issues in Drug Research and Development, New York: Marcel Dekker.

Gail, M.H. (1985). Eligibility exclusions, losses to follow-up, removal of randomized patients, and uncounted events in cancer clinical trials. Cancer Treat. Rep. 69(10): 1107-1112.

Hill, A.B. (1961). Principles of Medical Statistics, Seventh Edition. London: The Lancet.

Lagakos, S.W., Lim, L., and Robins, J.M. (1990). Adjusting for early treatment termination in comparative clinical trials. Statistics in Medicine 9: 1417-1424.

Lee, Y.J., Ellenberg, J.H., Hirtz, D.G., and Nelson, K.B. (1991). Analysis of clinical trials by treatment actually received: Is it really an option? Statistics in Med. 10: 1595-1605.

Lewis, J.A. and Machin, D. (1993). Intention-to-treat – Who should use ITT? Br. J. Cancer 68: 647-650.

Manski, C.F. (1990). Nonparametric bounds on treatment effects. American Economic Review, Papers and Proceedings 80: 319-323.

Meier, P. (1991). Comment (on a paper by Efron and Feldman). J. Am. Stat. Assoc. 86: 19-22.

Newell, D.J. (1992). Intention-to-treat analysis: Implications for quantitative and qualitative research. Int. J. Epidemiol. 21: 837-841.

Peduzzi, P., et al. (1993). Analysis as-randomized and the problem of non-adherence: An example from the Veterans Affairs randomized trial of coronary artery bypass surgery. Statistics in Med. 12: 1185-1195.

Peduzzi, P., et al. (1991). Intention-to-treat analysis and the problem of crossovers: An example from the Veterans Administration coronary bypass surgery study. J. Thorac. Cardiovasc. Surg. 101: 481-487.

Robins, J.M. (1989). The analysis of randomized and non-randomized AIDS treatment trials using a new approach to causal inference in longitudinal studies. In L. Sechrest, H. Freeman, and A. Mulley (Eds.) Health Service Research Methodology: A Focus on AIDS. NCHSR, U.S. Public Health Service.

Sackett, D.L. (1983). On some prerequisites for a successful clinical trial. In S.H. Shapiro and T.A. Louis (Eds.) Clinical Trials. New York: Marcel-Dekker.

Sackett, D.L. and Gent, M. (1979). Controversy in counting and attributing events in clinical trials. New Engl. J. Med. 301(26): 1410-1412.

Schwartz, D., Flamant, R., and Lellouch, J. (1980). Clinical Trials. London: Academic Press.

Schwartz, D. and Lellouch, J. (1967). Explanatory and pragmatic attitudes in therapeutic trials. J. Chron. Dis. 20: 637-648.

Sheiner, L.B. and Rubin, D.B. (1995). Intention-to-treat analysis and the goals of clinical trials. Clinical Pharmacol. & Therapeutics 57(1): 6-15.

Sommer, A. and Zeger, S.L. (1991). On estimating efficacy from clinical trials. Statistics in Med. 10: 45-52.

Stansfield, S.K., Pierre-Louis, M., Lerebours, G., and Augustin, A. (1993). Vitamin A supplementation and increased prevalence of childhood diarrhoea and acute respiratory infections. Lancet 341: 578-582.

CHAPTER 12

Estimating Clinical Effects

12.1 Introduction

A perspective on summarizing data from trials is necessary to understand some important experimental design issues. Because this book is not primarily about analyzing trials, the discussion here will be brief and will emphasize generating clinically helpful summaries of the data. Thorough accounting of the data from a clinical trial usually requires a number of skills beyond the scope of this book and concepts not covered in this chapter. The references cited can provide some help, but there is little substitute for further study and experience. For the reader with sufficient background and ambition, additional technical details can be found in Armitage and Berry [1994], Everitt [1989], and Campbell and Machin [1990]. Reporting guidelines are discussed in Chapter 14. Readers needing a more complete introduction to the analysis of survival data can consult Kleinbaum [1996]. The best substitute for analytic expertise is good experimental design and execution, which tend to simplify the data summary tasks.

Most clinical trials use more than one of the types of endpoints discussed in Chapter 6 and usually require several qualitatively different views of the data to address the basic research question. Informative analyses of data are based on several factors, including biological knowledge, the design of the study, proper counting of subjects and events to include, numeracy (understanding of numbers), familiarity with probability (and, in some cases, statistical models), and methods of inference. Applying these various concepts to clinical trials is usually not difficult.

12.1.1 Summarizing data requires structure

The design of a clinical trial imposes structure on the resulting data. In addition, the data analyst often assumes that other components of structure (e.g., a biological or population model) contribute to or underlie the observed data values. Provided these assumptions are reasonable and flexible, the results of the analysis are likely to be correct (at least approximately) and clinically useful. For example, in pharmacologic studies, blood samples are frequently used to display time concentration curves, which relate to simple physiologic models of drug distribution and/or metabolism. Accomplishing this requires investigators to specify a pharmacologic model and use statistical fitting methods to estimate the values of the parameters that best fit the data.

In SE trials of cytotoxic drugs, investigators are often interested in tumor response and toxicity of the drug or regimen. The usual study design permits estimating the unconditional probability of response or toxicity in patients who met the eligibility criteria. Additionally, the observed outcomes might be connected quantitatively to patient characteristics using simple statistical models. Comparative trials can yield formal tests of statistical hypotheses, but also usually provide more descriptive information about absolute probabilities of events and risk ratios in clinically important groups of patients.

For all types of studies, investigators must distinguish between those analyses, hypothesis tests, or other summaries of the data that are specified *a priori* and justified by the design of the trial and those which are exploratory. In many cases, the data themselves suggest certain comparisons or tests which, although biologically justifiable, may not be statistically reliable, because they were not anticipated in the study design. We would not want to focus on findings from such analyses as the principal result of a trial.

Example 24   *Suppose a series of patients meeting pre-defined eligibility criteria are given a six-week fixed-dose course of a new anti-hypertensive drug. The drug produces side effects in some individuals, which require dose reduction or discontinuation of the treatment. The design of this study suggests that the investigators are primarily interested in estimating the unconditional probability of benefit from the new drug and the proportion of patients who cannot tolerate the therapy. Suppose investigators also observe that patients who remain on the new drug have "significantly" lower blood pressure during the six-week study than those who are forced to resume their previous treatment. Although there may be biological reasons why the new treatment is superior, the study design and events do not permit reliably comparing it with standard therapy. In particular, the patients who experience side effects on the new treatment may be different in clinically important ways from those who tolerate the drug.*

12.1.2 Estimates of risk are natural and useful

Quantitative estimates of risk are natural and useful summaries of an important type of data. In horse racing, the ordinary betting odds is a commonly understood measure of risk and is used as a wagering guide. Unfortunately, it does not formally relate to the chances of a particular horse winning the race, but merely reflects the current allocation of money. In football and some other sports contests, quantitative estimates of team differences are often expressed as a "point spread". It is generally understood that the "point spread" equalizes the probability of winning a bet on either side. Thus, it is an indirect quantification of risk.

Table 12.1 Outcomes of Clinical Interest in Dose-Finding Studies Such as Phase I Trials

- Maximal tolerated dose
- Absorption rate
- Elimination rate
- Area under the curve
- Peak concentration
- Half life
- Correlation between plasma levels and side effects
- Proportion of patients who demonstrate evidence of efficacy

Although the quantification of risk in these cases seems useful for wagering, it would be of little help in medical studies because the true probability of success remains unknown. The analogous idea in clinical trials might be betting on which treatment in a trial will turn out to be superior, not a very useful activity. Instead, the clinician is most interested in estimating magnitude of differences, or relative differences, in risk.

Often in the clinical setting, we are interested in knowing the probability of a successful outcome, or the risk of failure, perhaps measured over time. When comparing treatments, changes or relative changes in risk are of primary interest. In a study comparing event times such as survival or disease recurrence/progression, group differences could be summarized as absolute differences in the probability of failure at some convenient point in time. In some cases, these same differences can be expressed as differences in median (or other convenient quantile) event times. When the hazard of failure is constant across time (or nearly so), a more efficient procedure is to summarize group differences as a ratio of hazards.

12.2 Dose-Finding Trials (Phase I Studies)

Obtaining clinically useful data from DF trials such as phase I studies is an extensive and complex endeavor. It depends on 1) evaluation of preclinical data, 2) knowledge of the physical and chemical properties of the drug and related compounds, 3) modeling drug absorption, distribution, metabolism, and elimination, and 4) judgment based on experience. Instead of a comprehensive mathematical presentation, I will discuss a few interesting points related to modeling and obtaining estimates of important pharmacokinetic parameters. Complete discussions of modeling and inferences can be found in Carson, Cobelli, and Finkelstein [1983] or Rubinow [1975].

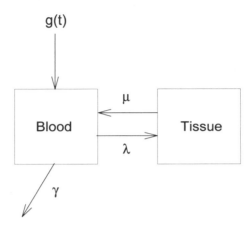

Figure 12.1 A simple two-compartment model for drug distribution.

12.2.1 Pharmacokinetic models are essential for analyzing DF trials

One of the principal objectives of phase I studies is to assess the distribution and elimination of drug in the body. Some specific parameters of interest are listed in Table 12.1. Pharmacokinetic (PK) models (or compartmental models) are a useful tool for summarizing and interpreting data from DF trials such as phase I studies. These models are helpful in study design, for example, to suggest the best times for blood or other samples to be taken. During analysis, the model is essential as an underlying structure for the data and permitting quantitative estimates of drug elimination. PK models have limitations because they are idealizations. No model is better than the data on which it is based. However when properly used, the model may yield insights that are difficult to gain from raw data. Some other objectives of phase I studies may not require modeling assumptions. Examples of these include secondary objectives, such as exploring the association between plasma drug levels and severity of side effects, or looking for evidence of drug efficacy. In any case, PK models are at the heart of using quantitative information from DF studies.

Drug absorption, distribution, metabolism, and excretion is not generally a simple process. However, relatively simple PK models can yield extremely useful information, even though they do not capture all of the complexities of the biology. In this chapter, I consider a simple but realistic PK model that facilitates quantitative inferences about drug distribution and elimination. An important consideration in assessing toxicity, especially in oncologic studies, is the area under the time-concentration curve in the blood (AUC). The model discussed below will permit study of the AUC.

12.2.2 A two-compartment model is simple but realistic

Consider a drug administered at a constant rate by continuous intravenous infusion. We assume that the drug is transferred from blood to a tissue compartment (and vice-versa) with first order kinetics, and eliminated directly from the blood, also by first order kinetics (Figure 12.1). This situation can be described by a two-compartment linear system in the following way. Suppose $X(t)$ and $Y(t)$ are the drug concentrations within blood and tissue, respectively, at time t and the drug is infused into the blood compartment with a rate of $g(t)$. Drug is transported from compartment X to Y at a rate λ, from Y back to X at a rate μ, and eliminated from X at a rate γ. The rate equations for the system are

$$\frac{dX(t)}{dt} = -(\lambda + \gamma)X(t) + \mu Y(t) + g(t), \qquad (12.1)$$

$$\frac{dY(t)}{dt} = \lambda X(t) - \mu Y(t), \qquad (12.2)$$

where $\frac{d}{dt}$ denotes the derivative with respect to time. The general solution of this system of differential equations is

$$X(t) = c_1(t)e^{\xi_1 t} + c_2(t)e^{\xi_2 t}, \qquad (12.3)$$

$$Y(t) = c_1(t)\frac{\xi_1 + \lambda + \gamma}{\mu}e^{\xi_1 t} + c_2(t)\frac{\xi_2 + \lambda + \gamma}{\mu}e^{\xi_2 t}, \qquad (12.4)$$

where

$$\xi_{1,2} = \frac{-(\lambda + \mu + \gamma) \pm \sqrt{(\lambda + \mu + \gamma)^2 - 4\mu\gamma}}{2} \qquad (12.5)$$

and $c_1(t)$ and $c_2(t)$ satisfy

$$\frac{dc_1(t)}{dt} = \frac{\xi_2 + \lambda + \gamma}{\xi_2 - \xi_1}g(t)e^{-\xi_1 t}, \qquad (12.6)$$

$$\frac{dc_2(t)}{dt} = -\frac{\xi_1 + \lambda + \gamma}{\xi_2 - \xi_1}g(t)e^{-\xi_2 t}. \qquad (12.7)$$

To get an explicit solution for the system, we must specify $g(t)$, the infusion rate as a function of time, and initial conditions $X(0)$ and $Y(0)$. An interesting special case is constant infusion for a fixed time period,

$$g(t) = \begin{cases} g_0, & t \le t_0 \\ 0, & t > t_0 \end{cases}. \qquad (12.8)$$

Then, substituting equations 12.5–12.8 into equation 12.3,

$$
X(t) = \begin{cases}
\frac{g_0}{r} + \frac{\xi_2 + \lambda + \gamma}{\xi_2 - \xi_1}\left(\frac{g_0}{\xi_1} + X(0)\right)e^{\xi_1 t} \\[2mm]
\quad - \frac{\xi_1 + \lambda + \gamma}{\xi_2 - \xi_1}\left(\frac{g_0}{\xi_2} + X(0)\right)e^{\xi_2 t}, & t \le t_0 \\[4mm]
\frac{\xi_2 + \lambda + \gamma}{\xi_2 - \xi_1}\left(\frac{g_0}{\xi_1} + X(0) - \frac{g_0}{\xi_1}e^{-\xi_1 t_0}\right)e^{\xi_1 t} \\[2mm]
\quad - \frac{\xi_1 + \lambda + \gamma}{\xi_2 - \xi_1}\left(\frac{g_0}{\xi_2} + X(0) - \frac{g_0}{\xi_2}e^{-\xi_2 t_0}\right)e^{\xi_2 t}, & t > t_0
\end{cases}
\tag{12.9}
$$

where the initial condition $Y(0) = 0$ has been incorporated. Here we have used the facts that $\xi_1 + \xi_2 = -(\lambda + \mu + \gamma)$ and $\xi_1 \xi_2 = \mu\gamma$. Hence, the area under the curve (AUC) for the first compartment is

$$
AUC_x = \int_0^{t_0} X(t)dt + \int_{t_0}^{\infty} X(t)dt = \frac{g_0 t_0 + X(0)}{\gamma}.
\tag{12.10}
$$

Sometimes it is helpful to express these models in terms of amount of drug and volume of distribution. Equation 12.10 can be rewritten

$$
AUC_x = \frac{D t_0 + W(0)}{\gamma V},
$$

where D is the dose of drug, V is the volume of distribution (assumed to be constant), $W(t) = V \times X(t)$ is the amount of drug, and γV is the "clearance". However, expressing AUC_x this way represents only a change of scale, which is not necessary for this discussion. Because drug "dose" is commonly expressed as weight of drug, weight of drug per kilogram of body weight, or weight of drug per square meter of body surface area, we can refer to $g_0 t_0 + X(0)$ as a dose, even though formally it is a concentration.

When the drug is infused constantly from time 0 to t_0 and $X(0) = 0$, $AUC_x = g_0 t_0/\gamma$. This is the ratio of total dose to the excretion rate. Another interesting case is when the drug is given as a single bolus, i.e., $t_0 = 0$, in which case $AUC_x = X(0)/\gamma$ which is also a ratio of total dose over excretion rate. The transport parameters λ and μ do not affect the AUC in the first compartment.

With similar calculations, we can find the solution for the second compartment,

$$
Y(t) = \begin{cases}
\frac{g_0 \lambda}{\mu\gamma} - \frac{\lambda}{\xi_2 - \xi_1}\left(\frac{g_0}{\xi_1} + X(0)\right)e^{\xi_1 t} \\[2mm]
\quad + \frac{\lambda}{\xi_2 - \xi_1}\left(\frac{g_0}{\xi_2} + X(0)\right)e^{\xi_2 t}, & t \le t_0 \\[4mm]
\quad - \frac{\lambda}{\xi_2 - \xi_1}\left(\frac{g_0}{\xi_1} + X(0) - \frac{g_0}{\xi_1}e^{-\xi_1 t_0}\right)e^{\xi_1 t} \\[2mm]
\quad + \frac{\lambda}{\xi_2 - \xi_1}\left(\frac{g_0}{\xi_2} + X(0) - \frac{g_0}{\xi_2}e^{-\xi_2 t_0}\right)e^{\xi_2 t}, & t > t_0
\end{cases}
\tag{12.11}
$$

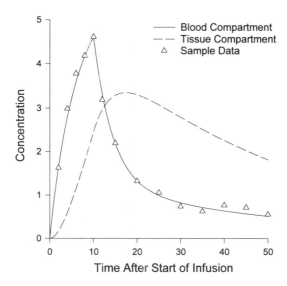

Figure 12.2 Time concentration curves and data from a two-compartment model. $T_0 = 10$, $\mu = 0.1$, $\gamma = 0.1$, $\lambda = 0.1$, **and** $g_0 = 1.0$.

and

$$AUC_Y = \frac{\lambda g_0 t_0 + \lambda X(0)}{\mu \gamma} = \frac{\lambda}{\mu} AUC_X. \qquad (12.12)$$

It is directly related to AUC in the first compartment and the transport rates λ and μ.

The behavior of this model is shown in Figure 12.2. Values for both compartments determined by numerical integration are shown with the tissue compartment peak lagging behind the vascular compartment peak as one would expect. When the infusion stops, the concentration in the blood begins to decline abruptly whereas the tissue curve shows an inflection point. Data points (with simulated error) that might be obtained from such a system are also shown in Figure 12.2.

12.2.3 PK models are used by "model fitting"

It is common in actual DF studies to have data that consist of samples from only the vascular compartment taken at various time points during the uptake or infusion of drug and during its elimination. The model in the form of equations 12.9 and 12.11 can be fitted to such data to obtain estimates of the rate constants which are the clinical effects of interest. An example of this for a continuous intravenous infusion of the anti-tumor drug cyclophosphamide in four patients is shown in Figure 12.3. For each study subject, the infusion was to last 60 minutes although the exact time varied. The value of g_0 was fixed at 10.0. Because of measurement error in the

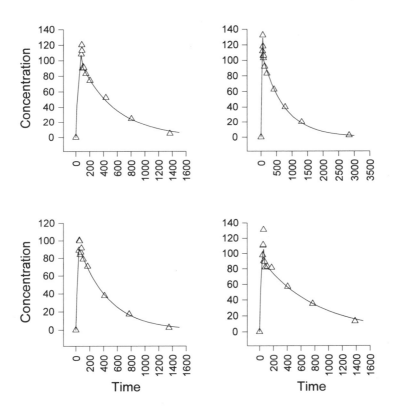

Figure 12.3 Sample data and model fits to time-concentration values from four patients in a DF trial. The triangles are observed serum levels and the solid lines are model fits.

infusion time and dosage, it is sometimes helpful to estimate both t_0 and g_0 (see Chapter 19). The fitted curves show a good agreement with the measured values. The estimated parameter values are shown in Table 12.2, along with the estimated AUCs. Of course, the quality of inference about such a drug would be improved by examining the results from a larger number of study subjects.

12.3   SE Studies

A common primary objective of SE studies is to estimate the frequency of side effects and the probability of success in treating patients with a new drug or combination. In oncology, the investigator is also usually interested in grading the toxicity seen and estimating overall length of survival. Often the outcome assessments for re-

Table 12.2 Estimated Rate Constants from Phase I Clinical Trial Data

#	t_0	$\widehat{\lambda}$	$\widehat{\gamma}$	$\widehat{\mu}$	$\widehat{AUC}$
1	85	.284	.015	.042	53,475
		(.0436)	(.0014)	(.0040)	
2	60	.250	.007	.057	78,876
		(.0190)	(.0004)	(.0065)	
3	50	.782	.012	.196	40,251
		(.9200)	(.0068)	(.1027)	
4	50	.239	.007	.061	63,509
		(.1684)	(.0044)	(.0275)	

Estimated standard errors are shown in parentheses.

sponse and toxicity are dichotomous, i.e., yes-no variables. Meeting these types of objectives requires estimating absolute probabilities.

12.3.1 Mesothelioma clinical trial example

To illustrate some clinically useful summaries of information from SE trials, consider data of the kind shown in Table 12.3. The patients on this (phase II) trial were all diagnosed with malignant mesothelioma, an uncommon lung tumor strongly related to asbestos exposure. Depending on the extent of disease at diagnosis, patients underwent one of three types of surgery: biopsy, limited resection, or extrapleural pneumonectomy (EPP), a more extensive operative procedure [Rusch, Piantadosi, and Holmes, 1991]. The goals of the SE trial were to determine the feasibility of performing EPP and to document the natural history of the disease. The complete data on 83 subjects are presented in Chapter 19.

Possibly important prognostic factors in patients with mesothelioma include sex, histologic subtype (hist), weight change at diagnosis (wtchg), performance status (ps), age, and type of surgery (surg). Disease progression is both an outcome of treatment and a potential predictor of survival. The progression and survival times are censored, i.e., some patients remained progression free or alive at the end of the study or cutoff date for analysis.

12.3.2 Summarize risk for dichotomous factors

Estimating the overall proportion of patients who progress is straightforward and will not be detailed here. Instead, we consider the relationships between disease progression as an intermediate outcome and the prognostic factors sex and performance status. In reality, progression is an event time, but will be treated as a dichotomous factor, temporarily, for simplicity. Both factors can be summarized in 2×2 tables (Table 12.4).

The probabilities and odds of progression are shown in Tables 12.5 and 12.6. Here the 95% confidence limits on the proportions are based on the binomial distribution. For dichotomous factors like those in Table 12.4, we are sometimes interested in

Table 12.3 Data from Mesothelioma SE (Phase II) Clinical Trial

Age	Sex	PS	Hist	Wtchg	Surg	PFS	Prog	Surv	Event
60	1	1	136	1	3	394	1	823	1
59	1	0	136	2	3	1338	0	1338	0
51	0	0	130	1	1	184	1	270	1
73	1	1	136	1	3	320	0	320	1
74	1	0	136	2	1	168	0	168	1
39	0	0	136	1	1	36	1	247	1
46	1	1	131	1	3	552	1	694	0
71	1	0	136	1	1	133	1	316	1
69	1	0	136	1	1	175	1	725	0
49	1	0	131	1	1	327	0	327	1
69	1	0	131	1	2	0	0	0	1
72	1	0	131	1	1	676	1	963	0
$\vdots$	$\vdots$	$\vdots$	$\vdots$	$\vdots$	$\vdots$	$\vdots$	$\vdots$	$\vdots$	$\vdots$

PFS is progression free time; Surv is survival time. Prog and Event are censoring indicator variables for progression and death, respectively. Performance status (PS) is dichotomized as high versus low.

absolute probabilities (or proportions). However, we are often interested in estimates of risk ratios such as the relative risk or odds ratio. If p_1 and p_2 are the probabilities of events in two groups, the odds ratio, θ, is estimated by

$$\widehat{\theta} = \frac{p_1}{1 - p_1} \div \frac{p_2}{1 - p_2} = \frac{ad}{bc} \, ,$$

where $p_1 = \frac{a}{a+c}, p = \frac{b}{b+d}$, etc. from the entries in a 2×2 table. For example, the odds ratio for progression in males versus females (Table 12.4) is $15 \times 14/(49 \times 5) = .857$. This can also be seen in Table 12.5. For odds ratios, calculating confidence intervals on a *log* scale is relatively simple. An approximate confidence interval for the log odds ratio is

$$\log\{\widehat{\theta}\} \pm Z_\alpha \times \sqrt{\frac{1}{a} + \frac{1}{b} + \frac{1}{c} + \frac{1}{d}} \, ,$$

where Z_α is the point on normal distribution exceeded with probability $\alpha/2$ (e.g., for $\alpha = 0.05$, $Z_\alpha = 1.96$). For the example above, this yields a confidence interval of $[-1.33, 1.02]$ for the log odds ratio or $[0.26, 2.77]$ for the odds ratio. Because the 95% confidence interval for the odds ratio includes 1.0, the male-female difference in risk of progression is not "statistically significant" using the conventional criterion.

The odds ratio is a convenient and concise summary of risk data for dichotomous outcomes and arises naturally in relative risk regressions such as the logistic model. However, the odds ratio has limitations and should be applied and interpreted with thought, especially in circumstances where it is important to know the absolute risk. For example, if two risks are related by $p' = p + \delta$, where δ is the difference in

Table 12.4 Progression by Sex and Performance Status (PS) for an SE Mesothelioma Trial

Progression	Overall	Sex		PS	
		Male	Female	0	1
No	20	15	5	10	10
Yes	63	49	14	42	21

absolute risks, the odds ratio satisfies

$$\theta \frac{p}{1-p} = \frac{1-(p+\delta)}{(p+\delta)}$$

or

$$\delta = \frac{p(1-\theta)(1-p)}{\theta(1-p)+p} .$$

This means that many values of p and θ are consistent with the same difference in risk. For example, all of the following (p, θ) pairs are consistent with an absolute difference in risk of $\delta = -0.2$: (0.30, 3.86); (0.45, 2.45); (0.70, 2.33); and (0.25, 6.33). As useful as the odds ratio is, it obscures differences in absolute risks that may be biologically important for the question at hand. Similar comments relate to hazard ratios (discussed below).

12.3.3 Non-parametric estimates of survival are robust

Survival data are unique because of censoring. Censoring means that some individuals have not had the event of interest at the time the data are analyzed or the study is over. For these people, we know only that they were at risk for a measured period of time and that the event of interest has yet to happen. Thus, their event time is censored. Using the incomplete information from censored observations requires some special methods which give "survival analysis" its statistical niche. The basic consequence of censoring is that we summarize the data using cumulative probability distributions rather than probability density functions, which are so frequently used in other circumstances.

In many clinical trials involving patients with serious illnesses like cancer, a primary clinical focus is the overall survival experience of the cohort. There are several ways to summarize the survival experience of a cohort. However, one or two frequently used methods make few, if any, assumptions about the probability distribution of the failure times. These "non-parametric" methods are widely used because they are robust and simple to employ. See Peto [1984] for a helpful review. For censored failure time data, the commonest analytic technique is the lifetable. Events (failures or deaths) and times at which they occur are grouped into convenient intervals (e.g., months or years) and the probability of failure during each interval is calculated.

Table 12.5 Probabilities and Odds of Progression by Sex for an SE Mesothelioma Trial

	Overall	Sex	
		Male	Female
Pr[progression]	0.24	0.23	0.26
95% CL	(0.154–0.347)	(0.138–0.357)	(0.092–0.512)
Odds of Progression	.317	0.306	0.357

Here I review the product limit method [Kaplan and Meier, 1951] for estimating survival probabilities with individual failure times. It is essentially the same as lifetable methods for grouped data. To avoid grouping of events into (arbitrary) intervals or to handle small cohorts, individual failure times are used. The method is illustrated in Table 12.7 using the SE mesothelioma trial data introduced above. First, the observed event or failure times are ranked from shortest to longest. At each event time, indexed by i, the number of subjects failing is denoted by d_i and the number of subjects at risk just prior to the event is denoted by n_i. By convention, censoring times that are tied with failure times are assumed to rank lower in the list. Unless there are tied failure times, the number of events represented by each time will be 0 (for censorings) or 1 (for failures).

For an arbitrary event time, the probability of failure in the interval from the last failure time is

$$p_i = \frac{d_i}{n_i} .$$

The probability of surviving the interval is $1 - p_i = 1 - \frac{d_i}{n_i}$. Therefore, the cumulative probability of surviving all earlier intervals up to the kth failure time is

$$\widehat{S(t_k)} = \prod_{i=0}^{k-1} \left(1 - \frac{d_i}{n_i}\right) = \prod_{t_i} \left(\frac{n_i - d_i}{n_i}\right), \qquad (12.13)$$

where the product is taken over all distinct event times. This calculation is carried through a few observations in Table 12.7.

For censored events, the previous product will be multiplied by 1 and, in the absence of an event, the survival estimate remains constant, giving the curve its characteristic step-function appearance. Although more complicated to derive, the variance of the product limit estimator can be shown to be [Greenwood, 1926]

$$Var\{\widehat{S(t_k)}\} = \widehat{S(t_k)}^2 \sum_{i=0}^{k-1} \frac{d_i}{n_i(n_i - d_i)} . \qquad (12.14)$$

The square roots of these numbers are shown in the last column of Table 12.7. Usually one plots $\widehat{S(t)}$ versus time to obtain familiar "survival curves", which can be done

Table 12.6 Probabilities and Odds Of Progression by Performace Status for an SE Mesothelioma Trial

	PS	
	0	1
Pr[progression]	0.19	0.32
95% CL	(0.096–0.325)	(0.167–0.514)
Odds of Progression	0.238	0.476

separately for two or more groups to facilitate comparisons. For the mesothelioma data, such curves are shown in Figure 12.4.

Investigators are frequently interested in the estimated probability of survival at a fixed time, which can be determined from the calculations sketched above. For example, the probability of surviving (or remaining event free) at 1 year is approximately 0.50 (Figure 12.4). When this estimate is based on a lifetable or product limit calculation, it is often called "actuarial survival". Sometimes clinicians discuss "actual survival", a vague and inconsistently used term. It usually means the raw proportion surviving, for example $\frac{25}{50} = 0.5$ or 50% at 1 year in the data above.

12.3.4 Parametric (exponential) summaries of survival are efficient

To discuss non-parametric estimates of survival quantitatively, it is necessary to agree on a reference point in time or have the entire survival curve available. This inconvenience can often be avoided by using a parametric summary of the data, for example, by calculating the overall failure rate or hazard. If we assume the failure rate is constant over time (i.e., the failure times arise from an exponential distribution), the hazard can be estimated by

$$\widehat{\lambda} = d / \sum_{i=1}^{N} t_i \, , \tag{12.15}$$

where d is the total number of failures and the denominator is the total follow-up or exposure time in the cohort. This estimate of the hazard was introduced in Chapter 7. It is the event rate per person-time (e.g., person-year or person-month) of exposure and summarizes the entire survival experience. More complicated procedures are necessary if the hazard is not constant over time or such an assumption is not helpful.

Because $2d\lambda/\widehat{\lambda}$ has a chi-square distribution with $2d$ degrees of freedom [Halperin, 1952], a $100(1 - \alpha)\%$ confidence interval for λ is

$$\frac{\widehat{\lambda}\chi^2_{2d,1-\alpha/2}}{2d} < \lambda < \frac{\widehat{\lambda}\chi^2_{2d,\alpha/2}}{2d} \, .$$

Table 12.7 Product Limit Estimates of Survival for Data from a SE Mesothelioma Clinical Trial (All Patients)

Event Time	Number of Events	Number Alive	Survival Probability	Failure Probability	Survival Std. Err.
t_i	n_i	d_i	$\widehat{S(t_i)}$	p_i	
0.0	1	83	1.0000	0	0
0.0	1	82	0.9880	0.0120	0.0120
4.0	1	81	0.9759	0.0241	0.0168
6.0	1	80	0.9639	0.0361	0.0205
17.0	1	79	0.9518	0.0482	0.0235
20.0	1	78	0.9398	0.0602	0.0261
22.0	1	77	0.9277	0.0723	0.0284
28.0	1	76	0.9157	0.0843	0.0305
⋮	⋮	⋮	⋮	⋮	⋮
764.0	1	12	0.2081	0.7919	0.0473
823.0	1	11	0.1908	0.8092	0.0464
948.0	1	10	0.1734	0.8266	0.0453
963.0	0	9	.	.	.
1029.0	0	8	.	.	.
1074.0	0	7	.	.	.
1093.0	0	6	.	.	.
1102.0	0	5	.	.	.
1123.0	0	4	.	.	.
1170.0	0	3	.	.	.
1229.0	1	2	0.1156	0.8844	0.0560
1265.0	1	1	0.0578	0.9422	0.0496
1338.0	0	0	.	.	.

When the sample size is large, $\widehat{\lambda}$ has an approximate normal distribution with mean λ and variance $\lambda^2/(d-1)$. Then, an approximate confidence interval is

$$\widehat{\lambda} - \frac{\widehat{\lambda} Z_{\alpha/2}}{\sqrt{d-1}} < \lambda < \widehat{\lambda} + \frac{\widehat{\lambda} Z_{\alpha/2}}{\sqrt{d-1}} .$$

Approximate confidence limits for the failure rate can also be calculated in the following way. It is easier to put confidence limits on the logarithm of the failure rate. In particular,

$$Var\{\log(\widehat{\lambda})\} = \frac{1}{d}$$

so that an approximate $(1-\alpha)\%$ confidence interval is

$$\log(\widehat{\lambda}) \pm Z_{1-\alpha} \times \frac{1}{\sqrt{d}} , \qquad (12.16)$$

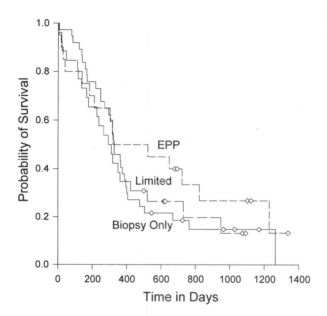

Figure 12.4 Non-parametric estimates of survival for a SE clinical trial in patients with mesothelioma.

where $Z_{1-\alpha}$ is the normal probability quantile for the width of the confidence interval (e.g., $Z_{.95} = 1.96$). The ends of the confidence interval on $\log(\widehat{\lambda})$ can be transformed back to the natural scale to produce the desired confidence limits. These simple parametric methods have been used on the data from Table 12.3 and the results are given in Table 12.8.

In many circumstances, one cannot reasonably assume that the hazard is constant over time. Certain parametric methods can still be employed if a good choice for an overall survival model is made or if there are intervals or epochs in which the hazard is approximately constant. Parametric methods can be very useful when studying subtle features of the data, for example, the tail of a survival distribution. In many cases, specialized computer software or methods of estimating model parameters are needed. A detailed discussion of this topic is given by Gross and Clark [1980]. Large or complex SE trials will likely employ descriptive or analytic methods similar to those given in the next section for comparative studies or in Chapter 13 for prognostic factor studies.

Table 12.8 Hazard Summary Data from a SE Mesothelioma Trial

Variable	Group	Exposure Time*	Number of Events	Hazard Rate	Approximate 95% CL
Overall	all	96.3	68	0.706	0.557 – 0.895
Sex	males	74.8	52	0.695	0.530 – 0.912
	females	21.5	16	0.743	0.455 – 1.213
PS	0	55.7	46	0.826	0.617 – 1.103
	1	40.6	22	0.541	0.356 – 0.822
Surgery	biopsy	41.2	32	0.776	0.549 – 1.098
	limited	26.5	21	0.792	0.516 – 1.215
	EPP	28.6	15	0.524	0.316 – 0.870

* Exposure time is measured in years.

12.4 Comparative Efficacy Trials (Phase III)

Developmental studies like DF and SE trials require mainly descriptive analysis. However, comparative trial designs encourage or require analyses that both describe the data and quantify the possible effects of chance on the observed treatment difference. A frequentist approach to the question of the effects of chance might be to test for "statistical significance", i.e., formally determine to what extent the observed differences between the treatment groups could be attributable to random variation. A Bayesian approach would be to derive a probability distribution for the treatment difference based on both prior information and the results of the trial.

In either case, the approach to questions of *clinical* significance depends partly on the endpoints being used. The approach also depends on the experimental unit. For example, when the experimental unit is a cluster, special methods for estimating event rates are needed [Donner and Klar, 1994]. Endpoints employed most frequently in comparative trials can be classified as continuous measures, binary outcomes, or event times. Each of these can be used to estimate absolute or relative effects and assess those effects for the play of chance. Most often, continuous measures are used to estimate treatment differences as opposed to risk ratios. Binary outcomes and event rates are measures of risk and are most frequently used in comparative studies to estimate risk ratios.

12.4.1 Examples of CTE trials used in this section

To discuss points of analysis about CTE trials, it is useful to have examples. I have selected two small but interesting trials that illustrate relevant concepts. One is a randomized trial testing whether or not a non-steroidal anti-inflammatory agent (sulindac) can reduce the number and size of colonic polyps in patients with Familial Ade-nomatous Polyposis (FAP) [Giardiello et al., 1993]. A second useful example, in which survival and disease recurrence are the primary statistical endpoints, is a ran-domized clinical trial comparing the benefit of cytoxan, doxorubicin, and platinum (CAP) as an adjuvant to radiotherapy for treatment of locally advanced non small-cell lung cancer following surgical resection [Lad, Rubinstein, Sadeghi, et al., 1988].

FAP prevention trial

FAP is an autosomal dominant genetic defect which predisposes those affected to de-velop large numbers of polyps in the colon, frequently at a young age. These polyps are prone to malignant changes and, if untreated, affected individuals may develop colon cancer. In addition to frequent screening and biopsy of polyps that form, pa-tients may require surgical procedures such as colectomy to prevent the formation of cancers. Serendipitous observations suggested that the drug employed in this clinical trial might benefit FAP patients. (This illustrates the role that observational studies can have in the early development of disease prevention strategies.) Sulindac and re-lated drugs inhibit the enzyme cyclo-oxygenase and may act beneficially to reduce polyp formation by enhancing pre-programmed cell death (apoptosis) as opposed to reducing proliferative rates.

In this trial, patients with FAP were randomly assigned to receive the drug as a preventive measure or a placebo. The primary endpoint was to examine the number and size of colonic polyps, as determined by colonoscopy, at 3, 6, 9 and 12 months after starting treatment. The analysis originally performed used relative changes over baseline in polyp number and size as the clinically relevant endpoints. This study was stopped at a planned interim analysis after approximately one-half of the fixed sample size was accrued, because the clinicians and trial methodologists felt that the evidence was ethically compelling in favor of treatment. Here we consider only the one-year data (Table 12.9). A complete listing of data is given in Chapter 19.

Lung cancer chemotherapy trial

This clinical trial tested the benefit of adding adjuvant chemotherapy to patients with surgically resected lung cancer. A total of 172 patients were randomized be-tween 1979 and 1985. The study illustrates an interesting collaboration between investigators applying the major modes of cancer treatment: radiotherapy, surgery, and chemotherapy. It was among the first to show the benefit of platinum based chemotherapy for non-small cell lung cancer.

In this trial, patients were followed for several years and substantial amounts of data were collected. Here we can only consider a portion of it, related to the primary endpoints and major prognostic factors. The data and analyses here differ slightly from the primary publication cited above because of additional follow-up informa-tion collected subsequently. However, the basic conclusions remain as previously reported. A data listing is given in Chapter 19. The methodology of this trial is noteworthy because of the careful intra-operative anatomic staging of the patients, a process that improves knowledge of the extent of disease and permits more accurate prognostication.

Table 12.9 Data from a CTE Clinical Trial in FamilialAdenomatous Polyposis

ID	Sex	Polyp Number at Month 0	Polyp Number at Month 12	Polyp Size at Month 0	Polyp Size at Month 12	Age	Treatment
1	0	7	.	3.6	.	17	1
2	0	77	.	3.8	.	20	0
3	1	7	4	5.0	1.0	16	1
4	0	5	26	3.4	2.1	18	0
5	1	23	16	3.0	1.2	22	1
6	0	35	40	4.2	4.1	13	0
7	0	11	14	2.2	3.3	23	1
8	1	12	16	2.0	3.0	34	0
9	1	7	11	4.2	2.5	50	0
10	1	318	434	4.8	4.4	19	0
11	1	160	26	5.5	3.5	17	1
12	0	8	7	1.7	0.8	23	1
13	1	20	45	2.5	3.0	22	0
14	1	11	32	2.3	2.7	30	0
15	1	24	80	2.4	2.7	27	0
16	1	34	34	3.0	4.2	23	1
17	0	54	38	4.0	2.9	22	0
18	1	16	.	1.8	.	13	1
21	1	30	57	3.2	3.7	34	0
22	0	10	7	3.0	1.1	23	1
23	0	20	1	4.0	0.4	22	1
24	1	12	8	2.8	1.0	42	1

12.4.2 Continuous measures estimate treatment differences

Continuous measures on each study subject are most often summarized as group averages or medians. A trial of blood pressure reducing drugs might compare the average diastolic blood pressure on each treatment. The actual level of the diastolic blood pressure might be less interesting than the differences between the groups. For example, a trial of human growth hormone in children with a deficiency as manifested by extremely short stature might compare the average height of the treatment groups. Here one would likely be interested in the group differences as well as the actual average heights in the treatment groups.

For these types of continuously distributed response measurements, an estimate of the effect of clinical interest might be $\widehat{\Delta}_{AB} = \overline{Y}_A - \overline{Y}_B$, where $\overline{Y}_A$ and $\overline{Y}_B$ are the average outcomes in the treatment groups. Not only are we interested in Δ_{AB}, the magnitude of the treatment difference, but we would also like to estimate its variability through a standard deviation or confidence interval. Although a p-value or other quantification of the play of chance will be interesting, it is likely that we would continue to study the treatment if $\widehat{\Delta}_{AB}$ is large enough, even if it is not "significantly different from zero".

In the FAP clinical trial, the average numbers of polyps after 12 months of treatment were 78 and 13 in the placebo and treatment groups, respectively. The average polyp sizes were 3.1 and 1.8 in the placebo and treatment groups, respectively. The difference in number of polyps between the treatment groups is not statistically significant using the t-test ($p = .15$) but the polyp size is significantly decreased ($p = .02$). Although the t-test applied to 12-month measurements is a valid procedure for testing the treatment effect based on the design of the trial, it does not use all of the available information from the study. Both baseline measurements and longitudinal assessments of polyp number and size are available and could contribute to information about the treatment effect. These are discussed below.

12.4.3 Baseline measurements can increase precision

There are many instances where we measure outcomes both at the beginning (baseline) and end of treatment on each patient. This occurs often in behavioral research, for example. In these circumstances, we could still estimate $\widehat{\Delta}_{AB}$ using only the values at end of treatment as in the FAP analysis above. However, it might be better to calculate each patient's *increment* over baseline after the treatment period, $\delta_i = Y_{i2} - Y_{i1}$, where the subscript i denotes patient and 1 and 2 denote baseline and end of treatment, respectively. Using the δ_i is sometimes called a gain-score analysis. The average increments in the treatment groups are $\overline{\delta}_A$ and $\overline{\delta}_B$, so that the effect of most clinical interest might be $\widehat{\Delta}_{AB} = \overline{\delta}_A - \overline{\delta}_B$, which is the difference of increments.

This approach, or one similar to it, is often more efficient than using only a single post-treatment measurement because the standard deviation of $\widehat{\Delta}_{AB}$ is probably reduced as the result of using two measurements from each study subject. Suppose that the variance of each of the measurements, Y_{ij}, is σ^2. Then

$$Var(\widehat{\Delta}_{AB}) = Var(\overline{\delta}_A) + Var(\overline{\delta}_B)$$

and

$$Var(\overline{\delta}_A) = \frac{Var(\delta_i)}{n} = \frac{\sigma^2 + \sigma^2 - 2 \times Cov(Y_{i1}, Y_{i2})}{n} = 2\frac{\sigma^2}{n}(1 - \rho), \quad (12.17)$$

where ρ is the within-subject correlation between baseline and post-treatment measurements. The covariance (correlation) of Y_{i2} and Y_{i1} is most likely positive (i.e., $\rho > 0$), reducing the variance of $\overline{\delta}_A$. The same applies to $\overline{\delta}_B$.

Example

Using the gain-score approach on the data from the FAP clinical trial, the average difference in the number of polyps between baseline and 12 months were 26.3 and -18.7 in the placebo and treatment groups, respectively. That is, on placebo, the number of polyps tended to increase whereas treatment with sulindac decreased the number of polyps. This difference was statistically significant ($p = .03$). For polyp size, the average change on placebo was -0.19 and on treatment was -1.52. This difference was also statistically significant ($p = .05$).

Analysis of covariance

An alternative approach using baseline information, which is probably better than a gain-score analysis [Laird and Aitkin, 1983], is an analysis of covariance (AN-COVA). This method employs the baseline measurements as covariates, which are used to adjust the end of treatment values using a linear regression model. In a simple case, the model takes the form

$$Y_{i2} = \beta_0 + \beta_1 Y_{i1} + \beta_2 T_i + \epsilon_i, \qquad (12.18)$$

where T_i is the treatment indicator variable for the ith person. β_2 is the treatment effect and the focus of interest for the analysis. One can show that the relative efficiency of the gain-score versus the linear model, as measured by the ratio of variances, is $2/(1 + \rho)$ in favor of the ANCOVA [Bock, 1975]. In any case, proper use of additional measurements on the study subjects can improve the precision or efficiency of the trial.

Example

In the FAP clinical trial, an analysis of covariance is shown in Table 12.10. The linear model used is as given above with the variables coded as in Table 12.9. The interpretation of the parameter estimates depends on the coding and on which terms are included in the model. Here β_0 is the sulindac effect, β_1 is the effect of the baseline measurement, and β_2 is the difference between the treatments. For polyp number, the first model is equivalent to the t-test above: the average number of polyps at 12 months is 13.0 on sulindac and the average *difference* between the treatments is 64.9 polyps ($p = .15$).

The second model shows that the number of polyps at 12 months depends strongly on the number at baseline ($p = .0001$) and that the difference between the treatments after accounting for the baseline number of polyps is 43.2, which is significant ($p = .04$). The results for polyp size are different, showing that the average polyp size at 12 months in the sulindac group is 1.83 and the *difference* in size of 1.28 attributable to the treatment is significant ($p = .02$). Also, the effect of treatment on polyp size does not depend on the baseline size.

12.4.4 Non-parametric survival comparisons

Above, I discussed the utility of non-parametric estimates of event time distributions. These are useful summaries, because they are relatively simple to calculate, can be generalized to more than one group, can be applied to interval grouped data, and require no assumptions about the distribution giving rise to the data. Methods that share some of these properties are widely used to *compare* event time distributions in the presence of censored data. One of the most common methods is the logrank statistic [Mantel and Haenszel, 1959]. To understand the workings of this statistic, consider a simple two-group (A versus B) comparison of the type that might arise in a randomized clinical trial.

Table 12.10 Analyses of Covariance for the Familial Adenomatous Polyposis Clinical Trial

Dependent Variable	Model Terms	Parameter Estimate	Standard Error	P-Value
Polyp number	β_0	13.0	30.8	–
	β_2	64.9	42.5	.15
Polyp number	β_0	−21.5	14.2	–
	β_1	1.1	0.1	.0001
	β_2	43.2	18.9	.04
Polyp size	β_0	1.83	0.37	–
	β_2	1.28	0.51	.02
Polyp size	β_0	1.13	0.90	–
	β_1	0.21	0.24	.40
	β_2	1.29	0.51	.02

All dependent variables are measured at 12 months.

As in the product limit method discussed above, the data are sorted by the event time from smallest to largest. At each failure time, a 2×2 table can be formed:

		Status:	
		Event	No Event
Group:	A	d_{iA}	$n_{iA} - d_{iA}$
	B	d_{iB}	$n_{iB} - d_{iB}$

where i indexes the failure times, the d's represent the numbers of events in the groups, the n's represent the number of subjects at risk, and either d_{iA} or d_{iB} is 1 and the other is 0 if all of the event times are unique. These tables can be combined over all failure times in the same way that 2×2 tables are combined across strata in some epidemiologic studies. In particular, we can calculate an overall "observed minus expected" statistic for group A (or B) as a test of the null hypothesis of equal event rates in the groups. This yields

$$O_A - E_A = \sum_{i=1}^{N} \frac{n_{iA} d_{iB} - n_{iB} d_{iA}}{n_i}, \qquad (12.19)$$

where $n_i = n_{iA} + n_{iB}$ and $d_i = d_{iA} + d_{iB}$. The variance can be shown to be

$$V_A = \sum_{i=1}^{N} \frac{d_i(n_i - d_i) n_{iA} n_{iB}}{(n_i - 1) n_i^2}. \qquad (12.20)$$

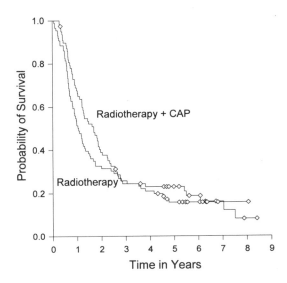

Figure 12.5 Survival by treatment group during a lung cancer clinical trial.

Then, the test statistic can be calculated as

$$Z = \frac{O_A - E_A}{\sqrt{V_A}} .$$

Z will have a standard normal distribution under the null hypothesis.

Example

For the lung cancer clinical trial introduced above, investigators were interested in testing the difference in disease recurrence rates and survival on the two treatment arms (Figures 12.5 and 12.6). When eligible patients are analyzed, the logrank statistic for survival calculated from equations 12.19 and 12.20 is 1.29 ($p = 0.26$) and for recurrence is 9.18 ($p = 0.002$).

12.4.5 Risk (hazard) ratios and confidence intervals are clinically useful data summaries

Although non-parametric methods of describing and comparing event time distributions yield robust ways of assessing statistical significance, they may not provide a concise clinically interpretable summary of treatment effects. For example, product-limit estimates of event times require us to view the entire recurrence curves in Figure 12.6 to have a sense of the magnitude of benefit from CAP. The problem of how to express clinical differences in event times concisely can be lessened by using hazard ratios (and confidence intervals) as summaries. These were introduced in the power

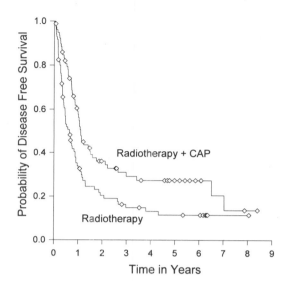

Figure 12.6 Disease Free Survival By Treatment Group During a Lung Cancer Clinical Trial.

and sample size equations in Chapter 7. The ratio of hazards between the treatment groups can be considered a partially parametric summary, because it shares characteristics of both parametric and non-parametric statistics. The hazard ratio is usually assumed to be constant over the course of follow-up, which is a parametric assumption. However, the ratio does not depend on the actual magnitude of the event times, only on their ranking. This is typical of non-parametric methods.

The hazard ratio is a useful descriptor, because it summarizes the magnitude of the treatment difference in a single number. Hazard ratios that deviate from 1.0 indicate increasing or decreasing risk depending on the numerical coding of the variable. It is also relatively easy to specify the precision of the hazard ratio using confidence intervals. Assuming a constant hazard ratio is likely to be at least approximately correct for the period of observation, even in many situations where the hazards are changing with time. In other words, the ratio may remain constant even though the baseline risk fluctuates. A fixed ratio is often useful, even when it is not constant over time. Furthermore, the ratio has an interpretation in terms of relative risk and is connected to the odds ratio in fundamental ways. Finally, the effects of both categorical and continuous prognostic factors can usually be expressed in the form of a hazard ratio, making it widely applicable.

Confidence intervals are probability statements about an estimate and not about the true treatment effect. For example, suppose the true hazard ratio has exactly the value we have estimated in our study. Then a 95 percent confidence interval indicates the region in which 95 percent of hazard ratio estimates would fall if we repeated the experiment. Informally, a confidence interval is a region in which we are confident that a true treatment effect or difference lies. Although incorrect, this notion is not too misleading. The value of confidence intervals is that they convey a sense of the precision with which an effect is estimated.

As indicated in Chapter 7, the estimated hazard from exponentially distributed event times has a chi-square distribution with $2d$ degrees of freedom. A ratio of chi-square random variables, i.e., the hazard ratio, has an F distribution with $2d_1$ and $2d_2$ degrees of freedom [Cox, 1953]. Therefore, a $100(1-\alpha)\%$ confidence interval for $\Delta = \lambda_1/\lambda_2$ is

$$\widehat{\Delta} F_{2d_1, 2d_2, 1-\alpha/2} < \Delta < \widehat{\Delta} F_{2d_1, 2d_2, \alpha/2}.$$

Here again, the calculations can be made more simple by using the approximate normality of $\log(\Delta)$.

Example

In the CAP lung cancer clinical trial, we can summarize the survival difference by saying that the hazard ratio is 1.22 with a 95% confidence interval of 0.87–1.70. The fact that the hazard ratio is near 1.0 tells us that the treatment offers little overall benefit on survival. The fact that this confidence interval includes 1.0 tells us that, even accounting for the minimal improvement in survival, the difference is not statistically significant at conventional levels. The hazard ratio for disease free survival is 1.72 with 95% confidence interval 1.21–2.47. Thus, the benefit of CAP for recurrence is clinically sizeable and statistically significant at conventional levels.

12.4.6 Statistical models are helpful tools

Statistical models are extremely helpful devices for making estimates of treatment effects, testing hypotheses about those effects, and studying the simultaneous influence of covariates on outcome. All models make assumptions about the data. Commonly used survival or relative risk models can be parametric, in which case they assume some specific distribution is the source of the event times, or partially parametric, in which case some assumptions are relaxed. Models can't be totally non-parametric, because this would be something of an oxymoron.

Here we view a small set of models principally as devices to facilitate estimating and comparing hazard ratios. As such, the proportional hazards (PH) model [Cox, 1972], is probably the most well-known and useful device. The essential feature of the model is that time, t, and the covariate vector (predictor variables), $\mathbf{X}$, enter the hazard function, $\lambda(t; \mathbf{X})$, in a way that conveniently factors,

$$\lambda(t; \mathbf{X}) = \lambda_0(t) e^{\beta \mathbf{X}},$$

where $\lambda_0(t)$ is the baseline hazard and β is a vector of regression coefficients to be estimated from the data. In other words, for an individual characterized by $\mathbf{X}$, the ratio of their hazard to the baseline hazard is $e^{\beta \mathbf{X}}$. We could write this relationship as

$$log \left\{ \frac{\lambda(t)}{\lambda_0(t)} \right\} = \boldsymbol{\beta} \mathbf{X} = \beta_1 X_1 + \beta_2 X_2 + \dots$$

to reveal its similarity to other covariate models. Thus, $\boldsymbol{\beta}$ is a vector of log hazard ratios. The model assumes that the hazard ratio is constant over time, and the covariates are also assumed to be constant over time. The effect of covariates is to multiply the baseline hazard, even for $t = 0$.

Estimating $\boldsymbol{\beta}$ is technically complex and not the subject of primary interest here. Computer programs for parameter estimation are widely available, enabling us to focus directly on the results. One advantage of the PH model is that the estimation can be stratified on factors that we have no need to model. For example, we could account for the effects of a risk factor by defining strata based on its levels, estimating the treatment effect separately within each level of the factor, and pooling the estimated hazard ratios over all strata. In this way, we can account for the effects of the factor without having to assume that its hazard is proportional because it is not entered into the model as a covariate.

When interpreting $\boldsymbol{\beta}$, we must remember that it represents the hazard ratio per unit change in the predictor variable. If the predictor is a dichotomous factor such as an indicator variable for treatment group, then a unit change in the variable simply compares the groups. However, if the variable is measured on a continuous scale such as age, then the estimated hazard ratio is per year of age (or other unit of measurement). For variables that are measured on a continuous scale, the hazard ratio associated with an n-unit change is Δ^n, where Δ is the hazard ratio. For example, if age yields a hazard ratio of 1.02 per year increase, then a 10-year increase will have a hazard ratio of $1.02^{10} = 1.22$.

For the CAP lung cancer trial, estimated hazard ratios and 95% confidence limits for predictor variables calculated from the PH model are shown in Table 12.11. Because of differences in the exact method of calculation, these might be slightly different from estimates that could be obtained by the methods outlined earlier in this chapter.

12.4.7 *P*-values do not summarize evidence

Not even a brief discussion of estimation and analysis methods for clinical trials would be complete without an appropriate de-emphasis of p-values as the proper currency for conveying treatment effects. There are many circumstances in which p-values are useful, particularly for hypothesis tests specified *a priori*. However, p-values have properties which make them poor summaries of clinical effects [Royall, 1986]. In particular, p-values do not convey the magnitude of a clinical effect. The size of the p-value is a consequence of two things: the magnitude of the estimated treatment difference and its estimated variability (which is itself a consequence of sample size). Thus, the p-value partially reflects the size of the experiment, which has no biological importance. The p-value also hides the size of the treatment difference, which does have major biological importance.

Table 12.11 Estimated Hazard Ratios from the Proportional Hazards Model for the CAP Lung Cancer Trial

Variable	Hazard Ratio	95% Conf. Bounds	P-Value
Survival Results			
treat='2'	1.22	.867 – 1.70	.26
cell type='2'	1.28	.907 – 1.81	.16
karn='2'	0.84	.505 – 1.40	.51
t='2'	0.94	.558 – 1.57	.80
t='3'	0.94	.542 – 1.63	.82
n='1'	1.09	.542 – 2.20	.81
n='2'	1.26	.691 – 2.30	.45
age	1.00	.984 – 1.02	.73
sex='1'	1.09	.745 – 1.58	.67
wtloss='1'	1.09	.602 – 1.98	.78
race='1'	1.21	.734 – 1.98	.46
Recurrence Results			
treat='2'	1.73	1.21 – 2.47	.003
cell type='2'	1.68	1.16 – 2.43	.006
karn='2'	0.72	.433 – 1.21	.22
t='2'	0.99	.576 – 1.71	.98
t='3'	0.89	.495 – 1.60	.70
n='1'	1.06	.499 – 2.26	.88
n='2'	1.30	.674 – 2.49	.44
age	1.00	.980 – 1.02	.96
sex='1'	0.93	.629 – 1.37	.71
wtloss='1'	1.48	.814 – 2.67	.20
race='1'	0.89	.542 – 1.48	.67

When faced with an estimated effect that is not statistically significant at customary levels, some investigators speculate "the effect might be statistically significant in a larger sample". This, of course, misses a fundamental point, because any effect other than zero will be statistically significant in a large enough sample. What the investigators should really focus on is the size and clinical significance of an estimated treatment effect rather than its p-value. In summary, p-values only quantify the type I error and incompletely characterize the biologically important effects in the data.

One of the weaknesses of p-values as summaries of strength of evidence can be illustrated in a simple way using an example given by Walter [1995]. Consider the following 2×2 tables summarizing binomial proportions:

	A	$\overline{A}$
B	1	7
$\overline{B}$	13	7

and

$$
\begin{array}{c|cc}
 & A & \overline{A} \\
\hline
B & 1 & 6 \\
\overline{B} & 13 & 6
\end{array}
$$

The column proportions are the same in both tables, although the first has more data and should provide stronger evidence than the second. For both tables, we can compare the proportions $\frac{1}{14}$ versus $\frac{1}{2}$ using Fisher's exact test [Agresti, 1996]. Doing so yields two-sided p-values of 0.33 and 0.26, respectively. In other words, the second table is more "statistically significant" than the first, even though it provides less evidence. This outcome is a result of discreteness and asymmetry. One should probably not make too much of it except to recognize that p-values do not measure strength of evidence.

To illustrate the advantage of estimation and confidence intervals over p-values, consider the recent discussion over the prognostic effect of peri-operative blood transfusion in lung cancer [Piantadosi, 1992]. Several studies (not clinical trials) of this phenomenon have been performed because of firm evidence in other malignancies and diseases that blood transfusion has a clinically important immunosuppressive effect. Disagreement about results of various studies has stemmed, in part, from too strong an emphasis on hypothesis tests instead of focusing on the estimated risk ratios and confidence limits. Some study results are shown in Table 12.12. Although the authors of the various reports came to different qualitative conclusions about the risk of blood transfusion because of differing p-values, the estimated risk ratios, adjusted for extent of disease, appear to be consistent across studies. Based on these results, one might be justified in concluding that peri-operative blood transfusion has a modest adverse effect on lung cancer patients. Interestingly, a randomized trial of autologous versus allogeneic blood transfusion in colorectal cancer has been reported recently [Heiss et al., 1994]. It showed a 3.5-fold increased risk attributable to the use of allogeneic blood transfusion with a p-value of 0.10.

12.5 Strength of Evidence Through Support Intervals

12.5.1 Support intervals are based on the likelihood function

Strength of evidence can be measured using the likelihood function [Edwards, 1972; Royall, 1997]. We can obtain a measure of the relative strength of evidence in favor of our best estimate versus a hypothetical value using the ratio of the likelihoods evaluated with each parameter value. Support intervals are quantitative regions based on likelihood ratios, that quantify the strength of evidence in favor of particular values of a parameter of interest. They summarize parameter values consistent with the evidence without using hypothesis tests and confidence intervals. Because they

Table 12.12 Summary of Studies Examining the Peri-Operative Effect of Blood Transfusion in Lung Cancer

Study	Endpoint	Hazard Ratio	95% Confidence Limits
Tartter et al.,1984	Survival	1.99	1.09 – 3.64
Hyman et al., 1985	Survival	1.25	1.04 – 1.49
Pena et al., 1992	Survival	1.30	0.80 – 2.20
Keller et al., 1988	Recurrence		
	Stage I	1.24	0.67 – 1.81
	Stage II	1.92	0.28 – 3.57
Moores et al., 1989	Survival	1.57	1.14 – 2.16
	Recurrence	1.40	1.01 – 1.94

All hazard ratios are transfused versus untransfused patients and are adjusted for extent of disease.

are based on a likelihood function, support intervals are conditional on, or assume, a particular model of the data. Like confidence intervals, they characterize a range of values which are consistent with the observed data. However, support intervals are based on values of the likelihood ratio rather than on control of the type I error.

The likelihood function, $\mathcal{L}(\Theta \mid \mathbf{D})$, depends on the observed data, $\mathbf{D}$, and one or more parameters of the model, Θ. We can view the likelihood as a function of the unknown parameter, conditional on the observed data. Suppose our best estimate of the unknown parameter is $\widehat{\Theta}$. Usually this will be the "maximum likelihood estimate". We are interested in the set of all values of Θ that are consistent with $\widehat{\Theta}$, according to criteria based on the likelihood ratio. We could, for example, say that the data (evidence) support any Θ for which the likelihood ratio relative to $\widehat{\Theta}$ is less than R. When the likelihood ratio for some Θ exceeds R, it is not supported by the data. This defines a support interval or a range of values for Θ which are consistent with $\widehat{\Theta}$. An example is given below.

12.5.2 Support intervals can be used with any endpoint

Support intervals can be constructed from any likelihood using any endpoint. If the purpose of our clinical trial is to estimate the hazard ratio on two treatments, we could employ a simple exponential failure time model. Let i denote an arbitrary study subject. We define a binary covariate, X_i, which equals 1 for treatment group A and 0 for treatment group B. The survival function is $S(t_i) = e^{-\lambda_i t_i}$ and the hazard function, λ_i, is assumed to be constant. Usually we model the hazard as a multiplicative function of covariates, $\lambda_i = e^{\beta_0 + \beta_1 X_i}$ (or $\lambda_i = e^{-\beta_0 - \beta_1 X_i}$), where

β_0 and β_1 are parameters to be estimated from the data, i.e., $\Theta' = \{\beta_0, \beta_1\}$. The hazard for a person on treatment A is $\lambda_A = e^{\beta_0 + \beta_1}$ and for a person on treatment B is $\lambda_B = e^{\beta_0}$. The hazard ratio is

$$\Delta_{AB} = e^{\beta_0 + \beta_1} / e^{\beta_0} = e^{\beta_1}.$$

Thus, β_1 is the log hazard ratio for the treatment effect of interest. (β_0 is a baseline log hazard which is unimportant for the present purposes.)

To account for censoring, we define an indicator variable Z_i which equals 1 if the ith person is observed to have an event and 0 if the ith person is censored. The exponential likelihood is

$$\mathcal{L}(\beta_0, \beta_1 \mid \mathbf{D}) = \prod_{i=1}^{N} e^{-\lambda_i t_i} \lambda_i^{Z_i} = \prod_{i=1}^{N} e^{-t_i e^{\beta_0 + \beta_1 X_i}} \left(e^{\beta_0 + \beta_1 X_i}\right)^{Z_i}.$$

If $\widehat{\beta}_0$ and $\widehat{\beta}_1$ are the MLEs for β_0 and β_1, a support interval for $\widehat{\beta}_1$ is defined by the values of θ which satisfy

$$
\begin{aligned}
R &> \frac{\prod_{i=1}^{N} e^{-t(_i e^{\widehat{\beta}_0 + \widehat{\beta}_1 X_i})} \left(e^{\widehat{\beta}_0 + \widehat{\beta}_1 X_i}\right)^{Z_i}}{\prod_{i=1}^{N} e^{-t_i(e^{\widehat{\beta}_0 + \theta X_i})} \left(e^{\widehat{\beta}_0 + \theta X_i}\right)^{Z_i}} \\[2mm]
&= \frac{e^{-\sum_{i=1}^{N} t(_i e^{\widehat{\beta}_0 + \widehat{\beta}_1 X_i})}}{e^{-\sum_{i=1}^{N} t(_i e^{\widehat{\beta}_0 + \theta X_i})}} \prod_{i=1}^{N} \left(\frac{e^{\widehat{\beta}_1 X_i}}{e^{\theta X_i}}\right)^{Z_i} \\[2mm]
&= e^{-\sum_{i=1}^{N} t_i (e^{\widehat{\beta}_0 + \widehat{\beta}_1 X_i} - e^{\widehat{\beta}_0 + \theta X_i})} \prod_{i=1}^{N} \left(e^{(\widehat{\beta}_1 - \theta) X_i}\right)^{Z_i}. \quad (12.21)
\end{aligned}
$$

Example

Reconsider the CTE lung cancer trial for which the estimated hazard ratio for disease free survival favored treatment with CAP chemotherapy. The log hazard ratio estimated using the exponential model is $(\widehat{\beta}_1 =) 0.589$ in favor of the CAP group. Using some software for fitting this model, it may be necessary to re-code the treatment group indicator variable as 0 versus 1, rather than 1 versus 2. Note that $e^{0.589} = 1.80$, which is similar to the hazard ratio estimated above from the PH model. The estimated baseline hazard depends on the time scale and is unimportant for the present purposes. However, from the exponential model, $\widehat{\beta}_0 = -6.92$.

Using these parameter estimates and applying equation 12.21 to the data, we can calculate support for different values of β_1 (Figure 12.7). The vertical axis is the likelihood ratio relative to the MLE and the horizontal axis is the value of β_1. For these data, values of β_1 between 0.322 and 0.835 fall within an interval defined by $R = 10$ and are, thus, strongly supported by the data. This interval corresponds to hazard ratios of 1.38 to 2.30. The 95% confidence interval for β_1 is $0.234 - 0.944$, which corresponds approximately to a support interval with $R = 12$.

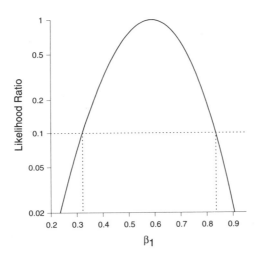

Figure 12.7 Support interval for the estimated hazard ratio for disease free survival in a lung cancer trial.

12.6 Special Methods of Analysis

When studying some biological questions, either the underlying disease, method of treatment, or the structure of the data requires an analytic plan that is more complicated than the examples given above. This tends to happen more in nonexperimental studies, because investigators do not always have control over how the data are collected. In true experiments, it is often possible to measure endpoints in such a way that simple analyses are sufficient. Even so, special methods of analysis may be needed to address specific clinical questions or goals of the trial. Some examples of situations that may require special or more sophisticated analytic methods are correlated responses, such as those from repeated measurements on the same individual over time or clustering of study subjects, pairing of responses such as event times or binary responses, covariates that change their values over time, measurement errors in independent variables, and accounting for restricted randomization schemes. Each of these can require generalizations of commonly used analytic methods to fully utilize the data.

Sometimes the hardest part of being in these situations is recognizing that ordinary or simple approaches to an analysis are deficient in one important way or another. Even after recognizing the problem and a solution, computer software to carry out the analyses may not be readily available. All of these issues indicate the usefulness of consulting a statistical methodologist during study design and again early in the analysis.

12.6.1 The bootstrap is based on re-sampling

Often, one of the most difficult tasks for the biostatistician is to determine how precise an estimate is. Stated more formally, determining the variance is usually more difficult than determining the estimate itself. When using statistical models with estimation methods like maximum likelihood, there are fairly simple and reliable ways of calculating the approximate variance of an estimate. Sometimes however, either the assumptions underlying the approximation are invalid or standard methods are not available. One example is placing confidence limits on the estimate of a median from a distribution.

In situations like this, one simple and reliable way to approximate the variance is to use a resampling method called the *bootstrap* [Efron and Tibshirani, 1986; 1993]. In the bootstrap, the observed data are resampled and the point estimate or other statistic of interest is calculated from each sample. The process is repeated a large number of times so that a distribution of possible point estimates is built up. This distribution, characterized by ordinary means, serves as a measure of the precision of the estimate. The sample at each step is taken "with replacement", i.e., any particular datum can be chosen more than once in the bootstrap sample.

Like randomization distributions, there are a large number of possible bootstrap samples. For example, suppose there are N observed values in the data and each bootstrap sample consists of M values. Then, there are N^M possible bootstrap samples. Some of these may not be distinguishable because of duplicate observations or sample points. Nevertheless, there are a large number of samples, in general, so that complete enumeration of the sample space is difficult. Therefore, the bootstrap distribution is usually approximated from a random sample of the N^M possibilities. A simple example should illustrate the procedure.

Suppose we have a sample of 50 event times and we are interested in placing confidence intervals on our estimate of the median failure time. The observed data plotted as a survival curve are shown in Figure 12.8. There are no censored observations in this example. Standard lifetable methods yield a ninety-five percent confidence interval for the median event time of (1.50–1.92). Samples of size 50 were taken with replacement and the bootstrap procedure was repeated 500 times. The medians and cumulative distribution from the bootstrap resamples actually obtained are shown in Table 12.13. 95% of the bootstrap medians fall between 1.49 and 1.92, in excellent agreement with standard methods. Calculations such as these are greatly facilitated by computer programs dedicated to the purpose. One example of a general resampling program is *Resampling Stats* [Resampling Stats, Inc., 1995].

Bootstrap methods can be used to validate modeling procedures. An example of its use in pharmacodynamic modeling is given by Mick and Ratain [1994].

12.6.2 Some clinical questions require other special methods of analysis

A book such as this can do little more than mention a few of the important statistical methods that are occasionally required to help analyze data from clinical trials. Here I briefly discuss some special methods that are likely to be important to the student

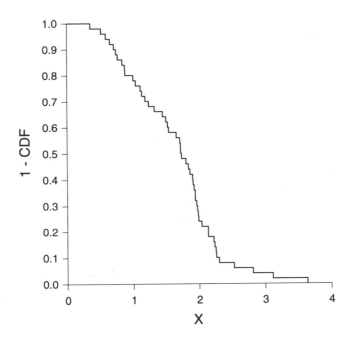

Figure 12.8 Survival distribution for bootstrap example.

of clinical trials. Most of these represent areas of active biostatistical research. For many of the situations discussed below, there are no widely applicable guidelines about the best statistical summary of the data to answer clinical questions. This results from the lower frequency with which some of these situations arise, and their greater complexity.

Longitudinal measurements

Because most clinical trials involve or require observation of patients over a period of time following treatment, investigators often record longitudinal assessments of outcomes, endpoints, and predictor variables. Using the additional information contained in longitudinal measurements can be difficult. For example, survival and disease progression are familiar longitudinal outcomes that require special methods of analysis. To the data analyst, the relationship between measurements taken in a longitudinal study are not all equivalent. For example, there is a difference between measurements taken within the same individual, which are correlated, and those taken from different individuals, which are usually uncorrelated or independent. Because most simple statistical approaches to analysis rely on the assumption of independent observations, coping with correlated measurements is an important methodologic issue.

Table 12.13 Cumulative Distribution of Medians Obtained from Bootstrap Simulation

Median	Number	Cum. %
1.254	1	0.2
1.280	1	0.4
1.342	1	0.6
1.385	1	0.8
1.411	1	1.0
1.448	3	1.6
1.473	1	1.8
1.486	2	2.2
1.494	2	2.6
1.498	9	4.4
1.511	2	4.8
⋮	⋮	⋮
1.912	3	95.2
1.915	11	97.4
1.920	3	98.0
1.921	1	98.2
1.922	1	98.4
1.924	1	98.6
1.931	2	99.0
1.931	1	99.2
1.939	1	99.4
1.940	1	99.6
1.941	1	99.8
1.974	1	100.0

When the primary data analysis tool is the linear model, such as for analyses of variance or linear regressions, correlated measurements are analyzed according to "repeated measures" or "longitudinal data" models. These types of data and models used to analyze them are increasingly used in studies of HIV and other diseases with repeated outcomes such as migraine, asthma, and seizure disorders. An in-depth discussion of statistical methods is given by Diggle, Liang, and Zeger [1994]. See also Zeger and Liang [1986], Zeger, Liang, and Albert [1988], and Liang and Zeger [1986]. These references also pertain to the analysis of other correlated outcomes.

Correlated outcomes

Longitudinal measures is not the only circumstance that gives rise to correlated observations. When the experimental unit is a cluster or group, outcomes may be correlated from individual to individual. This situation can arise if families are the experimental unit as in some disease prevention trials. For example, consider a clinical trial to assess the efficacy of treatments to eliminate *helicobacter pylori* in patients living in endemic areas. *Helicobacter pylori* has a causal association with peptic ulcer disease. After treatment with antibiotics and/or bismuth, patients may become re-infected because of environmental exposure or family contact. Therefore, it may be necessary to treat families as the experimental unit, in which case the outcomes between individuals in the same family will be correlated. In situations such as this, the analysis may need to employ methods to account for this dependency.

Other circumstances can also lead to correlated outcomes, e.g., when individuals have more than one outcome. For example, suppose recurrent pre-malignant or malignant lesions (e.g., skin cancers, bladder polyps, colonic polyps) are the clinical outcome of interest. We might be interested in the interval between such events, recognizing that prolongation of the between-lesion time could be the sign of an effective secondary preventive agent. Thus, each individual on study could give rise to two or more event times correlated with each other because they arise from the same person. Correlated dichotomous outcomes can arise in a similar way.

Individual study subjects can yield more than one endpoint as a consequence of the experimental design. This is the case for cross-over designs (discussed in Chapter ??) where each study participant is intentionally given more than one treatment. Estimating the difference in treatment effects within individuals while accounting for dependency is the major issue in the use of cross-over designs.

Time dependent covariates

Most of the prognostic factors (covariates) measured in clinical trials are fixed at baseline (start of treatment) and do not change during follow-up. Examples are severity of disease at diagnosis, age at diagnosis, sex, race, treatment group assignment, and pathologic type or class of disease. The methods of accounting for the influence of such prognostic factors in statistical regression models typically assume that their effects are constant over time. Statistical models usually assume that the effect of treatment as a prognostic factor is immediate following administration and constant over the follow-up period.

These assumptions are inadequate to describe the effects of all prognostic factors. First, disease intensity or factors associated with it can fluctuate following any clinical landmark such as beginning of treatment. Second, long-term prognosis may be a direct consequence of disease intensity or other time-varying prognostic factors measured at an earlier time. Third, some time-varying prognostic factors may be associated with outcome without being causal. In any case, we require statistical models that are flexible enough to account for the effects of predictor variables whose value changes over time. These type of variables are called "time dependent covariates" (TDC). TDCs are discussed in depth by Kalbfleisch and Prentice [1980] and Marubini and Valsecchi [1995].

It is helpful to distinguish between two basic types of TDCs. The first is *external*, implying that the factor can affect the individual's prognosis but does not carry information about the event time. External TDCs can be *defined* by a particular mechanism. An example is age, which is usually regarded as a fixed covariate (age at time 0), but may be considered as defined and time varying when prognoses change with the age of the study subject. TDCs can be *ancillary*, which indicates that they arise from a process not related to the individual. A second type of TDC is *internal*, a term that implies that a process within the individual, perhaps even the disease itself, gives rise to the prognostic factor. Extent of disease and response to treatment are examples of this. Cumulative dose of drug may also be an internal TDC if it increases because the patient survives longer.

Investigators should interpret the results of analyses employing TDCs with care. For internal TDCs in a treatment trial, the therapy may determine the value of the covariate. Adjusting on the TDC in such a case can "adjust away" the effect of treatment, making the prognostic factor appear significant and the treatment appear ineffective. This is almost never the correct description of the trial outcome.

Measurement error

Another usual assumption of most statistical modeling methods is that the predictor variables are measured without error. Although such models explicitly incorporate the effects of random error, it is usually assumed to be associated with the response measurement rather than with the predictor variables. This paradigm is clearly not applicable in all circumstances. For example, suppose we attempt to predict the occurrence of cancer from dietary factors, such as fat, calorie, and mineral content. It is likely that the predictor variables will be subject to measurement error as a consequence of recall error and inaccuracies converting from food substances to the components of interest.

Accounting for errors in predictor variables complicates statistical models and is not usually needed when analyzing clinical trials. Nonlinear models with predictor variables subject to measurement error are discussed by Carroll, Ruppert, and Stefanski [1995].

Random versus fixed effects

Most widely used statistical models assume that the effects of predictor variables are fixed (non-random). Sometimes, it makes more sense to model the influence of a predictor variable as a random effect. For example, in a multi-center study, the effect of interest may vary from institution to institution. Comparing two institutions may not be of interest. Also, testing the average treatment effect in different institutions may not be of interest because of systematic differences. In such a situation, investigators may be more interested in the relative size of the within and between institution variability.

A random effects model regards the study centers as a random sample of all possible institutions and accounts for variation both within and between centers. When using linear models or analyses of variance, such models are also called *variance components*. It will almost never be the case that centers participating in a trial can realistically be regarded as randomly chosen from a population of centers. However, this perspective may be useful for assessing the relative sizes of the sources of variation. An overview of random and mixed effects linear models is given by McLean, Sanders, and Stroup [1991]. Such models have been applied to longitudinal data [Laird and Ware, 1982]. See Taylor, Cumberland, and Sy [1994] for an interesting application to AIDS.

12.7   Exploratory or Hypothesis-Generating Analyses

12.7.1   Clinical trial data lend themselves to exploratory analyses

The data from clinical trials can and should be used to address questions in addition to those directly related to the primary objectives of the study. Such questions may be specified in advance of the trial, but are also often suggested by investigators after seeing the data. Because the structure of the experiment is usually not perfectly suited to answering such questions, the quality of evidence that results is almost always inferior to that arising from analyses of the primary objectives. Even so, it is scientifically important for investigators to use clinical trial data to explore new questions.

Usually we engage in this activity only after the primary questions have been answered, often in secondary publications or reports. Investigators make mistakes not because they perform exploratory analyses, but when they represent such findings as the primary results of the trial. It is essential to acknowledge the hypothetical nature of exploratory findings and recognize that the usual calculation of type I errors may be incorrect, especially when the data themselves suggest the hypothesis test. As a general rule, the same data should not be used both to generate a new hypothesis and to test it. Apart from the statistical pitfalls, investigators must guard against forcing the data to fit the hypotheses (data torturing) [Mills, 1993].

12.7.2   Multiple tests multiply errors

Data, in sufficient quantity and detail, can be made to yield nearly any effect desired by the adventuresome analyst performing hypothesis tests. They will almost certainly yield *some* effect if studied diligently.

> *There once was a biased clinician,*
> *Who rejected the wise statistician.*
> *By flogging his data*
> *With α and β,*
> *He satisfied all his ambition.*

A small thought experiment will illustrate effects of concern. Suppose we generate N observations sampled from a Gaussian distribution with mean 0 and variance 1. With each observation, we also randomly generate 100 binary indicator variables, $x_1, x_2, \ldots, x_{100}$, which can be used to assign the observation to either of two groups. We then perform 100 "group" comparisons defined by the x's, each at a specified α-level, e.g., $\alpha = 0.05$. Thus, the null hypothesis is true for all comparisons. Using this procedure, we would expect 5% of the tests to reject simply by chance. Of course, the type I error rate for the entire testing procedure greatly exceeds 5%. It equals $\alpha^* = 1 - (1 - \alpha)^{100} \approx 0.99$. In other words, we are virtually certain to find at least one "significant" difference based on partitioning by the x's.

Even if we ignore the problem of multiplicity of tests, what if we restrict our attention to only those differences which are large in magnitude? This corresponds to performing significance tests suggested by findings in the data. If we test only the ten largest group differences, presumably all five of the expected "significant" differences will be in this group. Thus, the expected type I error rate for each test will increase from the nominal 5% to $5/10 = 50\%$.

Investigators must be aware of these types of problems when performing exploratory analyses. Findings observed in such a setting, even if in accord with biological rationale, should be viewed as hypothesis-generating and have a high chance of being incorrect. In these cases, independent verification is essential, perhaps through another clinical trial.

12.7.3 Subset analyses are error prone

One of the easiest ways for the analysis of a clinical trial to follow an inappropriate direction occurs when investigators emphasize the findings from a particular subset of patients, especially when the results are different from the overall findings (i.e., an analysis including all randomized patients). These interesting results may be found in a particular subset of patients after an extensive search that is not based on any *a priori* biological hypothesis. Other times, an accidental observation in a subset may suggest a difference, which is then tested and found to be "statistically significant". If the investigators have prejudices or reasons from outside the trial to believe the findings, these circumstances could lead to a fairly firmly held belief in the validity of the results. Unfortunately, the potential for error in this scenario is high.

One example of how this type of error might occur, and be perpetuated, is illustrated by the enthusiasm some clinicians had in the 1980s and 1990s for the treatment of cancer patients with hydrazine sulfate. Hydrazine, H_2N-NH_2 (diamide or diamine), was discovered in 1887 and synthesized in 1907. However, it was not until World War II that interest developed in the compound as a rocket fuel. It is a powerful reducing agent and readily reacts with acids to form salts. Hydrazine is a known carcinogen in rodents and probably in humans [IARC, 1974]. It is metabolized by N-acetylation [Colvin, 1969] with varying rapidity according to acetylator phenotypes [Weber, 1987]. A condensed but well referenced review of hydrazine sulfate in cancer treatment can be found in the National Cancer Institute's final IND report to the FDA [NCI, 1993].

In the 1970s, there were suggestions that hydrazine sulfate could improve the survival of patients with advanced cancer [Gold, 1975]. Investigators suggested that the mechanism of action was by normalizing glucose metabolism in patients with cachexia. Cachexia is common in cancer patients and is a sign of poor prognosis. It may be due, in part, to tumor glycolysis. Although blocking glycolysis systemically is undesirable, inhibiting gluconeogenesis might be beneficial. Hydrazine sulfate is a non-competitive inhibitor of phosphoethanol pyruvate carboxykinase, the enzyme that catalyzes the conversion of oxaloacetate to phosphoenolpyruvate. This mechanism may explain observations that hydrazine sulfate inhibits tumor growth in animals [Gold, 1975].

Based on the possible biological actions suggested above and anecdotal case reports of human benefit, early uncontrolled trials of hydrazine sulfate were undertaken in the Soviet Union. The results were mixed. In 1990, a group of investigators reported results from a randomized clinical trial testing the effects of hydrazine sulfate in patients with advanced lung cancer [Chlebowski et al., 1990]. Although no statistically significant overall effect was found, a subset analysis revealed a group of patients that appeared to benefit from the drug. The subset of patients who seemed to have improved survival after treatment with hydrazine included those with the most advanced disease.

The analysis and report of this study emphasized the subset findings as primary results of the trial. Criticism of the trial report, suggesting that it might represent a type I error [Piantadosi, 1990], annoyed proponents of hydrazine sulfate. Commentary on the question in the well-known scientific forum afforded by *Penthouse* magazine suggested that patients were being denied a virtual cure for cancer and that unscrupulous researchers were profiting from continued denial of hydrazine's salutary effects:

> If you ... come down with cancer or AIDS ... you will probably be denied the one drug that may offer the best possibility of an effective treatment with the least side effects. It works for roughly half of all the patients who have received it and it's being deliberately suppressed ... [A] million Americans alone are being denied lifesaving benefits each year. ... [T]he apparent sabotaging of federally funded clinical trials of the drug deny the public access to it [Kamen, 1993].

The author of this article was said to be working on a book and a documentary film regarding hydrazine.

Scientists with no financial interests in the outcome of studies were performing large randomized clinical trials testing the effects of hydrazine in patients with lung and colon cancer. One clinical trial was conducted by the Cancer and Leukemia Group B (CALGB) and two others were done by the North Central Cancer Treatment Group (NCCTG) based at the Mayo Clinic. These studies were all published in the same issue of the *Journal of Clinical Oncology* in 1994 [Kosty et al., 1994; Loprinzi et al., 1994a; 1994b]. All of these studies showed hydrazine sulfate to be no better than placebo. Measurements of quality of life using standard methods of assessment also showed trends favoring placebo.

The findings at a planned interim analysis from one randomized trial suggested that hydrazine sulfate was nearly significantly *worse* than placebo [Loprinzi et al., 1994b]. This finding could have been due to chance imbalances in the treatment groups. In any case, the trial was terminated before its planned accrual target of 300 patients, because there was little chance that, given the interim results, hydrazine sulfate would be found to be beneficial. In addition to the rigorous design and analyses of these trials, the final reports emphasized only findings that were protected by the randomization.

Even with these methodologically rigorous findings in evidence, the proponents of hydrazine would not be silenced. Returning to *Penthouse*, they said

> The contempt of the Romanovs for their people has almost been rivaled in the United States by key figures in the American cancer establishment. These senior physicians have demonstrated their own brand of imperviousness to the suffering of millions by systematically destroying the reputation of an anticancer drug that has already benefited thousands and made life longer and easier for many more . . . [Kamen, 1994].

In 1993, because of the failure of hydrazine sulfate to demonstrate any benefit in large, randomized, double masked, placebo controlled clinical trials, the National Cancer Institute inactivated the IND for the drug. However, an editorial accompanying the publication of the results from the three NIH trials prophesied that the treatment might rise again [Herbert, 1994]. This was true, for in 1994, the General Accounting Office (GAO) of the U.S. Government began an investigation into the manner in which the three trials were conducted. The investigation was fueled by documents from the developer of hydrazine alleging that NCI had compromised the studies. In particular, questions were raised about the number of patients who might have received barbiturates or related drugs, said to interfere with the beneficial effects of hydrazine. A collection of new data (retrospectively) and re-analysis of the lung cancer trial supported the original conclusions [Kosty et al., 1995].

The final GAO report on the NCI hydrazine clinical trials appeared in September, 1995 [GAO, 1995]. After a detailed investigation of the allegations and research methods, the GAO supported conclusions by the study investigators and sponsors that hydrazine sulfate is ineffective. The GAO did criticize the failure to keep records of tranquilizer, barbiturate, and alcohol use, and the late analyses of such questions. These criticisms were dismissed by the Public Health Service in Appendix II of the GAO report. In any case, mainstream scientific and governmental opinion has converged on the view that hydrazine sulfate in not effective therapy for patients with cancer.

Lessons to be learned from hydrazine sulfate

The student of clinical trials can learn some very important general lessons by reading the scientific papers and commentaries cited above regarding hydrazine sulfate. With regard to subset analyses, power is reduced because of the smaller sample sizes on which comparisons are based. This tends to produce a high false negative rate. If investigators perform many such comparisons, the overall false positive rate will be increased. Thus, almost all findings are incorrect. Explorations of the data are worthwhile and important for generating new questions. However, one cannot test a hypothesis reliably using the same data that generated the question.

The hydrazine example also sketches implicitly some of the circumstances in which we need to maintain a cautious interpretation of clinical trial results. Even when there is *a priori biological justification for the hypothesis from animal studies*, interpretations and extrapolations of methodologically flawed human trials should be cautious before confirmatory studies are done. *Small trials* or those with *poor de-*

signs or analyses should be treated skeptically. The *results of subset analyses should not be emphasized* as the primary findings of a trial nor should *hypothesis tests suggested by the data*. When conducting exploratory analyses, *statistical adjustment* procedures can help interpret the validity of findings.

The reader of trial reports and other medical studies should be aware of the ways in which *observer bias* can enter trial designs or analyses. Aside from inappropriate emphasis, those analyzing or reporting a study should not have any *financial interests* in the outcome. Finally, apparent *treatment–covariate interactions* should be explored rigorously and fully.

12.8   Summary

The clinical effects of interest in phase I trials are usually drug distribution and elimination parameters and the association, if any, between dose and side effects. Pharmacokinetic models are essential for quantifying kinetic parameters such as elimination rate and half-life. These models are often based on simple mass action distribution of drug in a few idealized compartments. The compartments can often be identified physiologically as intravascular, extravascular, body fat, or similar tissues. Phase I trials usually provide useful dosage recommendations and usually do not provide evidence of efficacy.

SE clinical trials often focus on treatment feasibility and simple estimates of clinical efficacy or toxicity such as success or failure rates. More formally, these studies estimate the probability of success or failure (according to pre-defined criteria) when new patients are treated. Phase II studies in patients with life-threatening diseases can also provide estimates of survival and other event rates. Many other clinical or laboratory effects of treatment can be estimated from SE trials.

Comparative trials estimate relative treatment effects. Depending on the endpoint being used, the relative effect of two treatments might be a difference of means, a ratio, or a qualitative difference. Estimated risk ratios are important and commonly used relative treatment effects in phase III trials. Although not always required, statistical models can be useful when analyzing comparative trials to help estimate relative treatment effects and account for the possible influence of prognostic variables.

Besides statistical models, clinical trials often employ other special methods of analysis. These may be necessary for using the information in repeated measurements, when outcomes are correlated with one another, or when predictor variables change over time. The statistical methods for dealing with such situations are complex and require an experienced methodologist.

It is often important to conduct exploratory analyses of clinical trials, i.e., analyses that do not adhere strictly to the experimental design. In comparative trials, these explorations of the data may not be protected by the design of the study (e.g., randomization). Consequently, they should be performed, interpreted, and reported conservatively. This is true of results based on subsets of the data, especially when many such analyses are performed.

Table 12.14 Survival of Presidents, Popes, and Monarchs from 1690

Washington	10	Wilson	11		Leo XIII	25	
J. Adams	29	Harding	2		Pius X	11	
Jefferson	26	Coolidge	9		Ben XV	8	
Madison	28	Hoover	36		Pius XI	17	
Monroe	15	F. Roosevelt	12		Pius XII	19	
J.Q. Adams	23	Truman	28		John XXIII	5	
Jackson	17	Kennedy	3		Paul VI	15	
Van Buren	0	Eisenhower	16		John Paul	0	
Harrison	20	L. Johnson	9		John Paul II	18	+
Polk	4	Nixon	27				
Taylor	1	Ford	22	+	James II	17	
Fillmore	24	Carter	19	+	Mary II	6	
Pierce	16	Reagan	15	+	William III	13	
Buchanan	12				Anne	12	
Lincoln	4	Alex VIII	2		George I	13	
A. Johnson	10	Innoc XII	9		George II	33	
Grant	17	Clem XI	21		George III	59	
Hayes	16	Innoc XIII	3		George IV	10	
Garfield	0	Ben XIII	6		William IV	7	
Arthur	7	Clem XIII	11		Victoria	63	
Cleveland	24	Clem XIV	6		Edward VII	9	
Harrison	12	Pius VI	25		George V	25	
McKinley	4	Pius VII	23		Edward VIII	36	
T. Roosevelt	18	Greg XVI	15		George VI	15	
Taft	21	Pius IX	32		Elizabeth II	44	+

Survival in years from first taking office (see Lunn and McNeil, 1990).

Table 12.15 Results of a Double Masked Randomized Trial of Mannitol versus Placebo in Patients with Ciguatera Poisoning

ID	Signs and Symptoms Baseline	2.5 Hours	Treatment Group	Baseline Severity	Sex	Age	Time
1	10	3	M	18	F	24	330
2	10	7	M	12	M	12	270
3	12	8	M	21	F	18	820
4	12	6	M	24	M	11	825
26	5	0	P	9	M	37	910
28	4	4	P	9	M	41	2935
33	7	7	P	12	M	44	1055
37	10	10	P	23	M	46	1455
42	5	5	P	6	M	54	780
43	6	6	M	6	M	44	9430
50	11	11	M	16	F	46	390
51	7	7	M	12	F	27	900
59	7	7	M	12	M	46	870
94	12	6	M	19	M	44	80
95	14	14	M	27	M	45	490
98	14	7	M	34	F	34	415
116	8	7	M	12	F	25	605
117	8	5	M	20	F	18	650
118	16	11	M	27	F	16	645
501	3	0	P	3	F	27	2670
503	15	14	M	23	M	57	5850

Data from Palafox, Schatz, Lange, et al. [1997].

Table 12.16 Results of a Double Masked Randomized Trial of Mannitol Versus Placebo in Patients With Ciguatera Poisoning (Continued).

ID	Signs and Symptoms Baseline	Signs and Symptoms 2.5 Hours	Treatment Group	Baseline Severity	Sex	Age	Time
504	13	13	P	22	M	42	440
505	13	13	P	21	F	16	1460
512	13	1	P	31	F	14	545
513	5	0	M	29	F	30	670
514	17	8	P	37	M	40	615
515	25	24	M	54	F	19	645
516	21	20	M	27	F	29	1280
517	8	8	M	11	M	48	1500
613	12	1	P	34	M	9	740
615	11	8	M	45	M	9	415
701	11	0	P	11	M	40	540
705	12	12	M	14	F	38	1005
706	3	3	M	4	M	39	370
707	8	7	P	8	M	54	250
708	11	3	P	10	F	27	795
709	9	9	M	9	M	34	.
737	4	3	M	4	M	31	865
738	11	8	P	22	M	48	630
766	11	0	P	29	M	22	630
768	11	7	M	27	M	18	690
1000	6	6	P	11	M	50	795

Data from Palafox, Schatz, Lange, et al. [1997].

Table 12.17 Results of a Randomized Double Masked Trial of BCNU Polymer versus Placebo for Patients with Newly Diagnosed Malignant Gliomas

ID	Treat	Score	Sex	Age	Karn	GBM	Time	Status
103	1	25	M	65	1	0	9.6	1
104	1	25	M	43	1	0	24.0	0
105	1	19	F	49	0	1	24.0	0
107	1	17	M	60	0	1	9.2	1
203	1	21	F	58	0	0	21.0	1
204	1	26	F	45	1	1	24.0	0
205	1	27	F	37	1	0	24.0	0
301	1	23	M	60	1	1	13.3	1
302	1	26	F	65	0	1	17.9	1
306	1	24	F	44	0	1	9.9	1
307	1	24	F	57	0	1	13.4	1
402	1	27	M	68	1	1	9.7	1
404	1	27	M	55	0	1	12.3	1
407	1	10	M	60	0	1	1.1	1
408	1	23	M	42	0	1	9.2	1
412	1	27	F	48	1	0	24.0	0
101	2	26	F	59	1	1	9.9	1
102	2	14	F	65	0	1	1.9	1
106	2	21	M	58	1	1	5.4	1
108	2	21	F	51	0	1	9.2	1
109	2	22	F	63	1	1	8.6	1
201	2	17	F	45	0	1	9.1	1
202	2	20	F	52	0	1	6.9	1
303	2	26	M	62	1	1	11.5	1
304	2	27	M	53	1	1	8.7	1
305	2	25	F	44	1	1	17.1	1
308	2	24	M	57	0	1	9.1	1
309	2	25	M	36	1	1	15.1	1
401	2	27	F	47	1	1	10.3	1
403	2	27	M	52	1	1	24.0	0
405	2	18	F	55	0	1	9.3	1
406	2	26	F	63	0	1	4.8	1

Data from Valtonen et al. [1997].

12.9 Questions for Discussion

1. A new drug is thought to be distributed in a single, mostly vascular, compartment and excreted by the kidneys. Drug administration will be by a single IV bolus injection. What rate (differential) equation describes this situation? What should the time-concentration curve look like? Four hours after injection, 65% of the drug has been eliminated. What is the half-life? If the drug is actually distributed in two or more compartments, what will be the shape of the time-concentration curve?

2. The following event times are observed on a SE trial in patients with cardiomyopathy (censored times are indicated by a +): 55, 122, 135, 141+,144, 150, 153+, 154, 159, 162, 170, 171, 171+, 174, 178, 180, 180+, 200+, 200+, 200+, 200+, 200+. Construct a lifetable and estimate the survival at 180 days. Estimate the overall failure rate and an approximate 95% confidence interval.

3. In the mesothelioma SE trial, estimate the overall rate of progression and death rate. Are these rates associated with age, sex, or performance status? Why or why not?

4. In the CAP lung cancer trial, there are as many as $2 \times 2 \times 3 \times 3 \times 2 \times 2 \times 2 = 288$ subsets based on categorical factors (cell type, performance status, T, N, sex, weight loss, and race). The number of possible ways of forming subsets is even larger. Can you suggest a simple algorithm for forming subsets based on arbitrary classifications? Use your method to explore treatment differences in subsets in the CAP trial. Draw conclusions based on your analyses.

5. In the FAP clinical trial, test the treatment effect by performing gain score analyses on polyp number and polyp size. How do the results compare with analyses of covariance. Discuss. Can these analyses test or account for the effects of sex and age?

6. At one medical center, a new cancer treatment is classified as a success in 11 out of 55 patients. At another center using the same treatment and criteria, the success rate is 14 out of 40 patients. Using resampling methods, place a confidence interval on the *difference* in the success rates. What are your conclusions?

7. The data in Table 12.14 show the survival times in years measured from inauguration, election, or coronation for U.S. Presidents, Roman Catholic Popes, and British Monarchs from 1690 to the present [Lunn and McNeil, 1990]. (I have added censored observations to the list for individuals remaining alive in 1996.) Are there differences between the groups? Discuss your methods and conclusions.

8. Do this exercise without consulting the reference. The data in Tables 12.15 and 12.16 show the results of a double masked randomized clinical trial of mannitol infusion versus placebo for the treatment of ciguatera poisoning [Palafox, Schatz, Lange, et al., 1997]. The number of neurological signs and symptoms of poisoning at the start of treatment and 2.5 hours after treatment are given. Estimate the clinical effect and statistical significance of mannitol treatment. Discuss your estimate in view of the small size of the trial.

9. Do this exercise without consulting the reference. The data in Tables 12.16 and 12.17 show the results of a double masked randomized clinical trial of implantable biodegradable polymer wafers impregnated with (BCNU) versus placebo for the treatment of patients with newly diagnosed malignant gliomas [Valtonen, Timonen, Toivanen, et al. 1997]. Survival time (in weeks) following surgical resection is given for each patient. Estimate the clinical effect and statistical significance of BCNU wafer treatment. Discuss your estimate in view of the small size of the trial.

Chapter References

Agresti, A. (1996). An Introduction to Categorical Data Analysis. New York: John Wiley & Sons.

Armitage, P., and Berry, G. (1994). Statistical Methods in Medical Research, 3rd Edition. Oxford: Blackwell.

Bock, R.D. (1975). Multivariate Statistical Methods in Behavioral Research. New York: McGraw-Hill.

Campbell, M.J. and Machin, D. (1990). Medical Statistics. New York: John Wiley & Sons.

Carroll, R.J., Ruppert, D., and Stefanski, L.A. (1995). Measurement Error in Nonlinear Models. London: Chapman-Hall.

Carson, E.R., Cobelli, C., and Finkelstein, L. (1983). The Mathematical Modeling of Metabolic and Endocrine Systems. New York: John Wiley & Sons.

Chlebowski, R.T., Bulcavage, L., Grosvenor, M. et al. (1990). Hydrazine sulfate influence on nutritional status and survival in non-small cell lung cancer. J. Clin. Oncol. 8: 9-15.

Colvin, L.B. (1969). Metabolic fate of hydrazines and hydrazides. J. Pharm. Sci. 58: 1433-1443.

Cox, D.R. (1953). Some simple tests for Poisson variates. Biometrika 40: 354-360.

Cox, D.R. (1972). Regression models and life-tables (with discussion). J. Roy. Statist. Soc. (B) 34: 187-220.

Diggle, P.J., Liang, K.Y., and Zeger, S.L. (1994). Analysis of Longitudinal Data. Oxford: Oxford University Press.

Donner, A. and Klar, N. (1994). Methods for comparing event rates in intervention studies when the unit of allocation is a cluster. Am. J. Epidemiol. 140: 279-289.

Edwards, A.W.F. (1972). Likelihood. Cambridge: Cambridge University Press.

Everitt, B.S. (1989). Statistical Methods for Medical Investigations. New York: Oxford University Press.

GAO (1995). Cancer Drug Research: Contrary to Allegation, NIH Hydrazine Sulfate Studies Were Not Flawed. Washington, DC: General Accounting Office Publication GAO/HEHS-95-141.

Giardiello, F.M., Hamilton, S.R., Krush, A.J., Piantadosi, S., Hylind, L.M., Celano, P., Booker, S.V., Robinson, C.R., and Offerhaus, G.J.A. (1993). Treatment of Colonic and Rectal Adenomas with Sulindac in Familial Adenomatous Polyposis. N. Engl. J. Med. 328: 1313-1316.

Gold, J. (1975). Use of hydrazine sulfate in terminal and preterminal cancer patients: Results of investigational new drug (IND) study in 84 evaluable patients. Oncology 32: 1-10.

Greenwood, M. (1926). The errors of sampling of the survivorship tables, in Reports on Public Health and Statistical Subjects, no. 33. London: HMSO, Appendix 1.

Gross, A.J. and Clark, V.A. (1975). Survival Distributions: Reliability Applications in the Biomedical Sciences. New York: John Wiley & Sons.

Halperin, M. (1952). Maximum likelihood estimation in truncated samples. Ann. Math. Stat 23: 226-238.

Heiss, M.M., Mempel, W., Delanoff, C. et al. (1994). Blood transfusion-modulated tumor recurrence: First results of a randomized study of autologous versus allogeneic blood transfusion in colorectal cancer surgery. J. Clin. Oncol. 12: 1859-1867.

Herbert, V. (1994). Three stakes in hydrazine sulfate's heart, but questionable cancer remedies, like vampires, always rise again (editorial). J. Clin. Oncol. 12: 1107-1108.

Hyman, N.H., Foster, R.S., DeMeules, J.E., Costanza, M.C. (1985). Blood transfusions and survival after lung cancer resection. Am. J. Surg. 149: 502-507.

International Agency for Research on Cancer (IARC) (1974). Evaluation of carcinogenic risk of chemicals to man: Some aromatic amines, hydrazine and related substances, N-nitroso compounds and miscellaneous alkylating agents. Vol. 4. Lyon: IARC.

Kamen, J. (1993). Medical Genocide, Part 26: Hope, Heartbreak, and Horror. Penthouse, April.

Kamen, J. (1994). Stonewalled in the U.S.A. Penthouse, July.

Kalbfleisch, J.D. and Prentice, R.L. (1980). The Statistical Analysis of Failure Time Data. New York: John Wiley & Sons.

Kaplan, E.L., and Meier, P. (1958). Nonparametric estimation from incomplete observations. Am. Stat. Assoc. J. 53: 457-480.

Keller, S.M., Groshen, S., Martini, N., and Kaiser, L.R. (1988). Blood transfusion and lung cancer recurrence. Cancer 62(3): 606-610.

Kleinbaum, D.G. (1996). Survival Analysis: A Self-Learning Text. New York: Springer.

Kosty, M.P., Fleishman, S.B., Herndon II, J.E., et al. (1994). Cisplatin, vinblastine, and hydrazine sulfate in advanced, non-small cell lung cancer: A randomized placebo controlled, double blind phase III study of the Cancer and Leukemia Group B. J. Clin. Oncol. 12: 1113-1120.

Kosty, M.P., Herndon, J.E., Green, M. R., and McIntyre, O. R. (1995). Placebo-controlled randomized study of hydrazine sulfate in lung cancer (letter). J. Clin. Oncol. 13: 1529.

Lad, T., Rubinstein, L., Sadeghi, A. et al. (1988). The benefit of adjuvant treatment for resected locally advanced non-small cell lung cancer. J. Clin. Oncol. 6: 9-17.

Laird, N. (1983). Further comparative analyses of pretest posttest research designs. Amer. Statistician 37: 329-330.

Laird, N. and Ware, J.H. (1982). Random effects models for longitudinal data. Biometrics 38: 963-974.

Liang, K.Y., and Zeger, S.L. (1986). Longitudinal data analysis using generalized linear models. Biometrika 73: 13-22.

Loprinzi, C.L. Kuross, S.A., O'Fallon, J.R., et al. (1994). Randomized placebo controlled evaluation of hydrazine sulfate in patients with advanced colorectal cancer. J. Clin. Oncol. 12: 1121-1125.

Loprinzi, C.L., Goldberg, R.M., Su, J.Q., et al. (1994). Placebo controlled trial of hydrazine sulfate in patients with newly diagnosed non-small cell lung cancer. J. Clin. Oncol. 12: 1126-1129.

Lunn, A.D. and McNeil, D.R. (1991). Computer-Interactive Data Analysis. Chichester: John Wiley & Sons.

Mantel, N., and Haenszel, W. (1959). Statistical aspects of the analysis of data from retrospective studies of disease. JNCI 22: 719-748.

Marubini, E. and Valsecchi, M.G. (1995). Analysing Survival Data from Clinical Trials and Observational Studies. Chichester: John Wiley & Sons.

McLean, R.A., Sanders, W.L., and Stroup, W.W. (1991). A unified approach to mixed linear models. Am. Statistist. 45: 54-64.

Moores, D.W.O., Piantadosi, S., and McKneally, M.F. (1989). Effect of perioperative blood transfusion on outcome in patients with surgically resected lung cancer. Ann. Thorac. Surg. 47: 346-351.

National Cancer Institute (1993). Final Report to the Food and Drug Administration: Hydrazine Sulfate, NSC 150014, IND 33233. Private communication.

Palafox, N., Schatz, I., Lange, R., et al. (1997). Intravenous 20% mannitol versus intravenous 5% dextrose for the treatment of acute ciguatera: A randomized, placebo controlled, double masked trial. JAMA (submitted).

Pena, C.M., Rice, T.W., Ahmad, M., and Medendorp, S.V. (1992). Significance of perioperative blood transfusions in patients undergoing resection of stage I and II non-small cell lung cancers. Chest 102: 84-88.

Peto, J. (1984). The Calculation and Interpretation of Survival Curves. Chapter 21, in M.J. Buyse, M.J. Staquet, and R.J. Sylvester (Eds.), Cancer Clinical Trials, Oxford: Oxford University Press.

Piantadosi, S. (1990). Hazards of Small Clinical Trials (editorial). J. Clin. Oncol. 8(1): 1-3.

Piantadosi, S. (1992). The adverse effect of blood transfusion in lung cancer (editorial). Chest 102: 608.

Resampling Stats, Inc. (1995). Resampling Stats User's Guide. Arlington, Va.: Resampling Stats, Inc.

Royall, R.M. (1986). The effect of sample size on the meaning of significance tests. Am. Statistician 40: 313-315.

Royall, R.M. (1997). Statistical Evidence (A Likelihood Primer). London: Chapman and Hall (in press).

Rubinow, S.I. (1975). Introduction to Mathematical Biology. New York: John Wiley & Sons.

Rusch, V.W., Piantadosi, S. and Holmes, E.C. (1991). The role of extrapleural pneumonectomy in malignant pleural mesothelioma. J. Thoracic. Cardiovasc. Surg. 102: 1-9.

Tartter, P.I., Burrows, L., Kirschner, P. (1984). Perioperative blood transfusion adversely affects prognosis after resection of stage I (subset N0) non-oat cell lung cancer. J. Thorac. Cardvasc. Surg. 88: 659-662.

Taylor, J.M.G., Cumberland, W.G., and Sy, J.P. (1994). A stochastic model for longitudinal AIDS data. J. Am. Statist. Assoc. 89: 727-736.

Valtonen, S., Timonen, U., Toivanen, P., et al. (1997). Interstitial chemotherapy with carmustine-loaded polymers for high grade gliomas: A randomized, double-blind study. Neurosurgery, in press.

Walter, S.D. (1995). Methods of reporting statistical results from medical research studies. Am. J. Epidemiol. 141: 896-906.

Weber, W.W. (1987). The Acetylator Genes and Drug Response. New York: Oxford University Press.

Zeger, S.L., and Liang, K.Y. (1986). Longitudinal data analysis for discrete and continuous outcomes. Biometrics 42: 121-130.

Zeger, S.L., Liang, K.Y., and Albert, P. (1988). Models for longitudinal data: A generalized estimating equation approach. Biometrics 44: 1049-1060.

CHAPTER 13

Prognostic Factor Analyses

13.1 Introduction

Prognostic factor analyses (PFAs) are studies, often based on data that exist for other reasons, that attempt to assess the relative importance of several predictor variables simultaneously. The need to prognosticate is basic to clinical reasoning, but most of us are unable to account quantitatively for the effects of more than one or two variables at a time. Using the formality of a PFA, the additional structure provided by a statistical model, and thoughtful displays of data and effect estimates, one can extend quantitative accounting to many predictor variables. This is often useful when analyzing the data from clinical trials [Armitage, 1981].

The terms "predictor variables", "independent variables", "prognostic factors", and "covariates" are usually used interchangeably to describe the predictors. Prognostic factor analyses are closely related to methods that one might employ when analyzing a clinical trial, especially when adjusting for the effects of covariates on risk. In fact, the treatment effect in a designed experiment is a prognostic factor in every sense of the word. The statistical models employed for PFAs are the same as those used in clinical trials and the interpretation of results is similar. Furthermore, advanced planning is needed to conduct PFAs without making errors. Useful references discussing this subject include Byar [1982; 1984], George [1988], Harris and Albert [1991], Collett [1994], Marubini and Valsecchi [1995], and Parmar and Machin [1995].

PFAs differ from clinical trial analyses is some significant ways. Most importantly, PFAs are usually based on data in which investigators did not control the predictor variables or confounders as in experimental designs. Therefore, the validity of prognostic factor analyses depend on the absence of strong selection bias, on the correctness of the statistical models employed, and on having observed, recorded, and analyzed appropriately the important predictor variables. Accomplishing this requires much stronger assumptions than those needed to estimate valid effects in true experimental designs. Not only are the patients whose data contribute to PFAs often subject to important selection effects, but the reasons why treatments were chosen for them may also relate strongly to their prognosis. In fact, we expect that this will be the case if the physicians are effective in their work. Finally, a prognostic factor analysis does not permit certain control over unobserved confounders that can bias estimates of treatment effects. Similar concerns pertain to these types of analyses when used in epidemiologic studies, where they are also common.

After some preliminaries, I discuss methods for PFAs based on familiar statistical models. The discussion pertains to linear, logistic, parametric survival, and proportional hazards regression models. Finally, I discuss assessing prognostic factors using methods that are not based directly on statistical models.

13.1.1 Studying prognostic factors is broadly useful

A well-conceived study of prognostic factors can yield useful information about either the past, present, or future. PFAs can describe, explain, analyze, or summarize pre-existing data, e.g., those from a data base or comparative clinical trial. When results of PFAs are applied to new patients, they suggest information about the future of the individuals. All of these contexts are clinically useful.

One reason for studying prognostic factors is to learn the relative importance of several variables that affect, or are associated with, disease outcome. This is especially important for diseases that are treated imperfectly such as AIDS, cardiovascular disease, and cancer. A large fraction of patients with these diseases will continue to have problems or even die from them. Therefore, prognostication is important for both the patient and the physician. Examples of clinically useful prognostic factors in these settings are stage (or other extent of disease measures) in cancer and left ventricular function in ischemic heart disease. Predictions based on these factors can be individualized further, using other characteristics of the patient or the disease.

A second reason for studying prognostic factors is to improve the design of clinical trials. For example, suppose we learn that a composite score describing the severity of recurrent respiratory papillomatosis is strongly prognostic. We might stratify on disease severity as a way of improving the balance and comparability of treatment groups in a randomized study comparing treatments in this condition. Other studies may select only high- or low-risk subjects as determined by prognostic factors.

Knowledge of prognostic factors can improve our ability to analyze randomized clinical trials. For example, imbalances in strong prognostic factors in the treatment groups can invalidate simple comparisons. However, analytic methods that adjust for such imbalances can correct this problem. This topic is discussed later in this chapter. The same methods are essential when analyzing non-randomized comparisons.

Interactions between treatment and covariates or between prognostic factors themselves can be detected using the methods of PFAs [Byar, 1985]. Large treatment–covariate interactions are likely to be important, as are those which indicate that treatment is helpful in one subset of patients but harmful in another, so-called "qualitative" interactions. Detecting interactions depends not only on the nature of the covariate effects on outcome but also on the scale of analysis. For example, if covariates truly affect the outcome in a multiplicative fashion with no interactions, as in most non-linear models for survival and other endpoints, interactions are likely

Table 13.1 Hypothetical Effect Estimates Illustrating Interaction Between Two Factors On Different Scales of Measurement

Factor B	Factor A Present	
Present	No	Yes
No	10	20
Yes	30	60(40)

See text for explanation of the table.

to be found if an additive scale of analysis is used. Conversely, if the effect of co-variates is truly additive, interactions are likely to be observed if a multiplicative scale of analysis is used. Thus, interactions depend on the model being employed for analysis.

These effects are illustrated in Table 13.1, which shows hypothetical outcomes in 4 groups defined by 2 dichotomous prognostic factors. In the absence of both factors, the baseline response is 10. If the effect of factor A is to multiply the rate by 2 and the effect of B is to multiply the rate by 3, then a response of 60 in the yes-yes cell demonstrates no interaction. In contrast, if the effect of factor A is to add 10 to the baseline response and the effect of B is to add 20, then a response of 40 in the yes-yes cell demonstrates no interaction. Therefore, in either case there will be interaction on *some* scale of measurement, illustrating that interaction is model dependent.

Prognostic factors are also useful in assessing clinical landmarks during the course of an illness and deciding if changes in treatment strategy are warranted. This could be useful, for example, when monitoring the time course of CD4+ lymphocyte count in HIV positive patients. When the count drops below some threshold, a change in treatment may be indicated. A threshold such as this could be determined by an appropriate PFA.

13.1.2 Prognostic factors can be constant or time-varying

The numerical properties of prognostic factor measurements are the same as those for study endpoints discussed in Chapter 6. That is, prognostic factors can be continuous measures, ordinal, binary, or categorical. Most often, prognostic factors are recorded at study entry or "time 0" with respect to follow-up time and remain constant. These are termed "baseline" factors. The measured value of a baseline factor, such as sex or treatment assigned, does not change over time. Usually, when studying the effects of baseline factors, we assume that differences attributable to them happen instantaneously and remain constant over time.

Some prognostic factors may change their value over time, as discussed in Chapter 12. They would be assessed both at baseline and at several points following treatment as longitudinal measurements. For example, prostatic specific antigen (PSA) is a reliable indicator of disease recurrence in patients with prostate cancer. The PSA level may decrease to near zero in patients with completely treated prostate cancer, and the chance of detecting future cancer recurrence or risk of death may depend on recent PSA levels. Prognostic factors that change value over time are termed "time dependent covariates" (TDC) and special methods are needed to account for their effects on most outcomes.

There are two types of TDCs: intrinsic or internal, and extrinsic or external. Intrinsic covariates are those measured in the study subject, such as the PSA example above. Extrinsic TDCs are those that exist independently of the study subject. For example, we might be interested in the risk of developing cancer as a function of environmental levels of toxins. These levels may affect the patient's risk but exist independently. Both types of TDCs can be incorporated in prognostic factor models with appropriate modifications in the model equations and estimation procedures.

13.2 Model-Based Methods

One of the most powerful and flexible tools for assessing the effects of more than one prognostic factor simultaneously is a statistical model. These models describe a plausible mathematical relationship between the predictors and the observed endpoint in terms of one or more model parameters which have handy clinical interpretations. To proceed with this approach, the investigator must be knowledgeable about the subject matter and interpretation and: 1) collect and verify complete data, 2) consult an experienced statistical expert to guide the analysis, and 3) make a plan for dealing with decision points during the analysis.

Survival or time-to-event data constitute an important subset of prognostic factor information associated with clinical trials. Because of the frequency with which such data are encountered, statistical methods for analyzing them have been highly developed. Sources for the statistical theory dealing with these types of data are Lee [1992], Cox and Oakes [1984], and Kalbfleisch and Prentice [1980]. Recently, a new journal, *Lifetime Data Analysis*, has appeared as an international journal devoted to statistical methods for time-to-event data.

13.2.1 Models combine theory and data

A model is any construct which combines theoretical knowledge (hypothesis) with empirical knowledge (observation). In mathematical models, the theoretical component is represented by one or more *equations,* which relate the measured or observed quantities. Empirical knowledge is represented by *data,* that is, the measured quantities from a sample of individuals or experimental units. The behavior of a model is governed by its structure or functional form and unknown quantities or constants of nature called "parameters". One goal of the modeling process might be to estimate, or gain quantitative insight, into the parameters. Another goal might be to see if the data are consistent with the theoretical form of the model. Yet another goal might be to summarize large amounts of data efficiently, in which case the model need not be precise.

Statistical models generally have additional characteristics. First, the equations represent convenient biological constructs but are usually not fashioned to be literally true as in some biological or physical models. Second, statistical models often explicitly incorporate an error structure or a method to cope with the random variability which is always present in the data. Third, the primary purpose of statistical models is often to facilitate estimating the parameters so that relatively simple mathematical forms are most appropriate. Even so, the models employed do more than simply smooth data [Appleton, 1995]. A broad survey of statistical models is given by Dobson [1983].

If it has been constructed so that the parameters correspond to clinically interpretable effects, the model can be a way of estimating the influence of several factors simultaneously on the outcome. In practice, statistical models usually provide a concise way for estimating parameters, obtaining confidence intervals on parameter estimates, testing hypotheses, choosing from among competing models, or revising the model itself. Models with these characteristics include linear, generalized linear, logistic, and proportional hazards models. These are widely used in clinical trials and prognostic factor analyses and are discussed in more detail below.

13.2.2 The scale of measurements (coding) may be important

The first step in a PFA is to code the measurements (variable values) in a numerically appropriate way. All statistical models can be formulated by the numerical coding of variables. Even qualitative variables can be represented by the proper choice of numerical coding. There are no truly qualitative statistical models or qualitative variable effects. For this reason, the coding and scale of measurement which seems most natural clinically may not be the best one to use in a model. If an ordinal variable with three levels is coded 1, 2, 3 as compared with 10, 11, 12, the results of model fitting might be different. If a coding of 1, 10, 100 were used, almost certainly the results will be different. This effect can often be used purposefully to transform variables in ways that are clinically sensible and statistically advantageous.

Simple summary statistics should always be inspected for prognostic factor variables. These may reveal that some factors have highly skewed or irregular distributions, for which a transformation could be useful. Predictor variables do not have to have "normal", or even symmetric, distributions. Categorical factors may have some levels with very few observations. Whenever possible, these should be combined so that subsets are not too small.

Ordinal and qualitative variables often need to be re-coded as binary "indicator" or dummy variables that facilitate group comparisons. A variable with N levels requires $N-1$ binary dummy variables to compare levels in a regression model. Each dummy variable implies a comparison between a specific level and the reference level (which is omitted from the model). For example, a factor with three levels A, B, and C, would require two dummy variables. One possible coding is for the first variable to have the value 1 for level A and 0 otherwise. The second could have 1 for level B and 0 otherwise. Including both factors in a model compares A and B versus the reference group C. In contrast, if a single variable were coded 1 for level A, 2 for level B, and 3 for level C, for example, then including it in a regression would model a linear trend across the levels. This would imply that the A-B difference was

Table 13.2 Dummy Variables for a Four Level Factor with the Last Level Taken as a Reference

Factor	Dummy Variables		
Level	$x1$	$x2$	$x3$
A	1	0	0
B	0	1	0
C	0	0	1
D	0	0	0

the same as the B-C difference, which might or might not be appropriate. A set of three dummy variables for a factor with four levels is shown in Table 13.2.

13.2.3 Use flexible covariate models

The appropriate statistical models to employ in PFAs are dictated by the specific type of data and biological questions. Some models widely used in oncology (and elsewhere) are discussed by Simon [1984]. Regardless of the endpoint and structure of the model, the mathematical form will always contain one or more sub-models, which describe the effects of multiple covariates on either the outcome or a simple function of it. For example, most relative risk regression models used in failure time data and epidemiologic applications use a multiplicative form for the effects of covariates on a measure of relative risk. In the case of the proportional hazards regression model, the logarithm of the hazard ratio is assumed to be a constant related to a linear combination of the predictor variables. The hazard rate, $\lambda_i(t)$, in those with covariate vector $\mathbf{x}_i$ satisfies

$$\log\left\{\frac{\lambda_i(t)}{\lambda_0(t)}\right\} = \sum_{j=1}^{k} \beta_j \mathbf{x}_{ij} \ .$$

Because the covariates are additive on a logarithmic scale, the effects multiply the baseline hazard.

Similarly, the widely used logistic regression model is

$$\log\left\{\frac{p_i}{1 - p_i}\right\} = \beta_0 + \sum_{j=1}^{k} \beta_j \mathbf{x}_{ij} \ ,$$

where p_i is the probability of "success", $\mathbf{x}_{ij}$ is the value of the jth covariate in the ith patient or group, and β_j is the log-odds ratio for the jth covariate. This model contains and intercept term, β_0, unlike the proportional hazards model where the baseline hazard function, $\lambda_0(t)$, is arbitrary. In both cases, a linear combination of covariates multiplies the baseline risk.

Generalized linear models (GLMs) [Nelder and Wedderburn, 1972; McCullagh and Nelder, 1989] are powerful tools, which can be used to describe the effects of covariates on a variety of outcome data from the general exponential family of distributions. GLMs have the form

$$\eta_i = \beta_0 + \sum_{j=1}^{k} \beta_j \mathbf{x}_{ij}$$

$$E\{y_i\} = g(\eta_i),$$

where $g(\cdot)$ is a simple "link function" relating the outcome, y, to the linear combination of predictors. Powerful and general statistical theory facilitates parameter estimation in this class of models, which includes one-way analyses of variance, multiple linear regression models, log-linear models, logit and probit models, and others. For a comprehensive review, see McCullagh and Nelder [1989].

For both common relative risk models and GLMs, the covariate sub-model is a linear one. This form is primarily a mathematical convenience and yields models whose parameters are simple to interpret. However, more complex covariate models can be constructed in special cases such as additive models and those with random effects.

Models with random effects

All statistical models contain an explicit error term, which represents a quantity which is random, perhaps due to the effects of measurement error. Almost always, the random error is assumed to have mean zero and a variability that can estimated from the data. Most other effects (parameters) in statistical models are assumed to be "fixed", which means that they estimate quantities that are fixed or constant for all subjects. In some circumstances, we need to model effects which, like the error term, are random, but are attributable to sources other than random error. Random effects terms are a way to accomplish this and are used frequently in linear models. For a recent discussion of this topic in the context of longitudinal data, see Rutter and Elashoff [1994].

An example of a circumstance where a random effect might be necessary is a clinical trial with a large number of treatment centers and a patient population at each center that is somewhat different from one another. In some sense, the study centers can be thought of as a random sample of all possible centers. The treatment effect may be partly a function of study center, i.e., there may be clinically important treatment by center interactions. The effect of study center on the trial outcome variable might best be modeled as a random effect. A fixed-effect model would require a separate parameter to describe each study center.

13.2.4 Building parsimonious models is the next step

Quantitative prognostic factor assessment can be thought of as the process of constructing parsimonious statistical models. These models are most useful when 1) they contain a few clinically relevant and interpretable predictors, 2) the parameters or coefficients are estimated with a reasonably high degree of precision, 3) the predictive factors each carry independent information about prognosis, and 4) the model is consistent with other clinical and biological data. Constructing models that meet these criteria is usually not a simple or automatic process. We can use information in the data themselves (data-based variable selection), clinical knowledge (clinically based variable selection), or both. A useful tutorial on this subject is given by Harrell, Lee, and Mark [1996].

Don't use automated procedures

Using modern computing technology and algorithms, it is possible to automate portions of the model building process. This practice can be dangerous for several reasons. First, the criteria on which most automated algorithms select or eliminate variables for inclusion in the model may not be appropriate. For example, this is often done on the basis of significance levels (p-values) only. Second, the statistical properties of performing a large number of such tests and re-fitting models are poor when the objective is to arrive at a valid set of predictors. The process will be sensitive to noise or chance associations in the data. Third, an automated procedure does not provide a way to incorporate information from outside the model building mechanics. This information may be absolutely critical for finding a statistically correct and clinically interpretable final model. Fourth, we usually want more sophisticated control over the consequences of missing data values (an inevitable complication) than that afforded by automated procedures.

There are ways of correcting the deficiencies just noted. All of them require thoughtful input into the model building process from clinical investigators and interaction with a biostatistician who is familiar with the strengths and pitfalls. One statistical approach to prevent being misled by random associations in the data is to pre-screen prognostic factors based on clinical criteria. Many times prognostic factors are simply convenient to use rather than having been collected because of *a priori* interest or biological plausibility. Such factors should probably be discarded from further consideration.

An example of the potential difficulty with automated variable selection procedures is provided by the data in Table 13.3. The complete data and computer program to analyze them are given in Chapter 19. The data consist of 80 observed event times and censoring indicators. For each study subject, 25 dichotomous predictor variables have been measured. These data are similar to those available from many exploratory studies.

The first approach to building a multiple regression model employed a step-up selection procedure. Variables were entered into the regression model if the significance level for association with the failure time was less than 0.05. This process found X_1 and X_{12} to be significantly associated with the failure time.

A second model building approach used step-down selection, retaining variables in the regression only if the p-value was less than 0.05. At its conclusion, this method found X_3, X_{10}, X_{11}, X_{14}, X_{15}, X_{16}, X_{18}, X_{20}, X_{21}, and X_{23} to be significantly associated with the failure time (Table 13.4). It may be somewhat alarming to those unfamiliar with these procedures that the results of the two model building techniques do not overlap. The results of the step-down procedure suggest that the retention criterion could be strengthened. Using step-down variable selection and a p-value of 0.025 to stay in the model, *no* variables were found to be significant. This seems even more unlikely than the fact that nine variables appeared important after the step-down procedure.

Table 13.3 Simulated Outcome and Predictor Variable Data from a Prognostic Factor Analysis

#	Dead	Time	$X_1 - X_{25}$
1	1	7.38	1111111001110100010100101
2	1	27.56	1001100111001011001001110
3	1	1.67	1000110000111000011010010
4	1	1.82	1101001111011101100101101
5	0	10.49	0001110011110011111100101
6	1	14.96	1011111011000100101001011
7	1	0.63	0111001011101000010001111
8	1	10.84	1001010111111011110100101
9	1	15.65	1110010000001001110001100
10	1	4.73	0100100000011100101100000
11	1	14.97	0010111110010111110000010
12	1	3.47	0010111110011000000000000
13	1	4.29	1100110000101100010000001
14	1	0.11	1111110110111101000011000
15	1	13.35	0010101010110011010010011
⋮	⋮	⋮	⋮

These results are typical and should serve as a warning as to the volatility of results when automated procedures, particularly those based on significance levels, are used to build models without the benefit of biological knowledge. A second lesson from this example extends from the fact that the data were simulated such that all predictor variables were both independent from one another and independent from the failure time. Thus, all "statistically significant" associations in Table 13.4 are due purely to chance. Furthermore, the apparent joint or multivariable association, especially the second regression, disappears when a single variable is removed from the regression.

Resolve missing data

There are two alternatives for coping with missing covariate values. One could disregard prognostic factors with missing values. This may be the best strategy if the proportion of unknowns is very high. Alternatively, one can remove the individuals with missing covariates from the analysis. This may be appropriate for individuals who have missing values for a large fraction of the important covariates. Usually statistical packages have no way to cope with records that contain missing values for the variable being analyzed, other than to discard them.

Usually we do not have the luxury of analyzing perfectly complete data. Nearly all patients may have some missing measurements so that the number of records with complete observations is a small fraction of the total. If data are missing at random, i.e., the loss of information is not associated with outcomes or other covariates, it is

Table 13.4 Multiple Regressions Using Automated Variable Selection Methods Applied to the Data from Table 13.3

Model	Variables	Parameter Estimate	Standard Error	Wald χ^2	Pr $> \chi^2$	Risk Ratio
1	X_1	0.479	0.238	4.07	0.04	1.615
	X_{12}	−0.551	0.238	5.35	0.02	0.576
2	X_3	0.573	0.257	4.96	0.03	1.773
	X_{10}	−0.743	0.271	7.53	0.006	0.476
	X_{11}	0.777	0.274	8.06	0.005	2.175
	X_{14}	−0.697	0.276	6.38	0.01	0.498
	X_{15}	−0.611	0.272	5.06	0.02	0.543
	X_{16}	−0.670	0.261	6.57	0.01	0.512
	X_{18}	−0.767	0.290	7.01	0.008	0.465
	X_{20}	−0.610	0.262	5.42	0.02	0.544
	X_{21}	0.699	0.278	6.30	0.01	2.012
	X_{23}	0.650	0.261	6.20	0.01	1.916

best to disregard individuals with the missing variable. Loss of precision is the only consequence of this approach and we can still investigate the covariate of interest.

If missing data are more likely in individuals with certain outcomes (or certain values of other covariates), there may be no approach for coping with the loss of information that avoids bias. Removing individuals with missing data from the analysis in such a circumstance systematically discards certain influences on the outcome. For example, if individuals with the most severe disease are more likely to be missing outcome data, the aggregate effect of severity on outcome will be lessened. When we have no choice but to lose some information, decisions about how to cope with missing data need to be guided by clinical considerations rather than automated statistical procedures alone.

There is a third method of coping with missing values that can be useful. It is called *imputation*, or replacing missing data with values calculated in a way that allows other analyses to proceed essentially unaffected. This can be a reasonable alternative when relatively few data are missing, precisely the circumstance in which other alternatives are also workable. For example, missing values could be "predicted" from all the remaining data and replaced by estimates that preserve the overall covariance structure of the data. The effect of such procedures on the inferences that result must be studied on a case-by-case basis.

Screen factors for importance in univariable regressions

The next practical step in assessing prognostic factors is to screen all the retained variables in univariable regressions (or other analyses). It is important to examine the estimates of clinical effect (e.g., relative hazards), confidence intervals, and significance levels. Together with biological knowledge, these can be used to select a subset of factors to study in multivariable models. The most difficult conceptual part of this process is deciding which factors to discard as unimportant. The basis of this decision is threefold: prior clinical information (usually qualitative), the size of the estimated effect, and the statistical significance level. Strong factors, or those known to be important biologically should be retained for further consideration, regardless of significance levels.

The findings at this stage can help investigators check the overall validity of the data. For example, certain factors are known to be strongly prognostic in similar groups of patients. Investigators should examine the direction and magnitude of prognostic factor effects. If the estimates deviate from those previously observed or known, the data may contain important errors.

It is appropriate to use a relaxed definition of "significance" at this screening stage. For example, one could use $\alpha = 0.15$ to minimize the chance of discarding an important prognostic factor. This screening step usually reduces the number of factors to about $1/4$ of those started. The potential error in this process is the tendency to keep variables that are associated with the outcome purely by chance and/or that the modeling procedure may overestimate the effect of some factors on the outcome. The only way to prevent or minimize these mistakes this is to use clinical knowledge to augment the screening process.

Build multiple regressions

The next practical step in a PFA is to build a series of multivariable regression models and study their relative performance. To decrease the chance of missing important associations in the data, one should try more models rather than fewer. Consequently, step-down model building procedures may be better than step-up methods. Using step-down, all prognostic factors that pass the screening are included in a single multiple regression. The model is likely to be over-parameterized at the outset, in which case one or more factors will have to be removed to allow the estimation process to converge.

Following model fitting, we use the same evaluation methods outlined above to include or discard prognostic factors in the regression. After each change or removal of variables, the parameters and significance levels are re-estimated. The process stops when the model makes the most biological sense. It is satisfying when this point also corresponds to a local or global statistical optimum, e.g., when the parameter estimates are fairly precise and the significance levels are high.

Usually step-down variable selection methods will cause us to try more models than other approaches. In fact, there may be partially (or non-) overlapping sets of predictors that perform nearly as well as each other using model fitting evaluations. This is most likely a consequence of correlations between the predictor variables. Coping with severe manifestations of this problem is discussed below.

Some automated approaches can fit all possible subset regressions. For example, they produce all 1-variable regressions, all 2-variable ones, etc. The number of such regressions is large. For r predictor variables, the total number of models possible without interaction terms is

$$N = \sum_{k=1}^{r} \binom{r}{k}.$$

For 10 predictor variables, $N = 1023$. Even if all of these models can be fitted and summarized, the details may be important for distinguishing between them. Thus, there is usually no substitute for guidance by clinical knowledge.

Correlated predictors may be a problem

Correlations among predictor variables can present difficulties during the model building and interpretation process. Sometimes the correlations among predictor variables are strong enough to interfere with the statistical estimation process, in the same way that occurs with familiar linear regression models. Although models such as logistic and proportional hazards regressions are nonlinear, the parameter estimates are most often obtained by a process of iterated solution through linearization of estimating equations. Furthermore, covariates often form a linear combination in statistical models, as discussed above. Therefore, collinearity of predictors can be a problem in nonlinear models also.

Even when the estimation process goes well, correlated variables can create difficulties in model building and interpretation. Among a set of correlated predictors, any one will appear to improve the model prediction, but if more than one is included, all of them may appear unimportant. To diagnose and correct this situation, a number of models will have to be fitted and one of several seemingly "good" models selected as "best".

Clinicians are sometimes disturbed by the fact that statistical procedures are not guaranteed to produce one regression model that is clearly superior to all others. In fact, even defining this model on statistical grounds can be difficult, because of the large number of regressions which one would have to examine in typical circumstances. In any case, we should not be surprised that several models fit the data and explain it well, especially when different variables carry partially redundant information. Models cannot always be distinguished on the basis of statistical evidence because of our inability to compare non-nested models formally and the inadequacies of summary statistics like significance levels for variable selection. Nested models are those which are special cases of more complex ones. Nested models can often be compared with parent models using statistical tests such as the likelihood ratio (see Chapter 10).

The only reasonable way for the methodologist to solve these difficulties is to work with clinicians who have expert knowledge of the predictor variables, based on either other studies or preclinical data. Their opinion, when guided by statistical evidence, is necessary for building a good model. Even when a particular set of predictors appears to offer slight statistical improvement in fit over another, one should generally prefer the set with the most clear clinical interpretation. Of course, if the statistical evidence concerning a particular predictor or set of predictors is very strong, then these models should be preferred or studied very carefully to understand the mechanisms, which may lead to new biological findings.

13.2.5 Incompletely specified models may yield biased estimates

When working with linear models, it is well-known that omission of important predictor variables will not bias the estimated coefficients of the variables included in the model. For example, if Y is a response linearly related to a set of predictors, $\mathbf{X}$, so that

$$E\{Y\} = \beta_0 + \beta_1 X_1 + \beta_2 X_2 + \cdots + \beta_n X_n$$

is the true model and we fit an incompletely specified model, for example,

$$Y = \beta_0 + \beta_1 X_1 + \beta_2 X_2 + \beta_3 X_3 + \epsilon,$$

the estimates of β_1, β_2, and β_3 will be unbiased. The effect of incomplete specification is to increase the variances but not to bias the estimates [Draper and Smith, 1981].

In contrast, when using certain nonlinear models, the proportional hazards model among them, omission of an important covariate will bias the estimated coefficients, even if the omitted covariate is perfectly balanced across levels of those remaining in the model [Gail et al., 1984]. The same can be said for model-derived estimates of the variances of the coefficients [Gail et al., 1988]. The magnitude of the bias which results from these incompletely specified nonlinear models is proportional to the strength of the omitted covariate. For example, suppose we conduct a clinical trial to estimate the hazard ratio for survival between two treatments for coronary artery disease and that age is an influential predictor of the risk of death. Even if young and old patients are *perfectly* balanced in the treatment groups, failure to include age in a proportional hazards regression when using it to estimate the hazard ratio will yield a biased estimate of the treatment effect.

Although the existence of this bias is important for theoretical reasons, for situations commonly encountered in analyzing RCTs, there is not a serious consequence when important covariates are omitted, as they invariably are [Chastang et al., 1988]. The lesson to learn from this situation is that models are important and powerful conveniences for summarizing data, but they are subject to assumptions and limitations that prevent us from blindly accepting the parameters or significance tests they yield. Even so, they offer many advantages that usually outweigh their limitations.

13.2.6 Study second-order effects (interactions)

One advantage to using models to perform PFAs is the ability to assess interactions. For example, if response depends on both age and sex, it is possible that the sex effect is different in young, compared with old, individuals. In a linear model, an interaction could be described by the model

$$Y = \beta_0 + \beta_1 X_1 + \beta_2 X_2 + \gamma X_1 X_2 + \epsilon,$$

where γ represents the strength of the interaction between X_1 and X_2. Interactions of biological importance are relatively uncommon. Some interactions that seem to be important can be eliminated by variable transformations or different scales of analysis. However, large interactions may be important and regression models provide a convenient way to assess them.

One difficulty with using models to survey interactions is the large number of comparisons that have to be performed to evaluate all possible effects. If the model supports 6 prognostic factors, there are $6 + \binom{6}{2} = 21$ pair-wise interactions possible (each variable can interact with itself). Even if all estimated interaction effects are due only to chance, we might expect one of these to be "significant" using p-values as test criteria. The number of higher-order interactions possible is much larger. Usually we would not screen for interactions unless there is an *a priori* reason to do so or if the model does not fit the data well. Even then, we should employ more strict criteria for declaring an interaction statistically significant than for main effects to reduce type I errors.

It is important to include the main effects, or low-order terms, in the model when estimating interaction effects. Otherwise, we may mis-estimate the coefficients and wrongly conclude that the high-order effect is significant when it is not. This can be illustrated by a very simple example. Suppose we have the data shown in Figure 13.1 and the two models

$$E\{Y\} = \beta_0 + \beta_1 X_1$$

and

$$E\{Y\} = \beta_1^* X_1.$$

The first model has both a low-order effect (intercept) and a high-order effect (β_1). The second model has only the high-order effect β_1^*, i.e., the intercept is assumed to be zero. When fit to the data, the models yield $\beta_1 \approx 0$ and $\beta_1^* \neq 0$. In the first case, we obtain a correct estimate of the slope (Figure 13.1, dotted line). In the second case, we obtain an incorrect estimate of the slope because we have wrongly assumed that the intercept is zero (Figure 13.1, solid line). An analogous problem can occur when interaction effects are estimated assuming the main effects are zero (i.e., omitting them from the model).

13.2.7 PFAs can help describe risk groups

Information from a PFA can help clinicians anticipate the future course of a patient's illness as a function of several (possibly correlated) predictors. This type of prognostication is often done informally on purely clinical grounds, most often using a few categorical factors such as functional classifications or anatomical extent of disease. Stage of disease is a good example of a measure of extent from the field of cancer. Prognostication based only on simple clinical parameters can be sharpened considerably by using quantitative model-based methods.

Suppose we have measured two factors, X and Y, which are either present or absent in each patient and relate strongly to outcome. Patients could be classified into one of the following four cells: X alone, Y alone, both, or neither. It is possible that the prognoses of individuals in each of the four cells are quite different and that knowing into which "risk group" a patient is categorized would convey useful

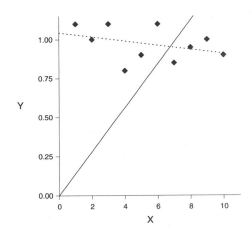

Figure 13.1 Hypothetical data for regression analyses with and without low-order effects.

information about his or her future. On the other hand, it might be that cells X and Y are similar, e.g., each representing the presence of a single risk factor, so that there are effectively only three risk levels. The three levels of risk would be characterized by one risk factor, two risk factors, or none.

When there are several prognostic factors, some of them possibly measured on a continuous scale rather than being dichotomous or categorical, these ideas can be extended using the types of models discussed above. Rather than simply *counting* the number of factors, the actual variable *values* can be combined in a weighted sum to calculate risk. The resulting values can then be ranked and categorized. The best way to illustrate the general procedure is with an actual example, discussed in detail in the next section.

Example

In patients with HIV infection, it is useful to have simple methods by which individual risk of clinical AIDS or death can be inferred. Many clinical parameters are known to carry prognostic information about time to AIDS and survival, including platelet count, hemoglobin, and symptoms [Graham et al., 1994]. Here I illustrate a risk set classification that is a combination of clinical and laboratory values for HIV positive patients from the Multi-Center AIDS Cohort Study (MACS) [Piantadosi, 1994]. The MACS is a prospective study of the natural history of HIV infection among homosexual and bisexual men in the United States. Details of the MACS study design and methods are described elsewhere [Kaslow et al., 1987].

From April 1984 through March 1985, 4954 men were enrolled in four metropolitan areas: Baltimore/Washington, DC, Chicago, Pittsburgh, and Los Angeles. There are 1809 HIV seropositive and 418 seroconverters in the MACS cohort. This risk set

analysis includes all HIV-1 seroprevalent men and seroconverters who used zidovudine prior to developing AIDS, and who had CD4+ lymphocyte data at study visits
immediately before and after the first reported use of zidovudine. The total number
of individuals meeting these criteria was 747.

Prognostic factors measured at baseline included age, CD4+ lymphocyte count,
CD8+ lymphocyte count, hemoglobin, platelets, clinical symptoms and signs, and
white blood cell count. The clinical symptoms and signs of interests were fever
(greater than 37.9 degrees C) for more than two weeks, oral candidiasis, diarrhea
for more than four weeks, weight loss of 4.5 kg, oral hairy leukoplakia, and herpes
zoster. There were 216 AIDS cases among individuals treated with zidovudine prior
to the cutoff date for this analysis and 165 deaths.

The initial step was to build to a multiple regression model for prediction of time
to AIDS or time to death using the proportional hazards regression model. After
model building, the log relative risk for each individual patient was calculated according to the equation

$$r_i = \sum_{j=1}^{p} \widehat{\beta}_j X_{ij} \, , \qquad (13.1)$$

where r_i is the aggregate relative risk for the ith patient, $\widehat{\beta}_j$ is the estimated coefficient for the jth covariate from the regression model, and X_{ij} is the value of the jth
covariate in the ith patient. Data values were then ordered from smallest to largest,
based on the value of r_i. Following this ordering based on aggregate estimated relative risk, individuals were grouped or categorized into discrete risk sets. The cut
points used for categorization and the number of groups were chosen empirically.
That is, they were chosen so that the groups formed would display the full range of
prognoses in the cohort. Usually this can be accomplished with three to five risk
groups.

Following the formation of risk groups, survival curves were drawn for individuals in each group. Finally, predicted survival curves were generated from the proportional hazards model and drawn superimposed on the observed curves as an informal
test of goodness of fit. The predicted survival curves in the risk groups cannot be
obtained directly from the original covariate regression. Instead, a second regression must be fit using a single covariate representing risk group. Because the risk
group classification is based only on covariates from the first regression, the second
regression a valid illustration of model performance based on the original predictors.

The units for expressing covariate values are shown in Table 13.5. The scale of
measurement is important because it directly affects the interpretation of risk ratio
estimates. For example, symptoms were coded as present or absent. Consequently,
the risk ratio for symptoms is interpreted as the increase in risk associated with any
symptoms. In contrast, change in CD4+ lymphocyte count was measured in units of
100 cells, so that its relative risk is per 100 cell increase.

For the time to AIDS endpoint, the final regression model shows significant effects for CD4 count, platelets, hemoglobin and symptoms (Table 13.6). When risk set
assignments are based on this model the resulting time to event curves are shown in
Figure 13.2. For time to AIDS, the first risk set was formed from individuals with the

Table 13.5 Coding of Covariate Values for AIDS Prognostic Factor Analysis

Variable Name	Measurement Units
CD4 Number	100 cells
CD8 Number	100 cells
Neopterin	mg/dl
Microglobulin	mg/dl
Platelets	25,000 cells
Hemoglobin	gm/dl
Symptoms	1 = yes, 0 = no

lowest risk of AIDS. This group constitutes 35% of the population. For the last risk set, the 15% with the highest risk was chosen. These individuals developed AIDS very rapidly, virtually all within the first 1.5 years after beginning zidovudine. The remaining risk sets were each formed from 25% fractions of the population. They indicate levels of risk intermediate between the most favorable and least favorable subsets. For the baseline variables model, equation 13.1 becomes

$$r_i = -0.373 \times CD4 + 0.020 \times CD8 - 0.071 \times Platelets \quad (13.2)$$
$$-0.168 \times Hemoglobin + 0.295 \times Symptoms.$$

The cut points used for these risk sets were: low risk, $r_i < -4.25$; low-intermediate risk, $-4.25 \leq r_i < -3.70$; high-intermediate risk, $-3.70 \leq r_i < -3.13$; and high risk, $r_i \geq -3.13$.

Regression models for survival time are shown in Table 13.7. For this endpoint, the proportions of individuals assigned to each risk set are slightly different than for time to AIDS (Figure 13.3). This was done to separate the highest and lowest risk subsets as much as possible. The first risk set for the baseline variables model was formed from the 30% of individuals with the lowest risk of death. For the last risk set, the 15% with the highest risk was chosen. These individuals had the poorest survival, living generally less than 1.5 years after beginning AZT. The remaining risk sets were each formed from 30% and 25% fractions of the population. They indicate levels of risk intermediate between the most favorable and least favorable subsets. For the baseline variables model, equation 13.1 becomes

$$r_i = -0.440 \times CD4 + 0.034 \times CD8 - 0.070 \times Platelets \quad (13.3)$$
$$-0.182 \times Hemoglobin + 0.030 \times Symptoms.$$

The cut points used for the risk sets were: low risk, $r_i < -4.73$; low-intermediate risk, $-4.73 \leq r_i \leq -3.95$; high-intermediate risk, $-3.95 < r_i \leq -3.29$; and high risk, $r_i > -3.29$.

The utility of these results lies in our ability to classify individuals into one of the risk groups on the basis of covariate values. This is fairly easily accomplished using the calculation defined by the linear combination in equation 13.2 or 13.3. A particular risk set is *heterogeneous* with respect to individual covariate values, but

Table 13.6 Proportional Hazards Multiple Regressions for Timeto AIDS

Variable	Relative Risk	95% CI	P-Value
CD4	0.69	0.63 – 0.75	0.0001
CD8	1.02	1.00 – 1.04	0.04
Platelets	0.93	0.89 – 0.97	0.0009
Hemoglobin	0.85	0.78 – 0.92	0.0001
Symptoms	1.34	1.08 – 1.67	0.008

homogeneous with respect to risk. Therefore, the character of a risk set does not have a simple interpretation in terms of covariates, but it does have a simple clinical interpretation, i.e., increased or decreased risk.

13.2.8 Power and sample size for PFAs

Sometimes we can conduct PFAs on a surplus of data and would like to know how few observations can be used to meet our objectives. Other times, we wish to know in advance how large a covariate effect must be to yield statistical significance. Both of these questions can be addressed by methods for determining power and sample size in PFAs. Calculating power for PFAs is difficult in general, but a few guidelines can be given.

Suppose we are studying a single binary predictor, denoted by X, in a time-to-event analysis analogous to the effect of treatment in a planned trial. The distribution of $X = 0$ and $X = 1$ in the study population will not be equal as it might have been if it actually represented an assignment to a randomized treatment group. Instead, X is probably going to be unbalanced. Furthermore, we are likely to be interested in the effect of X adjusted for other variables in the regression.

Under these assumptions, a sample size formula such as equation 7.21 might be used to determine the approximate number of observations needed in a proportional hazards regression model. To detect an adjusted hazard ratio of $\Delta = 1.5$ attributable to a binary covariate with 20% of the population having $X = 1$, with 90% power and using a type I error of 5%, we calculate

$$D = \frac{(r+1)^2}{r} \frac{(Z_\alpha + Z_\beta)^2}{[\log(\Delta)]^2} = \frac{(4+1)^2}{4} \frac{(1.96 + 1.282)^2}{[\log(1.5)]^2} = 240.$$

Therefore, we have a reasonable chance of detecting an adjusted risk ratio of 1.5 in a PFA using 240 subjects where 20% of them have $X = 1$ and 80% have $X = 0$. More precise methods for performing these types of calculations are available [Statistics and Epidemiology Research Co., 1993]. However, the general method is complex and not likely to be used frequently by clinical trial investigators. Consequently, it is not be discussed in detail here.

In any case, prognostic factor analyses most often utilize all of the data that bear on a particular question or analysis. Missing variables (incomplete records), interest in subsets, and highly asymmetric distributions of variable values tend to limit

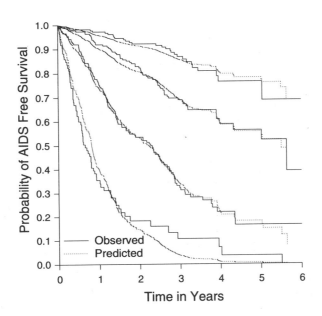

Figure 13.2 Observed and predicted AIDS-free survival of risk sets in the MACS cohort.

precision even when there appears to be a large database on which to perform analyses. For survival and time-to-event outcomes, the number of events is frequently the most restrictive characteristic of the data.

13.3 Adjusted Analyses of Comparative Trials

Covariates are also important purveyors of ancillary information in designed clinical trials. They facilitate validating the randomization, allow improved prognostication, can generate or test new hypotheses because of their associations with each other and with outcome, and may be used to improve (reduce the variance of) estimates of treatment effect. The possibility that estimates of treatment effect can be influenced or invalidated by covariate imbalance is one of the main reasons for studying the results of adjusted analyses.

Not all clinical trial statisticians agree on the need for adjusted analyses in comparative clinical trials. From a theoretical perspective, randomization and proper analysis guarantees unbiasedness and the correctness of type I error levels, even in the presence of chance imbalances in prognostic factors. However, randomized treat-

Table 13.7 Proportional Hazards Multiple Regressions for Timeto Death.

Variable	Relative Risk	95% CI	P-Value
CD4	0.64	0.59 – 0.71	0.0001
CD8	1.03	1.01 – 1.06	0.0009
Platelets	0.93	0.89 – 0.98	0.003
Hemoglobin	0.83	0.76 – 0.91	0.0001
Symptoms	1.35	1.08 – 1.69	0.01

ment assignment is not a guarantee that variability has not influenced the results of a particular study. The difference is the distinction between the *expectation* of a random process and its *realization* in a particular case. In some cases, adjustment can increase the precision of estimated treatment effects or control for the effects of unbalanced prognostic factors. The difference in estimated treatment effects before and after covariate adjustment often conveys useful biological information. Thus, although not strictly necessary for valid tests of the treatment effect, adjusted analyses may facilitate other goals of randomized clinical trials.

Suppose the analyst thought that the data from an RCT arose from an observational study rather than from an experimental design. The analysis would likely proceed much as it was sketched above for PFAs. Other investigators, knowing the true origins of the data, might not perform covariate adjustment. The conclusions of the two analyses could be different. Although we would prefer the analysis that most closely follows the paradigm of the study, it is not guaranteed to yield the best or most efficient estimate of the treatment effect. Thus, it seems we have little choice but to explore the consequences of covariate adjustment and emphasize the results that are most consistent with other knowledge.

13.3.1 What should we adjust for?

There are two sources of information to help in deciding which covariates should be used for adjusted analyses: the data and biological knowledge from outside the trial. An excellent discussion of using the observed data to decide which covariates should be studied in adjusted analyses is given by Beach and Meier [1989]. They conclude on the basis of some real-world examples and statistical simulations that only covariates associated with disparity (i.e., distributed differently in the treatment groups) and influence (i.e., distribution of outcomes across the covariate levels) are likely candidates for adjusted analyses. Specifically, the product of Z statistics for influence and disparity appears to govern the need for covariate adjustment, at least in simple cases.

Using these ideas, investigators might consider adjusting estimated treatment effects for prognostic factors that meet one of the following criteria:

1. Factors that (by chance) are statistically significantly unbalanced between the treatment groups,

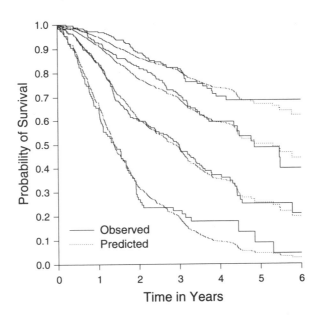

Figure 13.3 Observed and predicted survival of risk sets in the MACS cohort.

2. Factors that are strongly associated with the outcome, whether (significantly) unbalanced or not,

3. To demonstrate that a particular prognostic factor does not artificially create the treatment effect,

4. To illustrate and quantify the effects of factors of known clinical importance.

The philosophy underlying adjusting in these circumstances is to be certain that the observed treatment effect is "independent" of the factors. The quantitative measures of clinical interest after adjustment are changes in relative risk parameters rather than changes in -values. Therefore, some adjusted analyses will include statistically non-significant variables but will be informative in a broad context.

One should probably not routinely adjust estimated treatment effects for all of the covariates that are typically measured in comparative trials. Not only are large numbers of uninteresting covariates often recorded, but model building can produce spurious results. However, using clinical knowledge, preclinical data, and findings in the trial data, covariate adjustment can improve inferences from comparative trials.

13.3.2 Example

As an example of the utility of conducting adjusted analyses of treatment effects in randomized clinical trials, we consider a trial of BCNU impregnated implantable

Table 13.8 Proportional Hazards Regression Models Illustrating Adjusted Treatment Effects

Model	Variable	Hazard Ratio	95% Conf. Limits	P-Value
1	B vs. A	1.40	1.02 – 1.91	0.04
2	female vs. male	1.69	1.23 – 2.33	0.001
3	B vs. A	1.45	1.06 – 2.00	0.02
	female vs. male	1.74	1.26 – 2.40	0.001

polymers for the treatment of recurrent malignant gliomas [Brem et al., 1995]. Two-hundred-twenty-two patients were randomized with equal probability to receive either BCNU polymer or placebo polymer, implanted in the cavity remaining after surgical resection of recurrent tumors. The polymer released BCNU slowly over a three-week period to achieve higher local concentrations of drug than one could obtain with systemic administration. In this study, the randomization was not stratified to balance strong prognostic factors.

When the trial was analyzed, 215 patients had died of recurrent disease. The overall effect of BCNU polymer was to reduce the risk of death by approximately 18% (Figure 13.4). The estimated hazard ratio was 0.82 and the 95% percent confidence interval on the hazard ration was [0.45–1.03]. Thus, an analysis adhering strictly to the design of the trial and using the conventional interpretation of statistical significance would conclude that BCNU polymer was not of convincing benefit.

Interestingly, the pathological type of the tumor was a strong determinant of survival time, as were the previous use of nitrosureas, pathologically active versus quiescent cells, and other factors listed below. When the treatment effect was estimated stratified by pathologic type and adjusted for other factors, the precision of the estimate was improved and more convincing evidence of a beneficial effect of BCNU emerged. The adjusted regression analysis is shown in Table 13.9.

The primary purpose of the adjusted analysis was not to create statistical significance where none existed before. In fact, considerable evidence regarding the likely beneficial effect of BCNU already existed. The agent has shown activity in many studies when administered systemically. Furthermore, preclinical data for the polymer delivery system strongly supported its biological efficacy. Finally, the estimated hazard ratio for BCNU polymer did not change substantially after adjustment for the prognostic factors listed. Based on the findings of this trial and supporting data, biodegradable polymers impregnated with BCNU were approved by the Food and Drug Administration in 1996 for treatment of recurrent brain tumors.

This example illustrates the utility of adjusted analyses of comparative trials for reducing the variability of estimated treatment effects. Adjustment would also be useful for accounting for the effects of chance imbalances. Although there is a potential to use adjustment for data dredging and inappropriately enhancing statistical

Table 13.9 Proportional Hazards Multiple Regression Stratified by Pathologic Type of Tumor

Variable	Hazard Ratio	95% Conf. Limits	P-Value
BCNU polymer vs. placebo	0.69	0.52 – 0.91	0.01
Performance status ≥ 70 vs.< 70	0.66	0.49 – 0.91	0.01
Local vs. whole brain irradiation	0.59	0.42 – 0.83	0.003
Active vs. quiescent	1.93	1.26 – 3.78	0.02
Previous nitrosurea vs. none	1.53	1.13 – 2.08	0.006
White vs. other races	1.75	1.03 – 2.99	0.04
>75% resection vs. <75%	0.67	0.49 – 0.93	0.02
Age (per decade)	1.25	1.11 – 1.40	<0.001

significance, it is a valuable tool that can assist with the data analysis of randomized studies.

13.4 Non-Model-Based Methods for PFAs

Statistical models are flexible and informative tools that help estimate useful biological effects from experimental (and nonexperimental) study designs. Models derive their strengths from knowledge or assumptions about the error structure, covariate effects, and other mathematical relationships in the data. When these assumptions are incorrect, models may yield the wrong answers or may not utilize the information in the data efficiently. There are other approaches useful for examining structure and associations in data, which do not require all of the assumptions of statistical models. These approaches are quite general and as simple to apply as statistical models.

No statistical procedures are free of assumptions or pitfalls, including those which do not use structural models. Although the methods discussed here are relatively assumption-free, they do not necessarily yield inferences that are more clinically useful, relevant, accurate, or simple than statistical models. In some cases, they yield less information. These limitations will be discussed below. Interesting reviews and comparisons of model and non-model-based methods are given by Hand [1992] and Hadorn et al. [1992].

13.4.1 Recursive partitioning uses dichotomies

Recursive partitioning is a method for developing clinical prediction rules that uses dichotomies in prognostic variables to divide and subset the cohort. Its purpose is to form a small set of classes or categories, defined on several simple criteria, that have clinically significantly different outcomes. A new patient could be classified using the resulting scheme into a single category, and this classification would carry useful prognostic information.

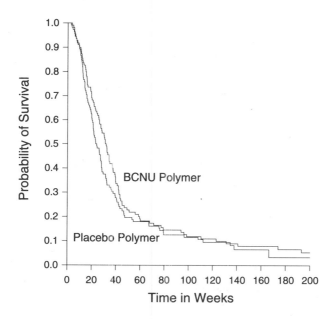

Figure 13.4 Observed survival following reoperation for malignant glioma.

Process

Recursive partitioning uses a stepwise approach to developing prediction rules. At each step, a bivariate analysis is performed to determine which predictive factor from the ones under consideration yields a partition of the data with the lowest false-positive and false-negative rates. Using some algorithms, the different types of errors can be assigned different weights. Then, each step partitions the data according to the lowest weighted probability of error. For each of the partitions that results, the same process is repeated using other prognostic variables. The result is a type of "tree", where each branch splits into two daughter branches based on a dichotomization of one predictor variable.

If this process is repeated enough times, the outcomes in one of the groups will all be the same, and no further partitioning of that group will be possible. Eventually, this will be true for all the remaining branches and the partitioning process stops. At this point, the classification tree can be "pruned" by re-combining branches that do not increase the classification error. This process is called *amalgamation*, giving the procedure its common name, "recursive partitioning and amalgamation" (RPA).

Practical use

The probabilities of correct classification from the partitioning tree can be used to guide therapeutic (or diagnostic) decisions. The trees that result from this process are clinically appealing because they are defined directly in terms of simple dichotomies of predictor variables. They require no computations to categorize patients and can yield reliable classifications.

Examples

Recursive partitioning has been used in a variety of clinical applications and is comparable to similar predictive methods based on discriminant or other models. RPA has been used to develop improved diagnostic capability for upper extremity fractures in children, where it appears to perform as well as a logistic discriminant function [McConnochie, Roghmann, and Pasternack, 1993]. Seleznick and Fries [1991] used RPA to detect prognostic factors for systemic lupus erythematosus. The technique has also been applied to prognosticating hospitalization for asthma [Li et al., 1995]. The classification methods have been extended to censored survival data [Clark et al., 1994; LeBlanc and Crowley, 1992; Segal, 1988] and have been used to study prognostic factors in breast cancer [Albain et al., 1992], ovarian cancer [Ansell, 1993], malignant gliomas [Curran et al., 1993], and childhood neuroblastoma [Shuster et al., 1992], to name a few examples.

13.4.2 Neural networks are used for pattern recognition

Neural networks are logically defined structures that are modeled after simple neuronal interconnections and were developed to assist with complex classification processes such as pattern recognition. Using data with known associations between the input variables and the outcomes (or output or classification variables), the network can be "trained" to yield a high probability of correct classification. This process involves modifying the strengths of internal associations to reinforce correct classifications and de-emphasize incorrect ones. A variety of algorithms can be used to optimize and error function. After training, the network is applied to new data, where it uses its internal rules to classify or predict outcomes from the input variables. In this way it can be used to make prognostic classifications similar to the model-based methods and recursive partitioning described above. See Warner and Misra [1996] for a recent review.

Neural networks are well suited to large complex problems such as pattern recognition. They have been used for speech synthesis and identifying military targets. However, they have also been successfully applied to diverse areas in the biological sciences such as predicting protein structure, diagnosis, and prognostication for patients with breast cancer. They can also be used to model censored survival data [Faraggi and Simon, 1995]. For a recent review of neural network applications to clinical data, see Minor and Namini [1996].

Structure

A simple neural network has three layers: input, hidden, and output (Figure 13.5). The input layer has one node for each input factor (variable, in the case of prognostication). Each of these nodes is connected to each node in the hidden layer, which typically contains fewer nodes than the input layer. Finally, each node in the hidden layer is connected to each output node. For simple prognostication (e.g., a binary response), the output layer can contain a single node.

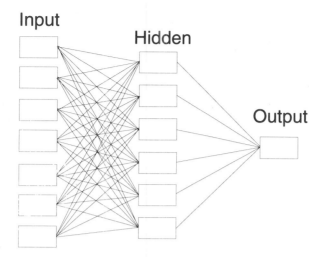

Figure 13.5 Connections in a basic neural network.

A consequence of this high degree of connectivity is that the network is complex and a large number of constants or parameters are required to specify its state. For example, a network with N inputs and N nodes in the hidden layer would have N^2 connections or weights that must be adjusted during training. This is considerably more parameters than a typical statistical model would require.

Practical use

Some practical aspects of using neural networks for prognostication are discussed by Clark et al. [1994] and Ravdin and Clark [1992]. Networks have been used for prognostication in cancer patients and appear to perform nearly as well as discrimination procedures such as logistic regression for predicting binary outcomes. However, neural networks do not seem to have been compared systematically and quantitatively to statistical models with a comparable number of parameters. For example, the interconnections in a neural network can only be described by using a relatively large number of parameters. This number may approximate n^2, where n is the number of nodes. In contrast, the typical statistical regression model usually employs much fewer than k parameters, where k is the number of variables.

Although developing prediction algorithms with neural networks is fairly simple, investigators may sacrifice some useful information when they give up more traditional model-based approaches. For example, it is difficult to quantify and formalize the degree of improvement that results from adding additional predictors to network models. There are no simple ways to quantify variability or precision in neural networks and no way to estimate risks or other clinical parameters attributable to individual prognostic factors. Thus, there is a trade-off between lack of assumptions and utility of the information that is produced by such methods.

13.5 Summary

An organized, detailed, quantitative study of prognostic factors usually provides valuable clinical information. These analyses help clinicians understand disease and select the best treatment for patients. They also provide a structure that can help to analyze clinical trials and design new studies. In some circumstances, there are biologically important interactions between risk factors or between treatment and predictors that can be illuminated by PFAs.

Statistical models, especially multiple regressions, provide a convenient and powerful way to conduct prognostic factor analyses. These models perform several useful services. They combine theory and data, provide structure to the data, allow estimation of clinically important quantities, and permit testing and revising of the model itself. To be useful, statistical models must be built on a foundation of good data, statistical expertise, and clinical judgment. Investigators should take particular care with numerical coding of predictors, selecting variables for multiple regressions, and assessing interactions.

The same methods used for PFAs can often help analyze and interpret the results of randomized clinical trials. In particular, these so-called adjusted analyses of treatment effect may be helpful when strong prognostic factors are not controlled in the execution of the study, to demonstrate that known predictors have not confounded the outcome, and to explore the data. It is not necessary to analyze comparative trials in this way routinely, but it can often help explain and illuminate the findings.

Besides statistical models, there are other useful ways for assessing the influence of prognostic factors on outcomes. These include recursive partitioning and neural network modeling. These methods tend to be operationally simple and yield clinically interpretable information about the effects of prognostic variables. The drawbacks to these techniques are that they do not quantify the effects of predictors or yield formal methods for revising the selection of variables.

13.6 Questions for Discussion

1. When two continuous covariates are studied on their natural scales, they appear to interact significantly. However, when they are both "transformed" using 0, 1, or 2 for levels <1, 1–10, and 10–100, respectively, no interaction is observed. How do you explain this?

2. Two prognostic factors have been previously observed to be strong predictors of outcome. In your analysis, however, they are only almost statistically significant, individually. When multiple regressions are constructed, the two predictors enter the model together (with opposite algebraic signs) and are highly significant. What might be going on and what should you do next?

3. Investigators using neural networks for assessing prognostic factors suggest that the method is superior than logistic regression for predicting outcome. Design and discuss a convincing method to compare the two methodologies in the same data. Assume that the data are plentiful and of high quality.

Chapter References

Albain, K.S., Green, S., LeBlanc, M., Rivkin, S., O'Sullivan, J. and Osborne, C.K. (1992). Proportional hazards and recursive partitioning and amalgamation analyses of the Southwest Oncology Group node-positive adjuvant CMFVP breast cancer data base: A pilot study. Breast Cancer Research Treat. 22: 273-284.

Ansell, S.M., Rapoport, B.L., Falkson, G., Raats, J.I., and Moeken, C.M. (1993). Survival determinants in patients with advanced ovarian cancer. Gyn. Oncol. 50: 215-220.

Appleton, D.R. (1995). What do we mean by a statistical model? Statistics in Med. 14: 185-197.

Armitage, P. (1981). Importance of prognostic factors in the analysis of data from clinical trials. Controlled Clin. Trials 1: 347-353.

Beach, M.L. and Meier, P. (1989). Choosing covariates in the analysis of clinical trials. Controlled Clin. Trials 10: 161S-175S.

Brem, H., Piantadosi, S., Burger, P.C. et al. (1995). Placebo-controlled trial of safety and efficacy of intraoperative controlled delivery by biodegradable polymers of chemotherapy for recurrent gliomas. Lancet 345: 1008-1012.

Byar, D.P. (1982). Analysis of Survival Data: Cox and Weibull Models with Covariates. Chapter 12, in Valerie Mike and Kenneth Stanley (Eds.), Statistics in Medical Research, New York: John Wiley & Sons.

Byar, D.P. (1984). Identification of Prognostic Factors, Chapter 24, in M.J. Buyse, M.J. Staquet, and R.J. Sylvester (Eds.), Cancer Clinical Trials, Oxford: Oxford University Press.

Byar, D.P. (1985). Assessing apparent treatment–covariate interactions in randomized clinical trials. Statistics in Med. 4: 255-263.

Chastang, C., Byar, D., and Piantadosi, S. (1988). A quantitative study of the bias in estimating the treatment effect caused by omitting a balanced covariate in survival models. Statistics in Med. 7, 1243-1255.

Clark, G.M., Hilsenbeck, S.G., Ravdin, P.M.,De Laurentiis, M., and Osborne, C.K. (1994). Prognostic factors: Rationale and methods of analysis and integration. Breast Cancer Research Treat. 32: 105-112.

Collett, D. (1994). Modelling Survival Data in Medical Research. London: Chapman and Hall.

Cox, D.R. and Oakes, D. (1984). Analysis of Survival Data. London: Chapman and Hall.

Curran, W.J., Jr., Scott, C.B., Horton, J., Nelson, J.S., Weinstein, A.S., Fischbach, A.J., Chang, C.H., Rotman, M., Asbell, S.O., Krisch, R.E., et al. (1993). Recursive partitioning analysis of prognostic factors in three Radiation Therapy Oncology Group malignant glioma trials. J. Nat. Cancer Instit. 85: 704-710.

Dobson, A.J. (1983). An Introduction to Statistical Modelling. London: Chapman and Hall.

Faraggi, D. and Simon, R. (1995). A neural network model for survival data. Statistics in Med. 14: 73-82.

Gail, M.H., Wieand, S., and Piantadosi, S. (1984). Biased estimates of treatment effect in randomized experiments with nonlinear regressions and omitted covariates. Biometrika 71(3): 431-44.

Gail, M.H., Tan, W.-Y., and Piantadosi, S. (1988). The size and power of tests for no treatment effect in randomized clinical trials when needed covariates are omitted. Biometrika 75(1): 57- 64.

George, S.L. (1988). Identification and assessment of prognostic factors. Sem. Onc. 15: 462-471.

Graham, N.M.H., Park, L.P., Piantadosi, S., Phair, J.P., Mellors, J., Fahey, J.L., and Saah, A.J. (1994). Prognostic value of combined response markers among human immunodeficiency virus infected persons: Possible aid in the decision to change zidovudine monotherapy. Clinical Infect. Dis. 20: 352-362.

Hadorn, D.C., Draper, D., Rogers, W.H., Keeler, E.B., and Brook, R.H. (1992). Cross-validation performance of mortality prediction models. Statistics in Med. 11: 475-489.

Hand, D.J. (1992). Statistical methods in diagnosis. Stat. Methods in Med. Research 1: 49-67.

Harrell, F.E., Jr., Lee, K.L., and Mark, D.B. (1996). Multivariable prognostic models: Issues in developing models, evaluating assumptions and adequacy, and measuring and reducing errors. Statistics in Medicine 15: 361-387.

Harris, E.K. and Albert, A. (1991). Survivorship Analysis for Clinical Studies. New York: Marcel Dekker.

Kalbfleisch, J.D. and Prentice, R.L. (1980). The Statistical Analysiis of Failure Time Data. New York: John Wiley & Sons.

Kaplan, E.L., and Meier, P. (1958). Nonparametric estimation from incomplete observations. Am. Stat. Assoc. J.: 53: 457-480.

Kaslow, R.A., Ostrow, D.G., Detels, R., et al. (1987). The Multicenter AIDS Cohort Study: Rationale, organization, and selected characteristics of the participants. Am. J. Epidemiol. 126: 310-318.'

LeBlanc, M. and Crowley, J. (1992). Relative risk trees for censored survival data. Biometrics 48: 411-425.

Lee, E.T. (1992). Statistical Methods for Survival Data Analysis, Second Edition. New York: John Wiley & Sons.

Li, D., German, D., Lulla, S., Thomas, R.G., and Wilson, S.R. (1995). Prospective study of hospitalization for asthma. A preliminary risk factor model. Am. J. Respir. Crit. Care Med. 151: 647-655.

Marubini, E. and Valsecchi, M.G. (1995). Analysing Survival Data from Clinical Trials and Observational Studies. Chichester: John Wiley & Sons.

McConnochie, K.M., Roghmann, K.J., and Pasternack, J. (1993). Developing prediction rules and evaluating patterns using categorical clinical markers: Two complementary procedures. Med. Decis. Making 13: 30-42.

McCullagh, P. and Nelder, J.A. (1989). Generalized Linear Models. London: Chapman and Hall.

Minor, J.M. and Namini, H. (1996). Analysis of clinical data using neural nets. J. Biopharmaceutical Statistics 6: 83-104.

Nelder, J.A. and Weddeburn, R.W.M. (1972). Generalized linear models. JRSS A 135: 370-384.

Parmar, M.K.B. and Machin, D. (1995). Survival Analysis: A Practical Approach. New York: John Wiley & Sons.

Piantadosi, S., Graham, N.M.H., Park, L., Saah, A., Kaslow, R., Detels, R. Rinaldo, C., and Phair, J. for the Multicenter AIDS Cohort Study (MACS). Risk sets for time to AIDS and survival based on pre- and post-treatment prognostic markers. First National Conference on Human Retroviruses and Related Infections, Am. Soc. Microbiology, December 12-16, 1993.

Ravdin, P.M. and Clark, G.M. (1992). A practical application of neural network analysis for predicting outcome of individual breast cancer patients. Breast Cancer Research Treat. 22: 285-293.

Rutter, C.M. and Elashoff, R.M. (1994). Analysis of longitudinal data: Random coefficient regression modeling. Statistics in Medicine 13: 1211-1231.

Segal, M.R. (1988). Regression trees for censored data. Biometrics 44: 35-47.

Seleznick, M.J. and Fries, J.F. (1991). Variables associated with decreased survival in systemic lupus erythematosus. Sem. Arthritis Rheum. 21: 73-80.

Shuster, J.J., McWilliams, N.B., Castleberry, R., Nitschke, R., Smith, E.I., Altshuler, G., Kun, L., Brodeur, G., Joshi, V., Vietti, T., and Hayes, F.A. (1992). Serum lactate dehydrogenase in childhood neuroblastoma. Am. J. Clin. Oncol. 15: 295-303.

Simon, R. (1984). Use of Regression Models: Statistical Aspects, Chapter 25, in M.J. Buyse, M.J. Staquet, and R.J. Sylvester (Eds.), Cancer Clinical Trials, Oxford: Oxford University Press.

Statistics and Epidemiology research Corporation (SERC). (1993). EGRET SIZ Reference Manual. Seattle: SERC.

Warner, B. and Misra, M. (1996). Understanding neural networks as statistical tools. Am. Statistiscian 50(4): 284-293.

CHAPTER 14

Reporting

14.1 Introduction

Reporting the results of a clinical trial is one of the most important and least studied aspects of clinical research. Investigators have an obligation to disseminate trial results in a timely and competent manner. Chalmers [1990] suggested that failure to publish a well-designed trial is a type of scientific misconduct. The goal of a clinical research report is to provide enough information to allow the reader to evaluate the authors' conclusions, i.e., whether or not they are justified within, and applicable outside, the specific study.

The overall utility of a trial report is a consequence of several components including the: 1) importance of the scientific question, 2) rigor of the study design and execution, 3) quality of the written report, and 4) external validity of the clinical trial. It may not be possible to judge the quality of the trial and appreciate the importance of the results if the report is poorly written. The way in which findings are described can have an impact on practitioner behavior [Bobbio, Demichelis, and Giustetto, 1994; Forrow, Taylor, and Arnold, 1992; Naylor, Chen, and Strauss, 1992]. Furthermore, the reporting methods and techniques can affect the reader's comprehension of the result [e.g., Elting and Bodey [1991].

Preparing the report of a clinical trial involves coordinating a number of independent tasks. These include resolving all questions about the data, finalizing the statistical analyses, interpreting the findings, building a consensus of investigator opinion, authoring the report, and responding to peer review and editorial feedback. These tasks can be extended in time as the data mature or additional questions arise. Each of these areas offers an opportunity for diverse opinions to be heard and possibly delay the reporting process. However, each area also represents an important opportunity to improve the quality of the final product by accommodating different views and criticisms. Failure of any link in this chain can cost the investigators much time and effort.

Frequently, results must be presented in more than a single forum such as an investigator's meeting, national society meeting, and journal. Also, reports must be tailored to the nature of the trial, the disease, and the audience. For example, the important issues will be different for disease prevention studies than for therapeutic trials. Similarly, papers written for a specialty journal may need to have a somewhat different emphasis from those for a more general audience.

A structured reporting style can reduce the opportunity for error during this last stage of research. The suggestions for reporting given in this chapter are typical of ones found in the literature for clinical trials and are intended to be flexible enough to apply to various trial types (e.g., Bailar and Mosteller [1988] and International Committee of Medical Journal Editors [1993]). Additional details have been given by the Standards of Reporting Trials Group [1994] and the Working Group on Recommendations for Reporting Clinical Trials in the Biomedical Literature [1994]. Also, knowledge of good reporting practices can help with critical reading and reviewing. For an in-depth discussion of evaluating the medical literature (with an epidemiologic orientation), see Gehlbach [1988].

14.1.1 Uniformity of reporting can improve comprehension

The most informative summaries and the amount of detail to report from a clinical trial depend on the nature of the clinical hypotheses being studied. We would not expect reports of single-institution pharmacologic trials to be similar to those from multi-center randomized trials. Furthermore, not all journal editors and reviewers will agree on the ideal content of reports. However, many features of good reports are similar for all types of trials and find widespread acceptance in journals. Some care must be taken so that uniform standards do not obscure important facts. See Walter [1995] for a discussion of this point in the context of confidence intervals.

One simple example of a uniform reporting criterion is a requirement to have all papers and presentations reviewed by the study principal investigator and the trial methodologist. This requirement is not likely to generate much controversy. A second simple example of uniformity relates to the protection of research subjects. Journals require affirmation that reports of research studies have been reviewed and approved by the investigators' Institutional Review Boards. Some other attempts at uniformity focus on the content of the report title and the content and structure of the abstract. Structured abstracts have been advocated by the Ad Hoc Working Group for Critical Appraisal of the Medical Literature [1987; Haynes et al., 1990] but are not universally employed.

Uniformity is helpful to readers, particularly to those who are the least familiar with the details of the disease or intervention under investigation. Uniformity of reporting is likely to become more of a priority in situations where the historical record, corporate memory, and detailed findings of particular studies become more distant in time, but remain vital to new research. The benefits of uniformity are evident in some chronic diseases like cancer, where standardized staging has improved trial design, reporting, and interpretation. Some cancer journals have called for a uniform reporting format [Weymuller and Goepfert, 1991] as have other specialty journals (e.g., Waldhausen and Localio [1996]).

Many journals have limitations on the length of research reports or at least discourage those that are long. Editors prefer short assertive papers without much speculation. Often, the methods section of papers are trimmed to meet such restrictions, causing important details to be omitted. One possible solution to this problem is to publish a separate methods paper for large or important clinical trials. Then, the results paper can contain only a summary of the key methodologic points. Because publishing a separate methods paper is usually not possible, investigators should provide complete and well-organized information in a single report.

14.2 Quality of the Literature

Ideally, published reports should inform the reader about all aspects of study design, conduct, analysis, and interpretation that are relevant for assessing the internal and external validity of the trial. Despite many years of published randomized comparative trials, the content and quality of trial reports in the literature remains remarkably inconsistent on these points. A few systematic studies of published papers highlight the variability of trial reports.

Mahon and Daniel [1964] examined 203 reports of drug trials published in the *Canadian Medical Association Journal* between 1956 and 1960. Only 11 of these reports were judged by the examiners to meet the criteria for a valid report. The most consistent deficiencies they noted were the absence of any type of control group (133 studies) and non-random allocation of controls (49 studies). More recently, Pocock, Hughes, and Lee [1987] examined 45 trial reports published during 1985 in three leading medical journals and found that the large majority did not provide sample size, misused confidence intervals, or tended to overestimate the efficacy of the treatment under investigation. Similar examinations of the published literature have shown deficiencies in descriptions of randomization [Altman and Doré, 1990; Gøtzsche, 1989; Schultz et al., 1994]. Although most attention regarding reporting has been given to randomized trials, phase I trials in oncology have also been found to be poorly described [Winget, 1995].

Traditionally, the information contained in a published report of a clinical trial has been determined entirely by the investigators and the journal editorial process. Some authors have given guides for reporting trial results [Grant 1989; Meinert, 1986; Mosteller, Gilbert, and McPeek, 1980; Simon and Wittes, 1985; Zelen, 1983]. In spite of these suggestions, trial reporting remains essentially unstructured. A few journals have also attempted to improve this area by publishing checklists and guidelines for reporting [Gardner, Machin, and Campbell, 1986; Gore, Jones, and Thompson, 1992; Murray, 1991], but most have not.

14.2.1 Peer review is the only game in town

The content of the medical literature reflects an imperfect editorial and peer review process. Limitations of peer review include unqualified, biased, tired, or inattentive referees and deficiencies in the management of submitted manuscripts. Some strengths of the process are discussed in Abby et al. [194]. Discussions of these and other aspects of peer review were undertaken at the Second International Congress on Peer Review in Biomedical Publication (Chicago, September 9–11, 1993). Many of the papers presented at the congress were published in Volume 272 of *JAMA* (No. 2). This journal issue provides a broad view of the peer review process. Several authors suggested quality rating instruments as a way to correct deficiencies in the peer review process [Cho and Bero, 1994; Feurer et al., 1994; Rochon et al., 1994].

Peer review has limitations and may be modified in the future because of its corruption, the growth of science, and electronic dissemination of information [Judson, 1994]. However, despite the current and future limitations of peer review, currently there are no good alternatives for judging the relative merits of scientific papers. Modifications in the process may improve timeliness, decrease bias, and correct other shortcomings, but peer review will not soon disappear. However, electronic publishing may stimulate replacing peer review in the near future with a quicker and more flexible alternative. Electronic media are attractive because they can potentially correct some of the deficiencies in a paper-based system. They can improve retrieval and linkages to related information, both for the reader and the author. As a consequence, papers can be more inclusive and detailed. Finally, electronic media can shorten the editorial and review process, perhaps even eliminate it, as the practice of posting preprints on electronic bulletin boards has done in some physics and biology groups.

Until peer review is eliminated, investigators have only the option of preparing reports in the traditional manner. A trial report may fail the initial test of peer review for a number of reasons. These include (see Kassirer and Campion [1994]): design flaws or consequential biases that prevent the question from being answered; deficiencies in presentation such as poor rationale or background, inappropriate omission or analysis of data, lack of objectivity, and poor writing; deficiencies in presentation of the results such as overemphasis on weak data, preliminary findings, or irrelevant data; and concerns about the importance or relevance of the work. Avoiding such errors usually permits the investigators to have an audience. What they do with the opportunity to have others read and review their work depends on some of the finer points of reporting.

14.2.2 Publication bias can distort impressions based on the literature

Publication bias is the name given to the tendency for studies with "positive" findings to be preferentially selected for publication over those with "negative" findings. It is a *selection bias* for studies that yield a particular type of result. This phenomenon has been convincingly demonstrated by several authors [e.g., Begg and Berlin, 1988]. An unsatisfactory but interesting study of publication bias has been discussed by Kemper [1990]. A paper that I helped to author was criticized by a peer reviewer because it was "not strongly positive". That journal rejected the paper, in large part, for this reason, although the manuscript was published in a different place. If the published literature is used as a basis for drawing conclusions about a treatment or group of related treatments from independent studies (as it should be), an impression biased in favor of the treatment could result. This effect is possible for both informal reviews of the literature and more quantitative ones such as overviews (discussed in Chapter 17).

In principle, publication bias should not be a problem. If an important therapeutic question is addressed by a trial, and the study has been conducted rigorously, and the report is properly written, the information will be useful to other investigators and practitioners. Therefore, it deserves to be published as much as studies that appear to show a therapeutic advance. However, investigators often lose enthusiasm for negative results because they seem less glamorous than positive ones and may be viewed as failures by the research team and sponsors. This can lead to weaker reports. Some journal editors prefer to publish positive studies because they seem to improve the stature of the journal. This is paradoxical because, if we assume that true treatment advances are uncommon, then positive reports are more likely to be in error than negative ones.

There is no completely satisfactory way for the reader to correct for publication bias when viewing a particular paper, although some analytic approaches to the problem have been suggested [Iyengar and Greenhouse, 1988]. One must recognize that selection bias exists and retain a little skepticism about positive results. In a few cases, readers may be aware of unpublished studies that contradict or fail to support a particular finding and these can be used to soften enthusiasm.. It may be useful to ask if the paper in question would have been published if it was a negative trial. In other words, is the quality of the study good enough to convey externally valid information consistent with no effect? Even so, there is no way to separate true positive results from false positive ones without replicating the study (several times). When conducting exhaustive quantitative overviews (Chapter 17), it is important to include data from both published and unpublished trials to counteract this bias.

Journal editors and reviewers can reduce publication bias in two ways. First, they must weight methodologic rigor and thorough reporting ahead of statistical significance when judging the merits of an article. Second, they must be willing to report negative findings from sound studies with as much enthusiasm as positive reports. Two other ideas might help correct this problem, although they seem unlikely to catch on. First, it would be helpful to have a peer-reviewed *Journal of Negative Trials* devoted to such results. This would encourage authors to complete and publish such studies, because they would obtain the same academic credit from them as from positive trials. Second, all journals should consider publishing shortened trial protocols for impending, well-designed studies. This practice is already done for a few large, selected, expensive, or otherwise high-profile trials. This would 1) alert the community to the conduct of a study, 2) make that fact available to literature searches, 3) encourage and shorten the results paper.

14.3 Contents of Clinical Trial Reports

There is considerable overlap in good reporting form and content for TM, DF, SE, CTE, and ES studies. The most comprehensive source for structure and content of trial reports is the International Conference on Harmonisation (ICH) consensus guideline [ICH, 1995]. This guideline requires over 40 pages to describe and contains a level of detail that exceeds what we would expect to find in the peer-reviewed literature. Nevertheless, it is an essential document from a regulatory perspective and illustrates aspects of study reporting that should be familiar to all investigators, even though a published report will be less extensive. In the remainder of this section, I discuss some specific statistical problems in reporting and then offer guidelines for specific types of trials.

14.3.1 Avoid statistical pitfalls

Standard notation should be used throughout the report. Although even good statistical notation can appear obscure to those unfamiliar with it, it usually helps clarify results and make them understandable to a larger audience. Similarly, using the proper summary or descriptive statistic is essential. For example, investigators sometimes use standard deviations and standard errors interchangeably. The standard deviation (or other measures of distributional spread such as interquartile range) should be used as a descriptive summary, whereas the standard error is intended to convey the uncertainty of an estimate, such as a mean. Confidence intervals, discussed in Chapter 12 also convey the precision of an estimate and are more informative than significance levels.

Reports of clinical trials often do not distinguish between clinical significance and statistical significance. Of these, clinical significance is the stronger notion and cannot be expressed in terms of statistical significance levels (p-values). It can be expressed in terms of the magnitude and direction of treatment effects or differences. Therefore, the currency of a trial report should be the size of treatment effects and the precision with which they are estimated. This is particularly important when assessing equivalence. Significance levels do not provide evidence of equivalence, whereas effect sizes do. Evidence of no difference is not the same as no evidence of difference [Altman and Bland, 1995].

14.3.2 Titles and abstracts should inform

Titles and abstracts need special attention, because they are the only part of many reports that some readers will see. The title should name both the drug, agent, regimen, test, device or therapy and the target disease or condition. Generic names for drugs should be given, along with trade names if a particular product has been used. The exact nature of the trial design (e.g., dose escalation, safety and efficacy, comparative efficacy) may be included in a subtitle.

Some journals require structured abstracts. Even when they do not, the abstract can usually be improved by paying attention to the following points. A good outline for an abstract recapitulates the text and includes the following points:

- Objectives of the study;
- Design of the trial;
- Setting or type of practices;
- Characteristics of the study population;
- Interventions used;
- Primary outcome measures;
- Principal result; and
- Conclusions.

Abstracts should be shorter than 250 words. Statistical methods are not usually included in an abstract.

14.3.3 Phase I trial reports need improvement

Although there is a large statistical literature on the merits of various designs for phase I drug trials, there has been little written about the methodological adequacy of published reports. One exception is the work by Winget [1996], who reviewed phase I studies of cytotoxic drugs for cancer therapy. Even in this highly specific and structured area, deficiencies can be found in the way that results are reported and drug doses selected for later clinical trials. From these observations in oncology, one would expect that early developmental trials in all disease areas are not documented optimally in the medical literature. Although the following discussion pertains to phase I, many of the points are also valid for TM and DF trials broadly.

Points to consider

Keeping in mind that the basic objectives of phase I drug trials are to observe pharmacokinetics, find a good therapeutic dose, assess toxicity, and look for evidence of efficacy, it is not difficult to outline a good phase I study report. The general categories to cover are 1) study design features, 2) characteristics of the study population, 3) estimates of clinically important pharmacokinetic parameters, 4) recommendations for the proper dose of drug to use in SE trials, 5) nature, severity, and reversibility of toxicity or side effects, and 6) evidence of treatment efficacy.

Design. Methods for phase I study designs are still actively evolving. In recent years, new designs have been suggested that appear to provide information efficiently and accurately about the dose-response or dose-toxicity function that underlies the observed outcomes. In reporting, it is important to describe the exact nature of the study design used because the quality of inference about the dose-response relationship can depend on it.

Patient characteristics. The outcome of developmental trials depends partly on the characteristics of the patients being treated. In cancer trials, patients who have been previously treated with cytotoxic therapy may have lower functional reserve in major organ systems due to toxicity. These patients may not experience side effects and responses similar to those in untreated patients. When major organ system toxicity is less of a concern, it may be satisfactory or advantageous to use a heterogeneous study population. In either case, it is essential to provide a sufficient level of detail regarding the patients' characteristics so that the reader can assess the external validity of the trial. It is common practice in oncology to use toxicity and side effect criteria that are widely agreed upon and well understood. Although more difficult in other disease settings, there are many circumstances where quantitative criteria can be used to describe side effects. Total number of deaths in the study population and those reasonably attributable to the treatment under study should be reported.

Pharmacokinetics. Pharmacokinetic models are useful devices for describing drug distribution and excretion. Investigators are usually interested in certain parameters of clinical importance, such as drug excretion rate, half-life, peak concentration, or area under the time–concentration curve (AUC). For many agents, cytotoxic drugs in particular, the frequency and severity of toxicity may relate strongly to parameters such as the AUC or the peak blood concentration. Estimates of these important pharmacokinetic parameters should be reported in the phase I publication, along with any empirical connections between them and actual toxicities observed. Pharmacokinetic estimates can depend on the model employed to analyze the data. Any such dependencies should also be reported.

Efficacy. It is relatively uncommon to have convincing objective evidence of efficacy during a phase I trial. However, it can occur and is an important finding when it does. For any sign of efficacy that might be attributable to the new therapy, investigators should report the type of (standard) response criteria used, the number of study subjects benefitting, and the duration of benefit. Many readers will also be interested in the cumulative dose (or dose intensity) used prior to observing responses, especially for cancer drugs. An important result from phase I studies is the recommended dose of drug to use in subsequent investigations. The study report should explicitly provide this recommendation, as well as the basis for it. In some cases, side effects may be more likely in older, younger, or more frail patients, requiring the dose to vary on the basis of baseline characteristics. Recommendations related to dose differences should also be explicitly stated in the phase I report.

Phase I report checklist

- Study design
    - experimental design (e.g., see Chapter 4)
    - inclusion and exclusion criteria
    - method for dose-finding
    - clinical and biological basis for the starting dose
    - reasons for stopping the trial
    - definition of the optimal dose
    - dose, route, and schedule of administration of the study drug and ancillary therapies
    - details of collection and modeling of pharmacologic data
- Patient characteristics
    - primary disease sites and extents of disease
    - extent of previous treatment
    - demographic summaries

- proportion of patients with poor prognosis based on objective criteria (e.g., performance status or functional index)
- Toxicity and side effects
- Recommendations for later trials

14.3.4 SE reports should minimize biases and overinterpretation

The clinical trials literature contains very little about reporting deficiencies, standards, or guidelines for SE clinical trials. However, investigators can anticipate these based on the purposes and potential weaknesses of these studies. The purposes of SE studies are to demonstrate treatment feasibility, to estimate success (efficacy), complication, and other event rates, and to facilitate informal comparisons with other therapies that might motivate comparative trials. SE trials also provide information about appropriate doses and scheduling of therapy for comparative trials.

Points to consider

Feasibility. With regard to feasibility goals, the SE report should present and quantify the frequency of problems that prevent the therapy from being carried out or require it to be modified (e.g., dosage reduced) because of side effects. To meet this goal effectively, investigators cannot permit "evaluability" or other clinical criteria to remove patients from the analysis who may represent evidence of non-feasibility. The report must have a complete accounting of the treatment histories for all patients who met the eligibility criteria. It is sometimes helpful to track and report patients who met the eligibility criteria but did not enter the trial. If this happens frequently, it may be a sign that the therapy is unacceptable to patients. It may also be necessary to distinguish between short- and long-term feasibility using appropriate criteria.

Efficacy and toxicity. Estimating success and complication rates requires a similar thorough accounting of patients. The criteria used to define a success should be reported. These criteria should use only information available at, or prior to, the specific clinical landmark. Successes defined in retrospect are suspect. The criteria used to establish a complication, toxicity, or side effect should also be contained in the report. Investigators should distinguish between major and minor side effects and define these terms in the report. In many chronic diseases, SE trials are designed to yield information about rates of disease progression, relapse, or death. Particularly for progression or relapse, the report should explain how they were defined. For relapse, presumably patients are found to be disease free by some criteria and then later found to have a relapse or recurrence. It is also helpful to describe the observed influence of prognostic factors on outcome, because this can provide evidence that the study population is similar to others that have been reported.

Treatment comparisons. SE trials permit, but usually don't encourage, comparisons with other treatments for the same population of patients. Some studies are carried out with the same or similar therapy at different institutions, again inviting comparisons. While such comparisons are error prone because of selection bias, they are natural and necessary. The SE trial report should recognize the potential for strong selection bias, qualify these types of comparisons (if they are made), and avoid definitive or overly enthusiastic statements about relative efficacy.

SE report checklist

- Introduction
    - background knowledge and literature review
    - basis for the investigation
    - principal question addressed by the trial
    - IRB review and approval
- Objectives
    - pre-specify a small set of primary objectives
    - identify which objectives are secondary
- Study design
    - type of trial
    - calendar time
    - planned sample size
    - early stopping and monitoring methods
    - clinical effects to be estimated
- Study setting
    - locations and types of institutions, hospitals, clinics, or community setting
    - characteristics of the patient population
    - referral patterns
- Patient characteristics
    - eligibility criteria
    - exclusion criteria
    - consent procedures
    - source of the study sample
- Treatments
    - generic and trade name of drug
    - dosage form and source
    - concomitant therapy
    - equipment or device manufacturers
    - treatment schedule and modifications permitted within the design
- Outcome measures
    - endpoints
    - laboratory measures
    - methods and frequency of active ascertainment
    - trial termination criteria
- Statistical methods

    – summary statistics for primary outcome
    – monitoring and interim analysis methods
    – control of prognostic factors such as stratification
    – methods for coping with data imperfections (e.g., intention-to-treat)
    – plans for subgroup analyses, if any
- Results
    – patient demographics and characteristics (by treatment group)
    – ineligible patients
    – non-complying patients and drop-outs
    – estimates of clinical effects (point estimates)
    – precision of clinical effect estimates
    – sensitivity of results to ineligible patients, drop-outs, and exclusions
- Discussion
    – biological strengths and weaknesses of results
    – consistency with data from outside the trial
    – implications for comparative trials

14.3.5 Employ a broad outline for completeness in CTE reporting

Structured reports for randomized controlled trials have been discussed by the Standards of Reporting Trials Group [1994], who recommend a checklist to assist in preparing or evaluating a trial report. Although heavily weighted toward statistical issues, these guidelines are also helpful for assessing the clinical merits of trial reports. The Standards of Reporting Trials Group divides trial reports into four content areas: 1) treatment assignment, 2) treatment masking, 3) subject follow-up, and 4) statistical analysis (methods and results). Considering the entire report, we should extend this outline to include other areas such as introduction, design, discussion, and tables.

Considerations for writing titles and abstracts for CTE trials are the same as those given above for developmental trials. The remainder of a workable outline for CTE trial reports is given below. Many of the points listed here may also pertain to some TM, DF, and SE trials.

Points to consider

Introduction and background. The introduction serves two purposes. First, it informs readers who are less knowledgeable than the authors about the specific subject matter of the disease and the trial. Second, it justifies the setting and the scientific hypothesis tested. Both objectives require concise summaries and current references. The introduction, like that for a protocol, should anticipate the specific objectives of the trial. For investigators focused on more subtle aspects of the investigation, these points will seem uninteresting. However, for readers who are new to the study, this introduction is vital and may dictate whether or not they continue reading.

Study design. There are many aspects of study design (discussed throughout this book) that are relevant to reporting the results of a CTE trial. Methods to control bias such as type of internal control and treatment masking should be described. In randomized trials, the method and administration of the randomization should be described to convince readers that it has been properly performed. Another source of error is the monitoring plan which must be especially carefully described if the trial was terminated before the fixed sample size design indicated. Publications from well-known multicenter groups may not require as much detail as those from single-institution or one-of-a-kind collaborations. However, when the trial is complex, controversial, high-profile, or otherwise of special interest, a separate design publication may be warranted.

Study sample and sites. Clinically relevant descriptions of both the study and target population should be reported. This includes stating the experimental unit unambiguously. For example, is the experimental unit the individual, a cluster or family, or a larger group? In some phase I trials, the unit of analysis may be the *treatment course* rather than the individual patient (appropriately or not). It may also be important to describe patients who met the eligibility criteria but chose not to participate in the trial, when this information is available. This may be especially helpful when patients from a large group are asked to participate, but many refuse. It may be difficult for readers to generalize from these situations to clinic populations that are available at their institutions. For non-randomized trials, referral and selection bias may make even detailed descriptions of the study group unsuitable or unconvincing to make comparisons with other studies. In any case, complete and accurate descriptions of the study population are essential so that the readers can assess the external validity of the results.

Treatment and eligibility failures. Eligibility for a trial is determined in advance of study entry from pre-entry criteria specified in the protocol. When ineligible patients are mistakenly placed on study, investigators often analyze only the subset of eligible patients (perhaps in addition to other analyses). The estimate of treatment effect obtained in this way is not biased by patient exclusions, because the selection factor (eligibility) affects both treatment groups equally. The trial report should describe those patients who were retrospectively found to have failed the eligibility criteria. Usually eligible patient analyses will be reported along with all randomized patient analyses. Similarly, the report should describe patients who did not complete the assigned treatment.

Sometimes a large fraction of patients complete the assigned therapy but receive additional therapy not specified by the protocol or design of the trial. For example, patients with esophageal cancer may undergo resection and chemotherapy, and have a variety of second line treatments if signs of disease progression or recurrence are observed. If some of these latter treatments are effective, the results of an initial treatment comparison based on recurrence or survival may be skewed. In general, it is difficult or impossible to use the statistical information in studies that permit "cross-overs" either to new treatments or to the other treatment arm, unless it is part of the study design. One might be able to use the information up to the time of stopping the assigned treatment using conventional methods of analysis.

Methods of treatment assignment and masking. Although treatment assignment methods in clinical trials are generally straightforward, studies of trial reports indicate that assignment methods for many trials are inadequately reported [Williams and Davis, 1994]. This seems to be true for both single-center and multi-center trials. To assure readers about the internal validity of the trial, investigators should report the methods by which treatment assignments were kept confidential.

Statistical methods and assumptions. Readers should be made aware of assumptions underlying the design and analysis of the trial (see checklist below). For a discussion of some practical issues, see DerSimonian et al. [1982]. Many clinicians understand the assumptions and limitations of common statistical procedures. However, readers should be convinced that the data analyst has verified all important assumptions and reported methods in detail for less well-known statistical procedures. Examples of assumptions that are often made in analysis, sometimes violated by the data, and also likely to be consequential are distributional assumptions underlying parametric hypothesis tests, error distributions in regression analyses, and proportionality of hazards in lifetable regressions.

Univariate analyses. It is likely that the data analyst will test the effect of all potentially important prognostic variables on the major outcomes. For these univariable analyses, investigators should report estimated treatment effects (odds ratios or hazard ratios), confidence intervals, and significance levels of tests of no treatment effect (p-values). This does not preclude presenting other displays of univariable analyses (e.g., survival curves or 2×2 tables) if these analyses are especially relevant to the goals of the study. However, the investigators should keep in mind that univariable analyses, particularly in uncontrolled studies, are subject to confounding. Consequently, these analyses need not be emphasized or presented in excessive detail.

Adjusted and multiple variable analyses. In most randomized trials, the univariable (unadjusted) comparison of treatment groups is a simple and valid summary of the treatment difference. However, many times it is useful to demonstrate that the treatment effect is not due to confounders. Evidence against confounding (by observed prognostic factors) can be obtained by using adjusted (multivariable) analyses. The best style of reporting multivariable analyses is the same or similar to that for univariate effects. However, the adjusted analyses reported are usually selected from a larger set of less informative or preliminary results. As an example, consider a lifetable regression model attempting to predict time to cancer recurrence. The "best" (most predictive but parsimonious) model might be built using a step-down procedure from a large set of potential prognostic factors. Each step in the analysis need not be reported, but the final model should be because it is a major objective of the analysis.

For multiple regression analyses, investigators usually report adjusted estimates of treatment effects, confidence intervals, and p-values. Not all prognostic factors retained in multiple regression models must be "statistically significant". It is often useful to keep non-significant effects in a multiple regression model to demonstrate convincingly that the treatment effect persists in their presence. See Chapter 13 for details regarding adjustment.

Negative findings. In non-comparative studies such as SE trials, investigators focus appropriately on the magnitude of clinical effects. Large or small effects can be judged in the context of the benefits of existing treatments, tempered by concerns about patient selection and confounding. One should not abandon this perspective in randomized comparisons. In comparative trials, the absence of a statistically significant difference is not the same as convincing evidence of no difference. In these studies, it is also important to focus on estimated treatment differences rather than hypothesis tests.

Between 1960 and 1977, Freiman et al. [1978] reviewed 300 studies reported in 20 journals. Of these, 71 randomized trials found no difference between the treatment groups. The authors found that most negative trials had low statistical power to detect a 25–50% relative difference in the treatment groups. A study of 102 negative trials from a set of 383 studies in 1994 had similar findings [Moher, Dulberg, and Wells, 1994].

When no statistically significant treatment effect or difference is found in a comparative trial, readers sometimes ask about the power of the study 1) against the original alternative hypothesis, and 2) to detect the observed difference. However, such power calculations are not usually helpful. This is true because, when the result is not significant, the treatment difference will usually be smaller than that on which the original power calculation was based. However, the study was not designed to detect this difference, making the power to detect the observed difference lower than the original power. Also, the original alternative hypothesis is no longer supported by the data. Therefore, the power against it, as well as other unsupported alternatives, is not very interesting.

Even so, it is sometimes helpful to report the motivations and assumptions behind the sample size employed in a trial. While knowing these may not affect interpretation of treatment differences when the study is complete, they may help in planning new or confirmatory trials. Helpful advice regarding these and other aspects of negative clinical trials is provided by Detsky and Sackett [1985].

Patient exclusions. Although the intention-to-treat principle should be followed for the principal analyses from designed experiments (Chapter 11), it is often helpful to conduct many other exploratory analyses. Exploratory analyses that violate the intention-to-treat principle may be particularly informative in large comparative studies, where the data are themselves a valuable resource. Examples of other types of analyses include eligible patients only, treatment received, and compliers only.

Most trial methodologists do not object to exploring the data, but take a fairly conservative view of what should be represented as the final primary result of the study. This is particularly true of analyses that exclude patients from consideration. If the intention-to-treat approach is not followed, for example, one should report differences between it and the results that investigators believe are more relevant. Then, readers of the literature can decide for themselves how consequential the different approaches are.

Statistical significance. P-values do not determine clinical or biological significance and, as discussed elsewhere in this book, are poor measures of strength of evidence. When basing inferences predominantly on p-values, an arbitrary level should not be the only criterion for a declaration of "statistical significance". When biological or clinical support is strong, effect estimates are large, and confidence intervals or p-values indicate significance near conventional levels, it seems appropriate to label the result as "statistically significant". Conversely, results with no biological or clinical support, or those which seem paradoxical, should be reported and interpreted with caution. Even when p-values are smaller than 0.05, these results can be type I errors.

Exploratory analyses. Exploratory or hypothesis-generating analyses should not be reported as the major findings of the trial. If subset or other exploratory analyses are performed, discrepancies between these and the major analyses of the clinical trial should be reported.

Biological consistency. The most reliable guides to the external validity of both primary study results and exploratory analyses are 1) confirmation of findings by similar studies and 2) consistency with established biological theory or findings. For clinical trials, exact replication is often not done and, even when supporting trials are undertaken, the results may take years to come out. Thus it is common to use preclinical data to support or refute the findings of trials. One should exercise caution in emphasizing findings that are unverified, seem counter to intuition, or contradict other seemingly well-established biological evidence. This is not to say that such findings shouldn't be reported. In fact, they may be vitally important. However, they should not generally be reported as the major findings of a study that was designed with other objectives in mind.

P-**values**. In Chapter 12, I discussed the inadequacy of p-values as summaries of evidence from data. Their well-known deficiencies should lead investigators to de-emphasize p-values as the most relevant summaries for published reports. In particular, the fact that repetitions of comparative clinical trials are unlikely to yield significance levels that resemble the original reports and the undesirable combining of effect size and precision implied by p-values should encourage investigators to de-emphasize them.

CTE report checklist

- Introduction
    - background knowledge and literature review
    - basis for the investigation
    - principal question or hypothesis addressed by the trial
    - IRB review and approval
- Objectives
    - pre-specify a small set of primary objectives
    - identify which objectives are secondary
- Study design
    - type of trial
    - calendar time
    - masking
    - method and administration of treatment allocation

- quantitative study design parameters
- early stopping and monitoring methods
- clinical effects to be estimated
- unit of randomization or treatment allocation
- Study setting

  - locations and types of institutions, hospitals, clinics, or community setting
  - characteristics of patient populations
  - referral patterns
- Patient characteristics

  - eligibility criteria
  - exclusion criteria
  - consent procedures
  - source of the study sample
- Treatments

  - generic and trade names of drugs
  - dosage forms and sources
  - concomitant therapy
  - equipment or device manufacturers
  - treatment schedule and modifications permitted within the design
- Outcome measures

  - endpoint definitions
  - laboratory measures
  - methods and frequency of active ascertainment
  - trial termination criteria
- Statistical methods

  - summary and test statistics for primary outcomes
  - unit of analysis
  - monitoring and interim analysis methods
  - control of prognostic factors such as stratification
  - methods for coping with data imperfections (e.g., intention-to-treat)
  - multi-variable methods such as adjustment
  - plans for multiple tests and subgroup analyses
  - definition of statistical significance
- Results

  - patient demographics and characteristics (by treatment group)
  - ineligible patients
  - non-complying patients and drop-outs
  - estimates of clinical effects (point estimates)
  - precision of clinical effect estimates
  - sensitivity of results to ineligible patients, drop-outs, and exclusions

- Discussion
  - strengths and weaknesses of trial results, based on design and analysis
  - consistency with data from outside the trial
  - consistency with other biological knowledge
  - implications for clinical practice
  - implications for future research
- Appendix
  - data listing
  - data collection instruments
  - analysis or other details
  - list of collaborators or contributors
- Tables and figures
  - limit decimal places and leading zeros
  - label axes and individual curves in graphs
- References and previous publications

14.4 Authorship

Listing authorship on papers is a difficult subject. Nearly all academic investigators require acknowledgment for career advancement in the form of peer-reviewed publications. For clinical investigators who do not have laboratory experiments to augment their original and methodological publication list, published reports of clinical trials are a critical measure of productivity.

In recent years, demands on authors have increased to the point where prior planning is necessary to decide on the details of the author list. In the past, it was common for authorship to be a "reward" for contributions to collaborative clinical trials. Physicians placing the most patients on study were often listed as authors of the report, even if they had little or nothing to do with the preparation or editing of the manuscript. This standard is no longer satisfactory. Most journal editors require all authors to have contributed substantially to the *report* and to agree with the material that it contains. Authors who do not help with the actual writing of the paper cannot give such assurances.

When conducting multi-center collaborative clinical trials, it is very helpful for investigators to agree on guidelines for authorship before initiating a trial or series of trials. Such a policy can minimize disagreement later. For example, the principal investigator of the study is often expected to be the first author. This individual will likely have played the greatest role in the formulation of the scientific question and protocol for the trial. For most SE and CTE trials, there is a strong rationale for making the study statistician second author. In a well-planned and executed study, the trialist helped formulate the study design, assured the timeliness and quality of the data, prepared the reports needed for assessing the outcome, and contributed greatly to the manuscript describing the results. This is a strong second position and one should expect this level of participation routinely by the methodologist for complex trials. Other authors should be determined in the order of their intellectual contribution to the study, including data gathering, interpretation, and manuscript writing.

Trial investigators do not seem to agree on the use of "group authorship", i.e., naming the *collaboration* as sole author rather than a few individuals. The merits of this approach are that it correctly emphasizes the collaboration and does not give disproportionate credit to a few investigators. The disadvantages of group authorship are that it does not recognize the high level of effort on the part of some investigators and it diffuses much needed academic credit to the point where essentially no one can receive it. Difficulty obtaining academic credit is a strong disincentive for young investigators to contribute to a collaboration.

Group authorship is not a good solution to the all of the problems surrounding multi-investigator collaborations. A good compromise is to indicate a few investigators who have prepared the report and list the collaborative group as the last author. One infrequently pursued option is to include everyone who contributed to the study in some reasonable order on the author list. An extreme example of this kind of excess is a recent report that lists 147 authors [Oliver, van der Aart, Agostoni-Carbone, et al., 1992]. Given the size of many collaborations, this option is also not especially feasible or informative.

14.5 Alternatives to Peer-Review

Peer-reviewed publication has its limitations and alternatives have been tried, some on a small but visible scale. Presentation of results in preliminary form at national or international society meetings is used concurrently with manuscript submission by many authors. This practice has evolved from the research setting, where such meetings can be used effectively to gain needed input from colleagues during the project, to clinical settings where results are disseminated more rapidly and incompletely than by printed media. Sometimes investigators deliberately use the popular press either to augment presentation at a meeting or entirely independently. Because the popular media only disseminate sketchy clinical research results, they are not truly an alternative to peer reviewed publication.

Another mechanism besides peer-reviewed publication for disseminating results is the so-called "clinical alert". This mechanism has been used by the National Institutes of Health since 1988 to make practitioners and researchers aware of trial results that appear to have great public health importance. The clinical alert is an abbreviated non-peer-reviewed report distributed to health professionals through direct mail or other means. The communication summarizes the trial design and results (there may be more than one study covered) and carries an implication that the conclusions are convincing enough to warrant a change in practice. This mechanism was first used in May 1988 to describe the results of three large trials in women with node-negative breast cancer that showed improvement in relapse-free survival [DeVita, 1991] and several times since then. This way of disseminating results has not been uniformly endorsed by the research community [Borgen, 1991]. See Hellman [1991], Macdonald [1990], Henderson [1990], Friedman [1990], and Wittes [1988] for different points of view.

14.6 Summary

There are many reasons for clinical investigators to focus considerable attention on the written reports of their trials. Because of the importance of the report and the complexity of the scientific issues, it is helpful to adopt standards for content and structure of the paper. The main theme for doing so is to use a logical structure that facilitates a complete and comprehensible paper. The report should allow the quality of the investigation to be evident. Otherwise, trials may not carry the weight of evidence that they should. Investigators cannot rely only on our imperfect peer review mechanism to produce reports of high quality.

The quality of phase I reports has been nearly neglected. They should document a basis for all of the important inferences that need to be made. This includes judging if the recommended dose is appropriate, learning about the pharmacologic or other behaviors of the treatment, and assessing side effects and efficacy. Because it is natural for readers to try to generalize and compare knowledge represented in SE trials, it is important for investigators to minimize the potential for bias and misinterpretation in these reports. This goal is facilitated by a complete accounting of eligible patients and acknowledgment of the limitations of the study design.

Readers of CTE trials will be most interested in the internal and external validity of the findings. Reports that do not facilitate both inferences may leave readers confused or ambivalent about the trial. If so, the findings may have little impact. Because of the strengths of design for most randomized trials, well-written reports of "negative" (no difference) results frequently carry as much or more useful information as "positive" results.

14.7 Questions for Discussion

1. Read or scan the following papers: Prostate Cancer Trialists' Collaborative Group, 1995; Greenberg et al., 1994; Fisher et al., 1989; Non-small Cell Lung Cancer Collaborative Group, 1995; Mountain and Gail, 1981; Sadeghi, Lad, Payne and Rubinstein, 1988; ISIS-4 Collaborative Study Group, 1995. Comment on the strengths and weaknesses of the authorship policy implied by each of them for primary outcome papers and how they are referenced in MedLine.

2. A small consortium of investigators is discussing their authorship policies as part of their formal organization meeting. An opinion is voiced that a biostatistician should be a major contributor to, and author of, all SE and III studies from the group and that this policy should be stated in the group's Constitution. Some clinicians disagree. Give your own opinion and help the

investigators resolve this question. Would your answer change depending on the experience and academic rank of the biostatistician?

3. Design a one-page checklist using the ideas in this chapter for assessing the quality of a published report from a CTE randomized trial. Try your checklist out on at least the following papers and discuss your findings: Rosell, Gomez-Codina, Camps et al., [1994]; Fisher, Agosti, Opal, et al., 1996; Villanueva, Balanzo, Novella, et al., 1996; Spector, McKinley, Lalezari, et al., 1996; Bhasin, Storer, Berman, et al., 1996.

4. Read Sokal [1996a; 1996b] (in that order) and comment on the papers from a peer review perspective.

Chapter References

Abby, M., Massey, M.D., Galandiuk, S., and Polk, H.C., Jr. (1994). Peer review is an effective screening process to evaluate medical manuscripts. JAMA 272: 105-107.

Ad Hoc Working Group for Critical Appraisal of the Medical Literature. (1987). A proposal for more informative abstracts of clinical articles. Ann. Intern. Med. 106: 598-604.

Altman, D.G., Gore, S., Gardner, M., and Pocock, S. (1983). Statistical guidelines for contributors to medical journals. Brit. Med. J. 286: 1489-1493.

Altman, D.G. and Bland, J.M. (1995). Absence of evidence is not evidence of absence. BMJ 311: 485.

Bailar, J. and Mosteller, F. (1988). Guidelines for statistical reporting for medical journals: Amplifications and explanations. Ann. Int. Med. 108: 266-273.

Begg, C. and Berlin, J. (1988). Publication bias: A problem in interpreting medical data (with discussion). J. R. Stat. Soc. A 151: 419-463.

Bhasin, S., Storer, T.W., Berman, N., et al. (1996). The effects of supraphysiologic doses of testosterone on muscle size and strength in normal men. New Engl. J. Med. 335: 1-7.

Bobbio, M., Demichelis, B., and Giustetto, G. (1994). Completeness of reporting trial results: Effect on physicians' willingness to prescribe. Lancet 343: 1209-1211.

Borgen, P.I. (1991). Reviewing peer review: The NCI clinical alert three years later. J. LA. State Med. Soc. 143(3): 39-41.

Chalmers, I. (1990). Underreporting research is scientific misconduct. JAMA 263: 1405-1408.

Cho, M.K. and Bero, L.A. (1994). Instruments for assessing the quality of drug studies published in the medical literature. JAMA 272: 101-104.

DerSimonian, R. Charette, L.J., McPeek, B., and Mosteller, F. (1982). Reporting on methods in clinical trials. New Engl. J. Med. 306: 1332-1337.

Detsky, A.S. and Sackett, D.L. (1985). When was a "negative" clinical trial big enough? Arch. Int. Med. 145: 709-712.

DeVita, V.T. (1991). Is a mechanism such as the NCI's clinical alert ever an appropriate alternative to journal peer review? Important Advances in Oncology : 241-246.

Elting, L.S. and Bodey, G.P. (1991). Is a picture worth a thousand medical words? A randomized trial of reporting formats for medical research data. Methods Inf. Med. 30: 145-150.

Feurer, I.D., Becker, G.J., Picus, D., Ramirez, E., Darcy, M.D., and Hicks, M.E. (1994). Evaluating peer reviews: Pilot testing of a grading instrument. JAMA 272: 98-100.

Fisher, B., Costantino, J., Redmond, C., et al. (1989). A randomized clinical trial evaluating tamoxifen in the treatment of patients with node-negative breast cancer who have estrogen-receptor-positive tumors. New Eng. J. Med. 320: 479-484.

Fisher, C.J., Agosti, J.M., Opal, S.M., et al., (1996). Treatment of septic shock with the tumor necrosis factor receptor:Fc fusion protein. New Engl. J. Med. 334: 1697-1702.

Forrow, L., Taylor, W.C., and Arnold, R.M. (1992). Absolutely relative: How research results are summarized can affect treatment decisions. Am. J. Med. 92: 121-124.

Freiman, J.A., Chalmers, T.C., Smith, H., and Kuebler, R.R. (1978). The importance of beta, the type II error, and sample size in the design and interpretation of the randomized controlled trial: Survey of 71 "negative" trials. New Eng. J. Med. 299: 690-694.

Friedman, M.A. (1990). If not now, when? JNCI 82: 106-108.

Gardner, M.J., Machin, D., and Campbell, M.J. (1986). Use of checklists in assessing the statistical content of medical studies. BMJ 292: 810-812.

Gehlbach, S.H. (1988). Interpreting the Medical Literature: Practial Epidemiology for Clinicians, Second Edition. New York: Macmillan.

Gore, S.M., Jones, G., and Thompson, S.G. (1992). The Lancet's statistical review process: Areas for improvement by authors. Lancet 340: 100-102.

Gøtzsche, P.C. (1989). Methodology and overt and hidden bias in reports of 196 double-blind trials of nonsteroidal anti-inflammatory drugs in rheumatoid arthritis. Controlled Clinical Trials 10: 31-56. Correction (1989) 10: 356.

Grant, A. (1989). Reporting controlled trials. Br. J. Obstet. Gynaecol. 96: 397-400.

Greenberg, E.R., Baron, J.A., Tosteson, T.D., et al. (1994). A clinical trial of antioxidant vitamins to prevent colorectal adenoma. New Engl. J. Med. 331: 141-147.

Haynes, R.B., Mulrow, C.D., Huth, E.J., Altman, D.G., and Gardner, M.J. (1990). More informative abstracts revisited. Ann. Intern. Med. 113: 69-76.

Hellman, S. (1991). Clinical alert: A poor idea prematurely used. Important Advances in Oncology : 255-257.

Henderson, I.C. (1990). Shouldn't we see the white flag before we cry victory? JNCI 82: 103-109.

International Committee of Medical Journal Editors. (1993). Uniform requirements for manuscripts submitted to biomedical journals. JAMA 269: 2282-6.

International Conference on Harmonisation (1995). Structure and Content of Clinical Study
Reports. Draft Consensus Guideline. Geneva: ICH Secretariat (c/o IFPMA).

ISIS-4 Collaborative Group (1995). ISIS-4: A randomized factorial trial assessing early captopril, oral mononitrate, and intravenous magnesium sulphate in 58,050 patients with
suspected acute myocardial infarction. Lancet 345: 669-685.

Iyengar, S. and Greenhouse, J.B. (1988). Selection models and the file drawer problem (with
discussion). Stat. Sci. 3: 109-135.

Judson, H.F. (1994). Structural transformations of the sciences and the end of peer review.
JAMA 272: 92-95.

Kassirer, J.P. and Campion, E.W. (1994). Peer review: Crude and understudied but indispensable.. JAMA 272: 96-97.

Kemper, K.J. (1990). Pride and prejudice in peer review. J. Clin. Epidemiol. 44: 343-345.

Macdonald, J.S. (1990). Sometimes a great notion. JNCI 82: 102-104.

Mahon, W.A. and Daniel, E.E. (1964). A method for the assessment of the reports of drug
trials. Can. Med. Assoc. J. 90: 565-569.

Meinert, C.L. (1986). Clinical Trials: Design, Conduct, and Analysis. Oxford: Oxford University Press.

Moher, D., Dulberg, C.S., and Wells, G.A. (1994). Statistical power, sample size, and their
reporting in randomized controlled trials. JAMA 272: 122-124.

Mosteller, F., Gilbert, J., and McPeek, B. (1980). Reporting standards and research strategies
for controlled clinical trials; agenda for the editor. Controlled Clin. Trials 1: 37-58.

Mountain, C.F. and Gail, M.H. (1981). Surgical adjuvant intrapleural BCG treatment for stage
I non-small cell lung cancer. Preliminary report of the National Cancer Institute Lung
Cancer Study Group. J. Thorac. Cardiovasc. Surg. 82: 649-657.

Murray, G.D. (1991). Statistical aspects of research methodology. Br. J. Surg. 78: 777-781.

Naylor, C.D., Chen, E., and Strauss, B. (1992). Measured enthusiasm: Does the method of
reporting trial results alter perception of therapeutic effectiveness? Ann. Intern. Med.
117: 916-921.

Non-small Cell Lung Cancer Collaborative Group (1995). Chemotherapy in non-small cell
lung cancer: A meta-analysis using updated data on individual patients from 52 randomised clinical trials. BMJ 311: 899-909.

Oliver, S.G., van der Aart, Q.J.M., Agostoni-Carbone, M. L., et al. (1992). The complete
DNA sequence of yeast chromosome III. Nature 357: 38-46.

Pocock, S.J., Hughs, M.D., and Lee, R.J. (1987). Statistical problems in the reporting of
clinical trials. New Engl. J. Med. 317: 426-432.

Prostate Cancer Trialists' Collaborative Group (1995). Maximum androgen blockade in advanced prostate cancer: An overview of 22 randomised trials with 3283 deaths in 5710 patients. Lancet 346: 265-269.

Rochon, P.A., Gurwitz, J.H., Cheung, M., Hayes, J.A., and Chalmers, T.C. (1994). Evaluating the quality of articles published in journal supplements compared with the quality of those published in the parent journal. JAMA 272: 108-113.

Rosell, R., Gomez-Codina, J., Camps, C., et al. (1994). A randomized trial comparing preoperative chemotherapy plus surgery with surgery alone in patients with non-small-cell lung cancer. New Engl. J. Med. 330: 153-158.

Sadeghi, A., Lad, T., Payne, D., and Rubinstein, L. and the Lung Cancer Study Group (1988). Combined modality treatment for resected advanced non-small cell lung cancer: Local control and local recurrence. Int. J. Radiat. Oncol. Biol. Phys. 15: 89-97.

Schulz, K.F., Chalmers, I., Hayes, R.J. and Altman, D.G. (1995). Empirical evidence of bias: Dimensions of methodologic quality associated with estimates of treatment effects in controlled trials. JAMA 273: 408-412.

Sokal, A.D. (1996a). Transgressing the boundaries: Toward a transformative hermeneutics of quantum gravity. Social Text 14: 217-251.

Sokal, A.D. (1996b). A physicist experiments with cultural studies. Lingua Franca: May/June.

Spector, S.A., McKinley, G.F., Lalezari, J.P., et al., (1996). Oral ganciclovir for the prevention of cytomegalovirus disease in persons with AIDS. Roche Cooperative Oral Ganciclovir Study Group. New Engl. J. Med. 334(23): 1491-1497.

Standards of Reporting Trials Group. (1994). A proposal for structured reporting of randomized controlled trials. JAMA 272: 1926-1931. Correction: 273: 776.

Villanueva, C., Balanzo, J., Novella, M.T., et al., (1996). Nadolol plus isosorbide mononitrate compared with sclerotherapy for the prevention of variceal rebleeding. New Engl. J. Med. 334: 1624-1629.

Waldhausen, J.A. and Localio, A.R. (1996). Notes from the editors. J. Thorac Cardiovasc. Surg. 112: 209-220.

Walter, S.D. (1995). Methods of reporting statistical results from medical research studies. Am. J. Epidemiol. 141: 896-906.

Weymuller, E.A. and Goepfert, H. (1991). Uniformity of results reporting in head and neck cancer (editorial). Head & Neck, July/August: 275-277. Reprinted in Laryngoscope 104: 784-785.

Williams, D.H. and Davis, C.E. (1994). Reporting of treatment assignment methods in clinical trials. Controlled Clin. Trials 15: 294-298.

Winget, M.D. (1996). Selected Issues Related to the Conduct, Reporting, and Analysis of Phase I Trials. Ph.D. Dissertation, Johns Hopkins University.

Wittes, R.E. (1988). Of clinical alerts and peer review (editorial). JNCI 80: 984-985.

Working Group on Recommendations for Reporting Clinical Trials in the Biomedical Literature (1994). Call for comments on a proposal to improve reporting of clinical trials in the biomedical literature: Position paper. Ann. Intern. Med. 121: 894-895.

Zelen, M. (1983). Guidelines for publishing papers on cancer clinical trials: Responsibilities of editors and authors. J. Clin. Oncol. 1: 164-169.

CHAPTER 15

Factorial Designs

15.1 Introduction

Factorial clinical trials are experiments that test the effect of more than one treatment using a design that permits an assessment of interactions among the treatments. The name arises because, historically, the control variables have been called *factors* rather than *treatments* as in most medical applications. A factor can have more than one *level*. For example, when studying drugs, a *factor* could be either a single drug or a combination of drugs. Different doses of the same drug would be factor *levels*. The essential feature of factorial designs is that all factors are varied systematically (i.e., some groups receive more than one treatment) and the experimental groups are arranged in a way that permits testing if the combination of treatments is better (or worse) than individual treatments. Some simple examples are given below.

The technique of varying more than one factor or treatment in a single study was used in agricultural experiments in England before 1900. The method did not become popular until developed further by R. A. Fisher [1935; 1960] and Yates [1935], but since then it has been used to great advantage in both agricultural and industrial experiments. Influential and more recent discussions of factorial experiments are given by Cox [1958] and Snedecor and Cochran [1980]. Factorial designs have been used relatively infrequently in medical trials, except recently in disease prevention studies.

Factorial designs offer certain advantages over conventional comparative designs, even those employing more than two treatment arms. The factorial structure permits certain comparisons to be made that cannot be achieved by any other design. In some circumstances, two treatments can be tested using the same number of subjects ordinarily used to test a single treatment. However, in spite of their potential advantages, factorial designs have important limitations. These must be understood before deciding if a factorial experiment is the best design to employ for a particular therapeutic question. More complete discussions of factorial designs in clinical trials can be found in Byar and Piantadosi [1985] and Byar, Herzberg, and Tan [1993]. For

388

Table 15.1 Four Treatment Groups and Sample Sizes in a 2×2 Balanced Factorial Design

Treatment	Treatment B		
A	No	Yes	Total
No	n	n	$2n$
Yes	n	n	$2n$
Total	$2n$	$2n$	$4n$

a discussion of such designs related to cardiology trials, particularly in the context of the ISIS-4 trial [Flather et al., 1994], see Lubsen and Pocock [1994].

15.2 Characteristics of Factorial Designs

15.2.1 Factorial designs are defined by their structure

The quickest way to learn the basic features of a factorial design is to study an example. The least complex factorial design has 2 treatments (A and B) and 4 treatment groups (Table 15.1). There might be n patients entered into each of the 4 treatment groups for a total sample size of $4n$ and a balanced design. One group receives neither A nor B, a second receives both A and B, and the other two groups receive one of A or B. This is called a 2×2 (two by two) factorial design. Although basic, this design illustrates many of the general features of factorial experiments. The design generates enough information to test the effects of A alone, B alone, and A plus B. The efficiencies in doing so will be presented below.

The 2×2 design generalizes to "higher-order" designs in a straightforward manner. For example, a factorial design studying 3 treatments, A, B, and C is the $2 \times 2 \times 2$. Possible treatment groups for this design are shown in Table 15.2. The design can also be depicted as a cubic array of treatment cells (Figure 15.1). The total sample size is $8n$ if all treatment groups have n subjects.

Aside from illustrating the factorial structure, these examples highlight some of the prerequisites necessary for, and restrictions on, using a factorial trial. First, the treatments must be amenable to being administered in combination without changing dosage in the presence of each other. For example, in Table 15.1, we would not want to reduce the dose of A in the lower right cell where B is present. The reasons for this will become more clear below. This requirement implies that the side effects of the treatments cannot be cumulative to the point where the combination would be impossible to administer.

Second, it must be ethically acceptable not to administer the individual treatments, or administer them at lower doses as the case may be. In some situations, this means having a no-treatment or placebo group in the trial. In other cases, A and B may be administered in addition to a "standard", so that all groups receive some treatment. Third, we must be genuinely interested in learning about treatment com-

Table 15.2 Eight Treatment Groups in a Balanced $2 \times 2 \times 2$**Factorial Design**

Group	A	B	C	Sample Size
	Treatments			
1	No	No	No	n
2	Yes	No	No	n
3	No	Yes	No	n
4	No	No	Yes	n
5	Yes	Yes	No	n
6	No	Yes	Yes	n
7	Yes	No	Yes	n
8	Yes	Yes	Yes	n

binations or else some of the treatment groups might be unnecessary. Alternatively, to use the design to achieve greater efficiency in studying two or more treatments, we must know that some interactions do not exist.

Fourth, the therapeutic questions must be chosen appropriately. We would not use a factorial design to test treatments that have exactly the same mechanisms of action (e.g., two ACE inhibitors for high blood pressure) because either would answer the question. Treatments acting through different mechanisms would be more appropriate for a factorial design (e.g., radiotherapy and chemotherapy for tumors). In some prevention factorial trials, the treatments tested also target different diseases.

15.2.2 Factorial designs are efficient

Although their scope is limited, factorial designs offer certain very important efficiencies or advantages when they are applicable. To illustrate this, consider the 2×2 design and the estimates of treatment effects that would result using an additive model for analysis (Table 15.3). Assume that the responses are group averages of some normally distributed response denoted by $\overline{Y}$. The subscripts on $\overline{Y}$ indicate which treatment group it represents. Note that half the patients receive one of the treatments (this is also true in higher-order designs). For a moment, further assume that the effect of A is not influenced by the presence of B.

There are two estimates of the effect of treatment A compared with placebo in the design, $\overline{Y}_A - \overline{Y}_0$ and $Y_{AB} - \overline{Y}_B$. If B does not modify the effect of A, it is sensible to combine (average) them to estimate the overall, or main, effect of A (denoted here by β_A),

$$\beta_A = \frac{(\overline{Y}_A - \overline{Y}_0) + (\overline{Y}_{AB} - \overline{Y}_B)}{2} . \tag{15.1}$$

Similarly,

$$\beta_B = \frac{(\overline{Y}_B - \overline{Y}_0) + (\overline{Y}_{AB} - \overline{Y}_A)}{2} . \tag{15.2}$$

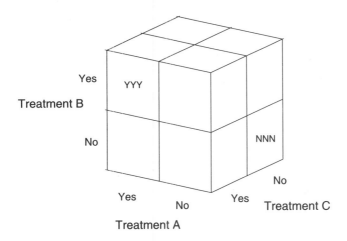

Figure 15.1 Structure of a $2 \times 2 \times 2$ factorial design. The cell with no treatments and the cell with all three treatments are labeled.

Thus, in the absence of interactions (i.e., the effect of A is the same with or without B and vice-versa), the design permits the full sample size to be used to estimate two treatment effects.

Now suppose that each patient's response has a variance σ^2 and that it is the same in all treatment groups. We can calculate the variance of β_A to be

$$Var(\beta_A) = \frac{1}{4} \times \frac{4\sigma^2}{n} = \frac{\sigma^2}{n} .$$

This is exactly the same variance that would result if A were tested against placebo in a single two-armed comparative trial with $2n$ patients in each treatment group. Similarly,

$$Var(\beta_B) = \frac{\sigma^2}{n} .$$

However, if we tested A and B separately, we would require $4n$ subjects in each trial or a total of $8n$ patients to have the same precision obtained from half as many patients in the factorial design. Thus, in the absence of interactions, these designs allow great efficiency in estimating main effects. In fact, in the absence of interaction, we get two trials for the price of one. Tests of both A and B can be conducted in a sin-

Table 15.3 Treatment Effects in a 2×2 Factorial Design

Treatment A	Treatment B	
	No	Yes
No	$\overline{Y}_0$	$\overline{Y}_B$
Yes	$\overline{Y}_A$	$\overline{Y}_{AB}$

gle factorial trial with the same precision as two single-factor trials using twice the sample size.

15.3 Interactions

We consider more general circumstances now where the effect of A might be influenced by the presence of B (or vice versa). In other words, there might be a *treatment interaction*. Some of the efficiencies just discussed will be lost. However, factorial designs are even more relevant in such cases.

15.3.1 Factorial designs are the only way to study interactions

One of the most consequential features of factorial designs is that they are the only type of trial design that permits study of treatment interactions. This is because the design has treatment groups with all possible combinations of treatments, allowing the responses to be compared directly. Consider again the two estimates of A in the 2×2 design, one in the presence of B and the other in the absence of B. The definition of an interaction is that the effect of A in the absence of B is different from the effect of A in the presence of B. This can be estimated by comparing

$$\beta_{AB} = (\overline{Y}_A - \overline{Y}_0) - (\overline{Y}_{AB} - \overline{Y}_B) \qquad (15.3)$$

with zero. If β_{AB} is near zero, we would conclude that no interaction is present. It is straightforward to verify that $\beta_{AB} = \beta_{BA}$.

When there is an AB interaction present, we cannot use the estimators given above for the main effects of A and B (equations 15.1 and 15.2) because they assume no interaction is present. Instead, we would employ

$$\beta'_A = (\overline{Y}_A - \overline{Y}_0) \qquad (15.4)$$

and

$$\beta'_B = (\overline{Y}_B - \overline{Y}_0). \qquad (15.5)$$

A more detailed look at estimators in the presence of interactions is given below.

In the $2 \times 2 \times 2$ design, there are three main effects and four interactions possible, all of which can be tested by the design. Following the notation above, the effects are

$$\beta_A = \frac{1}{4} \left[(\overline{Y}_A - \overline{Y}_0) + (\overline{Y}_{AB} - \overline{Y}_B) + (\overline{Y}_{AC} - \overline{Y}_C) + (\overline{Y}_{ABC} - \overline{Y}_{BC}) \right],$$
(15.6)

for treatment A,

$$\beta_{AB} = \frac{1}{2} \left[((\overline{Y}_A - \overline{Y}_0) - (\overline{Y}_{AB} - \overline{Y}_B)) + ((\overline{Y}_{AC} - \overline{Y}_C) - (\overline{Y}_{ABC} - \overline{Y}_{BC})) \right],$$
(15.7)

for the AB interaction, and

$$\beta_{ABC} = \left[(\overline{Y}_A - \overline{Y}_0) - (\overline{Y}_{AB} - \overline{Y}_B) - (\overline{Y}_{AC} - \overline{Y}_C) - (\overline{Y}_{ABC} - \overline{Y}_{BC}) \right]$$
(15.8)

for the ABC interaction.

When certain interactions are present, we may require an alternative estimator for β_A or β_{BA} (or for other effects). Suppose there is evidence of an ABC interaction. Then, instead of β_A, an estimator of the main effect of A would be

$$\beta'_A = \frac{1}{2} \left[(\overline{Y}_A - \overline{Y}_0) + (\overline{Y}_{AB} - \overline{Y}_B) \right],$$

which does not use β_{ABC}. Similarly, the AB interaction would be tested by

$$\beta'_{AB} = (\overline{Y}_A - \overline{Y}_0) - (\overline{Y}_{AB} - \overline{Y}_B)$$

for the same reason. Thus, when treatment interactions are present, we must modify our estimates of main effects and lower-order interactions, losing some efficiency. However, these designs are the only ones that permit treatment interactions to be studied.

15.3.2 Interactions depend on the scale of measurement

In the examples just given, the treatment effects and interactions have been assumed to exist on an additive scale. This is reflected in the use of sums and differences in the formulae for estimation. In practice, other scales of measurement, particularly a multiplicative one, may be useful. As an example, consider the response data in Table 15.4 where the effect of Treatment A is to increase the baseline response by 5 units. The same is true of B and there is no interaction between the treatments on this scale, because the joint effect of A and B is to increase the response by $5 + 5 = 10$ units.

In contrast, Table 15.5 shows data in which the effects of both treatments are to multiply the baseline response by 2.0. Hence, the combined effect of A and B is a fourfold increase, which is greater than the joint treatment effect for the additive case. If the analysis model were multiplicative, Table 15.4 would show an interaction, whereas if the analysis model were additive, Table 15.5 would show an interaction. Thus, to discuss interactions, we must establish the scale of measurement.

Table 15.4 Response Data from a Hypothetical Factorial Trial Showing No Interaction on an Additive Scale of Measurement

Treatment	Treatment B	
A	No	Yes
No	5	10
Yes	10	15

15.3.3 The interpretation of main effects depends on interactions

In the presence of an interaction in the 2×2 design, one cannot speak about an overall, or main, effect of either treatment. This is because the effect of A is different depending on the presence or absence of B. In the presence of a small interaction, where all patients benefit regardless of the use of B, we might observe that the magnitude of the "overall" effect of A is of some size and that therapeutic decisions are unaffected by the presence of an interaction. This is a so-called "quantitative" interaction, because it does not affect the direction of the treatment effect. For large quantitative interactions, it may not be sensible to talk about overall effects.

In contrast, if the presence of B reverses the effects of A, then the interaction is "qualitative", and treatment decisions may need to be modified. Here we would not talk about an overall effect of A, because it could be positive in the presence of B and negative in the absence of B, and could yield an average effect near zero.

15.3.4 Analyses can employ linear models

Motivation for the estimators given above can be obtained using linear models. There has been little theoretical work on analyses using other models. One exception is the work by Slud [1994], describing approaches to factorial trials with survival outcomes. Suppose we have conducted a 2×2 factorial experiment with group sizes given by Table 15.1. We can estimate the AB interaction effect using a linear model of the form

$$E\{Y\} = \beta_0 + \beta_A X_A + \beta_B X_B + \beta_{AB} X_A X_B, \qquad (15.9)$$

where the X's are indicator variables for the treatment groups and β_{AB} is the interaction effect. For example,

$$X_A = \begin{cases} 1, & \textit{for treatment group } A \\ 0, & \textit{otherwise} \end{cases}.$$

The design matrix has dimension $4n \times 4$ and is

$$\mathbf{X}' = \begin{bmatrix} 1 & \dots & 1 & \dots & 1 & \dots & 1 & \dots \\ 0 & \dots & 1 & \dots & 0 & \dots & 1 & \dots \\ 0 & \dots & 0 & \dots & 1 & \dots & 1 & \dots \\ 0 & \dots & 0 & \dots & 0 & \dots & 1 & \dots \end{bmatrix},$$

Table 15.5 Response Data from a Hypothetical Factorial Trial Showing No Interaction on a Multiplicative Scale of Measurement

Treatment A	Treatment B	
	No	Yes
No	5	10
Yes	10	20

where there are 4 blocks of n identical rows representing each treatment group and the columns represent effects for the intercept, treatment A, treatment B, and both treatments, respectively. The vector of responses has dimension $4n \times 1$ and is

$$\mathbf{Y}' = \{Y_{01}, \ldots, Y_{A1}, \ldots, Y_{B1}, \ldots, Y_{AB1}, \ldots\}.$$

Using ordinary least squares estimation, the solution to equation 15.9 is

$$\widehat{\boldsymbol{\beta}} = (\mathbf{X}'\mathbf{X})^{-1}\mathbf{X}'\mathbf{Y}.$$

When the interaction effect is omitted, the estimates will be denoted by $\widehat{\boldsymbol{\beta}^*}$. The covariance matrix of estimates is $(\mathbf{X}'\mathbf{X})^{-1}\sigma^2$, where the variance of each observation is σ^2.

We have

$$\mathbf{X}'\mathbf{X} = n \times \begin{bmatrix} 4 & 2 & 2 & 1 \\ 2 & 2 & 1 & 1 \\ 2 & 1 & 2 & 1 \\ 1 & 1 & 1 & 1 \end{bmatrix}, \qquad (\mathbf{X}'\mathbf{X})^{-1} = \frac{1}{n} \times \begin{bmatrix} 1 & -1 & -1 & 1 \\ -1 & 2 & 1 & -2 \\ -1 & 1 & 2 & -2 \\ 1 & -2 & -2 & 4 \end{bmatrix},$$

and

$$\mathbf{X}'\mathbf{Y} = n \times \begin{bmatrix} \overline{Y}_0 + \overline{Y}_A + \overline{Y}_B + \overline{Y}_{AB} \\ \overline{Y}_A + \overline{Y}_{AB} \\ \overline{Y}_B + \overline{Y}_{AB} \\ \overline{Y}_{AB} \end{bmatrix},$$

where $\overline{Y}_i$ denotes the average response in the ith group. Then,

$$\widehat{\boldsymbol{\beta}} = \begin{bmatrix} \overline{Y}_0 \\ -\overline{Y}_0 + \overline{Y}_A \\ -\overline{Y}_0 + \overline{Y}_B \\ \overline{Y}_0 - \overline{Y}_A - \overline{Y}_B + \overline{Y}_{AB} \end{bmatrix}, \qquad (15.10)$$

which corresponds to the estimators given above in equations 15.3–15.5. However, if the test for interaction fails to reject and the β_{AB} effect is removed from the model,

$$\widehat{\boldsymbol{\beta^*}} = \begin{bmatrix} \frac{3}{4}\overline{Y}_0 + \frac{1}{4}\overline{Y}_A + \frac{1}{4}\overline{Y}_B - \frac{1}{4}\overline{Y}_{AB} \\ -\frac{1}{2}\overline{Y}_0 + \frac{1}{2}\overline{Y}_A - \frac{1}{2}\overline{Y}_B + \frac{1}{2}\overline{Y}_{AB} \\ -\frac{1}{2}\overline{Y}_0 - \frac{1}{2}\overline{Y}_A + \frac{1}{2}\overline{Y}_B + \frac{1}{2}\overline{Y}_{AB} \end{bmatrix}.$$

The main effects for A and B are as given above in equations 15.1 and 15.2.

The covariance matrices for these estimators are

$$\widehat{Cov\{\boldsymbol{\beta}\}} = \frac{\sigma^2}{n} \times \begin{bmatrix} 1 & -1 & -1 & 1 \\ -1 & 2 & 1 & -2 \\ -1 & 1 & 2 & -2 \\ 1 & -2 & -2 & 4 \end{bmatrix}$$

and

$$\widehat{Cov\{\boldsymbol{\beta^*}\}} = \frac{\sigma^2}{n} \times \begin{bmatrix} \frac{3}{4} & -\frac{1}{2} & -\frac{1}{2} \\ -\frac{1}{2} & 1 & 0 \\ -\frac{1}{2} & 0 & 1 \end{bmatrix}.$$

In the absence of an interaction, the main effects of A and B are estimated independently and with higher precision than when an interaction is present. The interaction effect is relatively imprecisely estimated, indicating the larger sample sizes required to have a high power to detect such effects.

15.4 Examples of Factorial Designs

15.4.1 Important trials have used these designs

Several clinical trials conducted in recent years have used factorial designs (Table 15.6). The studies employing these designs tend to be prevention trials for reasons outlined above. One important study using a 2×2 factorial design is the Physicians' Health Study [Hennekens and Eberlein, 1985; Stampfer et al., 1985]. This trial has been conducted in 22,000 physicians in the U.S. and was designed to test the effects of 1) aspirin on reducing cardiovascular mortality, and 2) β-carotene on reducing cancer incidence. The trial is noteworthy in several ways, including its test of two interventions in unrelated diseases, use of physicians as subjects to report outcomes reliably, relatively low cost, and an all-male (high-risk) study population. This last characteristic has led to some criticism, which is probably unwarranted.

In January 1988, the aspirin component of the Physicians' Health Study was discontinued, because evidence demonstrated convincingly that it was associated with lower rates of myocardial infarction [Steering Committee of the Physicians' Health Study Research Group, 1989]. The question concerning the effect of β-carotene on cancer remains open and will be addressed by continuation of the trial. In the likely

Table 15.6 Some Recent Randomized Clinical Trials UsingFactorial Designs

Trial	Design	Reference
SWOG 8300	2×2	Miller et al., 1995
Physicians' Health Study	2×2	Hennekens and Eberlein, 1985
ATBC Prevention Trial	2×2	Heinonen et al., 1987
Desipramine	2×2	Max et al., 1992
Biofeedback/relaxation	2×2	Burish and Jenkins, 1992
ACAPS	2×2	ACAPS Group, 1992
Linxian Nutrition Trial	2^4 *	Li et al., 1993
Taxol	2×2	ten Bokkel Huinink et al., 1993
Retinitis pigmentosa	2×2	Berson et al., 1993
Artificial insemination	2^3	Karlstrom et al., 1993
Linxian Cataract Trial		Sperduto et al., 1993
Tocopherol/deprenyl	2×2	Parkinson Study Group, 1993
Womens' Health Initiative	2^3 *	Assaf and Carleton, 1994
Polyp Prevention Trial	2×2	Greenberg et al., 1994
Cancer/eye disease	2×2	Green et al., 1994
Cilazapril/hydrochlorthiazide	4×3	Pordy, 1994
Tropisetron	2^3	Hulstaert et al., 1994
Nebivolol	4×3	Lacourciere et al., 1994
WACS	2^3	Manson et al., 1995
Endophthalmitis vitrectomy	2×2	Endophth. Vitrectomy Study Group, 1995
Bicalutamide/flutamide	2×2	Schellhammer et al., 1995
Music/scents	3×3	Becker et al., 1995
ISIS-4	2^3	ISIS-4 Collaborative Group, 1996
Testosterone/exercise	2×2	Bhasin et al., 1996

* Denotes a partial replicate. The list is not comprehensive, but illustrates the scope of application.

absence of an interaction between aspirin and β-carotene, the second major question of the trial will be unaffected by the closure of the aspirin component.

Another interesting example of a 2×2 factorial design is the α-tocopherol β-carotene Lung Cancer Prevention Trial, conducted in 29,133 male smokers in Finland between 1987 and 1994 [Heinonen et al., 1987; The ATBC Cancer Prevention Study Group, 1994a]. In this study, lung cancer incidence is the sole outcome. It was thought possible that lung cancer incidence could be reduced by either or both interventions. When this trial was stopped in 1994, there were 876 new cases of lung cancer in the study population during the trial. Alpha-tocopherol was not associated with a reduction in the risk of cancer. Surprisingly, β-carotene was associated with a statistically significantly *increased* incidence of lung cancer [ATBC Cancer Prevention Study Group, 1994b]. There was no evidence of a treatment interaction. The unexpected findings of this study have been supported by the recent results of another large trial of carotene and retinol [Thornquist et al., 1993].

The Fourth International Study of Infarct Survival (ISIS-4) was a $2 \times 2 \times 2$ factorial trial assessing the efficacy of oral captopril, oral mononitrate, and intravenous magnesium sulphate in 58,050 patients with suspected myocardial infarction [ISIS-4 Collaborative Group, 1995; Flather et al., 1994]. No significant interactions among the treatments were found and each main effect comparison was based on approximately 29,000 treated versus 29,000 control patients. Among the findings was demonstration that captopril was associated with a small but statistically significant reduction in five week mortality. The difference in mortality was 7.19% versus 7.69% (143 events out of 4319), illustrating the ability of large studies to detect potentially important treatment effects, even when they are small in relative magnitude. Mononitrate and magnesium therapy did not significantly reduce five week mortality.

15.5 Partial (Fractional) Factorial Designs

15.5.1 Use partial factorial designs when interactions are absent

Partial, or fractional, factorial designs are those that omit certain treatment groups by design. A careful analysis of the objectives of an experiment, its efficiency, and the effects it can estimate may justify not using some groups. Because many cells contribute to the estimate of any effect, a design may achieve its intended purpose without some of the cells.

In the 2×2 design, all treatment groups must be present to permit estimating the interaction between A and B. However, for higher-order designs, if some interactions are known biologically not to exist, certain treatment combinations can be omitted from the design and still permit estimates of other effects of interest. For example, in the $2 \times 2 \times 2$ design, if the interaction between A, B, and C is known not to exist, that treatment cell could be omitted from the design and still permit estimation of all the main effects. The efficiency would be somewhat reduced, however. Similarly, the two-way interactions could still be estimated without $\overline{Y}_{ABC}$. This can be verified from the formulae above.

More generally, partial high order designs will produce a situation termed "aliasing" in which the estimates of certain effects are algebraically identical to completely different effects. If both are biologically possible, the design will not be able to reveal which effect is being estimated. Naturally, this is undesirable unless additional information is available to the investigator to indicate that some aliased effects are zero. This can be used to advantage in improving efficiency and one must be careful in deciding which cells to exclude. See Cox [1958] or Mason and Gunst [1989] for a discussion of this topic.

The Women's Health Initiative clinical trial is a $2 \times 2 \times 2$ partial factorial design study the effects of hormone replacement, dietary fat reduction, and calcium and vitamin D on coronary disease, breast cancer, and osteoporosis [Assaf and Carleton,

1994]. The study is expected to accrue over 64,000 patients and is projected to finish in the year 2007. The dietary component of the study will randomize 48,000 women, using a 3:2 allocation ratio in favor of the control arm and nine years of follow-up. Such a large and complex trial is not without controversy (e.g., Marshall, [1993]) and presents logistical difficulties, questions about adherence, and sensitivity of the intended power to assumptions that can only roughly be validated.

15.6   Incomplete Factorial Designs

15.6.1 Incomplete designs present special problems

Treatment groups can be dropped out of factorial plans without yielding a fractional replication. The resulting trials have been called "incomplete factorial designs" [Byar, Herzberg, and Tan, 1993]. In incomplete designs, cells are not missing by design intent, but because some treatment combinations may be infeasible. For example, in a 2×2 design, it may not be ethically possible to use a placebo group. In this case, one would not be able to estimate the AB interaction. In other circumstances, unwanted aliasing may occur, or the efficiency of the design to estimate main effects may be greatly reduced. In some cases, estimators of treatment and interaction effects are biased, but there may be reasons to use a design that retains as much of the factorial structure as possible. For example, they may be the only way to estimate certain interactions.

15.7   Summary

Factorial trial designs are useful in two circumstances. When two or more treatments do not interact, factorial designs can test the main effects of each using smaller sample sizes and greater precision than separate parallel groups designs. When it is essential to study treatment interactions, factorial designs are the only way to do so. The precision with which interaction effects are estimated is lower than that for main effects (in the absence of interactions), but these designs are the only ones that allow study of interactions.

When there are many treatments or factors, these designs require a relatively large number of treatment groups. In complex designs, if some interactions are known not to exist or are unimportant, it may be possible to omit some treatment groups, reduce the size and complexity of the experiment, and still estimate all of the effects of biological interest. Extra attention to the design properties is need to be certain that fractional designs will meet the intended objectives. Such fractional or partial factorial designs are of considerable use in agricultural and industrial experiments, but have not been applied frequently to clinical trials.

Ethical and toxicity constraints may make it impossible to apply either a full factorial or a fractional factorial design, yielding an incomplete design. The properties of incomplete factorial designs have not been studied extensively, but they may be the best design in some circumstances.

A number of important, complex, and recent clinical trials have used factorial designs. Because of the low potential for toxicity, these designs have been more frequently applied in studies of disease prevention. Examples include the Physicians' Health Study and the Womens' Health Trial. In medical studies, the design is employed usually to achieve greater efficiency, i.e., because the treatments are unlikely to interact.

15.8 Questions for Discussion

1. For the $2 \times 2 \times 2$ factorial design, repeat the calculation of least squares estimates from a linear model using a suitable design matrix. Do you obtain equations 15.6–15.8? Explain your findings.

2. Repeat the exercise omitting some or all interaction terms. Explain your findings.

3. Suppose a woman meets all of the eligibility criteria, except sex, for the Physicians' Health Study. Should she be treated with aspirin? Assume there are no contraindications and no other information about efficacy is available. Justify your answer.

4. Seasickness is a condition that is difficult to prevent and treat although many remedies have been suggested including drugs (e.g., oral meclizine and/or scopalamine patches), wrist bands, and applying tape over the navel (with or without an aspirin tablet!). Discuss the setting and a design for a trial testing these preventives. How will you control important factors such as age, history of previous episodes, diet, environmental factors, state of mind, and the placebo effect?

Chapter References

ACAPS Group. (1992). Rationale and design for the Asymptomatic Carotid Artery Plaque Study (ACAPS). Controlled Clin. Trials 13: 293-314.

Armitage, P., and Berry, G. (1994). Statistical Methods in Medical Research, 3rd Edition. Oxford: Blackwell.

Assaf, A.R. and Carleton, R.A. (1994). The Women's Health Initiative clinical trial and observational study: History and overview. Rhode Island Medicine 77: 424-427.

ATBC Cancer Prevention Study Group (1994a). The alpha-tocopherol beta-carotene lung cancer prevention study: Design, methods, participant characteristics, and compliance. Ann. Epidemiol. 4: 1-9.

ATBC Cancer Prevention Study Group (1994b). The effect of vitamin E and beta carotene on the incidence of lung cancer and other cancers in male smokers. New Engl. J. Med. 330: 1029-1034.

Becker, N., Chambliss, C., Marsh, C., and Montemayor, R. (1995). Effects of mellow and frenetic music and stimulating and relaxing scents on walking by seniors. Perceptual & Motor Skills 80: 411-415.

Berson, E.L., Rosner, B., Sandberg, M.A., Hayes, K.C., Nicholson, B.W., Weigel-DiFranco, C., and Willet, W. (1993). A randomized trial of vitamin A and vitamin E supplementation for retinitis pigmentosa. Arch. Ophthalmol. 111: 761-772.

Bhasin, S., Storer, T.W., Berman, N., et al. (1996). The effects of supraphysiologic doses of testosterone on muscle size and strength in normal men. New Engl. J. Med. 335: 1-7.

Burish, T.G. and Jenkins, R.A. (1992). Effectiveness of biofeedback and relaxation training in reducing the side effects of cancer chemotherapy. Health Psychol. 11: 17-23.

Byar, D.P. (1990). Factorial and reciprocal control designs. Statistics in Med. 9: 55-64.

Byar, D.P., Herzberg, A.M., and Tan, W-Y. (1993). Incomplete factorial designs for randomized clinical trials. Statistics in Med. 12: 1629-1641.

Byar, D.P., and Piantadosi, S. (1985). Factorial designs for randomized clinical trials. Cancer Treatment Rep 69: 1055-1063.

Cox, D.R. (1958). Planning of Experiments. New York: John Wiley & Sons.

Dodge, Y., and Afsarinejad, K. (1985). Minimal 2 connected factorial experiments. Comput Stat and Data Analysis 3: 187-200.

Endophthalmitis Vitrectomy Study Group (1995). Results of the Endophthalmitis Vitrectomy Study. A randomized trial of immediate vitrectomy and of intravenous antibiotics for the treatment of postoperative bacterial endophthalmitis. Archives Ophthalmol. 113: 1479-1496.

Fisher, R.A. (1935). The Design of Experiments. London: Collier Macmillan.

Fisher, R.A. (1960). The Design of Experiments, 8th Edition. New York: Hafner.

Flather, M., Pipilis, A., Collins, R. et al. (1994). Randomized controlled trial of oral captopril, of oral isosorbide mononitrate and of intravenous magnesium sulphate started early in acute myocardial infarction: Safety and haemodynamic effects. Eur. Heart J. 15: 608-619.

Freedman, L.S and Green, S.B. (1990). Statistical designs for investigating several interventions in the same study: Methods for cancer prevention trials. JNCI 82(11): 910-914.

Green, A., Battistitta, D., Hart, V., et al. (1994). The Nambour skin cancer and actinic eye disease prevention trial: Design and baseline characteristics of participants. Controlled Clinical Trials 15: 512-522.

Greenberg, E.R., Baron, J.A., Tosteson, T.D., et al. (1994). A clinical trial of antioxidant vitamins to prevent colorectal adenoma. New Engl. J. Med. 331: 142-147.

Heinonen, O.P., Virtamo, J., Albanes, D. et al. (1987). Beta carotene, alpha-tocopherol lung cancer intervention trial in Finland. In Proceedings of the XI Scientific Meeting of the International Epidemiologic Association, Helsinki, August, 1987. Helsinki: Pharmy.

Hennekens, C.H. and Eberlein, K. (1985). A randomized trial of aspirin and beta-carotene among U.S. physicians. Prev. Med. 14: 165-168.

Hulstaert, F., Van Belle, S., Bleiberg, H., et al. (1994). Optimal combination therapy with tropisetron in 445 patients with incomplete control of chemotherapy-induced nausea and vomiting. J. Clin. Oncol. 12: 2439-2446.

ISIS-4 Collaborative Group (1995). ISIS-4: A randomized factorial trial assessing early captopril, oral mononitrate, and intravenous magnesium sulphate in 58,050 patients with suspected acute myocardial infarction. Lancet 345: 669-685.

Karlstrom, P.O., Bergh, T., and Lundkvist, O. (1993). A prospective randomized trial of artificial insemination versus intercourse in cycles stimulated with human menopausal gonadotropin or clomiphene citrate. Fertil. Steril. 59: 554-559.

Lacourciere, Y., Lefebvre, J., Poirier, L., Archambault, F., and Arnott, W. (1994). Treatment of ambulatory hypertensives with nebivolol or hydrochlorthiazide alone and in combination. A randomized, double-blind, placebo-controlled, factorial-design trial. Am. J. Hypertension 7: 137-145.

Li, B, Taylor, P.R., Li, J.Y. et al. (1993). Linxian nutrition intervention trials. Design, methods, participant characteristics, and compliance. Ann. Epidemiol. 3: 577-585.

Lorenzen, T.J. and Anderson, V.L. (1993). Design of Experiments: A No-name Approach. New York: Marcel Dekker.

Lubsen, J. and Pocock, S.J. (1994). Factorial trials in cardiology (editorial). Eur. Heart. J. 15: 585-588.

Manson, J.E., Gaziano, J.M., Spelsberg, A., Ridker, P.M., Cook, N.R., Buring, J.E., Willett, W.C., and Hennekens, C.H. (1995). A secondary prevention trial of antioxidant vitamins and cardiovascular disease in women. Rationale, design, and methods. Ann. Epidemiology 5: 261-269.

Marshall, E. (1993). Women's Health Initiative draws flak. Science 262: 838.

Mason, R.L. and Gunst, R.L (1989). Statistical Design and Analysis of Experiments. New York: John Wiley & Sons.

Max, M.B., Zeigler, D., Shoaf, S.E. et al. (1992). Effects of a single oral dose of desipramine on postoperative morphine analgesia. J. Pain Symptom Manage. 7: 454-462.

Miller, T.P., Crowley, J., Mira, J., Schwartz, J.G., Hutchins, L., Baker, L., Natale, R., Chase, E.M., and Livingston, R. (1995). A randomized trial of treatment for localized inoperable non-small cell lung cancer comparing radiation alone to radiation plus chemotherapy and testing the efficacy of prophylactic whole brain radiation. International J. of Rad. Onc., Biol., Phys. (submitted).

Parkinson Study Group (1993). Effects of tocopherol and deprenyl on the progression of disability in early Parkinson's Disease. New Engl. J. Med. 328: 176-183.

Pordy, R.C. (1994). Cilazapril plus hydrochlorthiazide: improved efficacy without reduced safety in mild to moderate hypertension. A double-blind placebo-controlled multi-center study of factorial design. Cardiology 85: 311-322.

Schellhammer, P., Sharifif, R., Block, N., Soloway, M., Venner, P., Patterson, A.L., Sarosdy, M., Vogelzang, N., Jones, J., and Kiovenbag, G. (1995). A controlled trial of bicalutamide versus flutamide, each in combination with lutenizing hormone-releasing hormone analogue therapy, in patients with advanced prostate cancer. Casodex Combination Study Group. Urology 45(5): 745-752.

Slud, E.V. (1994). Analysis of factorial survival experiments. Biometrics 50; 25-38.

Snedecor, G.W. and Cochran, W.G. (1980). Statistical Methods, 7th Edition. Ames, IA: Iowa State University Press.

Sperduto, R.D., Hu, T.S., Milton, R.C., et al. (1993). The Linxian cataract studies. Two nutrition intervention trials. Arch. Ophthalmol. 111: 1246-1253.

Stampfer, M.J., Buring, J.E., Willett, W. et al. (1985). The 2×2 factorial design: Its application to a randomized trial of aspirin and carotene in U.S. physicians. Statistics in Med. 4: 111-116.

Steering Committee of the Physicians' Health Study Research Group (1989). Final report on the aspirin component of the ongoing physicians' health study. New Eng. J. Med. 321(3): 129-135.

ten Bokkel Huinink, W.W, Eisenhaur, E., and Swenerton, K. (1993). Preliminary evaluation of a multicenter, randomized comparative study of TAXOL (paclitaxel) dose and infusion length in platinum-treated ovarian cancer. Cancer Treat. Rev. 19 (Suppl. C): 79-86.

Thornquist, M.D., Owenn, G.S., Goodman, G.E., et al. (1993). Statistical design and monitoring of the carotene and retinol efficacy trial (CARET). Controlled Clin. Trials 14: 308-324.

Yates, F. (1935). Complex experiments (with discussion). J. Roy. Statist. Soc. B. 2: 181-247.

CHAPTER 16

Cross-Over Designs

16.1 Introduction

In the usual parallel or independent groups design, patients receive a *single* therapy (or combination of therapies) and the groups are treated concurrently. An alternative design, which is useful in some circumstances, is to administer each treatment to every patient at different times in the study as a way to permit within-patient comparisons of treatment effects. Because patients switch or cross over from one treatment to another using this strategy, these designs are called cross-over trials. Stated more formally, cross-over trials are those in which each patient is given more than one treatment, each at different times in the study, with the intent of estimating differences between them. Senn [1993, p. 3] defines them explicitly as trials

> in which subjects are given sequences of treatments with the object of studying differences between individual treatments (or sub-sequences of treatments).

In cross-over designs, the treatments are given during different time periods and all patients receive more than one treatment, though not usually simultaneously. These studies are the only commonly encountered clinical trials in which patients are not nested within treatments.

There is a large literature on cross-over designs, reflecting their instinctive appeal and dealing with limitations and controversies. Because the test for carry-over effects (discussed below) is inefficient, cross-over designs have not been well received by many statisticians. However, this situation may be changing. Brief but useful methodologic discussions of these designs can be found in Hills and Armitage [1979], Brown [1980], Fleiss [1986], Matthews [1988], and Grieve [1990]. A recent overview of the practical use of such designs is given by Cleophas and Tavenier [1995], and some aspects of optimal cross-over designs are explored by Jones and Donev [1996]. More specialized references will be mentioned in context later.

The simplest cross-over trial is the two-treatment (A and B) two-period design. In this type of study, there are two treatment periods and patients are randomized to receive either A followed by B or B followed by A. In the remainder of this chapter, I will refer almost exclusively to this AB/BA design, because it is the easiest cross-over to understand, and illustrates many of the important points about these types of trials. However, more complex cross-over trials may be employed in various clinical circumstances where the basic design is applicable. Extensions of this design include using more than one period for each treatment, a single treatment period for each of three or more treatments, or incomplete block designs, where not all patients receive all treatments. These more complex designs will not be covered here, but discussions of them can be found in Senn [1993] or Jones and Kenward [1989].

16.1.1 Other ways of giving multiple treatments are not cross-overs

There are other types of studies in which patients receive sequences of treatments. For example, in some cancer treatment trials, patients might be randomized between two groups: one that receives $A \rightarrow B \rightarrow C$ or one that receives $A \rightarrow B$, where A must be given first, B second, and C third. This study design as usually implemented is actually a test of the incremental effect of treatment C and not a test of the differences between the components. Most of these types of studies using sequences of treatments are not cross-over trials, because the experimental structure (and intent) does not permit assessing differences between the individual treatments. The sequence of administration of treatments is not a feature controlled by the experimenter and most of these trials are best viewed as parallel tests of treatment combinations.

In factorial designs, some patients also receive more than one treatment. However, basic cross-overs are different from these because some patients receive more than one treatment *simultaneously* in factorial trials. Even so, it is possible to construct factorial cross-overs. In such a trial, for example, there might be four treatment periods and four treatments for every patient: placebo, A, B, and $A + B$. The order in which a patient would receive the treatments in this type of trial could be determined by random assignment to permuted blocks. However, most factorial trials are not cross-overs and vice versa.

16.1.2 Treatment periods are randomly assigned

In a cross-over trial, subjects are not randomized to treatment in the same sense as they are in parallel group designs. This is even true of so-called "randomized" cross-over trials, because all participants receive all treatments. In these studies, only the *order* of administering the treatments is randomized. Because of this, the validity of the treatment comparison does not depend on the randomization as it might in parallel-groups designs. For example, randomization does not guarantee the expectation of an unbiased comparison of treatments in a cross-over trial. Instead, the validity of the treatment comparison depends on additional assumptions or findings described below.

At first, the diminished role of randomization in cross-over trials seems counter-intuitive or wrong. However, because these studies estimate within-patient differences in treatment effects, the balance of confounding factors like that induced by randomization in parallel-groups designs is not an issue. In other words, with respect to prognostic factors, the treatment groups are identical in cross-over trials, simply because the same individuals receive both treatments. In spite of this, the treatment groups are *not* identical in cross-over trials in other important ways. Specifically, the treatment groups differ with respect to their recent history of exposure to other potentially effective treatments.

This discussion highlights the primary source of difficulty with cross-over trials: the comparability of the treatment groups is not guaranteed by the structure of the trial alone. Comparability depends also on the treatment effects being confined to the period of their administration and follow-up. Investigators may not know at the start of the trial if such an assumption is warranted. Having comparable treatment groups appears to be partly a consequence of the outcome of the trial. This is quite different from a randomized, concurrent control, parallel-groups design, where the estimate of the treatment difference is valid regardless of whether either, both, or neither treatment is effective, and regardless of the duration of efficacy.

16.2 Advantages and Disadvantages

Based on the discussion so far, we can already anticipate some problems with the application, analysis, or interpretation of cross-over designs. However, there are circumstances where this type of design offers considerable advantages over a parallel-groups design. Investigators should fully understand the strengths and weaknesses of cross-over trials so they can be used effectively when the setting permits.

16.2.1 Cross-over designs can increase precision

The primary strength of cross-over trials is increased efficiency. Because each patient "serves as his or her own control", and the within-subject variability is usually less than the between-subject variability, the sample size for a cross-over trial will be lower than that for a comparable parallel-groups design. The cross-over design takes advantage of making treatment comparisons based on within- rather than between-subject differences. This allows the treatment difference to be estimated with greater precision, reducing the number of study subjects that are needed.

There are two effects that contribute to the greater efficiency of cross-over designs. First, because each patient receives both treatments, the trial needs only half as many subjects as an independent groups design to yield the same precision in the estimated treatment difference. Second, the sample size can often be reduced further, because within-subject responses to treatments are usually positively correlated. This also reduces the variance of the estimated treatment difference, further increasing efficiency.

For example, suppose treatment effects in a AB/BA design are estimated with variance σ^2 in each patient on each treatment and the average response on treatments

A and B are $\overline{Y}_A$ and $\overline{Y}_B$, respectively. Also, suppose there are no carry-over or period effects. If $\widehat{\Delta}_{AB} = \overline{Y}_A - \overline{Y}_B$ is the estimated treatment difference, then

$$Var(\widehat{\Delta}_{AB}) = \frac{\sigma^2}{n} + \frac{\sigma^2}{n} - 2Cov(\overline{Y}_A, \overline{Y}_B) \qquad (16.1)$$

$$= 2\frac{\sigma^2}{n}(1 - \rho_{AB}),$$

where n is the sample size in each group and ρ_{AB} is the within-subject correlation of responses on treatments A and B (assumed to be the same for all individuals).

In parallel-groups designs, the correlation of responses between the treatment groups is zero because the groups are composed of different individuals. In cross-over trials, the responses on the two treatments are correlated because they arise from the same patient. If the correlation between the responses for each individual is positive, as one might generally expect, the cross-over trial estimates Δ_{AB} with a smaller variance than an independent groups design would. If the correlation is zero, the variance of $\widehat{\Delta}_{AB}$ is the same as an independent groups design, which uses $2n$ total patients. If, for some reason the correlation between responses on A and B is large and negative (an unlikely circumstance), the cross-over trial could be less efficient, i.e., have a larger variance, than an independent groups design.

16.2.2 A cross-over design might improve recruitment

Another potential advantage of cross-over trials is that patient recruitment may be easier in some circumstances, because all patients receive all treatments under investigation. Sometimes patients may be unwilling to accept a no-treatment arm in a trial, but might be willing to delay therapy to the second treatment period. This could make it feasible to conduct a comparison that would otherwise be impractical for recruitment or be viewed as unethical.

For example, suppose we are interested in the effect of mild exercise (versus no intervention) on patients' sense of well-being in diseases like advanced cancer or AIDS. Although of unproven benefit, the intervention will probably sound like a good idea to many patients. When they find out it is being studied, they may prefer an exercise program over usual care. In a situation like this, a parallel-groups design may have many "drop-ins" in the exercise group, particularly among patients who already feel better or are more active. In a cross-over design, patients may be willing to postpone an exercise program to a second treatment period, knowing that they can derive benefit from it later, if it is effective. Thus, a two-period cross-over design could help recruitment and compliance in both treatment periods.

Administering two or more treatments to every patient may require more time or be more inconvenient, discouraging participation. This would certainly be the case if outcomes could only be assessed after diagnostic procedures such as X-rays, blood drawing, biopsies, lengthy questionnaires, or other tests. Acceptance might be greater if self-reports of symptoms are used. If the underlying disease is life threatening, diagnostic inconveniences might be unimportant to the patients. However, in chronic diseases, where cross-over trials may be more useful, factors that increase patient acceptance could be important determinants of accrual.

16.2.3 Carry-over effects are a potential problem

A potential problem with cross-over designs is the possibility that the treatment effect from one period might continue to be present during the following period. There are a number of ways in which this "carry-over" effect can happen. For example, the drug or treatment agent might physiologically persist during the second period. This could be prevented with a sufficiently long "washout" period between the treatment periods. The washout period is the interval between treatment periods, during which the previous treatment effect wears off and the patient's disease status returns to its baseline level.

Second, the first treatment could effect a permanent change or cure in the underlying condition of the patient. In this circumstance, the treatment given during the second period could look artificially superior. Finally, the underlying condition of the patient could change during the second period, and the treatment effect could depend on the patient's condition. This would constitute a true treatment by period interaction. Of course, this same type of temporal trend and treatment by time interaction can occur in parallel-groups designs, where it could also disturb the estimate of treatment effect.

The possibility of carry-over effects has been the focus of many concerns regarding cross-over trials. If there are differences in the carry-over effects in the two treatments (a likely situation unless both are zero), the design can yield biased estimates of the treatment effect, unless data from the second period are discarded [Freeman, 1989]. The basic design is very efficient at estimating within-subject differences in treatment main effects, but not very efficient at estimating carry-over effects. Some analytic approaches (discussed below) have suggested ways of estimating and dealing with carry-over effects. However, it is probably true that the data themselves from a cross-over trial are not very helpful in assessing carry-over effects. A better approach is to use the design of the study, particularly a washout period, to be certain that carry-over is not a problem.

A potential problem related to carry-over is *treatment by period interaction*. A treatment by period interaction means that the treatment effect is not constant in the different treatment periods (i.e., over time). In AB/BA cross-over trials, carry-over and treatment by period interaction are not distinguishable. More generally, however, they can be separated. Treatment by time interactions are not unique to cross-over studies and occur in other types of trials, e.g., parallel-groups designs. Carry-over effects can cause treatment by period interactions, which explains why there is concern over both in cross-over trials.

16.2.4 Drop-outs have strong effects

Two factors contribute to an increased likelihood of drop-outs in cross-over trials. First, the trial duration is longer than a comparable study using independent groups. This provides more opportunities for patients to drop out. Second, each participant is exposed to more drugs or treatments, increasing the chance of side effects that could contribute to dropping out.

The consequences of a drop-out in a cross-over trial may be more severe than in a parallel-groups design. If a participant drops out of a cross-over trial in the second study period, for example, simple analyses cannot use the data from only the first period. Thus, the data loss can be more significant than that from a single drop-out in a parallel-groups trial. Recently however, some authors have suggested ways of using incomplete observations in cross-over trials [Feingold and Gillespie, 1996].

16.2.5 Analysis is more complex than parallel-groups designs

Cross-over trials require more careful analysis than randomized parallel groups designs. The reason for added concern in cross-over trials is the possibility of carry-over effects and the need to determine that they have not confounded the estimates of treatment effect. Analytic approaches proposed for cross-over trials use either 1) a staged plan, where carry-over effects are studied in the first stage and, if none are found, the main effects are estimated in the second stage, or 2) baseline measurements in each period [Kenward and Jones, 1987] that can be used to test for carry-over.

More recently, Senn [1993] has suggested that analyses do not need to test for carry-over using a staged approach. Instead, carry-over should be actively controlled by the design of the trial. This and other details regarding analysis are discussed in the next section.

16.2.6 Prerequisites are needed to apply cross-over designs

Despite the potential benefits and efficiencies of the cross-over design, there are serious limitations to its widespread use. The first restriction is that investigators must have some knowledge of the sign and magnitude of the within-patient correlation between responses. As indicated above, a large negative value might make a cross-over design counterproductive, although this is unlikely to be the case.

Second, the underlying disease must have a constant intensity during all treatment periods. If the disease is cured by one of the treatments or can be expected to disappear in a short (relative to the treatment periods) time, the cross-over design will not be applicable. Also, if the condition is improving or worsening substantially, the treatment periods will not have the same baseline, and either the first or second one administered might artificially look better.

Third, the effect of the treatment needs to be restricted to the period in which it is applied. Equivalently, the treatment periods must be separated by a sufficient length of time for the effects of the earlier treatment to subside. If the washout period is too short, the latter treatment period will be biased by carry-over effects from the earlier treatment. If there is carry-over, the investigator will observe the simultaneous effect of two or more treatments, but attribute it only to the most recently administered one. Finally, cross-over trials can create added inconvenience for the patient and can present some challenging problem during analysis.

Investigators should be quite certain of the validity of the setting in which a cross-over trial is used and the expected view of such a trial by colleagues and regulators. For example, the potential for biased estimates of treatment effects from poor cross-over designs led the Food and Drug Administration in 1977 to conclude that such designs are a second choice to completely randomized or randomized block designs [FDA, 1977; O'Neill, 1978]. They stated

> [the cross-over design] is not the design of choice in clinical trials where unequivocal evidence of treatment effect is required ... in most cases, the completely randomized (or randomized block) design with baseline measurements will be the design of choice because it furnishes unbiased estimates of treatment effects without appeal to any modeling assumptions save those associated with the randomization procedure itself.

Although not suited to some studies of chronic disease like cancer, cross-over trials are well suited to other types of trials. For example, they might be a good design for bioavailability trials. For some diseases requiring chronic medication, like arthritis, angina, asthma, hypertension, or diabetes, cross-over trials might be an efficient way to compare treatments.

16.3 Analysis

In the last 30 years, a number of approaches have been suggested for analyzing cross-over trials or modifying their designs to cope with deficiencies. This section sketches some of these proposals and illustrates strengths and weaknesses of both the underlying design and the analytic strategies. The reader interested in more depth in the statistical details can refer to Senn [1993] or Jones and Kenward [1989]. Bayesian approaches to cross-over trials are discussed by Grieve [1985].

The classical approach to analyzing cross-over experiments was given by Grizzle [1965], who suggested conducting a preliminary test of carry-over. If the carry-over effect can't be ignored, the data from the first treatment period can be analyzed as though it arose from a parallel-groups design. The data from the second period are discarded. In the absence of carry-over effects, treatment effects are estimated from within-patient differences, using a linear model like the one discussed below.

An uncomplicated AB/BA design can be analyzed in a very straightforward manner. We calculate within-subject differences (treatment effects), $\delta = Y_A - Y_B$, and test for the effects of interest using appropriate averages of the δ's and their estimated standard error. The individual δ's are independent of one another. For example, a period effect implies that treatment effects are different in the two periods. In other words,

$$z = \frac{\bar{\delta}_1 - \bar{\delta}_2}{\sqrt{s.e.\{\bar{\delta}_1\} + s.e.\{\bar{\delta}_2\}}} \tag{16.2}$$

should differ only randomly from zero in the absence of a period effect. Therefore, z has a standard normal distribution under the null hypothesis. Similarly, the overall

Table 16.1 Cell Means Model for a Two-Period Cross-Over Trial

Treatments	Treatment Period	
	1	2
A then B	$\overline{Y}_{A1} = \beta_0$	$\overline{Y}_{B2} = \beta_0 + \beta_1 + \beta_2$
B then A	$\overline{Y}_{B1} = \beta_0 + \beta_1$	$\overline{Y}_{A2} = \beta_0 + \beta_2 + \beta_3$

treatment effect can be estimated by averaging the estimates from each period,

$$z = \frac{\overline{\delta}_1 + \overline{\delta}_2}{2\sqrt{s.e.\{\overline{\delta}_1\} + s.e.\{\overline{\delta}_2\}}} = \frac{\overline{\delta}}{\sqrt{s.e.\{\overline{\delta}\}}}. \tag{16.3}$$

Under the null hypothesis, this statistic also has a standard normal distribution. Although this serves as an introduction to the analysis of basic cross-over trials, more general approaches are based on linear models, discussed next.

16.3.1 Analysis can be based on a cell means model

Assume that individual responses arise from a linear model with error terms that are normally distributed. The group means for a two-period cross-over design with treatments A and B, one observation on each study subject in each period, and a possible carry-over effect can be parameterized as shown in Table 16.1. This parameterization allows the estimates to be summarized in a manner similar to that used in Chapter 15 for factorial designs. In this model, β_0 is the effect of treatment A alone, β_1 is the increment in treatment effect attributable to B, β_2 is the period effect, and β_3 is the carry-over effect. We cannot distinguish between carry-over and treatment by period interaction, because a term for the latter would appear in the model with, and not be separable from, β_3. Mean responses in each treatment-period cell are denoted by $\overline{Y}$ with appropriate subscripts.

Suppose that there is no treatment by period interaction, i.e., $\beta_3 = 0$. A non-zero period effect, $\beta_2 \neq 0$, means that the individual treatment effects are different in each period. Therefore, we can estimate β_2 by averaging the treatment effect differences in the two periods,

$$\widehat{\beta}_2 = \frac{1}{2}\left(\overline{Y}_{B2} - \overline{Y}_{B1} + \overline{Y}_{A2} - \overline{Y}_{A1}\right). \tag{16.4}$$

There are two estimates of the effect of treatment B compared with A, one from each period. They can be averaged to estimate β_1,

$$\widehat{\beta}_1 = \frac{1}{2}\left(\overline{Y}_{B2} - \overline{Y}_{A2} + \overline{Y}_{B1} - \overline{Y}_{A1}\right). \tag{16.5}$$

More generally, we must consider the possibility that $\beta_3 \neq 0$. A treatment by period interaction means that the incremental effects of treatment A (or B) in each period are not the same. We can estimate β_3 by

$$\widehat{\beta}_3 = \left(\overline{Y}_{A2} + \overline{Y}_{B1} - \overline{Y}_{B2} - \overline{Y}_{A1}\right). \qquad (16.6)$$

If β_3 is not zero, then we must estimate the treatment difference as

$$\widehat{\beta}_1 = \left(\overline{Y}_{B1} - \overline{Y}_{A1}\right),$$

i.e., using only the data from the first period.

Suppose each $\overline{Y}$ is estimated with variance σ^2/n and, in each treatment group, the within-person correlation of responses is ρ. Then, equation 16.1 can be used to calculate the variance of the difference between treatments in the same group. The formulae for $\widehat{\beta}_2$ and $\widehat{\beta}_1$ given above can be used to show that

$$Var\{\widehat{\beta}_2\} = Var\{\widehat{\beta}_1\} = \frac{\sigma^2}{n}(1-\rho).$$

In comparison, the variance of the interaction effect is

$$Var\{\widehat{\beta}_3\} = 4\frac{\sigma^2}{n}(1+\rho),$$

which is at least four times larger than $Var\{\widehat{\beta}_2\}$ for $\rho \geq 0$ (recall equation 16.1). Therefore, any cross-over trial designed to reliably detect main effects of treatment will have a less efficient test for the carry-over effect. However, the carry-over effect is critical to detect, because its presence affects both the analysis and interpretation of the trial. In the presence of clinically important carry-over effects, a cross-over design is no more efficient than an independent-groups trial. In fact, a cross-over design is relatively inefficient in testing the assumption of no carry-over effect, a conclusion supported by Brown [1980].

Some researchers feel that it is not necessary to establish definitively the absence of carry-over effects. Instead, the carry-over effect should be small in comparison to the treatment effect. This would seem to permit a test of the carry-over effect that has high power to rule out large values of β_3, but may not reject for smaller values. A perspective on this view is given by Poloniecki and Pearce [1983].

The carry-over effect can arise from more than one source. If the washout period is inadequate, the effect of the first treatment may persist into the second period. Also, the first treatment may alter the patient's condition permanently, perhaps without effecting a cure. Finally, the treatment effect may be proportional to the disease intensity. In a two-period cross-over trial, these complications are indistinguishable from one another and some or all of them must be assumed not to exist to utilize all of the data from the trial.

More general linear model approach

Assume a linear model with Gaussian errors for the AB/BA cross-over design of the form

$$E\{Y\} = \beta_0 + \beta_1 T + \beta_2 P + \beta_3 T \times P,$$

where Y is the response and T and P are indicator variables for treatment group and period, respectively. This model contains both a period effect and a treatment by period interaction (or carry-over effect). The design matrix, $\mathbf{X}$, for such an experiment with n subjects per group has dimensions $4n \times 4$ and can be written

$$
\mathbf{X} = \begin{bmatrix}
1 & \frac{1}{2} & \frac{1}{2} & \frac{1}{4} \\
1 & -\frac{1}{2} & -\frac{1}{2} & \frac{1}{4} \\
1 & \frac{1}{2} & \frac{1}{2} & \frac{1}{4} \\
1 & -\frac{1}{2} & -\frac{1}{2} & \frac{1}{4} \\
\vdots & \vdots & \vdots & \vdots \\
1 & \frac{1}{2} & -\frac{1}{2} & -\frac{1}{4} \\
1 & -\frac{1}{2} & \frac{1}{2} & -\frac{1}{4} \\
1 & \frac{1}{2} & -\frac{1}{2} & -\frac{1}{4} \\
1 & -\frac{1}{2} & \frac{1}{2} & -\frac{1}{4}
\end{bmatrix},
$$

where each pair of rows corresponds to the same subject treated with different treatments in different periods. In the design matrix, the successive columns correspond to an intercept, the treatment group, the period, and the treatment by period interaction (calculated by multiplying the treatment and period values). The treatment and period variable coding is chosen to be symmetric around zero and have a one-unit difference. This corresponds to the cell means approach discussed above. The vector of responses corresponding to this design matrix has length $4n$ and would be

$$
\mathbf{Y} = \begin{bmatrix}
Y_{A1} \\
Y_{B1} \\
Y_{A2} \\
Y_{B2} \\
\vdots
\end{bmatrix},
$$

where the subscripts indicate the treatment period and subject number.

Ordinary least squares cannot be used to estimate the model parameters, because each pair of responses is correlated, having arisen from the same individual. Instead, weighted least squares estimates must be obtained using

$$
\widehat{\boldsymbol{\beta}} = (\mathbf{X}'\boldsymbol{\Sigma}^{-1}\mathbf{X})^{-1}\mathbf{X}'\boldsymbol{\Sigma}^{-1}\mathbf{Y}, \tag{16.7}
$$

where $\boldsymbol{\Sigma}$ is the covariance matrix of responses [Draper and Smith, 1981]. If we assume that the variance of all responses is identical ($= \sigma^2$) and the within-subject covariances (or correlations) are equal ($= \gamma$), Σ has dimensions $4n \times 4n$ and

$$\Sigma = \begin{bmatrix} \sigma^2 & \gamma & 0 & 0 & \cdots \\ \gamma & \sigma^2 & 0 & 0 & \cdots \\ 0 & 0 & \sigma^2 & \gamma & \cdots \\ 0 & 0 & \gamma & \sigma^2 & \cdots \\ \vdots & \vdots & \vdots & \vdots & \ddots \end{bmatrix} = \sigma^2 \times \begin{bmatrix} 1 & \rho & 0 & 0 & \cdots \\ \rho & 1 & 0 & 0 & \cdots \\ 0 & 0 & 1 & \rho & \cdots \\ 0 & 0 & \rho & 1 & \cdots \\ \vdots & \vdots & \vdots & \vdots & \ddots \end{bmatrix}.$$

The block diagonal structure arises because pairs of responses are correlated within, but not between, individuals. In general, γ (ρ) will be positive because within-subject responses are positively correlated with one another. However, this is not absolutely required. In any case,

$$\Sigma^{-1} = \frac{1}{\sigma^4 - \gamma^2} \times \begin{bmatrix} \sigma^2 & -\gamma & 0 & 0 & \cdots \\ -\gamma & \sigma^2 & 0 & 0 & \cdots \\ 0 & 0 & \sigma^2 & -\gamma & \cdots \\ 0 & 0 & -\gamma & \sigma^2 & \cdots \\ \vdots & \vdots & \vdots & \vdots & \ddots \end{bmatrix}$$

$$= \frac{1}{\sigma^2(1 - \rho^2)} \times \begin{bmatrix} 1 & -\rho & 0 & 0 & \cdots \\ -\rho & 1 & 0 & 0 & \cdots \\ 0 & 0 & 1 & -\rho & \cdots \\ 0 & 0 & -\rho & 1 & \cdots \\ \vdots & \vdots & \vdots & \vdots & \ddots \end{bmatrix}.$$

In a model with a treatment effect, period effect, and a treatment by period interaction, the above matrices yield

$$(\mathbf{X}'\Sigma^{-1}\mathbf{X})^{-1} = \frac{\sigma^2}{n} \times \begin{bmatrix} \frac{1}{4}(1 + \rho) & 0 & 0 & 0 \\ 0 & 1 - \rho & 0 & 0 \\ 0 & 0 & 1 - \rho & 0 \\ 0 & 0 & 0 & 4(1 + \rho) \end{bmatrix},$$

which is the covariance matrix of the parameter estimates. Note the independence of the estimates using this variable coding (i.e., all covariances are zero) and that the treatment by period interaction is less precisely estimated (variance $= 4(\sigma^2 + \gamma)/n$) relative to the treatment difference (variance $= (\sigma^2 - \gamma)/n$). In other words, for a fixed sample size, the power to detect a treatment by period interaction of specified magnitude will be lower than that with which other effects can be detected. Then, the parameter estimates from equation 16.7 are

$$\hat{\beta} = \begin{bmatrix} \overline{Y}_{..} \\ \overline{Y}_{A.} - \overline{Y}_{B.} \\ \frac{1}{2}\{(\overline{Y}_{A1} - \overline{Y}_{B1}) - (\overline{Y}_{A2} - \overline{Y}_{B2})\} \\ (\overline{Y}_{A1} - \overline{Y}_{A2}) + (\overline{Y}_{B1} - \overline{Y}_{B2}) \end{bmatrix}.$$

EXAMPLE   415

The exact form of the estimates depends on the model parameterization. In this case, the treatment by period or carry-over effect is estimated by the sum of the period differences in the treatments. These estimates are the same, apart from algebraic sign, as those developed above from the cell means approach (equations 16.4–16.6).

16.3.2 Other issues in analysis

There are many other issues regarding cross-over trials and their analysis that cannot be covered in depth in this chapter. A few will be mentioned here to guide additional study. Baseline measurements taken at the beginning of each treatment period can be used in an analysis of covariance to improve effect estimates or the test of carry-over. Here we assume that baseline measurements at the second period are not affected by carry-over, i.e., there has been a sufficient washout. See Jones and Kenward [1989], Senn [1993], or Willan and Pater [1986] for discussions.

Much attention has been given to estimating carry-over effects from the data, despite the poor efficiency of such tests. The assessment of carry-over may depend on its magnitude relative to the treatment effect [Willan and Pater, 1986] or its direction [Lechmacher, 1991]. In any case, concern about carry-over effects can be reduced by using designs with more than two treatment periods [Laska, Meisner, and Kushner, 1983].

Cross-over trials may be indicated in many circumstances where binary or other responses arise. An overview of some proposed approaches is given by Kenward and Jones [1987]. Analysis of binary outcomes and drop-outs in multiple periods has been discussed by McKnight and Van Den Erden [1993]. Poisson responses are discussed by Layard and Arvesen [1978] and nonparametric tests of the data have been suggested [Senn, 1993]. Analyses can be approached from the perspective of multivariate response [Grender and Johnson, 1993].

16.4 Example

An interesting example of data arising from a two-period cross-over trial for the treatment of enuresis has been given by Hills and Armitage [1979]. Patients were treated with a new drug or placebo for 14 days. (The name and characteristics of the drug are not provided by the authors.) The number of dry nights out of 14 for each child is shown in Table 16.2. The study design and resulting data are not complicated and the authors used normal theory tests to assess the outcome of the trial.

The mean differences ($\pm$ s.e.m.) are 2.82 ($\pm$0.84) for group I and 1.24 ($\pm$0.86) for group II. The period effect is tested by equation 16.2 with standard error equal to $\frac{1}{2}\sqrt{0.84^2 + 0.86^2} = 0.60$. Thus, the test for period effect is

$$z = \frac{2.82 - 1.24}{2 \times 0.60} = 1.32,$$

Table 16.2 A Two-Period Cross-Over Trial: Treatment of Enuresis (Data from Hills and Armitage, 1979)

	Group I			Group II	
Patient Number	Period 1 Drug	Period 2 Placebo	Patient Number	Period 1 Drug	Period 2 Placebo
1	8	5	2	12	11
3	14	10	5	6	8
4	8	0	8	13	9
6	9	7	10	8	8
7	11	6	12	8	9
9	3	5	14	4	8
11	6	0	15	8	14
13	0	0	17	2	4
16	13	12	20	8	13
18	10	2	23	9	7
19	7	5	26	7	10
21	13	13	29	7	6
22	8	10			
24	7	7			
25	9	0			
27	10	6			
28	2	2			

which is not statistically significant. The test for overall treatment effect uses equation 16.3 or

$$z = \frac{2.82 + 1.24}{2 \times 0.60} = 3.38,$$

which is significant at the 0.01 level. Thus, the drug is effective at increasing the number of dry nights in a 14-day interval.

16.5 Summary

Cross-over trials are those in which study participants receive all treatments under investigation, each in a different study period. Between periods, a washout period is used to allow the effects of the previous treatment to disappear. Because the treatment effect is estimated within rather than between patients, cross-overs are more efficient than parallel groups designs. Although the design is not well suited to some acute diseases or types of outcomes, it is particularly well suited to investigations such as bioavailability trials.

Cross-over studies are subject to important limitations, particularly finding the proper clinical setting and actively determining that carry-over and treatment by period interactions do not destroy the applicability of the design. For two-treatment two-period cross-over trials, the effects of carry-over and treatment by period inter-actions are indistinguishable. Carry-over can be assessed by preliminary studies and eliminated by design. Statistical tests for carry-over after the data have been collected are inefficient and probably not helpful. Ancillary measurements, such as baseline covariates at the beginning of each treatment period, can improve the performance of cross-over designs.

16.6   Questions for Discussion

1. Instead of the design matrix given in section 16.1, suppose zero-one variable coding had been employed. What would happen to the covariance matrix of parameter estimates and the estimates themselves? Discuss the implications.
2. Describe the assumptions under the normal theory analysis of the enuresis two-period cross-over trial. Are the assumptions met by the data collected? Can you suggest at least two alternative approaches to the analysis?

Chapter References

Brown, B.W., Jr. (1980). The cross-over experiment for clinical trials. Biometrics 36: 69-79.

Cleophas, T.J.M. and Tavenier, P. (1995). Clinical trials in chronic diseases. J. Clin. Pharmacol. 35: 594-598.

Draper, N.R. and Smith, H. (1981). Applied Regression Analysis, Second Edition. New York: John Wiley & Sons.

Feingold, M. and Gillespie, B.W. (1996). Cross-over trials with censored data. Statistics in Med. 15: 953-967.

Fleiss, J.L. (1986). The Crossover Study. Chapter 10 in The Design and Analysis of Clinical Experiments. New York: John Wiley & Sons.

Fleiss, J.L. (1989). A critique of recent research on the two-treatment cross-over design. Controlled Clin. Trials 10: 237-243.

Freeman, P.R. (1989). The performance of the two-stage analysis of two-treatment, two-period crossover trials. Statistics in Medicine 8: 1421-1432.

Food and Drug Administration (1977). A report on the two-period crossover design and its applicability in trials of clinical effectiveness. Minutes of the Biometric and Epidemiology Methodology Advisory Committee (BEMAC) meeting.

Grender, J.M. and Johnson, W.D. (1993). Analysis of crossover designs with multivariate response. Statistics in Med. 12: 69-89.

Grieve, A.P. (1985). A Bayesian analysis of the two period cross-over design for clinical trials. Biometrics 42: 979-990. Corrigenda 42: 459 (1986).

Grizzle, J.E. (1965). The two-period change-over design and its use in clinical trials. Biometrics 21: 467-480. Corrigenda 30: 727 (1965).

Hills, M. and Armitage, P. (1979). The two-period cross-over clinical trial. British J. Clin. Pharmacol. 8: 7-20.

Jones, B. and Donev, A.N. (1996). Modelling and design of cross-over trials. Statistics in Med. 15: 1435-1446.

Jones, B. and Kenward, M.G. (1989). Design and Analysis of Cross-Over Trials. London: Chapman and Hall.

Kenward, M.G. and Jones, B. (1987). A log linear model for binary cross-over data. Appl. Statist. 36: 192-204.

Laska, E., Meisner, M., and Kushner, H.B. (1983). Optimal crossover designs in the presence of carryover effects. Biometrics 39: 1087-1091.

Layard, M.W.J. and Arvesen, J.N. (1978). Analysis of Poisson data in crossover trials. Biometrics 34: 421-428.

Lechmacher, W. (1991). Analysis of the cross-over design in the presence of residual effects. Statistics in Med. 10: 891-899.

Matthews, J.N.S. (1988). Recent developments in crossover designs. Intern. Statist. Rev. 56: 117-127.

McKnight, B. and Van Den Eeden, S.K. (1993). A conditional analysis for two-treatment multiple-period crossover designs with binomial or Poisson outcomes and subjects who drop out. Statistics in Med. 12: 825-834.

O'Neill, R.T. (1978). Subjects-own-control designs in clinical drug trials: Overview of the issues with emphasis on the two treatment problem. Presented at the Annual NCDEU Meeting, Key Biscayne, Florida.

Poloniecki, J.D. and Pearce, A.C. (1983). Letter to the editor. Biometrics 39: 789.

Senn, S. (1993). Cross-Over Trials in Clinical Research. Chichester: John Wiley & Sons.

Willan, A. and Pater, J. (1986). Carryover and the two-period cross-over clinical trial. Biometrics 42: 593-599.

Willan, A. and Pater, J. (1986). Using baseline measurements in the two-period cross-over clinical trial. Controlled Clin. Trials 7: 282-289.

CHAPTER 17

Overviews/Meta-Analyses

17.1 Introduction

An overview, or meta-analysis as it is often called, is a formal method for analyzing the results of several or many clinical trials for the purpose of combining, synthesizing, or integrating the findings. Of the terms "overview" or "meta-analysis" (or others such as data pooling, literature synthesis, etc.), the latter is the more widespread. "Overview" is more descriptive of the techniques used, but this term is often used to describe reviews that are not quantitative. The National Library of Medicine (NLM) has endorsed the term "meta-analysis". In 1989, the NLM began a MeSH heading for meta-analysis and named it a publication type in 1993.

Because of the ubiquitous problem of having to combine evidence from several studies, scientists have been engaging in this activity, formally or informally, for many years. Olkin [1995a; 1995b] gives an interesting historical perspective on meta-analyses and attributes early ones to Karl Pearson, R.A. Fisher, and other statisticians. Between 1930 and 1950, agriculture was a stimulus for combining evidence (and for developing other statistical methods). Between 1950 and 1970, there was little research on meta-analysis methods [Olkin 1995a].

An early proposal to minimize subjective analysis of similar experiments in the literature using a quantitative approach was given by Light and Smith [1971]. Several methods were used and discussed in the social sciences in the 1970s, but were not widely adopted. The term "meta-analysis" was first used by Glass [1976] to describe a statistical pooling method like that commonly used now. Glass defined meta-analysis as

> ... the statistical analysis of a large collection of analysis results from individual studies for the purpose of integrating the findings. It connotes a rigorous alternative to the casual, narrative discussions of research studies which typify our attempts to make sense of a large volume of research literature.

419

While the definitions do not necessitate using randomized studies, this is the context in which the clinically most reliable and important meta-analyses are conducted. The discussion in this chapter refers principally to meta-analyses of randomized trials.

Clinicians have been engaged informally in statistical overviews for many years. Formal efforts to develop the field in recent times spread from the social sciences [Hedges and Olkin, 1985] to medicine in the 1980s, especially oncology and epidemiology. One of the earliest statistical overviews in medicine was that of Chalmers, examining the effect of warfarin on myocardial infarction outcomes [Chalmers et al., 1977]. Useful reviews of meta-analysis are given by Dickersin and Berlin [1992] and Finney [1995]. An excellent source for depth and diversity of opinion is the proceedings of the Potsdam International Consultation on Meta-Analysis published in the *Journal of Clinical Epidemiology* [Volume 48(1), 1995].

One of the principal reasons why meta-analyses are helpful to clinical researchers today is the large number of similar trials being conducted. For example, the number of randomized clinical trials approaches 10,000 per year. Synthesizing results informally from many studies can be difficult and confusing. Also, researchers are frequently interested in small treatment differences (one of the main reasons for performing randomized comparisons), because they can have major public health importance when applied to common diseases. Important differences may be obscured by the variability of individual studies, which is why results in the literature often appear to disagree. However, combining evidence frequently shows consistency and permits one to estimate small but clinically significant effects.

The earliest meta-analyses required only information in the published trial reports. While this made overviews accessible to many readers, it is now clear that more than the published information is usually necessary to perform rigorous overviews. The meta-analysts usually need to obtain and analyze the actual patient data from each trial to produce a credible result. Because individual patient data are not published routinely, additional effort is required to conduct a proper overview.

17.1.1 Overviews increase precision

The primary purpose of an overview is analytic rather than descriptive. The analyst looks for consistency in studies, especially similar randomized clinical trials (RCTs), that may not be readily apparent from selective or casual reading. Also, the analyst looks to explain heterogeneity or differences in studies. There are several reasons why this activity is useful. First, RCTs are large and expensive and we would like to gain as much information from them as possible. Second, we intuitively expect well-performed RCTs to "agree with" one another. Third, RCTs tend to be externally valid with respect to relative treatment effects, even if selection bias has made the comparison groups atypical for the diseased population.

An expert's review of the field is one alternative to a formal overview. However, the typical clinical review can be subjective and incomplete. When there is uncertainty about the consistency of the findings in different studies, incompleteness and subjectivity is a disadvantage. For example, if the effects of treatment are small, or go against the prevailing theory, or if the expert focuses only on the statistical significance of findings (rather than the magnitude of the effects), this type of review could mislead. Despite the limitations of expert reviews, meta-analyses will not and should not replace them.

Meta-analysis attempts to counteract these deficiencies by 1) basing data on a comprehensive literature review, sometimes even using relevant data that have not yet been published or negative findings that could not be published, and 2) using formal methods for combining estimates of treatment effect from the studies. However, we must always ask if the question posed by a meta-analysis is well defined so that its apparent precision is useful.

In addition to a firm base for inference, the statistical tools employed in the typical meta-analysis are rigorous and more reliable than those used in other types of reviews. Formal methods are used to combine various types of endpoints such as group means, odds ratios, and hazard ratios. Also, some methods using random effects models attempt to account explicitly for study-to-study variability. Finally, the statistical power of meta-analyses is often very high. Small treatment differences can be estimated with a high degree of precision and can yield highly statistically significant results. The high statistical power results from combining large amounts of data. In cases where the disease under study is common, the public health importance of even small treatment benefits can be large.

17.2   A Sketch of Meta-Analysis Methods

17.2.1 Meta-analysis necessitates prerequisites

Meta-analysis, like all formal research methods, needs to proceed from a foundation of planning and design. The basic steps required are 1) formulation of a purpose and specification of an outcome for the analysis, 2) identification of relevant studies, 3) establishing inclusion and exclusion criteria for studies, 4) data abstraction and acquisition, 5) data analysis, and 6) dissemination of results and conclusions. Weaknesses in any of these steps can compromise the validity and strength of the meta-analysis.

Because meta-analyses require so much effort, they should not be undertaken casually or without clear purpose. A difficult but essential part of meta-analysis, like a clinical trial, is choosing an important feasible question to address. This chapter can be of little help in selecting a question, except to emphasize that both clinical and methodological knowledge is required to assess the importance and feasibility of the study plan.

17.2.2 Many studies are potentially relevant

Retrieval

Having been stimulated by an appropriate question, the meta-analysis investigator will use several sources to identify trials on which to base the study. Personal knowledge is an important source of information but will usually be incomplete. Experts in the field can be consulted but may miss, or be unaware of, some relevant clinical trials. Experts are an important and reliable way to gather information about trials that have not yet appeared in traditional media.

Usually a large number of relevant and important trials can be found using computerized searches of literature databases. Such searches are possible in most medical libraries at minimal cost and can be accomplished quickly. The reference lists from selected publications are an important additional source for identifying relevant trials. Additional expertise may be required to be sure that foreign language studies are identified by computerized searches. Human recollections and computer retrievals may miss recently published trials. Therefore, it may be important to search for recent publications by hand.

Limitations of retrieval

The methods just outlined have unavoidable limitations. "Publication bias" can result when the medical literature is used as a source for studies. The published literature is neither a complete repository nor a random sample of trials actually performed. For example, studies that do not show statistically significant differences or treatment effects, so-called "negative" trials, are less likely to appear in the literature than "positive" ones, creating publication bias. It is our scientific nature to be attracted more to "progress" than to its apparent absence. Furthermore, the literature probably contains a higher proportion of results that are type I errors than statistical significance levels would suggest.

Publication bias is a serious concern for meta-analyses. Several authors have discussed the implications of publication bias and suggested methods for compensating for it [Begg and Berlin, 1988; Dear and Begg, 1992; Hedges, 1992]. Complete ascertainment of unpublished trials is an important step, as is an emphasis on the magnitude of treatment effects rather than their statistical significance.

Some sources of information may not be covered by the computerized searches discussed above. This "fugitive literature" includes government reports, book chapters, dissertations, and conference proceedings. Studies published in languages other than English can escape notice easily, as can those conducted or published outside the time window in which the meta-analyst searches. Finally, we must consider the difficulty of dealing with non-randomized studies. If they are excluded from the meta-analysis, important evidence may be lost. If they are included, there is a risk of introducing another source of bias.

Information retrieval for meta-analyses in the future would benefit from two improvements today. The first is prospective registration of trials when they are initiated in a comprehensive database. A database of this type would facilitate meta-analyses later and would be an important source of information about clinical trials as a method of investigation. If used properly, it could also improve policy decisions by regulators and sponsors. The Cochrane Collaboration [Chalmers, 1993] comes close to this goal. A second area for improvement is complete reporting of trial results, which might be facilitated by formal guidelines [Standards of Reporting Trials Group, 1994].

17.2.3 Select studies

Eligibility criteria for study inclusion

Meta-analysts establish specific eligibility criteria for including clinical trials in their study. The purpose of these criteria is to reduce bias in the selection of trials and to increase the reproducibility of the findings. When drafting such inclusion criteria, investigators must consider the specific treatment employed in each trial. To include a trial in the meta-analysis, we must be able to justify that its test of treatment effect is similar in design to those from other studies selected. Often this means selecting studies of only a specific agent, combination, or modality, but sometimes it permits a broader definition of "treatment". For example, the Early Breast Cancer Trialists Collaborative Group (EBCTCG) performed a large and important meta-analysis looking at the benefit of chemotherapy in breast cancer [EBCTCG, 1990]. For some of these analyses, the chemotherapy combination did not have to be identical or be given at the same dose. Nevertheless, the results showed clearly the benefit of treatment.

Many clinical trials yield more than one publication. However the principal endpoint paper will usually be most relevant to the meta-analysis. Sometimes it may be reasonable to exclude trials employing a very small sample size or those with limited follow-up. Trials with low power may be methodologically weak in other ways, and therefore of questionable validity. In any case, small studies are not likely to influence the results of a meta-analysis greatly.

Abstracting data

It may be helpful to use a data abstraction form to organize and collect the information from each clinical trial included in the meta-analysis. Using this method, investigators can help control the selection and removal of patients from the analysis, resolve questions about ancillary treatments, determine the clinical outcome for each patient, and identify and collect information on important prognostic factors. The reliability and reproducibility of these steps may be increased by a suitable data abstraction form. Also, investigator bias can be reduced using masking and by separating data collection tasks in appropriate ways.

17.2.4 Plan the statistical analysis

The main issues in planning the statistical analysis are choosing an effect estimate, deciding on the unit of analysis (trial versus individual patient), quality scoring of studies, and selecting the specific statistical methods to use. The estimate of treatment effect can be an average effect size calculated from all the studies. Examples of effect sizes used in meta-analyses include mean differences (standardized), risk ratios, correlations, and p-values. Some quantitative issues are discussed by Greenland [1987].

Observed minus expected frequencies is a commonly used summary of effect (illustrated below). This method may not be optimal when effects are present [Greenland and Salvan, 1990], but it is relatively simple and illustrates the principles of analysis. In any case, the overall effect estimate can also be adjusted for prognostic factors. Adjustment may be indicated if the prognostic factor composition of the trial cohorts are very different. Like individual clinical trials, investigators must plan for subgroup analyses and deal with treatment non-adherence and losses to follow-up. It may be useful to cumulate the results chronologically rather than show each study individually. Olkin [1995b] gives an interesting example of this.

A quality rating system for the trials included has been suggested as a way to improve the strength of evidence coming from meta-analyses. For example, the analysis could be stratified or weighted according to the perceived quality. A "sensitivity analysis", using quality scoring as an indicator to include or exclude each trial, could help validate the findings obtained in this way. There is a tendency for more recently conducted studies to be higher quality than old ones, because of methodologic improvements and having more experienced and knowledgeable investigators. However, there are exceptions to this rule. Also, errors or scientific misconduct by some individuals associated with a particular trial do not necessarily reduce the quality of all the data. In spite of the potential utility of quality scales in conducting meta-analyses, they are subjective and their reliability and validity remains unknown.

17.2.5 Summarize the data using observed and expected

A widely used statistical method for meta-analyses is based on calculating the deviation of the observed result in the treatment group within each trial from the result expected under a null hypothesis. This is "observed minus expected" or $O - E$. Observed and expected calculations can be based on statistics such as number of events, survival rates, or other appropriate clinical endpoints. The $O - E$ method avoids comparing results from one trial with those from another. The sum of the deviations is divided by an estimate of its variability to yield an overall test of the null hypothesis. If there is no treatment effect, the $O - E$ values are equally likely to be positive or negative, and their sum will differ only randomly from 0.

When the null hypothesis is not true, the $O - E$ method may not be the optimal one for assessing the risk ratio. However, it is not difficult to calculate and illustrates the important characteristics of the method.

Suppose that number of events is the primary outcome measure for studies comparing treatment versus control. In the ith study, the total number of participants is N_i, the number in the treatment group is n_i, and the total number of events observed is K_i. Define the overall event rate to be $p_i = K_i/N_i$. The null hypothesis states that the treatment has no effect, i.e., treatment assignment and outcome are independent. Randomization, and independence of treatment assignment and outcome, means that we can view the n_i individuals assigned to the treatment group as a simple random sample of all N_i participants.

Under these assumptions, the number of events observed in the treatment group, O_i, follows a hypergeometric distribution [Johnson and Kotz, 1969]. The hypergeometric probability distribution is specified by

$$\Pr\{O_i = x\} = \frac{\binom{K_i}{x}\binom{N_i - K_i}{n_i - x}}{\binom{N_i}{n_i}} ,$$

where $\max\{0, n_i - (N_i - K_i)\} \le x \le \min\{K_i, n_i\}$. The expected value of this distribution is $\mathcal{E}\{O_i\} = E_i = n_i p_i$ and the variance is

$$Var\{O_i\} = n_i p_i (1 - p_i)\frac{N_i - n_i}{N_i - 1} = f_i K_i (\frac{N_i - K_i}{N_i - 1})(1 - f_i),$$

where $f_i = n_i/N_i$. These formulae allow us to calculate an overall test statistic from M studies using the sum of $O - E$ and its variance (E is not a random variable),

$$Z = \frac{\sum_{i=1}^{M}(O_i - E_i)}{\sqrt{\sum_{i=1}^{M} Var\{O_i\}}},$$

which will have a standard normal distribution under the null hypothesis. Large negative values of Z imply that the treatment reduces the expected number of events.

17.2.6 Example

The methods sketched above are illustrated in the meta-analysis of long-term antiplatelet therapy discussed by Peto, Collins, and Gray [1995], and the Antiplatelet Trialists' Collaboration [1994]. In the 11 randomized trials conducted, therapy consisted of aspirin (ASA), dipyramidole, sulphinpyrazone, or combinations and the endpoints were vascular events defined as myocardial infarction, stroke, or vascular death. The data from the trials and meta-analysis calculations are summarized in Table 17.1. The individual and overall odds ratios with 99% confidence limits are shown in Figure 17.1. The aggregate effect is an odds ratio of 0.75 ($p < 0.00001$), demonstrating the efficacy of antiplatelet drugs in reducing vascular events. The strength and consistency of these findings are greater than one would be likely to find with either an informal review or examination of only a few of the trials. Even though 8 of the 11 trials have confidence intervals that include an odds ratio of 1.0, the aggregate evidence from the meta-analysis in favor of treatment is compelling.

17.3   Other Issues

17.3.1 Meta-analyses have practical and theoretical limitations

Researchers do not universally agree on the theoretical validity of meta-analysis, its practical application, or interpretation. A number of problems are illustrated by Feinstein [1995]. Bailar [1995] suggests that improperly conducted meta-analyses can, and have, produced misleading results and provides some examples. Difficulties in practical applications include selecting studies of high quality and properly executing and interpreting the analysis. Greenland [1994] cautions against uncritical acceptance of some widely used meta-analytic methods, such as graphical summaries, random effect models, and quality scores. These concerns are discussed from a more fa-

Table 17.1 Randomized Trials of Prolonged Antiplatelet Therapy

Trial	Therapy	Treatment	Control	$O - E$	Var
Cardiff I	ASA	58/615	76/624	-8.5	29.9
Cardiff II	ASA	129/847	185/878	-25.2	64.2
PARIS I	ASA or ASA+Dip.	244/1620	77/406	-12.7	43.3
PARIS II	ASA+Dipyridamole	154/1563	218/1565	-31.9	82.0
AMIS	ASA	395/2267	427/2257	-16.9	168.2
CDP-A	ASA	88/758	110/771	-10.2	43.1
GAMIS	ASA	39/317	49/309	-5.6	18.9
ART	Sulphinpyrazone	102/813	130/816	-13.8	49.8
ARIS	Sulphinpyrazone	38/365	57/362	-9.7	20.7
Micristin	ASA	65/672	106/668	-20.8	37.3
Rome	Dipyridamole	9/40	19/40	-5.0	4.6
All	Any	1321/9877	1685/9914	-160.1	562.0

Odds ratios and 99% confidence limits are shown in Figure 17.1. From Peto, Collins, and Gray [1995].

vorable perspective by Olkin [1994] in his commentary. Meta-analysis methods have been proposed for observational studies, a topic viewed dimly by Shapiro [1994]. He provides examples of such studies that are of questionable validity.

We must keep in mind that meta-analyses are observational studies subject to the limitations and potential biases of such methods. They are not the same as confirmed randomized trials, but are weaker or stronger depending on the studies that comprise them, the definition of "treatment", and the methods used to synthesize the results. It is likely that more experience with methods and more attention to reporting of clinical trials will be needed for meta-analyses to reach their full potential.

When planning or interpreting meta-analyses, investigators should keep in mind limitations of the method. As with all types of studies, there is sometimes a discrepancy between statistical and clinical significance. Often the confidence intervals placed on the overall treatment effects in meta-analyses do not account for sources of variability in the studies. For example, if the confidence intervals are calculated assuming that the individual treatment effects are "randomly" sampled from a homogeneous population of treatment effects, they may be optimistically narrow. Like poor-quality data undermine a clinical trial, no meta-analysis method can validate combining evidence from flawed trials. Khan, Daya, and Jadad [1996] emphasize the importance of trial quality on the final overview. Finally, clinical investigators should not be encouraged to perform (small) under-powered randomized trials with the hope of combining them later in a meta-analysis.

17.3.2 Meta-analysis has taught useful lessons

Despite limitations and continued development of methods, meta-analyses have already provided researchers with some important lessons. They provide a quantitative

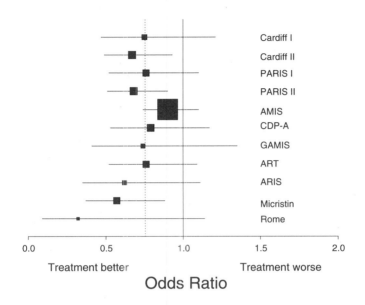

Figure 17.1 Meta-analysis of antiplatelet therapy. Observed odds ratios and 99% confidence limits from 11 randomized clinical trials. The dotted line shows the overall odds ratio (= 0.75). Data are presented in Table 17.1.

method for synthesizing the results from more than one study that can establish a basis for policy decisions. Meta-analyses have highlighted and improved the quality of reporting clinical trials in medical journals and have suggested ways in which the methodology of trials can be improved. They are a resource for planning new investigations and can suggest if a trial is not needed because of the weight of existing evidence or if a new study may be informative. Finally, meta-analyses provide a historical perspective on treatment issues and create a comprehensive quality controlled database that may be useful for other questions in the future.

Meta-analyses can also directly affect treatment decisions. When used for this purpose, they will sometimes generate controversy. One example is the assessment of mortality in patients with cardiovascular disease who are taking calcium channel blockers [Furberg, Psaty, and Meyer, 1995; Opie and Messerli, 1995; Kloner, 1995; Yusuf, 1995]. The overview suggested that such drugs (nifedipine, in particular) may cause increased mortality.

Investigators are also use meta-analyses to assist in the design and monitoring of clinical trials. This is a natural role for studies that synthesize the available evidence regarding a treatment. An in-depth perspective on the use of meta-analyses for this purpose was provided by the Conference on Meta-Analysis in the Design and Monitoring of Clinical Trials, published in *Statistics in Medicine* [Vol. 15(12), 1996].

17.4 Summary

Meta-analysis is a formal quantitative process for combining the evidence about treatment effect from more than one clinical trial. Because the data from many similar studies can be combined using the method, meta-analyses have the potential to demonstrate treatment effects with a high degree of precision. This high precision can demonstrate small, but clinically important, treatment effect convincingly. Because of the varied content and quality of clinical trial reports, meta-analyses should be performed only on patient-level data. Careful planning, comprehensive data collection, and a formal approach to statistical methods is necessary for a high-quality meta-analysis.

Meta-analyses have important weaknesses. Meta-analyses are not experimental designs and their validity relies on retrieving existing data and on the quality of the studies that generated the data. Incomplete retrieval of trials or data can bias the result. Because positive trial results are probably more likely to appear in the literature than negative ones (publication bias), meta-analyses can overestimate the benefits of treatment.

Meta-analyses have had a positive impact on the quality of clinical trials and their publications.

17.5 Questions for Discussion

1. When an expert conducts a review of a particular issue, he or she may do so without the formal statistical methods of a meta-analysis. Compare and contrast this to a meta-analysis and discuss the advantages and disadvantages of each approach.
2. Discuss the similarities and differences between a cumulative meta-analysis and a sequential randomized trial.

Chapter References

Bailar, J.C. (1995). The practice of meta-analysis. J. Clin. Epidemiol. 48: 149-157.

Begg, C.B. and Berlin, J.A. (1988). Publication bias: A problem in interpreting medical data. J. R. Stat. Soc. A 151: 419-463.

Boden, W.E. (1992). Meta-analysis in clinical trials reporting: Has a tool become a weapon? (editorial). Am. J. Cardiology 69: 681-686.

Chalmers, I. (1993). The Cochrane Collaboration: Preparing , maintaining, and disseminating systematic reviews of the effects of health care. Ann. N. Y. Acad. Sci. 703: 156-165.

Chalmers, T.C. (1991). Problems induced by meta-analyses. Statistics in Med. 10: 971-980.

Chalmers, T.C. (1993). Meta-analytic stimulus for changes in clinical trials. Statist. Methods in Med. Research 2: 161-172.

Chalmers, T.C., Matta, R.J., Smith, H., Jr., and Kunzler, A.M. (1977). Evidence favoring the use of anticoagulants in the hospital phase of acute myocardial infarction. New Engl. J. Med. 297: 1091-1096.

Cook, D.J., Guyatt, G.H., Ryan, G., et al. (1993). Should unpublished data be included in meta-analyses? Current convictions and controversies. JAMA 269: 2749-2753.

Cook, D.J., Sackett, D.L., and Spitzer, W.O. (1995). Methodologic guidelines for systematic reviews of randomized control trials in health care from the Pottsdam Consultation on Meta-Analysis. J. Clin. Epidemiol. 48: 167-171.

Dear, K.B.G. and Begg, C.B. (1992). An approach for assessing publication bias prior to performing a meta-analysis. Stat. Sci. 7: 237-245.

Dickersin, K. and Berlin, J.A. (1992). Meta-analysis: State-of-the-science. Epidemiologoc Reviews 14: 154-176.

Doll, R. (1994). The use of meta-analysis in epidemiology: Diet and cancers of the breast and colon. Nutr. Rev. 52: 233-237.

Early Breast Cancer Trialists' Collaborative Group (1990). Treatment of Early Breast Cancer, Vol. 1: Worldwide Evidence 1985–1990. Oxford: Oxford University Press.

Feinstein, A.R. (1995). Meta-analysis: Statistical alchemy for the 21st century. J. Clin. Epidemiol. 48: 71-79.

Finney, D.J. (1995). A statistician looks at met-analysis. J. Clin. Epidemiol. 48: 87-103.

Furberg, C.D., Psaty, B.M., and Meyer, J.V. (1995). Nifedipine: Dose-related increase in mortality in patients with coronary heart disease. Circulation 92: 1326-1331.

Glass, G.V. (1976). Primary, secondary, and meta-analysis of research. Educ. Research 5: 3-8.

Greenland, S. (1987). Quantitative methods in the review of the epidemiologic literature. Epidem. Reviews 9: 1-30.

Greenland, S. (1994). A critical look at some popular meta-analytic methods. Am. J. Epidemiol. 140: 290-296 (with discussion).

Greenland, S., and Salvan, A. (1990). Bias in the one-step method for pooling study results. Statist. in Med. 9: 247-252.

Hedges, L.V. (1992). Modeling publication selection effects in meta-analysis. Stat. Sci. 7: 246-255.

Hedges, L.V. and Olkin, I. (1985). Statistical Methods for Meta-Analysis. Orlando, FL: Academic Press.

Johnson, N.L. and Kotz, S. (1969). Distributions in Statistics, Discrete Distributions. New York: John Wiley & Sons.

Jones, D.R. (1995). Meta-analysis: Weighing the evidence. Statistics in Med. 14: 137-149.

Kloner, R.A. (1995). Nifedipine in ischemic heart disease. Circulation 92: 1074-1078.

Khan, K.S., Daya, S., and Jadad, A.R. (1996). The importance of quality of primary studies in producing unbiased systematic reviews. Arch. Intern. Med. 156: 661-666.

Light, R.J. and Smith, P.V. (1971). Accumulating evidence: Procedures for resolving contradictions among different research studies. Harvard Educ. Rev. 41: 429-471.

Meinert, C.L. (1989). Meta-analysis: Science or religion? Controlled Clin. Trials 10: 257S-263S.

Moher, D., Fortin, P., Jada, A.R., et al. (1996). Completeness of reporting of trials published in languages other than English: Implications for conduct and reporting of systematic reviews. Lancet 347: 363-366.

Oakes, M. (1993). The logic and role of meta-analysis in clinical research. Stat. Methods in Med. Research 2: 147-160.

Olkin, I. (1994). Invited commentary re: A critical look at some popular meta-analytic methods. Am. J. Epidemiol. 140: 297-299.

Olkin, I. (1995a). Statistical and theoretical considerations in meta-analysis. J. Clin. Epidemiol. 48: 133-146.

Olkin, I. (1995b). Meta analysis: Reconciling the results of independent studies. Statistics in Med. 14: 457-472.

Opie, L.H. and Messerli, F.H. (1995). Nifedipine and mortality: Grave defects in the dossier. Circulation 92: 1068-1073.

Petitti, D.B. (1994). Meta-Analysis, Decision Analysis, and Cost-Effectiveness Analysis. Synthesis in Medicine. New York: Oxford University Press.

Peto, R. (1987). Why do we need systematic overviews of randomized trials? Statistics in Med. 6: 233-240.

Peto, R., Collins, R., and Gray, R. (1995) Large-scale randomized evidence: Large simple trials and overviews of trials. J. Clin. Epidemiol. 48: 23-40.

Shapiro, S. (1994). Meta-analysis/shmeta-analysis. Am. J. Epidemiol. 140: 771-778.

Spitzer, W.O. (1995). The challenge of meta-analysis. J. Clin. Epidemiol. 48: 1-4.

Standards of Reporting Trials Group. (1994). A proposal for structured reporting of randomized controlled trials. JAMA 272: 1926-1931. Correction: 273: 776.

Stewart, L.A. and Clarke, M.J. (1995). Practical methodology of meta-analyses (overviews) using updated individual patient data. Statistics in Med. 14: 2057-2079.

Wachter, K.W. (1988). Disturbed by meta-analysis? Science 241: 1407-1408.

Yusuf, S. (1995). Calcium antagonists in coronary artery disease and hypertension: Time for reevaluation? Circulation 92: 1079-1082.

CHAPTER 18

Fraud and Misconduct in Clinical Research

18.1 Introduction

Falsifications and fabrications in science have a long history, even if one considers only well-documented cases. Allegations of data fabrication or falsification and other actions that would be unacceptable by today's standards have been made against Ptolemy, Galileo, Newton, Dalton, Mendel, and others. For example, Ptolemy is said to have used the astronomical observations of Hipparchus of Rhodes and claimed them as his own in formulating his theories. Newton apparently fudged calculations in his *Principia* to agree with his gravitational theory, and used his presidency of the Royal Society to discredit Leibniz's credible claim of having invented the calculus. Investigation and re-analysis of Mendel's work strongly suggests falsification of data to correspond with theory. This case is particularly interesting to statisticians [Fisher, 1936].

Manipulating data to reinforce theory may not be uncommon in the history of science. In the 19th century, Charles Babbage, the inventor of the calculating machine, lamented the widespread practices of data "trimming", "cooking", and "forgery" in the sciences [Babbage, 1836]. For a somewhat controversial but sobering review of these and other cases of possible misconduct, including more modern ones, see Broad and Wade [1982], Kohn [1986], or Miller and Hersen [1992]. Friedlander [1995] reviews a number of cases in the biological and basic sciences, particularly in the context of situations on the fringes of science.

Although many of the historical instances are arguable either way because of lack of evidence, recent instances clearly involve misconduct. The circumstances surrounding the discovery of Piltdown man is an interesting and prominent example from the 20th century, which involved outright fraud or trickery. In 1912, a human skull and the jaw of an ape were planted in a gravel pit on Piltdown Common, near

Lewes, England, to suggest that the earliest human was from Great Britain. Belief in the legitimacy of the artifacts extended over many years and fooled many knowledgeable scientists. It was not until 1953 that the bones were proven to be crudely faked, although some scientists suspected and attempted to expose it much earlier [Matthews, 1981; Kohn, 1986]. It was not until 1996 that solid evidence about the identity of the perpetrator was published [Gardiner and Currant, 1996].

There have been many well-documented instances of misconduct from the basic medical sciences. One example is the work of Spector on the protein kinase cascade leading to the phosphorylation of sodium-potassium ATPase [McKean, 1981]. The findings could not be replicated by several scientists who attempted it and were discovered to be at least partly fraudulent [Broad and Wade, 1982; Kohn, 1986; Racker and Spector, 1981]. A second example is the human Hodgkin's disease cell lines of Long, found to actually be from the owl monkey [Harris et al., 1981; Wade, 1981]. One of the most controversial, interesting, and unfortunate cases in recent times is that of Thereza Imanishi-Kari, who was accused of misconduct when she worked with Nobel Laureate David Baltimore, but later exonerated on appeal. The best concise summary of this complex case is given by Kevles [1996]. In 1996, five papers related to the genetics of leukemia were retracted after an admission of data fabrication by a graduate student. The senior author on these papers was the director of the National Center for Human Genome Research. These more recent cases indicate that historical instances of misconduct are not a consequence of lack of sophistication on the part of the scientific community.

In the clinical sciences, there have been extensive and painful episodes of misconduct in recent times [Engler et al., 1987; Relman, 1983]. Today, there seems to be an increase in reports of fraud or misconduct in many areas of science. Discussions in the context of nursing can be found in Morrison [1990], Denham [1993], and Chop and Silva [1991]. The true incidence depends on our definition of misconduct (discussed below). However, there is much more activity in science now than in the past, and most cases of possible fraud are treated with more openness and public scrutiny than they were even 25 years ago. The incidence may be no higher than in the past but the number of events and our awareness may be greater. Heightened awareness and vigilance, as discussed below, may actually have decreased the frequency of misconduct cases today.

Relatively little has been written about misconduct related to statistical methods other than fabrication and falsification of data. One exception is the discussion of fraudulent statistical methods in the context of risk assessment by Bross [1990]. Bross defines a fraudulent statistical method as one that gives false or misleading results and is intended to deceive. He places certain quantitative risk assessment methods in this category, a notion that might make many biostatisticians uncomfortable.

18.1.1 Integrity and accountability are critically important

In recent years, public officials have increasingly questioned the ability of the scientific community to ensure integrity in the conduct of research. Clinical trials have not been free from this increasing scrutiny. The trend is both a consequence of highly visible instances of misconduct by scientists and changing public perceptions about the research process. Along with the increase in the magnitude and influence of the research enterprise in recent years, scientists have been asked for greater accountability when using public funds. Also, research efforts are becoming more complex and require collaborations between institutions and investigators that may necessitate greater accountability. Finally, many research efforts are commercialized rapidly or are sponsored by industry, even if they take place in academic settings, leading to demands for more careful review [Schwartz, 1991]. Not only do these situations increase public awareness, but they also contribute to an evolving standard for integrity.

Scientific research is basically a creative enterprise, but one that relies on trust. It is paradoxical that this scientific process of balanced skepticism must ultimately rely on a foundation of trust. Because it does, violations of that trust through misconduct or fraud threaten science in the most fundamental way. A well-rounded discussion from this perspective is given by Fuchs and Westervelt [1995]. The violation of trust may explain the disproportionate publicity and attention that misconduct cases often receive. Those engaged in science have taken the issue of misconduct seriously. Extensive studies and recommendations have been made by the Institute of Medicine [IOM, 1989] and the National Academy of Sciences [NAS, 1992a; 1992b] in addition to the attention given by the Public Health Service (discussed below).

Although not less important, the basis of trust in science is distinctly different from that in other creative activities such as art, music, or literature. Historically, clinical researchers have relied upon trust, honesty, objectivity, and the error-correcting nature of the scientific method to guarantee the integrity of research. Peer review, both in funding of research and publication of results has been a major component of the process. Unfortunately, personal or group ambition sometimes conflicts with scientific ethic. When objectivity is lost for this or any other reason, the research process is prone to breakdown. All types of error become more likely: honest error, self-deception, sloppiness, dishonesty, and criminal behavior.

Many views of fraud, its consequences, detection, and prevention are taken from the perspective of basic science research. It may be more important to detect fraud in clinical trials than in basic research, for several reasons. First, basic research may be more self-correcting than clinical trials by its very nature, particularly because many fundamental experimental findings are replicated independently. Second, clinical trials usually have greater or more immediate consequences for the public health and welfare than basic research. Finally, clinical trials often have a higher public profile than basic research. In any case, being able to conduct clinical trials is a privilege granted to investigators by both the patient participants in their studies and the public. This trust is violated by any acts that are disrespectful of the study participants or the research process.

18.1.2 Fraud and misconduct are difficult to define

"Fraud" is a term that is often informally applied to dishonest acts or intentional deception. However, the legal interpretation of the term "fraud" in the United States implies injury or damage to victims. Because this criterion is often not applicable to scientific research, the term "misconduct" is probably more appropriate to describe deviant scientific behavior. Unfortunately, "misconduct" can also be applied appropriately to a variety of actions by researchers, some of which are not especially consequential or relevant to the objectives of scientific research (e.g., sexual harassment). Although difficult to define satisfactorily (see below), misconduct, like pornography, is often easy to identify. An exception that illustrates the difficulty in defining misconduct is theft of intellectual property. There is a fine line between this and the appropriate dissemination of new ideas. Several authors have discussed this point [Judson, 1994; McCutchen, 1991; Rennie, Flanagin, and Glass, 1991; Relman, 1984; Swazey, Anderson, and Lewis, 1993].

Science is somewhat unique, in that the scientific method *is* the integrity of the discipline. This orientation toward process has evolved mostly since the 18th century but has been applied to clinical trials only in the last 40 years. The concept of ethics in science can become distorted by the idea that science is composed of a fixed set of rules. The only "rule" in science is the search for truth, a goal that is merely ancillary to most other human endeavors. In fact, the scientific ethic is determined by the structure of the process rather than the outcome [Friedlander, 1995].

Questions about the definition of scientific integrity and misconduct are, therefore, questions about what elements of the process are integral to the scientific method. In other words, the meaning of scientific integrity depends on the meaning of science. The general norms of science are: 1) intellectual integrity (honesty) and objectivity, 2) tolerance, 3) doubt of certitude, 4) recognition of error, 5) unselfish engagement, and 6) communal spirit [Bulger, 1994; Cournand, 1977; Denzin and Lincoln, 1994]. These also apply to clinical investigators. In clinical trials, the question is further complicated by the ethics of the practitioner–patient relationship. Concern and respect for the patient may not always be coincident with scientific goals.

One could define misconduct as significant deviations from these norms. However, misconduct is usually defined more in terms of a lack of intellectual integrity and objectivity. There have been formal definitions offered for scientific misconduct or fraud by at least four organizations: The National Academy of Sciences (NAS), The Public Health Service (PHS), the National Science Foundation (NSF), and The Royal College of Physicians (RCP). Even though all these definitions are sensible, I will use the National Academy of Sciences definition and avoid the term *fraud,* except in the informal sense of the word.

National Academy of Sciences

The NAS Panel that studied the integrity of the research process in the U.S. [National Academy of Sciences, 1992a] distinguished between three types of inappropriate behavior by scientists: 1) misconduct in science, 2) questionable research practices, and 3) other misconduct. These are summarized in Table 18.1.

The NAS defined misconduct in science as data fabrication, data falsification, or plagiarism, but did not include errors of judgement, differences of opinion, or mistakes in the recording, selection, or analysis of data. Questionable research practice is conduct that goes against, and may be detrimental to, traditional values underlying the research process. These can include failing to maintain records, exploiting research subordinates or subjects, and using inappropriate analytic methods to enhance the significance of research findings. There are no clear standards of behavior regarding questionable research practices and no general agreement as to the seriousness of such actions. Other forms of misconduct are not unique to science, but can occur in the process of any type of research. These include harassment of individuals, misuse of funds, and conflicts of interest. Conflicts of interest are common and do not necessarily constitute misconduct. However, because they can affect scientific objectivity, conflicts of interest need to be treated openly, and occasionally will disqualify the opinions of some investigators.

Public Health Service

The Public Health Service has regulations defining misconduct in science and guiding approaches to allegations of misconduct. Government agencies such as NIH, the Centers for Disease Control and Prevention, and the FDA are covered by these regulations. In 1989, the PHS defined scientific misconduct as

> fabrication, falsification, plagiarism, or other practices that seriously deviate from those that are commonly accepted within the scientific community for proposing, conducting, or reporting research. It does not include honest error or honest differences in interpretations or judgments of data [DHHS, 1989, p.32447].

Unfortunately, the regulations do not explicitly define fabrication, falsification, or plagiarism. Furthermore, they do not define deviations from commonly accepted practice.

The practical application of this rule has resulted in a number of actions being seen as misconduct by the PHS. These include: failure to perform research supported by PHS while claiming progress in reports; naming authors on publications without their knowledge; selective reporting of primary data; unauthorized use of data from another researcher; false reporting of patient status in clinical research; use of improper and faulty statistical methods.

National Science Foundation

The NSF defined misconduct as 1) fabrication, falsification, plagiarism, or other serious deviation from accepted practices, or 2) retaliation against whistleblowers who act in good faith [NSF, 1987; 1991]. Additionally, the NSF extended the definition to non-research activities such as education and outlined procedures and actions to be taken in cases of possible misconduct. Full investigations take place only if an initial inquiry finds it necessary. Procedures for inquiries are discussed below in the section on institutional approaches to misconduct. If misconduct is found, penalties

Table 18.1 Elements of Misconduct in Science as Defined by the National Academy of Sciences

MISCONDUCT IN SCIENCE

- Data fabrication (making up data)
- Data falsification (changing data values)
- Plagiarism

QUESTIONABLE RESEARCH PRACTICES

- Failing to retain important data for a reasonable period of time
- Inadequate research records
- Refusing to allow reasonable access to data by others
- Using inappropriate statistical methods to enhance the significance of findings
- Exploiting or inadequately supervising research subordinates
- Naming authors without regard to significant contribution to the research reported

OTHER MISCONDUCT

- Sexual and other harassment
- Misuse of funds
- Gross negligence
- Vandalism
- Violation of research regulations
- Conflict of commitment or interest

can range from a letter of reprimand to prohibiting individuals from participating in certain research activities sponsored by NSF.

Royal College of Physicians

In England, the RCP defined "misconduct" as piracy, plagiarism, and fraud [Royal College of Physicians, 1991]. They define *piracy* as taking ideas from others without acknowledgment. *Plagiarism* is the copying of ideas, data, or text without credit. *Fraud* is defined as "deliberate deception, usually the invention of data".

Overview of definitions

It is interesting that none of the current definitions of misconduct or fraud explicitly mention the intent of the perpetrator. However, it is commonly understood that misconduct is a purposeful act, unlike error, which is inadvertent. Often, the motive for misconduct can be established. The absence of a motive does not disprove misconduct, but is more typical of error. Thus, we demand more stringent evidence to label an act as misconduct and little evidence to call it an error. Although there is significant overlap in these definitions, problem areas remain. Some discussed be-

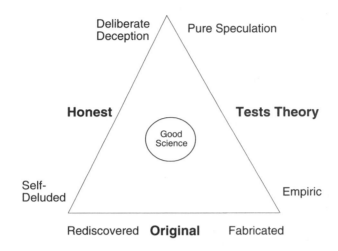

Figure 18.1 Balance of factors characteristic of good science.

low include the definition of due process and review, the role of whistleblowers, and how to cope with false accusations of misconduct.

18.2 Research Practices

Research practices in science are influenced in six major ways, which include: 1) scientific norms, 2) specific disciplines, 3) individuals and teams, 4) institutions, 5) government, and 6) society. Scientists and clinical researchers share common training, values, and experiences, which help to establish scientific norms, at least within the discipline. Even so, it is not clear to what extent individual researchers adhere to the norms because of competing pressures such as research funding and competition for academic recognition and positions. A perspective on this is given in a series of short articles by by Cohen, Marshall, and Taubes [1995]. Specific disciplines assist in establishing good research practices through both specific guidelines and diffuse practices such as peer review. In clinical trials, good research practices are outlined in places such as the Helsinki Declaration and the Belmont Report (Chapter 3).

Individual scientists and research teams are important determinants of good research practices through the process of "mentoring" or training young scientists. Mentoring helps encourage important values such as creativity and collaboration. Similarly, institutional policies are strong determinants of the environment in which research is conducted. In fact, universities and other research institutions may be the most important elements in fostering integrity in scientific research [Danforth and Schoenhoff, 1992]. Some academic institutions have adopted guidelines that they expect faculty to observe when conducting research [National Academy of Sciences, 1992b]. Even so, many institutions have no formal guidelines regarding authorship and mentoring. Because of specific and highly public instances of scientific misconduct, most institutions have adopted policies for handling such cases. They are required by the federal government to have policies for handling misconduct to be eligible for federally sponsored research grants. Additionally, institutions must submit an assurance that they will follow the policies.

In contrast, government agencies have policies that regulate many areas of research. These include informed consent in clinical trials, animal research, and laboratory safety. Policies and procedures to regulate the treatment of alleged misconduct do not have wide agreement. The history of the development of the Office of Research Integrity (ORI) is an example of such differences of opinion [Office of Research Integrity, 1993]. Societal concerns about waste, mismanagement, and fraud in the use of government funds has translated into requirements for greater accountability from research scientists. Similarly, worries about real or imagined ethical abuses, such as those surrounding the use of human subjects for radiation experiments during the early years of the Cold War, highlight the public's concern for accountability [Committee on Human Radiation Experiments, 1995].

18.2.1 Misconduct has been uncommon

By most published estimates, the frequency of cases of scientific misconduct is low. The actual number of cases is probably higher than that reported [Swazey, 1993]. Between 1980 and 1990, there were fewer than 100 recognized cases of misconduct in science [National Academy of Sciences, 1992a]. Although given the number of research investigators and research grants, this number appears to be small, it is likely that the number of true cases is under-reported, because of those allegations that were investigated by other means. From detailed studies of investigated cases, it appears that plagiarism is the most common type of scientific misconduct. For example, it accounted for half of the 41 allegations reviewed by the National Science Foundation in 1990 [National Science Foundation, 1990]. There have been publicized cases of misconduct in other countries as well, including Great Britain [Freestone and Mitchell, 1993; Lock, 1988; Lock, 1995; Wells, 1992], Australia [Lock, 1990], India [Jayaraman, 1991], and Germany [Eisenhut, 1990; Foelsing, 1984]. A noteworthy case from Australia is connected with lawsuits over Bendectin, a drug manufactured and used in the U.S. for nausea and vomiting during pregnancy [Humphrey, 1992; Skolnick, 1990].

In the U.S., reviews of publicly reported cases have been done by Woolf [1981; 1986; 1988]. In 1988, there was a NSF/AAAS survey of 392 deans of graduate studies at institutions affiliated with the Council of Graduate Schools. Forty percent of the responders indicated they were aware of *possible* cases of misconduct. Other reports and surveys concerning misconduct are given in the NAS report [National Academy of Sciences, 1992a].

Currently, the frequency of misconduct can only be determined approximately. Data are available for Public Health Service Research in the U.S. through the Office of Research Integrity (ORI). Between 1991 and 1995, the number of misconduct cases closed by the ORI has varied between 30 and 60 per year. The total case load includes institutional inquiries, institutional investigations, ORI inquiries, and ORI investigations. At least half of all cases appear to result in findings of misconduct. The ORI does not report the number of research projects under its jurisdiction. In 1995 for example, 41 investigations were closed by ORI and/or institutions with the finding of 24 cases of misconduct. Some cases are carried over from year-to-year and not all findings are upheld on appeal.

18.2.2 Causes of misconduct

There are several factors that can contribute to the occurrence of misconduct. These include academic pressure to publish, financial gain, professional vanity, lack of understanding of the research process, and psychiatric illness. Of these, academic pressure is widely regarded as a common contributing cause that may come from diverse sources. Appointment and promotions often depend as much on the quantity of publication as on their quality. Productivity also contributes greatly to obtaining and keeping research grants. Closely related to this type of academic pressure is professional vanity and ego. Recognition by peers is greatly prized by researchers and comes with many tangible and abstract rewards.

Financial gain may not be a common cause of misconduct, at least among academic investigators. They are usually not in a position to profit financially from a particular research project. With increasing technology transfer out of academic centers into commercial enterprises, the opportunity for investigators to realize personal financial gain is greater now than in the past. It is possible that more cases of misconduct motivated by money will arise in the future.

There are very few data regarding the role of psychiatric illness in scientific misconduct. Response to stress and self-expectations are likely to be important determinants. The egregiousness of some of the cases of misconduct reported, however, suggests that more than just academic pressures are at work. These can easily explain an isolated incident, but many cases of misconduct illustrate long-term patterns of behavior, attitudes, and a lack of integrity that would be out of place in any professional setting. There has been little or no psychological work in this area, partly because such cases are so uncommon. General discussions are given by Miller [1992] and Thelen and DiLorenzo [1992].

Clinical research and clinical trials have characteristics that may increase pressures on investigators. There is constant pressure to accrue patients to meet the temporal and scientific objectives of the trial. Eligibility and exclusion criteria might be perceived as an obstacle in such circumstances. Similarly, the specifications of the protocol may occasionally conflict with the needs of an individual patient. While there is never a need to conform to the protocol if the physician does not believe it is in the patient's best interest, a conflict can create pressure to falsify data items to give the appearance of conformity.

18.3 General Approach to Allegations of Misconduct

18.3.1 Government

The first systematic public discussion of reports of fraud in biomedical research was in the 1980 Congressional hearings of the Oversight and Investigations Subcommittee of the House Science and Technology Committee. The hearings were in response to public disclosure of instances of misconduct at four major research centers. In 1985, Congress required Public Health Service (PHS) grantees to adopt administrative procedures for reviewing reports of scientific fraud (public law 100-504). Guidelines for doing so were issued by the PHS in 1986. By 1989, most institutions receiving more than 100 PHS awards had adopted such procedures. However, nearly 80% of institutional grantees had no guidelines. Final regulations requiring institutional guidelines were published by PHS in 1989 (42 CFR 50). The PHS consists of the National Institutes of Health, the Centers for Disease Control and Prevention, the Food and Drug Administration, the Substance Abuse and Mental Health Services Administration, the Health Resources Services Administration, the Agency for Health Care Policy and Research, the Agency for Toxic Substances and Disease Registry, and the Indian Health Service.

Investigating allegations of scientific misconduct requires a two-stage process: an inquiry and an investigation. The inquiry is usually confidential and within the institution. The extent of the inquiry may be determined locally. Institutions may elect to perform an inquiry formally or informally, using existing committees. An institutional inquiry can determine that an allegation of misconduct lacks merit, at which time the matter is closed. If the inquiry determines that an investigation is warranted, a formal process of investigation must be initiated. The inquiry itself cannot determine guilt. If an investigation is required, the institution must notify the sponsoring agency. The investigation is usually performed by a special appointed panel of objective experts. In the event that the institution lacks the resources to be thorough, fair, and objective, it can request that the PHS conduct its own investigation through the Office of Research Integrity.

A principal component of PHS handling of allegations of scientific misconduct is the Office of Research Integrity (ORI). The background of this Office is as follows: In 1989, the Office of Scientific Integrity (OSI) was formed in the NIH Director's Office and the Office of Scientific Integrity Review (OSIR) was formed in the Office of the Assistant Secretary for Health in the PHS. The OSIR was responsible for establishing PHS policies for misconduct in science, while the OSI was to implement the policies and conduct investigations. In 1992, the OSI and OSIR were merged into a single office called the ORI, under the Assistant Secretary, making these activities independent of PHS funding agencies. In June, 1993, the ORI became independently established by statute within the Department of Health and Human Services (HHS) with the director reporting to the Secretary of HHS. In 1995, the ORI was placed in the Office of Public Health and Science, which is headed by the Assistant Secretary for Health.

The National Science Foundation (NSF) has a policy similar to the PHS. The responsible entity is the Office of the Inspector General (OIG), established by Congress in 1989 [Inspector General Act Amendments, 1988]. The OIG is also responsible for auditing grants and contracts awarded by the NSF. The policy of the NSF is to make research institutions responsible as much as possible for dealing with all aspects of alleged misconduct in science. In response to allegations of misconduct, institutions must conduct investigations that the OIG deems fair and complete.

Role of the Office of Research Integrity

The role of the ORI is defined in PHS regulations. Its responsibilities include: to 1) assure that all PHS grantees have appropriate mechanisms for dealing with allegations of misconduct, 2) oversee the conduct of institutional investigations, 3) conduct investigations when necessary (e.g., within PHS), 4) defend findings of misconduct before the Departmental Appeals Board when required, 5) develop regulations and policies to assure fairness and due process, and 6) promote research integrity. In cases where ORI determines that an investigation of allegations was not in accordance with regulations, it may initiate a new, separate investigation. In addition to its other activities, the ORI publishes a quarterly newsletter, which provides details on closed cases, and publishes an annual report (e.g., ORI [1995]) where additional information can be found.

Although the ORI can become involved in misconduct cases through a variety of mechanisms, their formal role is subject to certain limitations. For example, the ORI has authority only in cases involving Department of Health and Human Services funding (PHS, NIH, etc.). Furthermore, the types of misconduct on which it may rule are restricted by the regulatory definition (above). Since 1992, DHHS has had a hearing mechanism (Departmental Appeal Board [DAB]) by which findings of misconduct can be reviewed formally and legally at the departmental level. When this happens, findings such as data fabrication must be demonstrated to be "material" (i.e., substantive), and the ORI must prove intent for the findings to stand. If an assessment of misconduct is affirmed, the actions that ORI can take are limited to debarring the investigator from receiving federal funds and/or serving on advisory committees for a limited period of time.

Despite the limited-sounding nature of these actions, investigation by an institution and/or the ORI is difficult for all associated with the case. The cases cast a shadow on scientific work, consume time and resources of both the accused and investigating staff, and may leave lingering questions about different but seemingly related matters. In some high-profile cases, many individuals, locally and nationally, not directly involved in the study may experience a significant impact from an investigation.

In clinical trials, investigation by ORI is motivated by concerns about the health of the public, public and media awareness of the issue, and the need to correct potential scientific errors. Because clinical trials are often large, expensive, and not likely to be repeated in the same form, there is concern that they are not as self-correcting as other scientific enterprises. Also, the ORI cannot easily conduct an investigation without the cooperation and assistance of the trial coordinating center and local institution. For multi-center trials, the institution being investigated, the coordinating center, the trial sponsor, and ORI must work together. This consumes considerable resources. These activities affect the patients on the trials, the investigators, and the science community at large.

18.3.2 Institutions

Like the PHS, most medical institutions have a structured, staged approach to examining allegations of scientific misconduct. The following sketch is based on policies and procedures at one institution, independent of, but in conformance with, recommended PHS procedures. The preliminary inquiry into good-faith allegations of misconduct is performed by an advisory committee appointed by the Dean, which maintains strict confidentiality. The purpose of the preliminary inquiry is to determine if the allegations have merit. If the inquiry finds the allegations were without merit, the process is terminated. The implicated person or persons and the accuser will be notified of the findings and dismissal of the allegations no later than when the preliminary inquiry is completed. The case is then considered closed and no notification of outside organizations is required.

If the allegations of misconduct appear to have merit based on the preliminary inquiry, a full investigation takes place by an ad hoc committee. If this committee finds that misconduct has taken place, a full report is made for adjudication by a Standing Committee on Discipline. This Committee is responsible for initiating any immediate actions outside the university that are required by the findings, such as notification of journals, sponsors, or the public. The Standing Committee reports its finding to the Advisory Board of the Medical Faculty, which will consider what appropriate disciplinary actions are needed.

At the end of this chapter, an example of formal misconduct guidelines are given. These come from faculty policies for *Procedures for Dealing with Issues of Professional Misconduct* of the Johns Hopkins University School of Medicine [Johns Hopkins, 1995]. The university, like most, also has separate formal faculty policies for conflict of commitment, rules and guidelines for responsible conduct of research, and grievance procedures.

18.3.3 Problem Areas

Defining and dealing with deviant behavior by scientists is a difficult problem. Doing so raises questions about defining and recognizing such behavior, double standards for scientists compared with other professionals, and personal loyalties. There seems to be no consensus among scientists, research sponsors, or the public on these issues. An interesting perspective on the lack of consensus is given by Dyson [1993]. One can also raise serious questions about what role, if any, government should play in dealing with scientific misconduct [Hansen and Hansen, 1991; Klein, 1993].

Despite progress and agreement in formally defining misconduct in science, guidelines for how to approach specific allegations, and steps for prevention, there are a number of areas in which current standards can be improved. The *definition of mis-*

conduct finds no universal agreement, especially concerning areas such as incompetence and reckless or extremely biased interpretation of results. *Requirements for evidence of misconduct* is another area for potential disagreement. Careless error and poor judgement might be considered by some, but not by others, as evidence of misconduct. It is probably true that all clinical trials contain data errors and circumstances of poor judgement. However, one must ascertain the motives and intent of the investigators before misconduct can be established. There is *no universal standard of proof* applied by research institutions or the PHS/NSF.

The appropriate nature and extent of *due process* for those accused of misconduct is another difficult area. The consequences of a finding of misconduct are potentially serious. Investigators can be prevented from receiving funding for a period of years and have their reputations damaged. There is often disagreement about the nature of an appropriate process for adjudication and appeal. The case cited at the beginning of this chapter regarding Thereza Imanishi-Kari illustrates both the consequences of allegations and the impact of lack of due process. In June, 1996, a federal appeals board cleared Imanishi-Kari of charges of misconduct, an action which did little to satisfy critics on both sides of the debate [Singer, 1996; Weiss, 1996]. One should also read the account of this case by Healy [1996] for a perspective on this issue. Similarly, the *role of the courts* is not well defined, leaving the possibility that some findings could be challenged on legal grounds.

Not all institutions are able to provide the same quality of investigation for allegations of misconduct. This *lack of uniformity* could create injustices. The quality of ORI investigations is sometimes criticized, and it is not clear whether or not they should conduct investigations. Also, we must consider the possibility that whistleblowers may face reprisals by individuals or institutions exposed. However, the possibility exists that *false accusations* could be made to damage the reputations of good scientists and that whistleblowing may be a convenient posture for such accusers to take.

In many cases, researchers who are not a party to the case may be interested in the findings of investigations. This is sometimes true for cases in which no finding of misconduct is made. Despite the *Freedom of Information Act*, some information is held confidential by ORI. This restriction can present problems for those trying to understand more about the nature and extent of misconduct, or use the information in other appropriate ways. The role, if any, of *peer review* in detecting or controlling misconduct is controversial. Study of many cases suggests that it is an inadequate mechanism with which to detect misconduct. However, other structures, such as authorship guidelines and requirements for IRB approval, seem like sensible steps to discourage misconduct.

18.4 Characteristics of Some Misconduct Cases

There are many misconduct cases that one could choose that highlight important points about scientific integrity and how these problems are examined and resolved. Many detailed descriptions are provided by Broad and Wade [1982], Kohn [1986], and Miller and Hersen [1992]. Two cases of misconduct are particularly interesting. The first is noteworthy because of its extensiveness, boldness, and relevance to many aspects of the problem of scientific misconduct. It is a "modern" case, amplified by the power of medical journals to disseminate information. The second is recent and more directly related to the conduct, analysis, and interpretation of clinical trials. It is also "modern" because the sensationalism of the episode was created or distorted by the media. Both cases have useful lessons for clinical investigators reflecting on the integrity of the scientific process.

Anticipating the details below, it is interesting and disturbing to see the extent to which retrospective views of these high-profile cases by review committees find faults with the supervision of the individuals in question. Frequently there are clues that falsification is taking place, particularly when seen after the fact. At the time, however, with the limited information available to any one collaborator or supervisor, the evidence may not be sufficient to question the basis of trust, which is so fundamental to the scientific process.

18.4.1 Darsee case

An extensive case of misconduct came to light in 1981, when a 34-year-old clinical investigator, John R. Darsee, M.D., was found by colleagues at Harvard to have fabricated data in one study. Evidence subsequently developed showed that Darsee had fabricated data, beginning when he was an undergraduate student at Notre Dame, continuing through his residency and fellowship at Emory, and into his fellowship at Brigham and Women's Hospital, an affiliate of Harvard. Details of this extensive case can be found in an editorial by Relman [1983] and a review by Culliton [1983].

Chronology of events

The index act of fabrication took place on May 21, 1981, during a laboratory experiment on dogs. Dr. Darsee was seen obtaining data over a few hours but labeling them to make it appear that they had been collected over a period of two weeks. The action took place within plain sight of co-workers. An internal investigation of Dr. Darsee's research was begun by his supervisor. At first, there was no evidence of more extensive fabrication and Darsee was allowed to continue participating in an NIH collaborative study. Even so, the offer of a faculty position was withdrawn and his NIH fellowship was terminated.

In November, 1981, the fabrications and falsifications appeared to extend to a major NIH collaborative study. The data from Harvard were found to be strongly different from those obtained at other sites in the multi-institutional study. At this time, an external committee was appointed by the Dean of Harvard to investigate.

In December, 1981, NIH appointed a second panel to conduct an independent audit and, after six months, another group, composed of senior NIH staff, was asked to review the panel's findings. Subsequently, investigations at Emory and even of undergraduate days at Notre Dame were performed. Extensive problems were found in Darsee's work from Emory [Knox, 1983].

Findings

At least 17 published papers and 53 abstracts written or coauthored by Darsee were ultimately retracted because of fraud or fabrication. In some cases, his coauthors had too little contact with the research to realize that fabrications had taken place, while in others, Darsee invented the data and published without the knowledge of the coauthors. In a few circumstances, Darsee insisted that individuals be listed as coauthors, over their objections, because they had been helpful in the past. In retrospect, some of the reports in the medical literature were incredible.

For example, one paper, published in 1981 in the *New England Journal of Medicine*, studied taurine levels in myocardial tissue [Darsee and Heymsfield, 1981]. It was based on a family of 43 members and stated that twice-yearly blood samples were drawn from each person on two consecutive days after fasting overnight. Additionally, 24-hour urine samples were said to have been collected on everyone. One patient was a 2-year-old child. Claims were made regarding tissue samples which, in hindsight, were highly questionable. The paper states that myocardial tissue was obtained within four hours of death from three patients and that cardiac biopsies were done before pacemaker insertions. These claims were considered unlikely by investigators, in retrospect. For these procedures (and many other of Darsee's clinical studies) no IRB approvals were requested. In this paper, Darsee acknowledged help from three individuals who probably did not exist. Thus, the fabrication extended beyond falsifying data to include inventing collaborators.

Perspective

Because of the length of time involved and extensiveness of the fabrications, it is evident than little can be done to stop an unscrupulous scientist, even when he or she collaborates with knowledgeable and reasonably attentive colleagues. This, then, is the first lesson to be learned from the Darsee affair. A second and third lesson are to see the extent to which science is not self-correcting with fraudulent data and the inability of peer review to detect it. Most of Darsee's work was peer reviewed by good editorial processes and was able to pass without suspicion.

With special regard to clinical trials, a fourth lesson is the need for explicit guidelines and oversight for collection, maintenance, and analysis of data. The fifth feature of the Darsee case, and one that has contributed to widespread improvement in the last decade, is a focus on the responsibilities and contributions of coauthors. To be a coauthor requires substantial input into study design, analysis, interpretation, and writing of the research report. Finally, it is evident from this case that misconduct investigations may need to examine a researcher's entire work over many years. Patterns there may be important for verifying true misconduct.

18.4.2 Poisson (NSABP) Case

The National Surgical Adjuvant Breast and Bowel Project (NSABP) is a large multi-center collaborative oncology clinical trials group that has pioneered, among other treatments, breast conserving surgical treatment for breast cancer in the United States. The NSABP has been headquartered in Pittsburgh under the leadership of Dr. Bernard Fisher, involves as many as 5,000 physicians at 484 institutions in North America, and has been funded by the National Cancer Institute (NCI) since about 1960. The data falsification by a single investigator within the NSABP produced enormous controversy from various perspectives and taught many lessons to clinical trialists. A detailed look at the chronology of events is essential to understanding the facts and consequences of the case. Additional details can be found in NCI Press Releases [1994a–f], Goldberg and Goldberg [1994], Angell and Kassire [1994], Cohn [1994], and an exchange of letters in the *New England Journal of Medicine* [Vol. 330, pp. 1458–1462].

Chronology of events

In June, 1990, an NSABP data manager noted discrepancies in data received from one institution, L'Hôpital Saint-Luc in Montreal, Canada. The principal investigator at L'Hôpital Saint-Luc was Roger Poisson, M.D. This institution was soon audited twice, in September and December, 1990, by representatives of the NSABP Coordinating Center. As a result of findings in the audits, the NSABP suspended accrual by that institution in February, 1991, and notified the NCI that problems had been found. The NCI notified the Office of Scientific Integrity (soon to be ORI) and the Food and Drug Administration (FDA), after which both agencies began independent investigations of the matter.

In May, 1991, Dr. Poisson was listed in the Public Health Service alert system and was disqualified for life by the FDA from receiving investigational drugs. The ORI filed a formal complaint against him in September, 1991. While the administrative proceedings were happening, NCI and NSABP officials were not allowed to comment publicly on the investigation. The NSABP re-analyzed the clinical trials under suspicion internally after deleting the questionable data, and found the new results to be nearly identical to those published originally. Both NCI and ORI were convinced that continuing to rely on the previously published results would pose no risk to the public health.

By December, 1992, the ORI completed its report, released it to the NSABP and L'Hôpital Saint-Luc in February, 1993, and published the findings in the *ORI Newsletter* [ORI, April, 1993] and the *Federal Register* [DHHS, June, 1993]. A notice also appeared in the *NIH Guide for Grants and Contracts* [NIH, June 25, 1993]. The case did not come to public attention until well after these events had taken place, as a consequence of newspaper articles published in the *Chicago Tribune*, beginning March 13, 1994. The media and public attention seemed surprising to many individuals knowledgeable about the case, because the investigation had been closed and published for nearly a year, and because government and academic officials knew that the research findings were not sensitive to the inclusion or exclusion of data from the Montreal institution. These facts were slower to be disseminated than the anxiety over the fabrications.

Since March, 1994, other instances of irregularities in NSABP studies came to light including concern over patient consents and data quality at the Memorial Cancer Research Foundation of Southern California and audits were undertaken at institutions in Louisiana, New York, and California. On March 28, 1994, Dr. Fisher was forced to resign as head of the NSABP, and on April 13, 1994 Congressman John D. Dingell, chair of the Subcommittee on Oversight and Investigations of the House of Representatives, held investigations focused on the NIH's response to the events. Dr. Fisher was sharply criticized by Mr. Dingell. In July, 1994, Fisher filed a lawsuit against the University of Pittsburgh for violating his rights to due process when he was forced to resign. On March 6, 1995, Fisher filed suit against NCI because 148 of his papers had been labeled with "scientific misconduct" warnings on computer listings. After a hearing in March, 1995, the labels were removed, pending a final judgement on the suit.

Findings

The ORI was able to document 115 instances of data falsification or fabrication in data arising from 99 patients at L'Hôpital Saint-Luc. Dr. Poisson had participated in 22 NSABP clinical trials, placing about 1500 patients on study. The fabrications, some using duplicate records to avoid detection, involved 7% of the patients. Fourteen of the 22 trials had been published. Research subjects with falsified data were included in four publications from the NSABP. Study B-06 compared lumpectomy with or without radiation therapy to mastectomy for the treatment of early stage breast cancer. Study B-13 compared chemotherapy to no further treatment among women with surgically resected node negative, ER negative disease. Study B-14 compared Tamoxifen to placebo in women with surgically resected node negative, ER positive cancer. Protocol B-16 compared Tamoxifen plus chemotherapy to Tamoxifen alone among postmenopausal women with node positive breast cancer.

The fabrications and falsifications found were consequential for patient eligibility but not outcome. There was documentation of falsified estrogen receptor (ER) values in some patients, alterations of dates of surgery and biopsy to meet eligibility requirements, and accrual of ineligible patients. Consent forms could not be found for three patients who were placed on study protocols. The ORI deemed all data from L'Hôpital Saint-Luc unreliable on the basis of these findings. They recommended that all future NSABP trials be published without such data, that the group publish a re-analysis of previous studies without the questionable data, and that Dr. Poisson be prevented from receiving federal funds. At NCI's request, Dr. Poisson was replaced as Saint-Luc's principle investigator in March, 1991. NCI asked Dr. Fisher to publish a manuscript re-analyzing the studies after excluding data from Saint-Luc. Since the initial findings, some irregularities in data from 11 other institutions participating in NSABP trials were found.

Perspective

The NSABP case is remarkable from a variety of perspectives. From the first perspective, we see the blatant fabrication of data in important clinical trials by an experienced and respected researcher. Dr. Poisson's violation of the public and scientific trust was dealt with quickly by government and academic authorities. The penalties imposed were appropriate. From a second perspective, only eligibility criteria were fabricated and there was no evidence of harm to individuals or to the quantitative findings of the trials. These facts make this episode of misconduct appear to have less impact than many other cases. Nevertheless, its very existence makes it consequential. Dr. Poisson seemed unable to get past this point [Poisson, 1994].

Third, the case touches on the responsibilities of clinical investigators, sponsors, regulators, and the media when they uncover evidence of misconduct. Dr. Fisher was criticized for failing to publish revised manuscripts quickly, according to requests by NCI and others. The NSABP's misjudgment of the need for this and the disproportionate public response to the case can surely be considered honest error. Many officials knew the quantitative unimportance of the data falsifications on the study results and the fact that numerous other well-performed clinical trials strongly supported the findings of the NSABP studies B-06, B-13, B-14, and B-16. They could probably have alleviated much public concern by emphasizing this.

Readers wishing to obtain a detailed perspective on the NSABP case and useful references in as compact a form as possible should read the *New England Journal of Medicine* editorial by Angell and Kassirer [1994], and replies in the correspondence section of the same issue. The case is made there that journal editors are among those who need to know when findings of misconduct are made and changes to the published literature may be required. The journal also argues that they should be notified during the investigation. This is clearly problematic, because many investigations do not result in a finding of misconduct.

Finally, we must consider the forces that can transform a misconduct case into front-page news after it has been closed for a year. Even after two years of investigation, an additional year following closure by the ORI, and the fact that considerable knowledge was in hand concerning the lack of impact of the findings on the public health and results of the trial, a large amount of tension and anxiety was created among all the parties involved with the case. One has to consider the possibility of political or other forces being at work and expect that the final chapter in this misconduct case has yet to be written.

Impact of the NSABP case

At the time of this writing, the impact of the NSABP case is still being felt in the clinical trials community. There have been formal procedural changes in the way that NCI and ORI disseminate information about misconduct cases. In particular, journals will be automatically notified of such findings in the future [Broder, 1994; Bivens and Macfarlane, 1994]. Many NIH sponsored clinical trials coordinating centers have examined their methods for data quality control and monitoring in the light of some criticism [e.g., Cohen, 1994; Weiss et al., 1993]. Interestingly, NCI sponsored studies are already among the most carefully monitored. It seems likely that monitoring of NIH sponsored trials, particularly the role and conduct of the DSMC, will be more formal and uniform in the future (see Chapter 10). There is likely to be increased attention to quality control procedures, particularly auditing, in the future despite its dubious value in suppressing misconduct [Shapiro and Charrow, 1989].

However, there is probably little that an audit can do to discourage a determined and unscrupulous investigator who maintains duplicate records to avoid detection.

Clinical trials are naturally messy, though not fraudulent because of it. It would be unfortunate to see too much effort used to thoroughly clean up data errors in clinical trials without knowing if this would improve their validity. Excessive auditing or other quality control procedures could increase the cost of trials and thereby reduce their size or number. It is probably true that all trials have a range of error in them, but provided the error rate is low, it is unlikely that it has much impact on their validity. Scientific integrity demands that investigators try to get the most reliable answers they can and not spend resources unless it will help correct a significant problem. For trial designers, it is important to have only eligibility criteria which are truly necessary.

Two other issues come into sharp focus upon reviewing the NSABP case. First is the rather poor treatment that NSABP officials have received throughout the affair by some government and university officials. At times, the trialists seemed to be treated like those who perpetrated the misconduct rather than uncovered it. As of December 1996, the ORI had not closed cases involving NSABP officials. Perhaps institutions and/or the ORI could promote standards for civility and collaboration when performing these investigations. Furthermore, it is difficult to find trustworthy, innovative, experienced clinical researchers like most of the NSABP members. The NSABP has contributed greatly over the years to clinical science, but was judged quickly and harshly by some. All trialists feel vulnerable with regard to the actions of their collaborators, making the Poisson case very sobering.

It is not obvious that re-analyses of clinical trials in question because of misconduct should discard all the data from the institution where misconduct was found. In the NSABP case, the violations were in eligibility criteria and not outcomes, making it debatable as to whether or not any of the ineligible patients should be excluded. Consider the discussion in Chapter 4 concerning design validity compared with biological validity. In a survey of opinions about falsified data, many trial participants stated that they would like to see the analysis include problem records [McIntyre, Kornblith, and Coburn, 1996]. For example, if the eligibility criteria had been violated through honest error, the "all patients randomized" analysis would include them and would be a valid comparison of the treatments. If the misconduct had been solely financial, for example, we would probably not consider discarding data. While, in the NSABP case, it seems prudent to exclude the cases, we think this way, in part, because we know that the results remain unaffected by our action. What if the study results depended on the presence or absence of those participants?

Misconduct cases such as the NSABP experience bring into sharp focus the different frameworks in which the actions of scientists will be viewed. Scientists tend to view their own actions, misconduct or not, in a purely scientific framework. However, suspicion or proof of misconduct forces us to view and manage the situation from perspectives that may be primarily non-rational. A larger relevant perspective is that of the public's health, safety, and perception. When dealing with allegations of misconduct, researchers need to appreciate the consequences of their actions when viewed publicly. This is often the most important perspective. Some actions, which are (only) scientifically correct, might be seen as arrogant by the public. Openness, conservatism in dealing with risks, efficiency, and a willingness to make changes in process are non-scientific attributes that can greatly reassure the public.

18.4.3 Recognizing fraud or misconduct

In most of the well-known cases of scientific misconduct, the improper actions took place over a prolonged period, and came to light after a single precipitating event. Usually the published reports cannot be distinguished from legitimate science, except in retrospect and with the awareness of other questionable or improper actions by the researcher. In fact, as in the Poisson case, the published reports may still accurately convey much quantitative information. The peer review publication process is not an efficient way to recognize improper behavior.

It is unusual to question findings after they appear solely on the basis of information contained in the published report. An interesting exception in the basic sciences is the paper by Kuznetsov [1989], supposedly containing molecular biological evidence against evolution, and a critique of the work by Larhammar [1994; 1995]. Kuznetsov reported finding an "antievolutionary factor" that functioned through messenger RNA. His work was published in a somewhat unusual place for its evolution-related conclusions. Larhammar became skeptical enough to study it only after seeing the paper cited by a creationist.

In reviewing Kuznetsov's work, Larhammar noted a number of discrepancies: the methods were unusual and poorly documented; the report contained unusual precision and consisted mostly of tables and numbers; biological inconsistencies were ignored; non-existent journals were cited several times; two references were cited by the author himself but the journals could not be found, and the papers were not even on his own list of publications; an article attributed to another researcher in a known journal did not exist; and many papers cited had grammatically incorrect and illogical titles. Larhammar suggests that the paper by Kuznetsov contains fabricated data and references. If so, it is unusual in that it could have been detected by a knowledgeable and skeptical review.

Falsification is more likely in some areas

In the clinical conduct of trials, falsifications are more likely for certain source data. This can be a consequence of having some data sources supervised by individuals who are pressured to keep schedules and accruals up to date and/or who may not share the clinical and scientific ethic that discourages falsification. Support staff and junior faculty members may not have sufficient ethics training to help them resolve problems caused by this kind of pressure. The first potential problem area in data is eligibility and exclusion criteria. Known disqualifying characteristics of the patient may be ignored or falsified. Age, dates of clinical landmarks, or other numerical data can be easily altered. Similarly, previous treatments or events in the medical history may be suppressed.

When the protocol calls for serial measurements or documentation of diagnostic tests, reports from previous clinic visits may be propagated as current. Biopsy, blood, urine, or other specimens may be carried along or replaced with those from other patients. Entire clinical visits can be fabricated or dates changed to meet protocol specifications. Pill counts or medication diaries can be altered. This type of behavior may be common among patients (on or off studies) who wish to appear compliant with the rules of the study. Unfortunately, all of these areas are also subject to honest error. Although it is difficult to distinguish between error and falsification on the basis of a few events, investigators should be aware of and suspicious about a pattern of "mistakes".

Detecting problems

Some circumstances are so unlikely that they suggest misconduct. Although it is a matter of judgment as to how unusual circumstances are, investigators may be alerted to possible misconduct by observing the following points: Although pleasing, high accrual rates (combined with low rejection rates) may represent a problem, especially if eligibility is not documented in a timely fashion. Real patients and clinic visits are prone to stretch or violate the rigid criteria of the protocol. If this appears not to happen because the need for exceptions or variances never arises, but the data are carefully and completely recorded, there may be a problem.

Discrepancies between source documents and the data base can also be a sign of trouble. There may be source documents missing or clinic logs may be different from the data recorded. These and other similar problems may be noted by quality assurance or audit personnel. Auditing is an important tool for assuring data quality, but may not be sufficient when used without additional measures [Shapiro and Charrow, 1989; Weiss et al., 1993]. Collaborative groups of investigators have no universal audit policy [Cohen, 1994]. Finally, certain behavior is suspicious. This includes an individual frequently scheduling patient visits when no supervisors are present (e.g., after hours), refusing to have colleagues cover for him or her, or refusing to undergo quality assurance checks. Allegations (formal or informal) or suspicions by other staff members may be a response to suspicious behavior.

18.4.4 Misconduct cases yield other lessons

When reviewing the process and findings of many misconduct cases, some common themes emerge that seem to characterize the cases, perhaps even contributing to the findings. Not all of these occur in each case of misconduct, but they can help us to understand the roots of inappropriate behavior by researchers. One potential problem area is the use of questionable or *unverifiable data* such as those transmitted orally or in an interview. Data arising in this fashion may be more subject to error and bias of all types than objectively collected ones. For the same reason, they may be more prone to falsification and should be avoided, if possible. However, there are circumstances in which it is worth collecting and using such data. It is up to the designers and administrators of the study to anticipate and minimize problems. *Unconventional research methods or design* may contribute to, or be associated with misconduct. Of course, such methods may also be associated with breakthroughs and innovation. In either case, unconventional methods probably deserve more scrutiny than methods that are well-known.

Plagiarism of ideas or words is explicitly defined as misconduct and is some-times associated with a more widespread and long-term pattern of inappropriate behavior. Many times, the discovered incident of misconduct is not the first, and a careful review reveals a more extensive history of repeated plagiarism. Some misconduct cases originate with, or are perpetuated by, a *lack of respect for or rapport* among colleagues. Manifestations of this might include more acrimonious, personal, extensive, emotional, and longer-term disagreements than those typical of scientific debate. Evidence for a lack of respect may need to be viewed in light of its potential association with misconduct.

Many investigations of misconduct have one or more *collections of data* as a focus. Often, the data themselves are the main issue. In other cases, questions about origination, authenticity, or quality of the data are central to the issue of misconduct. Thus, documentation, organization, and quality control procedures for data are vital in both review of allegations and prevention of misconduct. Individuals responsible for data need proper technical and ethical training. They should not work alone or without adequate supervision, be overworked, or placed under undue pressure to meet performance guidelines. Extra risk of inappropriate conduct is probably present if problems with interpersonal relationships occur in conjunction with such pressures.

Finally, investigators should take particular care with *politically high-profile research* or when using *controversial drugs or devices*. Scientific misconduct is not more probable in such cases, perhaps being even less likely than elsewhere. However, any instances of questionable practice in these situations are likely to be examined in a forum that amplifies errors and discourages impartial discourse. In these settings, guilt may be assumed before an adequate review of allegations can be accomplished.

18.5 Clinical Investigators' Responsibilities

Clinical investigators have responsibilities for both patient care and the integrity of the research process. In specific research areas, investigators may have additional responsibilities beyond those discussed here, to ensure the correctness and quality of their findings. An investigator may comply with standards as an individual or, in the case of many academic environments, the department or university may furnish some critical components as part of a general support for research. In many cases, cooperative mechanisms are in place to assist or support some basic needs. In any case, the investigator must assume the final responsibility for all aspects of the research.

There are a few written guidelines outlining the investigator's responsibilities, particularly in collaborative research projects or those subject to governmental oversight. For example, when investigators hold Investigational New Drug (IND) licenses, they are subject to rules and regulations promulgated by the Food and Drug Administration (FDA). Similarly, NIH and individual institutions have requirements in specific cases. NIH and institutions will hold investigators responsible for standards of research practices. Ignorance of the requirements is not an adequate defense for deficiencies.

In recent years, some multi-center clinical trial protocols are prepared by companies or other sponsoring organizations without naming a principal investigator (PI). This may make some aspects of study development more rapid or convenient. Presumably, the sponsor expects to perform all of the duties of the PI. While the PI role is a difficult and time consuming one and research sponsors actually do much of the work, failing to name a principal investigator creates many problems. Important responsibilities (see below) are diffused and could be overlooked. Because there is no identified focus for responsibility, participating institutional investigators may not be able to obtain all the information they require from a single source. Decisions that need to be made during the conduct of the study could be delayed. Failure to name an experienced clinician as principal investigator is an unnecessary and serious shortcoming.

18.5.1 General responsibilities

At least implicitly, clinical investigators assume, as a minimum, the following responsibilities for clinical trials under their supervision:

1. Developing a clinical hypothesis and a feasible approach to answer the study questions.
2. Establishing statistically valid endpoints for the clinical objectives of the study.
3. Defining the data to be collected.
4. Documenting the feasibility and scientific rationale for the approach.
5. Constructing record keeping forms and systems.
6. Maintaining a data system for timely, complete, and accurate recording of data elements, which are necessary to meet the objectives of the study. The data should be accessible to authorized investigators at all times for quality control purposes (but not necessarily to the clinical investigators).
7. Performing and documenting quality assurance procedures and results. This includes participation in audits based on predefined standards. Multi-center collaborations often come with these requirements.
8. Providing a mechanism for timely and objective review of safety, pathological review of specimens, and subjectively derived data by a Data Safety and Monitoring Board or other appropriate mechanism.
9. Timely and complete detection and reporting of unexplained deaths on study and/or adverse drug reactions or other side effects of treatment.
10. Accounting for investigational drugs and devices.
11. Assuring and documenting that the project complies with regulatory requirements and other oversight. These can come from the institution, the hospital, the study sponsor, NIH, or the FDA.
12. Certifying the clinical and research competence of co-investigators and other physicians or health professionals participating in the project.
13. Data ownership, access, information systems, and storage of data for time periods required by NIH or institutions.

18.5.2 Additional responsibilities related to INDs

When the investigator is using an unlicensed drug for research purposes, an IND approval from the FDA is required. Thus, the investigator must submit the IND application to the agency. The application and approval process requires:

1. Documentation on Form 1572 of co-investigators and participating investigators (those treating patients on the study but not listed as co-investigators). This requires names, addresses, location of the study and the Institutional Review Board (IRB) that is responsible for the research.

2. The co-investigators must report adverse experiences and deaths to the principal investigator (PI), so that they may be included in an annual report.

3. The PI must collect curriculum vitae from all participating investigators and documentation of education, training, and experience.

4. The PI must name or serve as a study monitor to oversee all aspects of the investigation.

5. During the study, adverse events must be reported to the FDA within ten days of the event. An annual progress report to the FDA is required and, at study termination, a final report is sent to the FDA and IRB.

6. For NIH studies, Form 310 (IRB review documentation) is required. Similarly, the PI must maintain documentation of all collaborating IRBs and assure that the consent forms contain necessary information about risks, benefits, and treatment alternatives.

7. The PI is responsible for timely distribution to all investigators, in writing, of all study amendments.

8. None of the federal reporting requirements substitute for local institutional requirements.

18.5.3 Sponsor Responsibilities

Some of the responsibilities sketched above may be met, in part, by the investigator's institution or sponsor. When an individual investigator submits an IND application to the FDA, he or she is the sponsor. These might include:

1. Expertise and timely consulting regarding:
   (a) Study design and performance
   (b) Biostatistical support for study design and analysis
   (c) Regulatory and policy issues

2. Support for clinical research functions too complex for single investigators, including:
   (a) Audit process and certification of study performance
   (b) Maintenance of an accurate, quality controlled, flexible, and powerful database
   (c) Expert and collegial peer review of research project development

3. Efficient research support services, including:

      (a) Patient registration/randomization

      (b) Eligibility checking

      (c) IND administration

      (d) Repository and tracking of consent documents

      (e) Files of study protocol documents

4. Data management/coordination support

5. Preparation of files for statistical analysis

6. Statistical analysis

18.6 Summary

Scientific misconduct has a long history, but its origins, causes, and exact frequency are obscure. Because funding for research is scarce, public oversight of science is more attentive than it has been at many times in the past. Prominant instances of misconduct by scientists also increase public awareness and scrutiny.. Unfortunately, peer review and replication of results are not sufficient safeguards against misconduct.

Workable definitions of misconduct are difficult because it is hard to define the norms of science. These include, but may not be limited to, honesty and objectivity, tolerance, doubt of certitude, recognition of error, unselfish engagement, and communal spirit. Significant departures from any of these norms would likely be seen as misconduct. In the U.S., a widely held view of the definition of scientific misconduct comes from the National Academy of Sciences. They define misconduct as plagiarism, data fabrication, and data falsification, but also delineate questionable research practices and other forms of misconduct.

Research institutions and sponsors have formal procedures for dealing with allegations of misconduct. For research funded by the U.S. Public Health Service, misconduct cases are handled by the Office of Research Integrity (ORI), which ensures that institutions have adequate mechanisms for dealing with allegations, oversees institutional investigations, or conducts its own investigations. The National Science Foundation has an entity with a similar role.

Review of the circumstances surrounding some misconduct cases in the clinical sciences suggests that investigators can learn some valuable lessons about preventing or detecting misconduct. First is the benefit of increased awareness of the potential for problems and maintaining a healthy skepticism about unusual findings. Individuals with little supervision and a great deal of responsibility and pressure are more likely to behave inappropriately. Subjective or unverifiable data may be more prone to error, including dishonest mistakes. Recurrent irregularities can also be a sign of an underlying cause. Finally, investigators should be more attentive to unconventional research methods, individuals with interpersonal difficulties or other stress, and controversies over data, methods, or treatments.

18.7 Questions for Discussion

1. Discuss the role of "whistleblowers" in identifying and investigating scientific misconduct. You might consult the report by Rossiter [1992]. Is the role for such a person the same as or different from their role in other areas such as financial impropriety?

2. Discuss your views on due process for scientists accused of misconduct. What are the required elements of the process you favor (e.g., investigation, defense, judgment, appeal) and where should they be located?

3. Discuss changes in the peer review process that might discourage or detect data fabrication or falsification. How practical are your suggestions?

4. Discuss the role of didactic education in preventing scientific misconduct. Give examples if you can find them.

5. Read Hill [1995] and discuss ways in which it might be applicable to peer review of manuscripts.

18.8 Appendix: Procedures for Dealing with Misconduct

The following procedures illustrate a university approach to dealing with professional misconduct. They are taken from the pamphlet titled *Faculty Policies of the Johns Hopkins University School of Medicine: Procedures for Dealing with Issues of Professional Misconduct.*

18.8.1 Introduction

The School of Medicine is an institution dedicated to truth in pursuit of knowledge, through biomedical research, to the transmission of knowledge through teaching, and to the application of medical knowledge to patient care. A spirit of mutual respect and a broad trust that all faculty members, students, and staff share this dedication to the truth are essential to the functioning of the School. Nevertheless, from time to time some members of the community may appear to have disregarded accepted norms of professional behavior. The procedures outlined here were developed to provide a fair and orderly means of handling issues of suspected professional misconduct.

"Professional misconduct", for the purpose of this document, means deception in scholarship, research, patient care, or in the supervision or administration of research, or intentional disregard of established norms of conduct in these activities. The term "professional misconduct" encompasses "research fraud" within the meaning of the University's Policy on Integrity in Research, which defines research fraud as "the intentional falsification or fabrication of data or results, plagiarism, misconduct in the application of research procedures so as to bias results, or other deceptive research or reporting procedures." Established norms of conduct are more fully described in the Report of the Association of American Universities Committee on the Integrity of Research. Disregard of established norms of conduct may be intentional or may be inadvertent. In either case, public trust and the pursuit of scientific truth are endangered, and the School has an obligation to act. It may be appropriate, however, for the School to respond differently to different acts of misconduct.

The following procedures recognize that it may be difficult to determine whether misconduct has occurred, and that the process of inquiry or investigation must be sufficiently flexible to permit early termination of the proceedings when it becomes clear that charges are unjustified or that the issue can be resolved appropriately by other expeditious means. For this reason, the procedure for determining whether professional misconduct has occurred has been divided into three major stages: Preliminary Inquiry, Investigation, and Adjudication.

Moreover, as the goal of these procedures is to assure that fairness is afforded each person alleged to have committed an act of professional misconduct, every preliminary inquiry and subsequent investigation shall be based on a presumption of innocence until proven otherwise. It is not intended that the proceedings be adversarial in nature. Rather, it is intended that all stages of this procedure be conducted in the spirit of peer review. The University and School of Medicine will not have legal counsel present during meetings of inquiring, investigative, or deliberative bodies, and no person accused and no accuser may appear before an inquiring, investigative, or deliberative body with legal counsel. The School firmly believes that duly constituted boards and committees of the faculty should be free to meet directly with their colleagues on the business of the School without presence of counsel.

18.8.2 I. The Advisory Committee on Professional Misconduct

The Advisory Committee on Professional Misconduct shall consist of three senior faculty members appointed by the Dean. The committee shall advise, in a confidential manner, any member of this academic community who suspects that misconduct by a School of Medicine faculty member, student, or staff member, has occurred but who may be uncertain as to whether the acts in question constitute professional misconduct; or who requires guidance about the manner in which professional misconduct should be reported; or who may be uneasy about approaching a department director, division director, or the dean with a serious allegation. A person who suspects misconduct has the option of consulting with the Advisory Committee before taking other steps. If a person feels assured, after consultation with the Advisory Committee, that there has been no professional misconduct, he or she should take no further action in the matter. In the event that a person alerts the Advisory Committee to a possible instance of professional misconduct but declines to pursue the issue further contrary to that committee's advice, the Advisory Committee is obligated by its knowledge of the alleged misconduct to report the allegation to the department or division director or the dean. Withholding the identity of the person bringing the matter to the attention of the Advisory Committee cannot be guaranteed, since this person may be an important witness or source of information.

Since a charge of misconduct, even if unjustified, may seriously damage an individual's career, it is desirable for any issue of misconduct to be handled in as confidential a manner as possible under the circumstances. As few people as possible should be involved at any stage of the procedure. Normally an inquiry or investigation should be commenced as promptly as possible, and continued in an expeditious manner, with full attention to the interests of all individuals involved.

18.8.3 II. Preliminary Inquiry

Any faculty member, student, or staff member who suspects that professional misconduct has occurred has an obligation to report that suspicion to the director of the department or division affected or to the Dean of the School of Medicine. There must be no recriminations for a person bringing an allegation in good faith, and persons who have acted in good faith will be protected from retaliatory conduct.

The purpose of the preliminary inquiry is to provide prompt termination of accusations of misconduct that are erroneous, frivolous, or malicious. The question is: Do the initial allegations warrant investigation? The department or division director must initially determine whether or not it is appropriate for him or her to conduct the preliminary inquiry. If the department or division director is personally associated to any degree with the research or for any other reason is unable to conduct the preliminary inquiry in an impartial manner, or if the initial allegation of misconduct is received by the Dean, then the preliminary inquiry shall be conducted by the Dean or his designee. Otherwise, the department inquiry shall be conducted by the Dean or his designee. Otherwise, the department or division director will review the matter personally or with the help of a departmental ad hoc committee. The purpose of the review is to identify serious accusations and to put to rest frivolous, patently unjustified or mistaken allegations.

A preliminary inquiry also may be initiated at the insistence of the Dean upon information that has come to his attention from any source whatsoever.

The person accused of misconduct must be notified of the inquiry no later than the time that the outcome of the inquiry is reported. The department or division director or Dean shall determine whether and to what extent it is necessary or appropriate to involve the person accused in the inquiry at an earlier stage for clarification purposes.

If the department or division director decides that there are no grounds for a charge of misconduct and that no further action is necessary, a written report of the matter should be submitted to the Dean and the chairman of the Standing committee on Discipline. Where the department or division director believes that extraordinary circumstances exist that make written communication inappropriate and that a departure from normal practice is necessary to protect innocent parties, the submission of the report to the Dean and the chairman of the Standing committee on Discipline may be oral. Alternatively, if the Dean or his designee decides that there are no grounds for a charge of misconduct and that no further action is necessary, a written report of the matter should be submitted to the chairman of the Standing Committee on Discipline. However, where the Dean or his designee believes that extraordinary circumstances exist that make written communication inappropriate and that a departure from normal practice is necessary to protect innocent parties, the submission of the report to the chairman of the Standing Committee on Discipline may be oral. If no written report is submitted to the Dean or to the Chairman of the Standing Committee on Discipline, the department or division director or Dean, as appropriate, shall establish a confidential, sequestered file stating the findings of the inquiry, including the reasons for not submitting a report to the Dean or the Standing Committee on Discipline.

If the department or division director decides on the basis of information gathered during the inquiry that there is reason to suspect that misconduct has occurred, he shall report his findings to the Dean and the chairman of the Standing Committee on Discipline. If the Dean or his designee decides on the basis of information gathered during the inquiry that there is reason to suspect that misconduct has occurred, he shall report his findings to the chairman of the Standing Committee on Discipline. An early oral notification is encouraged, but this should be followed immediately by a written notification.

At the conclusion of the inquiry, the department or division director or Dean shall advise the person initiating the investigation of the disposition of the matter.

If, following preliminary inquiry, there appears to be grounds for a charge of professional misconduct, the Dean will initial a formal investigation into the matter and notify the Provost of the pending investigation.

18.8.4 III. Investigation

The purpose of the investigation is to assemble all relevant evidence relating to the alleged misconduct from documentation, from interviews with those involved, and from interviews with those knowledgeable about the activities under investigation. This procedure of data collection by peers is to objective, independent, unbiased, thorough, and non-judgmental. The investigation should determine whether there was fabrication, dishonesty, or such significant disregard of the norms of professional conduct as to call into question the reliability of research, the credibility of reported results of clinical or non-clinical activities, or the propriety of any conduct which, if subjected to scrutiny, would adversely affect the integrity and reputation of the academic and research activities of the University and its faculty. The Ad Hoc Committee will conduct a careful review of the allegations, employing procedures appropriate to the nature of the inquiry and designed to afford a fair opportunity to all concerned individuals to present their information and views to the committee. Consideration should be given to review of all research or patient care with which the accused is involved. Throughout the investigation, the accused and any collaborators or supervisors whose role in the alleged misconduct is under scrutiny should be afforded the opportunity to respond to questions related to their own performance and conduct and to provide additional information relevant to the subject matter of the inquiry.

The investigation will be conducted by an ad hoc committee appointed by the Dean and consisting of one or more disinterested members of the Standing committee on Discipline and additional faculty members as may be appropriate under the circumstances.

At this stage, the following steps must be taken by the Dean or his designee (if they have not been taken earlier).

1. The person accused of misconduct must be informed in writing of all of the charges against him, the source of the accusation, and that an investigation is taking place. The person accused shall be informed promptly of any amendment to the original charges.

2. The person accused will be notified of the identity of the members of the Ad Hoc Committee appointed by the Dean to conduct the investigation. The person accused may request that the Dean direct the substitution of a member of the Ad Hoc Committee for reasons of bias or potential conflict of interest.

3. The Ad Hoc Committee shall provide the accused with written notification of the place, time and date of a meeting at which his appearance is requested. Every effort shall be made to schedule such meetings at a mutually convenient time. Unless waived by the accused, no initial meeting between the accused and the Ad Hoc committee shall take place less than seven (7) days after the receipt of the Ad Hoc Committee's notification. The accused may request a rescheduling of the meeting(s) with the Ad Hoc Committee for good cause. The failure or refusal of the accused to meet with the Ad Hoc Committee shall not deter the progress of the investigation. If the person accused is no longer a member of the Johns Hopkins academic community, the requirements of written notice and an opportunity to answer to the charge of misconduct shall be observed as far as is practicable, but a failure of the person accused to respond or to make himself available to those with investigatory responsibilities shall not deter the inquiry and investigation.

4. All relevant materials and documents must be secured in the office of the Dean at the earliest opportunity.

5. At the beginning of the investigation stage, the person accused will be afforded the opportunity to consult with an uninvolved senior faculty member of his choice (e.g., a former member of the Committee on Discipline, who is knowledgeable about the proceedings), who will serve as "ombudsman" to the person accused throughout the proceedings. The role of the ombudsman will be to offer advice and guidance regarding the procedural aspects of the investigation. This individual will be appointed subject to approval by the person accused, and will subsequently remain uninvolved in any adjudication proceedings, and will be available throughout the investigation and subsequent stages to the accused individual, and may, upon request, accompany the person accused to meetings with investigating or adjudicating committees.

6. All meetings of the Ad Hoc Committee with the accused and persons interviewed shall be recorded verbatim. Copies of the recordings may be furnished the accused upon request.

7. The accused may present relevant evidence for examination and consideration by the Ad Hoc Committee. The accused may request that the Ad Hoc Committee interview certain individuals with relevant information concerning the matter under investigation. Whenever feasible, the accused will be afforded the opportunity to question the accuser at a meeting of the Ad Hoc

Committee before the Ad Hoc Committee completes its final report. If, in the judgement of the Dean, this would impose undue hardship on individuals involved, the face-to-face meeting may be waived. The accused may suggest to the Ad Hoc Committee any avenues of inquiry he believes are likely to produce relevant evidence.

8. The accused shall be afforded an opportunity to present a written statement at the inception and close of the Ad Hoc Committee's investigation.

9. The accused shall be furnished with a copy of the Ad Hoc Committee's report. Such report shall identify the persons interviewed, a summary of the interview, a description of the documents, data and other evidence examined by the Ad Hoc Committee, and the Committee's conclusion regarding each of the allegations.

10. Any granting agency that is supporting the research in question must be informed that an investigation is taking place. This may be done, consistent with the applicable agency rules, without identifying individuals. The agency shall be kept informed of progress throughout the investigation in accordance with its particular requirements.

11. At any stage of the investigation the Dean, after consultation with the Ad Hoc Committee, may take steps to notify other parties who, in his judgement, should be informed of the on-going investigation or its conclusion, and whether interim administrative action is necessary.

If the Ad Hoc Committee's investigation concludes that no professional misconduct has occurred, and if the Dean concurs with these findings, the matter shall be closed, with attention to full restoration of the reputation of those under investigation. The Dean shall retain the records of the investigation including the findings of the Ad Hoc Committee in a confidential, sequestered file. A copy of the Ad Hoc Committee's findings shall be sent to the chairman of the Standing Committee on Discipline.

If the allegations of misconduct are found by the Ad Hoc Committee to have been maliciously motivated or based on fraudulent evidence, appropriate disciplinary action may be initiated against those responsible in accordance with normal procedures. If, in the judgement of the Ad Hoc Committee, the allegations, however incorrect, appear to have been made in good faith, no retaliatory or disciplinary action shall be taken against the accusers from retaliation.

If the Ad Hoc Committee concludes that professional misconduct has occurred, it shall report its findings to the Standing Committee on Discipline, to the Dean, and to the accused.

18.8.5 IV. Adjudication by Standing Committee on Discipline

The role of the Standing Committee on Discipline is to review the investigation report in the context of any written material submitted by those alleged to have engaged in misconduct, and then to make judgemental recommendation concerning the future course of action. The questions are: Should the matter be dropped in whole or in part? Should there be further investigation? should the matter be referred to the Advisory Board for review and recommended disciplinary action?

Interested parties such as the accused and the accuser(s) shall be extended an opportunity to appear before and to submit written comments on the report of the Standing committee on Discipline indicating why the report to the Ad Hoc Committee should be accepted or rejected in whole or in part, or otherwise modified. Comments by interested parties on the report of the Ad Hoc Committee should be received by the office of the Dean within ten days of their receipt of the report.

The Standing Committee on Discipline shall review the report(s) of the Ad Hoc Committee together with any written comments submitted by interested parties. The Standing Committee on Discipline may (1) accept or reject the report in whole or in part, and recommend to the Advisory Board of the Medical Faculty those sanctions and remedial actions, if any, which the Standing Committee may consider appropriate to the circumstances; or (2) return the matter to the Ad Hoc committee for additional investigation or modification of its report. The Standing Committee's recommendations to the Advisory Board of the Medical Faculty may include one or more of the following: (1) withdrawal or correction of papers and abstracts, (b) notification directed to editors of journals where fraudulent or suspect research has been published, (c) notification of sponsoring agencies, (d) termination or alteration of employment status of persons whose misconduct is substantiated, (e) release of information about the incident to the public, particularly when public funds were used to support the fraudulent or suspect research, or (f) any other action deemed appropriate to the circumstances.

18.8.6 V. Advisory Board of the Medical Faculty

The Standing Committee on Discipline shall forward the report and its recommendations to the full Advisory Board (ABMF) which shall, in executive session, consider and decide the disciplinary action to be taken, if any. Before the Advisory Board reaches its decision, it may request the appearance of the accused and the accused shall be given an opportunity to appear before it and to submit any written statement or materials relevant to the matter under consideration . The ABMF shall report its decision to the Dean and to the accused. All records of the proceedings shall be maintained by the Dean.

If the ABMF determines that further investigation is necessary, it may return the matter to the Standing Committee on Discipline.

18.8.7 VI. Appeals

The appeal mechanism is limited to addressing the adherence to established procedure and the appropriateness of the disciplinary action. Following receipt of the decision of the ABMF, the accused, an accuser or any member of an investigation committee may take an appeal of that decision to the Dean within fourteen days. In the event of an adverse decision by the Dean, the accused, an accuser or any member of an investigation committee may take an appear of that decision to the Provost of the University within fourteen days. Review by the Dean and the Provost shall be limited to the adequacy of the procedures followed and to the appropriateness of the disciplinary action taken.

18.8.8 VII. Office of the General Counsel

The responsibilities of the Office of the General Counsel shall include:

1. ensuring compliance with all applicable laws and regulations;
2. monitoring the progress of the resolution of each allegation of professional misconduct to ensure adherence to the established School and University procedures;
3. general supervision of proceedings for the purpose of affording procedural fairness to the accused, the accuser and witnesses.

The Office of the General Counsel will not act as the prosecutor of the accused or defender of the accused, but will act as an impartial legal advisor to the Administration of the School of Medicine and University. Procedural questions from the accused, accuser and or prospective witnesses should be referred to the Office of the Dean and, when necessary, referred thereafter to the Office of the General Counsel.

The Office of the General Counsel is available to render advice to department or division directors, the Dean or his designee, the Advisory Committee on Professional Misconduct, the Standing Committee on Professional Misconduct, ad hoc committees, and the ABMF at any step of the proceedings. Individuals serving in any of these capacities are encouraged to seek legal guidance regarding any procedural question, particularly in connection with the preparation of written reports of actions taken, or before any action is taken with respect to any person believe to have made an accusation of professional misconduct in bad faith. Any contact or inquiry to the University or School of Medicine from a lawyer outside the University, including contacts and inquiries emanating from legal representatives of any Federal, State or local agency, must be referred to the Office of the General Counsel.

18.8.9 VIII. Exclusivity of Procedure

This procedure for the resolution of allegations of professional misconduct is the exclusive mechanism within the School of Medicine for adjudication of questions of this nature. A person sanctioned under this procedure may not invoke the School's grievance procedure in an effort to gain a readjudication of the charge.

Chapter References

Advisory Committee on Human Radiation Experiments, Final Report (1995). Washington, DC: Government Prnting Office.

Angell, M. and Kassire, J.P. (1994). Setting the record straight in the breast cancer trials (editorial). New Engl. J. Med. 330: 1448-1450.

Babbage, C. (1830/1970). Reflections on the Decline of Science in England. (New York: Augustus Kelley).

Bivens, L.V. and Macfarlane, D.K. (1994). Fraud in breast cancer trials. New Engl. J. Med. 330: 1461.

Broad, W. and Wade, N. (1982). Betrayers of the Truth. New York: Simon and Schuster.

Broder, S. (1994). Fraud in breast cancer trials. New Engl. J. Med. 330: 1460-1461.

Bross, I.D. (1990). How to eradicate fraudulent statistical methods: Statisticians must do science. Biometrics 46: 1213-1225.

Bulger, R.E. (1994). Toward a statement of the principles underlying responsible conduct in biomedical research. Academic Medicine 69(2): 102-107.

Chop, R.M. and Silva, M.C. (1991). Scientific fraud: Definitions, policies, and implications for nursing research. J. Prof. Nursing 7: 166-171.

Cohen, J. (1994). Clinical trial monitoring: Hit or miss? Science 264: 1534-1537.

Cohen, J., Marshall, E., and Taubes, G. (1995). Conduct in science. Science 268: 1705-1720.

Cohn, I. (1994). Whither NCI and NSABP? (editorial). Arch. Surg. 129: 1005-1009.

Cournand, A. (1977). The code of the scientist and its relationship to ethics. Science 198: 699-705.

Culliton, B.J. (1983). Coping with fraud: The Darsee case. Science 220: 31-35.

Danforth, W.H. and Schoenhoff, D.M. (1992). Fostering integrity in scientific research. Academic Medicine 67: 351-356.

Darsee, J.R. and Heymsfield, S.B. (1981). Decreased myocardial taurine levels and hypertaurinuria in a kindred with mitral valve-valve prolapse and congestive cardiomyopathy. New Engl. J. Med. 304: 129-135.

Denham, S.A. (1993). Stemming the tide of disreputable science: Implications for nursing. Nursing Forum 28: 11-18.

Denzin, N. and Lincoln, Y. (1994). Handbook of Qualitative Research. Newbury Park, CA: Sage Publications.

Department of Health and Human Services (DHHS) (1989). Responsibilities of PHS awardee and applicant institutions for dealing with and reporting possible misconduct in science: Final rule. Fed. Regist. 54 (August 8): 32446-32451.

Department of Health and Human Services (DHHS) (1993). Findings of scientific miscon-
    duct: Roger Poisson, M.D., St. Luc Hospital, Montreal, Canada. Fed. Regist. 58(117):
    33831.

Dyson, F.J. (1993). Science in trouble. American Scholar 62: 513-525.

Eisenhut, L.P. (1990). Universität prüft Anschuldigungen gegen Professorin. Kolner Stad-
    tanzeiger (October 24).

Engler, R.L., Covell, J.W., Friedman, P.J., Kitcher, P.S., and Peters, R.M. (1987). Misrepresen-
    tation and responsibility in medical research. New Engl. J. Med. 317: 1383-1389.

Fisher, R.A. (1936). Has Mendel's work been rediscovered? Ann. Sci. 1: 115-137.

Foesling, A. (1984). Der Mogelfaktor. Hamburg, 20-21.

Friedlander, M.W. (1995). At the Fringes of Science. Boulder: Westview Press.

Fuchs, S. and Westervelt, S.D. (1995). Fraud and trust in science. Persp. Biol. and Med. 39:
    248-269.

Gardiner, B. and Currant, A. (1996).

Goldberg, K.B. and Goldberg, P. (Eds..) (1994). NCI apologizes for mismanagement of NS-
    ABP, says Fisher resisted criticism. Cancer Letter 20 (16): April 22.

Hansen, K.D. and Hansen, B.C. (1991). Scientific fraud and the Public Health Service Act:
    A critical analysis. News 5: 2512-2515.

Hansen, B.C. and Hansen, K.D. (1995). Academic and scientific misconduct: Issues for nurs-
    ing educators. J. Prof. Nursing 11: 31-39.

Harris, N., Gang, D.L., Quay, S.C., Poppmea, S., Zamecnik, P.C., Nelson-Rees, W.A., and
    O'Brien, S.J. (1981). Contamination of Hogdkin's disease cell cultures. Nature 289:
    228-230.

Healy, B. (1996). The dangers of trial by Dingell. New York Times, July 3.

Hill, T.P. (1995). The significant-digit phenomenon. Am. Math. Monthly 102: 322-327.

Humphrey, G.F. (1992). Scientific fraud: The McBride case. Med. Sci. Law 32: 199-203.

Inspector General Act Amendments (1988). Public Law 100-504 (102 Stat. 2515).

Institute of Medicine (IOM) (1989). The Responsible Conduct of Research in the Health
    Sciences. Washington, DC: National Academy Press.

Jayaraman, K.S. (1991). Gupta faces suspension. Nature 349: 645.

Johns Hopkins University School of Medicine (1995). Procedures for Dealing with Issues of
    Professional Misconduct, in Faculty Policies, p. 15-23. Baltimore: Johns Hopkins
    University School of Medicine.

Judson, H.F. (1994). Structural transformation of the sciences and the end of peer review.
    JAMA 272: 92-94.

Kevles, D.J. (1996). The assault on David Baltimore. New Yorker, May 27, 1996.

Klein D.F. (1993). Should the government assure scientific integrity? Acad. Med. 68 (Suppl.): S56-S59.

Knox, R.A. (1983). Deeper problems for Darsee: Emory probe. JAMA 249: 2867-2874.

Kohn, A. (1986). False Prophets. Oxford: Basil Blackwell.

Kuznetsov, D.A. (1989). In vitro studies of interactions between frequent and unique mR-NAs and cytoplasmic factors from brain tissue of several species of wild timber voles of Northern Eurasia, Clethrionomys glareolus, Clethrionomys fratter, and Clethrion-omys gapperi: A new criticism to a modern molecular-genetic concept of biological evolution. Int. J. Neurosci. 49: 43-59.

Larhammar, D. (1994). Lack of experimental support for Kuznetsov's criticism of biological evolution (letter). Int. J. Neurosci. 77: 199-201.

Larhammar, D. (1995). Severe flaws in scientific study criticizing evolution. Skeptical Inquirer, 19: 30-31.

Lock, S. (1988). Scientific misconduct. Brit. Med. J. 297: 1531-1535.

Lock, S. (1990). Medical Misconduct: A Survey in Britain. In J. Bailar et al. (Eds.), Ethics and Policy in Scientific Publication. Bethesda, MD: Council of Biology Editors.

Lock, S. (1995). Lessons from the Pearce affair: Handling scientific fraud. BMJ 310: 1547-1548.

Matthews, L.H. (1981). Piltdown Man: The missing kinks. New Scientist April 30, 1981: 282-282 (ten-part series).

McCutchen, C.W. (1991). Peer review: Treacherous servant, disastrous master. Technol. Rev. October 1991: 28-360.

McIntyre, O.R., Kornblith, A.B., and Coburn, J. (1996). Pilot survey of opinions on data falsification in clinical trials. Cancer Invest. 14(4): 392-395.

McKean, K. (1981). A scandal in the laboratory. Discover November, 1981: 18-23.

Miller, D. J (1992). Personality Factors in Scientific Fraud and Misconduct. Chapter 7 in D.J. Miller and M. Hersen (Eds.), Research Fraud in the Behavioral and Biomedical Sciences. New York: John Wiley & Sons.

Morrison, R.S. (1990). Disreputable science: Definition and detection. J. Adv. Nursing 15: 911-913.

National Academy of Sciences (NAS) (1992a). Responsible Science: Ensuring the Integrity of the Research Process, Vol. I. Washington, DC: National Academy Press.

National Academy of Sciences (NAS) (1992b). Responsible Science: Ensuring the Integrity of the Research Process, Vol. II. Washington, DC: National Academy Press.

NCI Press Office (1994a). Press release. March 24.

NCI Press Office (1994b). Press release. March 29.

NCI Press Office (1994c). Press release. April 12.

NCI Press Office (1994d). Press release. April 21.

NCI Press Office (1994e). Press release. April 22.

NCI Press Office (1994f). Press release. May 2.

NIH (1993). Final findings of scientific misconduct: Roger Poisson, M.D., St. Luc Hospital, Montreal, Canada. NIH Guide for Grants and Contracts. Vol. 22, No. 23, June 25, 1993: 3.

National Science Foundation (NSF) (1987). Misconduct in science and engineering research: Final regulations. Fed. Reg. 52 (July 1): 24466-24470.

National Science Foundation (NSF) (1990). Semiannual Report to the Congress. Number 3. Washington, DC: Office of the Inspector General, NSF.

National Science Foundation (NSF) (1991). Misconduct in science and engineering research: Final rule. Fed. Reg. 56 (May 14): 22286-22290.

Office of Research Integrity (ORI) (1993). Office of Research Integrity: An Introduction. Rockville: Department of Health and Human Services.

Office of Research Integrity (ORI) (1993). Case Summary: Fabricated and falsified clinical trial data. Office of Research Integrity Newsletter, Vol. 1, No. 2. April, 1993: 2.

Office of Research Integrity (ORI) (1995). Annual Report 1995. Rockville, MD: Office of Research Integrity.

Racker, E. and Spector, M. (1981). The Warburg effect revisited: Merger of biochemistry and molecular biology. Science 213: 303-307.

Relman, A.S. (1983). Lessons from the Darsee affair. New Eng. J. Med. 308: 1415-1417.

Relman, A.S. (1984). Dealing with conflicts of interest. New Engl. J. Med. 311: 405.

Rennie, D., Flanagin, A., and Glass, R.M. (1991). Conflicts of interest in the publication of science. JAMA 266: 266-267.

Rossiter, E.J.R. (1992). Reflections of a whistle-blower. Nature 357: 434-436.

Royal College of Physicians (1991). Fraud and misconduct in medical research. J Royal College Physicians London 25: 89-94.

Schwartz, R.P. (1991). Maintaining integrity and credibility in industry-sponsored clinical research. Controlled Clin. Trials 12: 753-760.

Shapiro, M.F. and Charrow, R.P. (1989). The role of data audits in detecting scientific misconduct. JAMA 261: 2505-2511.

Singer, M. (1996). Assault on science. Washington Post, June 26.

Skolnick, A. (1990). Key witness against morning sickness drug faces scientific fraud charges. JAMA 263: 1468-1473.

Society of University Surgeons (1991). Misconduct and fraud in research: Social and legislative issues symposium of the Society of University Surgeons. Surgery 110: 1-7.

Swazey, J.P., Anderson, M.S., and Lewis, K.S. (1993). Ethical problems in academic research. Am. Sci. 81: 542-553.

Thelen, M.H. and DiLorenzo, T.M. (1992). Academic Pressures. Chapter 9 in D.J. Miller and M. Hersen (Eds.), Research Fraud in the Behavioral and Biomedical Sciences. New York: John Wiley & Sons.

Wade, N. (1981). A diversion of the quest for truth. Science 211: 1022-1025.

Weiss, R. (1996). Proposed shifts in misconduct reviews unsettle many scientists. Washington Post, June 30.

Weiss, R.B., Vogelzang, N.J., Peterson, B.A. et al. (1993). A successful system of scientific data audits for clinical trials. JAMA 270: 459-464.

Woolf, P.K. (1981). Fraud in science: How much, how serious? Hastings Center Report 11 (October): 9-14.

Woolf, P.K. (1986). Pressure to publish and fraud in science. Annals of Internal Medicine 104: 254-256.

Woolf, P.K. (1988). Deception in scientific research. Jurimetrics Journal 29: 67-95.

CHAPTER 19

Data and Programs

19.1 Introduction

The data used in this book and computer programs for analyzing them are described in detail in this chapter. The programs are written using software packages or languages available for IBM compatible personal computers. Most use the *Statistical Analysis System* (SAS) for Windows [SAS Institute, 1985] or *MLAB* [Civilized Software, 1996]. In some cases, *S-PLUS* [Statistical Sciences, 1995] programs are also provided. Each of the programs has been developed and run on a computer using a 166 megahertz Pentium processor, where they typically take only a few seconds to run. All the data and programs are available on the computer disk that accompanies this book. The same analyses described here, or ones similar to them, could be accomplished in a variety of ways. However, I have chosen uncomplicated methods that are available to many readers using common software and hardware. Readers interested in other data sets useful for practice or examples can consult Andrews and Herzberg [1985] or Hand et al. [1994].

MLAB (*M* odeling *LAB* oratory) may be less familiar to some readers and therefore requires a few words of explanation. *MLAB* was originally developed at the National Institutes of Health for interactive use in constructing and testing mathematical models. In the late 1980s, it was rewritten, expanded, and improved for the microcomputer platform and is currently available for DOS, Windows, and Mac. As a development tool, it contains some ideal features. For example, it is command driven with a natural, mathematically oriented syntax. It allows flexible function definitions by the user, including differential equation defined models, and incorporates full matrix and graphics capabilities. It is particularly useful and fast for fitting sophisticated models (e.g., systems of nonlinear differential equations) to data. It is exceptionally well suited to tasks where model development, as contrasted with parameter estimation, is the primary focus.

19.2 Phase I Trial from Chapter 12

19.2.1 Program

The following computer code is an $MLAB$ program to fit the pharmacokinetic model from Chapter 12 to data from four patients. Because the model is relatively over-parameterized for the number of data points, it is helpful to perform the fits in a staged fashion, i.e., fitting only some of the parameters at each stage with others held fixed. When the estimates at each stage converge, all can be optimized together. This process takes a little additional time but greatly improves the convergence.

```
delete X,Y,g,w;
"Initial conditions";
initial X(0)=0;
initial Y(0)=0;
"Differential equation model";
function X diff t(t)=-(lam+gam)*X+mu*Y+g(t);
function Y diff t(t)=lam*X-mu*Y;
"Infusion function";
function g(t)=if t<t0 then g0 else 0;
"Optional weight function; not used here";
"Because it always equals 1";
function wgt(z)=1;
"Begin fitting";
DATA1=read("f:DATA1.DAT",15,2);
q=wgt on DATA1 col 2;
del w;
"Draw data points";
draw DATA1 line 0,pt 2;
"Starting guesses";
t0=85;
lam=0.21;
mu=0.04;
gam=0.01;
g0=10;
"Fit in steps";
fit(lam,gam,mu),X to DATA1, weight q;
fit(t0,lam,gam,mu,g0),X to DATA1, weight q;
ksread();
"Solve the system with estimated parameters";
a=integrate(X diff t, 0:1500:5);
"Draw solution";
draw a col(1,2) line 2;
del DATA1;
"Output results in file result.lst";
print "DATA1" in result;
```

```
print t0, lam, mu, gam, g0 in result;
view;
"Repeat process for next patient's data";
DATA2=read("f:DATA2.DAT",15,2);
q=wgt on DATA2 col 2;
del w;
draw DATA2 line 0,pt 2;
t0=60;
lam=0.21;
mu=0.04;
gam=0.01;
g0=10;
fit(lam,gam,mu),X to DATA2, weight q;
fit(t0,lam,gam,mu,g0),X to DATA2, weight q;
ksread();
a=integrate(X diff t, 0:3000:5);
draw a col(1,2) line 2;
del DATA2;
print "DATA2" in result;
print t0, lam, mu, gam, g0 in result;
view;
DATA3=read("f:DATA3.DAT",15,2);
q=wgt on DATA3 col 2;
del w;
draw DATA3 line 0,pt 2;
t0=50;
lam=0.21;
mu=0.04;
gam=0.01;
g0=10;
fit(lam,gam,mu),X to DATA3, weight q;
fit(t0,g0),X to DATA3, weight q;
fit(lam,gam,mu),X to DATA3, weight q;
fit(t0,g0),X to DATA3, weight q;
fit(lam,gam,mu),X to DATA3, weight q;
fit(t0,g0),X to DATA3, weight q;
fit(lam,gam,mu),X to DATA3, weight q;
fit(t0,g0),X to DATA3, weight q;
fit(t0,lam,gam,mu,g0),X to DATA3, weight q;
ksread();
a=integrate(X diff t, 0:1500:5);
draw a col(1,2) line 2;
del DATA3;
print "DATA3" in result;
print t0, lam, mu, gam, g0 in result;
view;
```

```
DATA4=read("f:DATA4.DAT",15,2);
q=wgt on DATA4 col 2;
del w;
draw DATA4 line 0,pt 2;
t0=50;
lam=0.21;
mu=0.04;
gam=0.01;
g0=10;
fit(lam,gam,mu),X to DATA4, weight q;
fit(t0,g0),X to DATA4, weight q;
fit(lam,gam,mu),X to DATA4, weight q;
fit(t0,g0),X to DATA4, weight q;
fit(lam,gam,mu),X to DATA4, weight q;
fit(t0,g0),X to DATA4, weight q;
fit(lam,gam,mu),X to DATA4, weight q;
fit(t0,g0),X to DATA4, weight q;
fit(t0,lam,gam,mu,g0),X to DATA4, weight q;
ksread();
a=integrate(X diff t, 0:1500:5);
draw a col(1,2) line 2;
del DATA4;
print "DATA4" in result;
print t0, lam, mu, gam, g0 in result;
view;
```

19.2.2 Data

The phase I study time-concentration values for four patients are shown in Table 19.1.

Table 19.1 Phase I Trial Data

	Time	Conc.		Time	Conc.
Data1:	0	0.00	Data3:	0	0.00
	79	108.26		45	88.94
	85	120.36		50	100.60
	87	113.11		53	99.78
	95	90.41		60	84.10
	105	91.89		72	86.79
	115	90.80		80	91.52
	145	83.30		105	78.97
	205	74.40		170	70.76
	435	52.53		415	37.74
	805	24.78		771	17.33
	1365	4.92		1350	2.65
	1365	4.92			
Data2:	0	0.00	Data4:	0	0.00
	53	111.79		46	97.89
	60	132.38		50	110.28
	62	118.16		53	111.32
	70	105.96		58	131.14
	80	103.00		60	90.22
	90	105.93		73	89.34
	118	92.16		83	81.96
	191	83.14		113	82.96
	420	62.75		175	81.60
	778	40.00		408	57.19
	1310	20.04		770	35.12
	2835	2.30		1383	13.30

19.3 SE Trial from Chapter 12

19.3.1 Data and analysis

The data can be read and analyzed with the following SAS program. The complete data are listed in Tables 19.2 and 19.3. Frequencies and lifetables are generated with simple calls to the relevant SAS procedures and the hazard calculations and confidence intervals are performed using a custom macro. The macro requires a grouping variable, hence the use of a dummy value always equal to 1 to calculate the overall statistics.

```
/* SAS Program To Analyze */
/* SE Clinical Trial */
/* Used in Chapter 11 */
options nodate ps=55;
title 'Mesothelioma SE Trial';
data one;
file 'c:\sas\phase2.dat';
input age sex ps hist wtchg
surg ptime prog stime dead;
proc freq data=one;
tables dead prog ps sex hist wtchg surg;
/* non-parametric survival estimates */
proc lifetest data=one;
time stime*dead(0);
proc lifetest data=one;
time ptime*prog(0);
/* the following macro calculates hazards */
/* and confidence intervals for event time data */
%macro screener(data=_LAST_,group=,time=,event=,by=);

proc sort data=&data;
by &by &group;
data screen;
set &data;
if &group=" then delete;
data screen;
set screen;
by &by &group;
keep &by &group _time_ _events_
_lambda_ _number_ _low95_ _high95_;
retain _time_ _events_ _number_;
if first.&group then do;
_number_ = 0;
_time_ = 0;
_events_ = 0;
```

```
end;
add=1;
if &time=. or &event=. then do;
&time=0;
&event=0;
add=0;
end;
_time_ = _time_ + &time;
_events_ = _events_ + &event;
_number_ = _number_ + add;
if last.&group then do;
_time_ = _time_;
_lambda_ = _events_/_time_;
std = 1.0/sqrt(_events_);
_low95_ = exp(log(_lambda_)-1.96*std);
 _high95_ = exp(log(_lambda_)+1.96*std);
output;
end;
data screen;
set screen;
by &by;
retain denom;
%if &by^= %then %do;
if first.&by then denom=.;
%end;
if &group=" then return;
if denom=. and _lambda_>0.0 then denom=_lambda_;
_ratio_ = _lambda_/denom;
proc print data=screen;
by &by;
var _number_ _time_ _events_
_lambda_ _low95_ _high95_ _ratio_;
id &group;
%mend; /* end of macro */
/* a dummy group variable is used */
/* to generate overall statistics */
%screener(data=one,group=dummy,time=stime,event=dead,by=);
title 'Overall';
%screener(data=one,group=sex,time=stime,event=dead,by=);
title 'By Sex';
%screener(data=one,group=ps,time=stime,event=dead,by=);
title 'By PS';
%screener(data=one,group=surg,time=stime,event=dead,by=);
title 'By Type of Surgery';
run;
```

Table 19.2 Data from Mesothelioma SE Clinical Trial

Age	Sex	PS	Hist	Wtchg	Surg	PFS	Prog	Surv	Event
60	1	1	136	1	3	394	1	823	1
59	1	0	136	2	3	1338	0	1338	0
51	0	0	130	1	1	184	1	270	1
73	1	1	136	1	3	320	0	320	1
74	1	0	136	2	1	168	0	168	1
39	0	0	136	1	1	36	1	247	1
46	1	1	131	1	3	552	1	694	0
71	1	0	136	1	1	133	1	316	1
69	1	0	136	1	1	175	1	725	0
49	1	0	131	1	1	327	0	327	1
69	1	0	131	1	2	0	0	0	1
72	1	0	131	1	1	676	1	963	0
44	0	0	130	2	2	223	1	265	1
45	1	0	136	2	2	184	1	237	1
57	1	0	132	1	2	145	1	176	1
60	0	1	131	1	1	316	0	316	1
22	1	1	131	1	2	87	1	310	1
46	0	1	131	1	1	135	1	166	1
60	1	0	131	1	3	1	1	28	1
72	1	0	131	1	2	199	1	730	1
65	1	0	131	1	3	39	0	39	1
65	1	1	131	1	2	61	1	116	1
60	1	0	131	1	3	17	0	17	1
64	1	0	131	2	3	799	1	1229	1
61	1	0	131	2	1	61	1	294	1
38	1	0	131	1	1	176	1	322	1
65	1	1	136	1	3	6	0	6	1
73	0	1	131	1	2	292	1	422	1
74	1	0	136	2	2	22	1	22	1
76	1	0	136	1	1	106	1	375	1
57	1	1	131	1	3	248	1	302	1
60	0	0	.	1	1	63	1	365	1
56	1	0	136	1	1	145	1	387	1
62	0	0	136	1	1	104	1	327	1
60	1	0	131	1	1	20	1	247	1
67	0	0	131	1	1	181	1	669	1
64	1	0	131	1	2	89	1	948	1
67	1	1	136	1	1	0	1	400	1
56	0	1	131	1	2	724	1	1074	0
52	1	0	160	2	1	62	1	137	1
56	1	0	131	1	3	93	1	210	1
44	1	0	136	1	3	402	1	648	1

Table 19.3 Data from Mesothelioma SE Clinical Trial (Cont'd)

Age	Sex	PS	Hist	Wtchg	Surg	PFS	Prog	Surv	Event
50	0	0	136	2	2	141	1	520	1
63	1	0	.	2	1	156	1	304	1
68	1	1	131	1	2	265	1	349	1
50	1	0	.	2	3	305	1	317	1
41	0	1	131	1	1	181	1	395	1
60	1	0	131	1	1	274	1	503	1
65	1	0	136	2	2	20	1	20	1
47	1	1	131	1	3	411	1	679	0
46	1	1	131	1	2	624	0	624	0
70	1	1	131	1	2	278	1	617	0
58	1	0	136	1	1	20	1	85	1
57	1	1	132	1	3	112	1	139	1
75	1	0	132	2	2	47	1	47	1
66	1	1	136	1	3	294	1	523	1
77	1	0	.	1	1	126	1	157	1
65	0	0	.	2	1	117	1	545	0
46	0	0	131	1	1	63	1	218	1
71	0	1	132	2	1	139	0	139	1
61	1	0	136	1	1	538	1	1170	0
58	1	0	131	1	3	390	1	722	1
49	1	1	136	1	3	1102	0	1102	0
50	1	0	136	1	3	166	1	182	1
73	1	0	136	1	2	58	1	136	1
44	1	0	136	1	1	406	0	406	1
47	0	1	131	1	3	1123	0	1123	0
68	1	0	136	1	1	1009	1	1029	0
66	1	0	132	1	2	37	1	112	1
46	1	1	131	1	1	104	1	764	1
56	1	1	136	1	2	33	1	225	1
68	1	1	136	1	1	20	1	122	1
59	1	0	136	1	2	73	1	165	1
58	0	0	131	1	1	4	0	4	1
66	1	1	132	2	2	205	1	361	1
82	1	0	160	1	1	78	0	78	1
73	1	0	131	1	1	1265	0	1265	1
57	0	0	130	1	2	273	1	318	1
72	1	1	136	2	1	2	1	362	1
69	1	1	.	1	2	1093	0	1093	0
64	0	1	130	1	1	475	0	475	1
65	1	1	130	1	2	292	0	292	1
72	1	1	130	1	2	324	1	499	0

19.4 CTE Polyposis Trial from Chapter 12

19.4.1 Data and analysis

The data can be read and analyzed with the following SAS program. The complete data are listed in Tables 19.4 and 19.5.

```
title 'Polyposis RCT';
data one;
input id sex polyp0 polyp3 polyp6
polyp9 polyp12 size0 size3 size6
size9 size12 surg age treat;
cards;
proc glm;
class treat;
model polyp12=treat/solution;
proc glm;
class treat;
model polyp12=polyp0 treat/solution;
run;
```

Table 19.4 Data from Polyposis CTE Clinical Trial

ID	Sex	Polyp0	Polyp3	Polyp6	Polyp9	Polyp12
1	0	7	6	.	.	.
2	0	77	67	71	63	.
3	1	7	4	4	2	4
4	0	5	5	16	28	26
5	1	23	16	8	17	16
6	0	35	31	65	61	40
7	0	11	6	1	1	14
8	1	12	20	7	7	16
9	1	7	7	11	15	11
10	1	318	347	405	448	434
11	1	160	142	41	25	26
12	0	8	1	2	3	7
13	1	20	16	37	28	45
14	1	11	20	13	10	32
15	1	24	26	55	40	80
16	1	34	27	29	33	34
17	0	54	45	22	46	38
18	1	16	10	.	.	.
21	1	30	30	40	50	57
22	0	10	6	3	3	7
23	0	20	5	1	1	1
24	1	12	8	3	4	8

Table 19.5 Data from Polyposis CTE Clinical Trial (Cont'd)

ID	Size0	Size3	Size6	Size9	Size12	Surg	Age	Treat
1	3.6	3.4	.	.	.	1	17	1
2	3.8	2.8	3.0	2.8	.	1	20	0
3	5.0	2.6	1.2	0.8	1.0	1	16	1
4	3.4	3.6	4.0	2.8	2.1	1	18	0
5	3.0	1.9	1.0	1.0	1.2	1	22	1
6	4.2	3.1	5.6	4.6	4.1	1	13	0
7	2.2	-	0.4	0.2	3.3	1	23	1
8	2.0	2.6	2.2	2.2	3.0	1	34	0
9	4.2	5.0	5.0	3.7	2.5	1	50	0
10	4.8	3.9	5.6	4.4	4.4	1	19	0
11	5.5	4.5	2.0	1.3	3.5	1	17	1
12	1.7	0.4	0.6	0.2	0.8	1	23	1
13	2.5	2.3	2.7	3.2	3.0	1	22	0
14	2.3	2.8	3.7	4.3	2.7	1	30	0
15	2.4	2.2	2.5	2.7	2.7	1	27	0
16	3.0	2.3	2.9	2.5	4.2	1	23	1
17	4.0	4.5	4.2	3.6	2.9	1	22	0
18	1.8	1.0	.	.	.	1	13	1
21	3.2	2.7	3.6	4.4	3.7	0	34	0
22	3.0	3.0	0.6	1.1	1.1	0	23	1
23	4.0	1.1	0.6	0.4	0.4	0	22	1
24	2.8	1.1	0.1	0.4	1.0	0	42	1

19.5   CTE Lung Cancer Trial from Chapter 12

19.5.1 Data and analysis

The data can be read and analyzed with the following SAS program. An *S-PLUS* program is also provided on the disk. The coding of the variable values is given in Table 19.6. The complete data (eligible patients only) are listed in Tables 19.7 through 19.11.

```
data one;
infile "a:/lung/lung.dat" firstobs=2;
input celltype karn t n treat
surv dead dfs event age race
elig wtloss sex;
if elig=0;
proc lifetest data=one;
time surv*dead(0);
strata treat;
proc lifetest data=one;
time dfs*event(0);
strata treat;
run;
```

Table 19.6 Coding of Variables for Randomized Phase III Lung Cancer Clinical Trial

Tx:	1	Radiotherapy + CAP	Sex:	0	female
	2	Radiotherapy		1	male
T:	Tumor status		Elig:	0	eligible
				1	not eligible
N:	Nodal status		PS:	1	performance status 5-7
				2	performance status 8-10
Age:	age in years		Surv:	survival, in days	
Cell:	1	squamous	Dead:	0	alive
	2	non-squamous		1	dead
Wt:	Weight loss 0 $< 10\%$		Dfs:	disease free survival, in days	
	1 $\geq 10\%$				
Race:	0	other	Event:	0	alive
	1	white		1	recurrence, second primary, or death

Table 19.7 Data from a Randomized CTE Lung Cancer Clinical Trial

Cell	PS	T	N	Tx	Surv	Dead	DFS	Event	Age	Race	Elig	Wt	Sex
1	2	1	0	2	1046	1	413	1	70	1	0	1	1
1	2	2	2	1	342	1	342	0	67	1	0	1	1
1	2	2	2	2	54	1	18	1	61	1	0	0	1
1	2	2	2	1	303	1	264	1	52	1	0	0	1
1	2	1	2	2	295	1	248	1	59	0	0	0	1
2	1	3	2	2	88	1	59	1	39	0	0	0	0
2	2	2	2	2	241	1	241	0	46	0	0	0	0
2	2	1	2	2	567	1	252	1	44	0	0	0	1
2	2	2	2	1	286	1	211	1	38	0	0	1	0
2	2	2	1	1	265	1	262	1	62	1	0	0	1
2	2	1	2	2	224	1	133	1	61	1	0	0	0
2	2	3	1	1	1314	0	1314	0	45	0	0	0	0
2	2	2	2	2	1900	0	113	1	53	1	0	1	0
2	2	2	2	1	1819	0	1819	0	65	1	0	0	1
2	2	2	2	1	1710	0	1710	0	40	0	0	0	0
2	2	3	0	2	1669	1	475	1	55	1	0	0	1
2	2	2	2	2	986	1	63	1	55	1	0	0	1
2	1	1	2	2	210	1	45	1	65	1	0	0	1
2	2	3	2	2	2023	0	63	0	59	0	0	0	1
1	1	3	2	2	731	1	436	1	52	0	0	0	1
1	2	3	2	2	607	1	330	1	58	1	0	0	1
1	2	3	1	2	1520	1	757	1	69	1	0	0	1
1	2	2	2	1	441	1	441	0	64	1	0	0	1
1	2	2	2	1	328	1	295	1	66	1	0	0	1
1	2	3	0	2	192	1	27	1	70	1	0	0	1
2	1	3	2	1	853	1	640	1	71	1	0	0	1
2	2	1	2	2	248	1	248	0	69	1	0	0	1
2	2	2	2	1	1011	1	115	1	70	1	0	0	0
2	2	2	2	1	358	1	154	1	40	1	0	0	0
2	2	1	2	2	354	1	165	1	70	1	0	0	0
2	2	1	2	1	1977	1	1977	0	63	1	0	0	1
2	2	2	2	2	2318	0	2318	0	57	1	0	0	1
2	2	2	2	1	2740	1	277	1	49	1	0	0	0
2	2	2	2	1	742	1	551	1	59	1	0	0	1

Table 19.8 Data from a Randomized CTE Lung Cancer Clinical Trial (Cont'd).

Cell	PS	T	N	Tx	Surv	Dead	DFS	Event	Age	Race	Elig	Wt	Sex
1	1	3	0	1	206	1	190	1	65	1	0	1	1
2	1	3	1	1	1743	0	1743	0	68	0	0	1	1
1	1	2	2	2	37	1	28	1	58	0	0	0	1
1	2	2	2	1	475	1	361	1	70	1	0	0	0
1	2	2	2	1	2875	0	2875	0	59	1	0	0	0
1	2	3	0	2	388	1	388	0	58	1	0	0	1
1	2	2	2	1	1390	1	966	1	46	1	0	0	1
1	2	2	2	2	2481	0	2286	0	59	1	0	0	1
1	2	2	2	2	1744	1	973	1	47	1	0	0	1
1	2	2	1	1	2293	0	2135	0	52	1	0	1	1
1	2	2	2	1	2049	0	2049	0	56	1	0	0	1
1	2	2	2	2	636	1	351	1	53	1	0	0	1
1	2	3	2	1	970	1	384	1	55	1	0	0	1
1	2	2	2	1	406	1	352	1	66	1	0	0	1
1	2	3	1	2	226	1	56	1	59	1	0	0	1
2	1	2	2	1	454	1	414	1	68	1	0	0	0
2	1	2	2	2	116	1	105	1	57	1	0	0	0
2	2	1	2	2	1321	1	1087	1	53	1	0	0	1
2	2	2	2	2	400	1	266	1	65	0	0	0	0
2	2	2	2	1	150	1	97	1	68	1	0	0	1
2	2	2	2	1	1018	1	807	1	63	1	0	0	1
2	2	3	2	2	303	1	127	1	65	1	0	1	1
2	2	2	2	2	166	1	125	1	64	1	0	0	1
2	2	2	2	1	371	1	255	1	65	1	0	0	1
2	2	3	2	2	215	1	125	1	59	1	0	0	1
2	2	2	1	1	331	1	316	1	66	1	0	0	1
2	2	2	2	2	81	1	30	1	65	1	0	0	0
2	2	2	2	1	469	1	342	1	58	1	0	0	0
2	2	2	2	1	662	1	392	1	62	1	0	0	1
2	2	2	2	2	639	1	142	1	71	1	0	0	1
2	2	2	2	1	699	1	580	1	43	1	0	0	0
2	2	2	2	2	1577	0	1577	1	56	1	0	0	1
2	1	3	2	2	79	1	79	1	67	1	0	0	0
2	2	2	2	2	255	1	97	1	47	1	0	0	1
2	2	1	2	2	427	1	165	1	41	1	0	0	1

Table 19.9 Data from a Randomized CTE Lung Cancer Clinical Trial (Cont'd).

Cell	PS	T	N	Tx	Surv	Dead	DFS	Event	Age	Race	Elig	Wt	Sex
1	1	1	2	2	1289	1	1289	0	57	1	0	0	1
1	1	3	2	2	1651	1	245	1	51	0	0	0	0
1	1	3	1	1	1897	0	1897	0	48	1	0	0	1
1	1	2	2	2	1389	1	1388	1	71	1	0	0	1
1	2	1	1	2	1664	0	679	1	54	1	0	0	1
1	2	3	0	1	3067	0	3067	0	60	1	0	0	1
1	2	2	2	2	916	1	700	1	57	1	0	0	1
1	2	3	2	1	438	1	147	1	50	1	0	0	1
1	2	1	2	2	533	1	317	1	41	1	0	0	1
1	2	2	2	2	325	1	234	1	45	1	0	0	1
1	2	1	2	1	817	1	515	1	64	1	0	0	0
1	2	3	1	1	2218	0	2218	0	59	1	0	0	1
1	2	1	2	2	974	1	961	1	61	1	0	0	0
1	2	2	1	1	616	1	376	1	60	1	0	0	1
1	2	2	2	1	153	1	81	1	64	1	0	.	1
1	2	2	2	2	229	1	97	1	64	1	0	0	1
1	2	2	2	2	330	1	330	1	56	1	0	0	1
1	2	3	1	1	231	1	231	0	63	1	0	.	1
1	2	2	2	2	554	1	364	1	68	1	0	0	1
1	2	2	2	2	325	1	149	1	49	1	0	.	1
1	2	1	2	1	826	1	772	1	58	1	0	0	1
1	2	3	0	2	2209	0	2209	0	67	1	0	.	0
1	2	3	2	1	680	1	680	0	58	1	0	0	0
1	2	2	2	1	162	1	162	0	69	1	0	0	1
1	2	2	2	2	359	1	57	1	67	1	0	0	0
1	2	2	2	2	1949	0	1949	0	63	1	0	0	1
1	2	2	2	1	302	1	271	1	57	1	0	0	1
1	2	3	1	2	185	1	172	1	59	1	0	0	1
1	2	2	1	2	23	1	23	0	62	1	0	0	1
1	2	2	2	1	292	1	292	0	58	1	0	0	0
1	2	3	2	2	2252	0	2252	0	65	1	0	0	0
1	2	3	2	2	215	1	175	1	58	1	0	0	1
1	2	2	2	1	1669	0	1669	0	59	1	0	0	1

Table 19.10 Data from a Randomized CTE Lung Cancer Clinical Trial (Cont'd).

Cell	PS	T	N	Tx	Surv	Dead	DFS	Event	Age	Race	Elig	Wt	Sex
2	1	2	2	1	941	0	382	1	65	1	0	0	1
2	1	3	2	2	234	1	164	1	54	1	0	0	0
2	1	1	2	1	633	1	53	1	52	1	0	1	1
2	2	2	2	2	273	1	55	1	57	1	0	0	0
2	2	3	0	2	243	1	62	1	74	1	0	0	1
2	2	2	1	1	439	1	402	1	53	1	0	0	1
2	2	3	2	1	144	1	103	1	51	1	0	0	1
2	2	2	2	2	36	1	36	1	56	1	0	0	1
2	2	3	0	2	183	1	25	1	57	1	0	0	1
2	2	1	2	1	378	1	367	1	55	1	0	0	1
2	2	3	1	2	1026	1	1026	0	46	1	0	0	1
2	2	3	1	1	129	1	22	1	64	0	0	1	1
2	2	3	1	1	538	1	538	0	72	1	0	0	1
2	2	2	2	2	167	1	57	1	65	1	0	1	0
2	2	2	1	1	231	1	167	1	39	0	0	0	0
2	2	2	2	2	491	1	423	1	33	1	0	0	0
2	2	2	2	2	2940	0	2940	0	52	1	0	0	0
2	2	2	2	2	362	1	273	1	61	1	0	0	1
2	2	3	2	1	461	1	313	1	71	0	0	0	0
2	2	2	2	1	2452	0	2375	1	52	1	0	0	1
2	2	2	2	1	130	1	94	1	46	1	0	0	0
2	2	3	1	2	432	1	301	1	50	1	0	0	1
2	2	2	2	2	298	1	116	1	68	1	0	0	1
2	2	2	2	1	2007	1	1248	1	48	1	0	0	0
2	2	2	2	2	269	1	189	1	56	1	0	0	1
2	2	2	2	2	256	1	206	1	32	0	0	0	0
2	2	3	2	1	716	1	716	0	67	1	0	0	1
2	2	2	1	1	106	1	76	1	64	1	0	.	0
2	2	3	1	1	259	1	217	1	55	1	0	.	1
2	2	2	1	2	343	1	85	1	60	1	0	0	1
2	2	2	2	2	873	1	612	1	42	1	0	0	0

Table 19.11 Data from a Randomized CTE Lung Cancer Clinical Trial (Cont'd).

Cell	PS	T	N	Tx	Surv	Dead	DFS	Event	Age	Race	Elig	Wt	Sex
2	2	3	1	1	616	1	540	1	49	1	0	0	0
2	2	1	2	1	591	1	205	1	48	1	0	0	1
2	2	3	2	1	524	1	410	1	61	1	0	1	1
2	2	3	2	2	97	1	57	1	66	1	0	0	1
2	2	2	2	2	234	1	146	1	60	1	0	0	1
2	2	3	2	1	224	1	126	1	39	1	0	0	1
1	2	3	0	1	931	1	931	0	51	1	0	0	1
1	2	2	2	1	872	1	403	1	42	1	0	0	1
1	2	2	2	2	444	1	395	1	46	1	0	0	0
1	2	2	1	1	670	1	266	1	62	1	0	0	1
1	2	2	0	2	1717	0	473	1	62	0	0	0	1
1	2	3	1	1	1114	1	1089	1	68	0	0	0	1
1	2	2	2	1	943	1	943	0	55	1	0	0	0
2	2	3	0	2	478	1	114	1	56	1	0	1	1
2	2	2	2	1	2569	1	2566	1	40	1	0	0	1
2	2	3	0	2	182	1	174	1	60	1	0	0	1
2	2	2	2	2	115	1	115	0	46	1	0	0	1
2	2	2	2	1	104	1	35	1	57	1	0	0	0
2	2	3	1	1	683	1	448	1	59	1	0	0	1
2	2	3	1	2	2316	0	317	1	71	0	0	0	0
2	2	2	2	1	213	1	114	1	48	1	0	0	0
2	2	2	2	2	2305	0	2305	0	74	1	0	0	1
2	2	2	2	1	234	1	211	1	57	1	0	0	1
2	2	2	2	2	440	1	232	1	57	0	0	0	1
2	2	2	2	1	121	0	121	0	51	1	0	1	1
2	2	3	0	2	378	1	125	1	63	1	0	1	1
2	2	2	2	2	1995	0	131	0	43	1	0	0	0
1	1	3	1	1	241	1	9	1	56	0	0	0	1
1	1	2	2	2	206	1	96	1	56	1	0	1	1
2	1	3	1	2	457	1	109	1	56	0	0	0	1
2	2	3	0	1	2220	1	2220	0	59	0	0	0	1

19.6 Bootstrap Example from Chapter 12

19.6.1 Data and analysis

The event time data are shown in Table 19.12. The following SAS program reads the data file and performs the bootstrap simulations to determine the confidence limits on the median event time.

```
data one;
input c x;
/* standard lifetable analysis */
proc lifetest data=one;
time x;
/* bootstrap samples */
/* change seed for a new sample */
data two;
retain seed 8545613;
do sample=1 to 500;
do i=1 to 50;
call ranuni(seed,u);
u=1+u*50;
c=int(u);
output;
end;
end;
/* count the frequencies that each */
/* observation was chosen */
proc freq noprint data=two;
by sample;
tables c/out=three;
proc sort data=three;
by c;
/* replicate data the required */
/* number of times */
data two;
merge three one;
by c;
keep x count sample;
proc sort data=two;
by sample;
data two;
set two;
keep x sample;
do i=1 to count;
output;
end;
```

```
/* determine the median of each */
/* bootstrap sample */
proc univariate noprint data=two;
output out=four median=median;
by sample;
/* output results */
proc print data=four;
proc freq data=four;
tables median;
proc univariate data=four;
var median;
run;
```

Table 19.12 Event Times for Bootstrap Confidence Intervals.

N	Time	N	Time
1	0.59	26	1.86
2	0.84	27	0.87
3	1.11	28	0.74
4	1.71	29	1.92
5	1.32	30	1.73
6	1.80	31	1.54
7	1.94	32	0.88
8	1.91	33	2.30
9	2.53	34	1.99
10	1.04	35	1.72
11	2.25	36	2.22
12	0.77	37	1.84
13	1.45	38	0.71
14	1.52	39	1.98
15	1.72	40	2.14
16	3.11	41	1.90
17	1.94	42	2.23
18	1.96	43	1.50
19	0.51	44	1.00
20	3.64	45	1.65
21	2.81	46	0.65
22	1.18	47	0.35
23	2.26	48	2.04
24	2.14	49	1.24
25	1.97	50	1.13

19.7 Prognostic Factor Analysis Example from Chapter 13

19.7.1 Data and analysis

The following SAS program reads the data file and performs the analyses. The data are listed in Tables 19.13–19.14.

```
data one;
retain seed 31491711;
keep surv dead x1-x25;
nobs = 80;
pcen = 0.1;
hazard = 0.1;
p = 0.5;
ct=2*(1-pcen)/hazard;
do i=1 to 10;
  f=(1-exp(-hazard*ct))/(hazard*ct)-pcen;
 f1=exp(-hazard*ct)/ct-(1-exp(-hazard*ct))/
(hazard*ct*ct);
  ct=ct-f/f1;
end;
do j=1 to nobs;
call ranuni(seed,u);
atime=ct*u;
call ranuni(seed,u);
dtime=(-log(u))/hazard;
dead=1;
surv=dtime;
if dtime+atime>ct then do;
  surv=ct-atime;
  dead=0;
end;
array x25;
do i=1 to dim(x);
  xi = 0;
  call ranuni(seed,u);
  if u<p then xi = 1;
end;
output;
end;
proc phreg data=one;
model surv*dead(0)=x1-x25/selection=s sle=.05 sls=.05;
proc phreg data=one;
model surv*dead(0)=x1-x25/selection=b sle=.05 sls=.05;
```

```
proc phreg data=one;
model surv*dead(0)=x1-x25/selection=b
 sle=.025 sls=.025;
run;
```

Table 19.13 Data from a Prognostic Factor Analysis.

#	Dead	Time	$X_1 - X_{25}$
1	1	7.38	1111111001110100010100101
2	1	27.56	1001100111001011001001110
3	1	1.67	1000110000111000011010010
4	1	1.82	1101001111011101100101101
5	0	10.49	0001110011110011111100101
6	1	14.96	1011110110001001010010111
7	1	0.63	0111001011101000010001111
8	1	10.84	1001010111110111101001011
9	1	15.65	1110010000001001110001100
10	1	4.73	0100100000011100101100000
11	1	14.97	0010111100101111100000010
12	1	3.47	0010111110011000000000000
13	1	4.29	1100110000101100010000001
14	1	0.11	1111110110111101000011000
15	1	13.35	0010101010110011010010011
16	1	12.95	0000001100111101000000100
17	1	5.51	0110110001100010011010111
18	1	16.23	0110000000010010111111001
19	1	14.93	1100010111010000011110011
20	1	5.32	1011101000010001101100111
21	1	2.32	1010111100011001001001111
22	1	16.75	1100000110011111001010010
23	1	20.07	0101010111100100000100010
24	1	8.70	1111000010001001011011111
25	1	4.52	1001001100110000101101010
26	1	9.60	1110100111101100100000000
27	1	32.17	0001010011111101101101011
28	1	12.88	1011111101110111101111011
29	1	14.79	1010101110001010111111010
30	1	0.67	1011000010011001011110010
31	1	28.57	1100010000111100111000001
32	1	0.96	0110011111100011011010101
33	1	45.49	0111101011110001011100000
34	1	1.02	1010101110000010001111011
35	1	16.57	1000101011010001000001001
36	1	0.97	1110011111101110010100110
37	1	6.93	1000111100101100111000110
38	1	12.55	0000000000011010010010111
39	1	2.03	0110010001000111011010111
40	1	4.29	1110101011101001011010101

Table 19.14 Data from a Prognostic Factor Analysis.

#	Dead	Time	$X_1 - X_{25}$
41	1	14.29	0010100011101011100001010
42	1	16.49	0100011011001100101110001
43	1	4.53	1111000110011001010100000
44	1	8.57	1010100101111101001001100
45	0	14.54	0111111111100011111000111
46	1	15.80	0111111011011001100000010
47	1	2.47	0011000110000011101111110
48	1	9.88	1001011000010010111010011
49	1	10.42	1100001101110111110110100
50	1	21.71	0111010101110110111110000
51	1	11.64	0000101100100011101100000
52	0	23.50	0100101010010110111101110
53	1	1.25	1100100110110000001001001
54	1	1.59	1110001011000100011111110
55	1	3.62	0010100110000011100110100
56	1	15.11	1010111110000100101111010
57	1	2.20	1100100101100000011110000
58	1	2.86	1001011001100110111100110
59	1	0.67	0101011110010000001010000
60	1	1.96	1010110110000011010001010
61	1	14.85	0101100111011011110011000
62	1	25.07	1101101111110101000111101
63	1	38.84	0110000101011111011010000
64	1	10.07	1001010101110010001011011
65	1	32.52	1111001101010010000100011
66	1	8.07	1100011001111000010000111
67	1	8.63	0110011100010100110010110
68	1	7.18	0110101011111101100100001
69	1	3.54	1101101010101100001100100
70	1	31.21	0000001010001011010110101
71	1	12.24	0000000101011010001111101
72	1	7.38	1110100010000011010001101
73	1	7.40	1011110010100111001110111
74	1	5.16	0110110100111111110110110
75	1	29.97	1000010001010101101001011
76	1	3.01	1110101001000001101001100
77	1	13.00	0111010000000111100011011
78	1	19.47	0010110001000110101111110
79	1	1.37	0011001010100001110011010
80	1	0.95	0011011001101000101011001

19.8   CTE Trial from Chapter 13

19.8.1   Data and analysis

The following SAS program reads the data file and performs the analyses. The coding of the data variables on 222 patients is given in Table 19.15. The data themselves are given in Tables 19.16–19.21. An *S-PLUS* program is also provided on the disk.

```
/* SAS Program To Read and Analyze */
/* CTE Brain Tumor Clinical Trial Data */
/* Used in Chapter 12 */
data one;
infile 'a:\brain\brain.dat' firstobs=2;
input treat resect75 age interval
karn race local male nitro weeks
event path grade;
age10=age/10;
/* stratified proportional hazards model */
proc phreg data=one;
strata path;
model weeks*event(0)=treat karn local grade
nitro race resect75 age10;
/* non-parametric survival estimates */
proc lifetest data=one;
time weeks*event(0);
run;
```

Table 19.15 Coding of Variables for Randomized CTE Brain Tumor Clinical Trial.

Tx:	0	placebo	Sex:	0	female
	1	polymer		1	male
R75:	0	< 75% recection	Nitro:	0	no
	1	> 75% resection		1	yes
Age:	age in years		Weeks:	survival in weeks	
Dx:	years from diagnosis		Event:	0	alive
				1	dead
PS:	0	< 70	Path:	1=	Glioblastoma
	1	≥ 70		2=	Anaplastic Astrocytoma
				3=	Oligodendroglioma
				4=	Other
Race:	0	other	Grade:	0=	Quiescent
	1	white		1=	Active

Table 19.16 Data from a Randomized CTE Brain Tumor Clinical Trial.

Num	Tx	R75	Age	Dx	PS	Race	RT
1	0	1	38	0.9	1	0	1
2	1	1	41	1.6	1	1	0
3	0	0	57	1	1	1	1
4	1	1	50	0.9	1	1	0
5	0	1	60	1	0	1	0
6	1	1	55	1.2	1	1	1
7	0	1	30	3.3	1	0	1
8	0	1	60	0.7	1	1	1
9	0	1	28	1.9	1	1	1
10	1	1	61	1.5	1	1	1
11	1	1	37	1.2	1	1	1
12	0	1	47	2	1	1	0
13	1	1	42	0.8	1	1	1
14	1	1	38	5.6	1	1	1
15	0	1	36	4.7	1	1	1
16	0	1	28	1.8	1	1	1
17	1	1	38	1.6	1	1	1
18	0	1	43	1.5	0	1	1
19	1	1	31	8.4	1	1	1
20	1	1	42	0.8	1	1	1
21	0	1	48	1.6	1	1	1
22	0	1	52	0.3	0	1	0
23	1	1	45	1	1	1	1
24	0	1	65	0.5	1	1	1
25	0	1	27	2.1	1	1	0
26	1	1	46	0.9	0	1	1
27	1	1	73	0.4	1	1	0
28	1	1	49	1.2	1	1	1
29	0	1	47	0.7	1	1	1
30	0	1	42	5.5	0	1	1
31	0	1	39	0.8	1	1	1
32	0	1	37	0.6	1	1	1
33	1	1	54	1.1	1	0	1
34	1	1	61	0.5	1	1	1
35	1	1	32	1	1	1	1
36	0	0	42	0.9	1	1	1
37	1	0	42	1.9	0	1	1

Table 19.17 Data from a Randomized CTE Brain Tumor Clinical Trial (Cont'd).

Num	Sex	Nitro	Weeks	Event	Path	Grade
1	1	0	42.57	1	3	1
2	1	1	23.14	1	1	1
3	1	1	9.57	1	1	1
4	1	1	15.00	1	1	1
5	0	0	19.86	1	1	1
6	1	0	37.00	1	1	1
7	0	0	137.86	1	1	1
8	1	0	13.71	1	1	1
9	1	0	31.43	1	1	1
10	1	0	58.86	1	4	0
11	1	1	31.86	1	1	1
12	0	1	11.14	1	1	1
13	1	0	110.57	1	2	1
14	1	0	193.43	0	3	1
15	1	0	23.14	1	1	1
16	1	0	12.43	1	1	1
17	1	0	71.43	1	1	1
18	1	1	2.71	1	1	1
19	1	0	141.00	1	1	1
20	0	0	123.14	1	2	1
21	1	0	79.43	1	2	1
22	1	0	15.29	1	1	1
23	1	1	173.29	0	3	1
24	1	0	21.14	1	1	1
25	0	0	67.29	1	2	1
26	1	0	34.29	1	1	1
27	0	0	42.14	1	2	1
28	0	1	42.14	1	1	1
29	1	0	43.43	1	1	1
30	1	0	16.71	1	1	1
31	0	1	26.14	1	1	1
32	1	0	19.43	1	1	1
33	1	1	25.86	1	1	1
34	1	0	42.43	1	1	1
35	0	0	44.00	1	2	1
36	1	1	15.86	1	1	1
37	1	1	15.29	1	3	1

Table 19.18 Data from a Randomized CTE Brain Tumor Clinical Trial (Cont'd).

Num	Tx	R75	Age	Dx	PS	Race	RT
38	0	0	51	0.5	1	1	1
39	1	0	36	0.5	1	1	1
40	0	1	42	0.3	1	1	1
41	1	0	34	2.2	1	1	1
42	1	0	54	0.7	0	0	1
43	0	0	36	1.5	1	1	0
44	0	1	38	4.9	0	1	1
45	1	1	57	1.9	1	1	1
46	1	1	57	1	0	1	1
47	0	1	45	1.5	1	1	1
48	0	0	59	1.2	0	1	1
49	1	1	51	0.8	1	1	1
50	0	1	55	0.3	0	1	1
51	0	1	61	0.6	0	1	1
52	1	1	70	0.7	1	1	1
53	0	1	44	0.2	1	1	0
54	0	0	68	0.6	1	1	0
55	1	0	50	0.8	1	0	0
56	1	1	35	3.9	1	0	1
57	1	1	43	1.7	1	1	0
58	1	1	43	4.7	1	1	0
59	0	0	24	3.8	0	1	1
60	0	0	59	0.8	0	1	1
61	1	1	51	7.5	0	0	0
62	1	1	59	0.3	0	1	0
63	0	0	33	1.4	1	1	1
64	0	1	24	8.2	1	0	1
65	0	1	38	9	1	1	1
66	1	1	63	0.6	0	1	1
67	1	1	42	2.7	1	1	1
68	0	1	26	0.9	1	1	1
69	0	1	64	1.4	0	1	0
70	1	1	33	1.5	1	1	1
71	0	0	32	0.5	0	1	1
72	0	1	33	0.4	1	1	1
73	1	0	54	0.6	0	1	1
74	1	1	49	0.6	1	1	1

Table 19.19 Data from a Randomized CTE Brain Tumor Clinical Trial (Cont'd).

Num	Sex	Nitro	Weeks	Event	Path	Grade
38	0	0	27.14	1	3	1
39	0	1	37.14	1	4	1
40	1	0	54.57	1	3	1
41	1	1	96.43	1	2	1
42	1	1	27.43	1	1	0
43	1	0	35.86	1	3	1
44	0	1	24.43	1	1	1
45	1	0	193.14	1	3	1
46	1	0	34.86	1	1	1
47	1	0	21.14	1	3	1
48	0	0	3.29	1	2	1
49	1	0	77.57	1	4	1
50	0	0	15.00	1	1	1
51	0	0	20.14	1	1	1
52	1	0	41.14	1	3	1
53	0	0	45.29	1	1	1
54	1	0	19.86	1	3	0
55	0	0	37.71	1	1	1
56	1	0	68.00	1	3	1
57	0	0	39.71	1	1	1
58	0	0	117.71	0	3	1
59	1	0	31.57	1	3	1
60	1	0	27.86	1	2	1
61	1	0	39.71	1	4	1
62	0	0	11.86	1	1	1
63	1	0	46.57	1	1	1
64	0	1	75.86	1	3	1
65	1	0	136.29	0	1	1
66	1	1	98.57	1	1	0
67	1	1	39.14	1	1	1
68	1	1	117.57	0	3	0
69	1	1	4.14	1	1	1
70	1	0	94.00	1	1	1
71	1	1	24.00	1	1	1
72	0	1	22.86	1	2	1
73	1	1	21.86	1	1	1
74	1	1	30.29	1	1	1

Table 19.20 Data from a Randomized CTE Brain Tumor Clinical Trial (Cont'd).

Num	Tx	R75	Age	Dx	PS	Race	RT
75	1	1	51	1.7	1	1	1
76	0	1	48	0.9	0	1	1
77	0	1	36	0.5	1	0	1
78	1	1	41	5.1	0	1	1
79	0	1	50	8.5	1	1	1
80	0	1	25	0.3	0	1	1
81	1	1	62	1.1	1	1	1
82	1	1	45	0.9	0	1	1
83	0	1	62	0.8	1	1	1
84	1	1	46	0.8	0	1	1
85	0	1	38	0.4	1	1	1
86	1	1	57	1.4	1	1	1
87	0	1	64	1.6	1	1	1
88	0	1	58	0.4	0	1	1
89	1	1	65	1.9	1	1	1
90	0	1	57	7.6	0	1	.
91	0	1	44	6	1	0	1
92	1	0	29	0.6	0	1	0
93	1	1	39	2.8	1	1	0
94	0	1	54	1.1	1	1	0
95	1	1	54	0.9	1	1	0
96	1	0	56	0.5	0	1	1
97	0	0	59	0.6	0	1	0
98	1	0	57	1.3	0	1	0
99	1	1	43	0.6	1	1	0
100	0	1	50	1.2	0	1	1
101	0	1	57	5.8	1	1	1
102	1	1	38	0.7	1	1	1
103	0	1	40	2.1	0	0	1
104	0	0	62	2.2	0	1	1
105	0	1	69	0.5	0	1	1
106	1	0	72	0.6	0	1	1
107	1	1	45	2.2	0	1	1
108	1	0	50	0.8	0	1	1
109	0	1	47	14.8	1	1	0
110	0	0	48	1.2	1	1	1
111	1	1	63	0.7	0	1	0

Table 19.21 Data from a Randomized CTE Brain Tumor Clinical Trial (Cont'd).

Num	Sex	Nitro	Weeks	Event	Path	Grade
75	1	1	60.29	1	1	1
76	0	0	17.29	1	1	1
77	1	0	156.29	0	4	1
78	1	1	31.14	1	1	1
79	0	0	36.43	1	3	1
80	0	0	134.71	1	2	1
81	1	1	5.57	1	1	1
82	0	1	25.57	1	1	1
83	1	1	39.57	1	3	0
84	0	0	3.57	1	3	1
85	1	0	116.43	0	2	1
86	1	0	11.14	1	1	0
87	1	1	7.29	1	1	1
88	1	0	9.43	1	1	0
89	0	1	11.00	1	1	1
90	1	0	166.43	1	1	1
91	0	0	76.43	1	3	1
92	1	1	31.14	1	1	1
93	1	0	193.29	0	3	1
94	1	1	37.71	1	2	1
95	1	1	16.00	1	1	1
96	1	0	26.29	1	1	1
97	1	0	12.00	1	1	0
98	1	1	28.14	1	1	1
99	1	0	26.29	1	1	0
100	1	1	5.14	1	1	1
101	1	0	169.00	0	4	0
102	1	1	5.43	1	1	1
103	1	1	108.71	0	1	1
104	1	1	18.00	1	1	1
105	1	1	40.57	1	3	1
106	1	1	30.71	1	1	1
107	0	1	30.14	1	1	1
108	0	1	16.71	1	1	1
109	0	1	12.71	1	3	1
110	1	1	21.00	1	2	1
111	1	1	11.71	1	2	1

Table 19.22 Data from a Randomized CTE Brain Tumor Clinical Trial.

Num	Tx	R75	Age	Dx	PS	Race	RT
112	0	1	62	0.6	0	1	1
113	1	1	73	0.7	0	1	1
114	0	0	59	1.5	1	1	1
115	1	0	36	0.5	1	1	1
116	0	1	60	0.9	0	1	1
117	1	0	33	1.8	0	1	1
118	1	0	30	7.9	0	1	1
119	0	1	57	0.9	0	1	1
120	0	1	47	1.9	0	1	1
121	1	0	37	6.9	0	1	1
122	1	1	32	0.6	0	1	1
123	0	1	39	2.4	0	0	1
124	0	1	30	7.2	0	1	0
125	1	0	54	1.2	0	1	1
126	1	1	75	1	0	1	1
127	0	1	65	3.6	0	1	1
128	1	1	57	1	0	1	1
129	0	1	26	2.5	0	1	1
130	0	1	67	0.4	0	1	1
131	1	1	46	1.8	0	1	1
132	0	1	28	3.8	0	1	1
133	1	1	48	0.4	0	1	1
134	0	0	26	0.7	0	1	1
135	1	0	65	0.5	0	1	0
136	0	1	58	0.7	0	1	1
137	1	0	58	1.2	0	1	1
138	1	1	30	1.7	1	1	1
139	1	1	67	0.9	0	1	1
140	0	0	33	1	1	1	1
141	1	1	56	6.1	1	1	1
142	0	1	46	0.6	1	1	1
143	1	1	33	1	1	1	0
144	0	1	52	2.2	0	1	0
145	1	1	35	5.2	1	1	0
146	0	1	57	0.8	0	1	1
147	0	1	23	0.8	1	1	1
148	1	1	31	0.3	1	1	0

Table 19.23 Data from a Randomized CTE Brain Tumor Clinical Trial (Cont'd).

Num	Sex	Nitro	Weeks	Event	Path	Grade
112	1	0	67.43	1	1	1
113	1	1	21.00	1	1	1
114	1	1	32.57	1	2	1
115	0	1	9.29	1	1	1
116	0	1	22.14	1	4	1
117	0	0	42.57	1	1	1
118	1	1	39.43	1	1	1
119	1	1	10.57	1	1	1
120	0	1	27.14	1	1	1
121	0	1	37.57	1	1	1
122	0	0	16.14	1	1	1
123	1	1	96.57	1	2	1
124	0	1	21.57	1	1	1
125	1	1	12.71	1	1	1
126	0	0	24.14	1	1	1
127	0	1	11.57	1	1	1
128	0	1	45.14	1	1	0
129	0	0	26.29	1	1	0
130	0	0	27.29	1	1	1
131	1	1	43.43	1	1	1
132	0	1	14.14	1	2	1
133	1	1	43.43	1	1	1
134	0	0	15.86	1	1	1
135	0	0	39.86	1	1	1
136	1	1	10.57	1	1	1
137	1	1	16.14	1	1	1
138	0	0	59.71	1	1	1
139	1	0	34.29	1	1	1
140	0	1	23.00	1	1	0
141	1	0	131.43	1	4	1
142	1	1	34.57	1	1	1
143	0	0	20.14	1	1	1
144	0	1	16.43	1	1	1
145	1	0	170.29	0	3	1
146	1	0	6.71	1	1	1
147	1	0	14.14	1	1	1
148	1	0	49.29	1	1	1

Table 19.24 Data from a Randomized CTE Brain Tumor Clinical Trial (Cont'd).

Num	Tx	R75	Age	Dx	PS	Race	RT
149	0	1	39	0.9	1	1	1
150	1	1	59	0.8	1	0	1
151	0	0	45	0.8	0	1	1
152	1	1	54	3.5	0	1	1
153	0	0	53	4.2	1	1	1
154	1	1	63	1.8	1	1	1
155	0	1	55	0.5	0	1	1
156	1	0	60	0.7	0	1	1
157	0	1	53	0.5	0	1	1
158	0	1	62	.	1	1	1
159	0	0	77	0.5	0	1	1
160	1	0	43	0.5	0	1	1
161	0	1	59	0.9	0	1	1
162	1	1	27	2.3	1	1	1
163	1	1	49	1.3	1	1	0
164	0	1	31	0.6	1	1	0
165	1	1	34	1.1	1	1	1
166	0	1	68	0.6	1	1	1
167	0	0	39	0.2	0	1	1
168	0	0	38	3.6	0	1	1
169	0	1	60	0.2	0	1	1
170	1	1	46	0.5	0	1	1
171	1	1	54	3.2	0	1	1
172	0	1	42	1.4	0	0	1
173	1	0	49	0.6	0	1	1
174	0	1	66	0.5	0	1	1
175	1	0	45	2.4	1	1	1
176	0	1	43	3	1	1	1
177	1	1	57	0.8	1	1	1
178	0	1	37	3.4	1	1	1
179	1	1	32	0.8	1	1	1
180	0	0	50	1.8	1	1	1
181	1	1	51	0.8	0	0	0
182	0	1	60	4.4	0	1	1
183	0	0	19	0.5	1	1	0
184	0	0	47	1.1	0	1	0
185	1	1	64	1.3	0	1	0
186	1	1	64	0.4	1	1	0

Table 19.25 Data from a Randomized CTE Brain Tumor Clinical Trial (Cont'd).

Num	Sex	Nitro	Weeks	Event	Path	Grade
149	1	0	47.43	1	1	1
150	0	0	79.29	1	1	1
151	1	1	8.29	1	1	1
152	0	0	174.00	1	3	1
153	1	0	112.29	1	1	1
154	1	1	15.29	1	1	1
155	0	0	12.86	1	1	1
156	0	0	22.71	1	1	1
157	0	0	28.29	1	1	1
158	0	1	28.00	1	1	1
159	1	1	21.71	1	1	1
160	1	1	4.71	1	1	1
161	1	1	108.14	1	1	0
162	1	1	194.57	0	1	1
163	1	0	32.57	1	1	1
164	1	0	40.86	1	1	1
165	1	1	196.14	0	2	1
166	1	0	11.00	1	1	1
167	1	0	29.43	1	1	1
168	1	1	32.14	1	1	1
169	1	0	26.00	1	1	1
170	1	0	21.71	1	3	1
171	1	1	12.29	1	1	1
172	1	0	138.14	0	3	1
173	0	0	24.71	1	1	1
174	0	1	21.29	1	1	1
175	1	0	45.29	1	1	1
176	0	1	14.43	1	1	1
177	0	1	15.86	1	1	1
178	1	0	53.43	1	1	1
179	1	1	7.71	1	1	1
180	1	1	5.86	1	1	1
181	0	0	28.43	1	1	1
182	0	0	91.29	0	3	1
183	0	0	42.14	1	3	1
184	1	0	10.14	1	1	1
185	1	0	18.86	1	1	1
186	1	0	9.57	1	1	1

Table 19.26 Data from a Randomized CTE Brain Tumor Clinical Trial (Cont'd).

Num	Tx	R75	Age	Dx	PS	Race	RT
187	1	1	41	1.2	0	1	1
188	1	0	44	12.2	1	1	1
189	0	0	52	0.5	0	1	0
190	0	0	24	0.9	1	1	0
191	0	0	57	0.8	0	1	0
192	1	0	30	3.1	0	0	0
193	1	0	43	0.5	0	1	0
194	1	1	58	0.8	0	0	1
195	0	1	64	0.4	0	1	1
196	0	0	80	0.3	0	1	1
197	1	1	31	14	1	1	1
198	1	1	56	0.8	0	1	1
199	0	1	50	0.9	1	1	1
200	0	1	62	0.7	0	1	0
201	1	1	58	1.1	0	1	0
202	1	1	50	1.9	1	0	0
203	0	1	63	1.1	1	1	0
204	0	1	27	1.4	0	0	0
205	1	0	37	4	0	1	1
206	1	1	32	1.1	1	1	1
207	0	0	32	18	1	1	1
208	0	1	53	4.6	1	1	0
209	1	1	68	0.8	1	1	1
210	0	1	41	0.8	1	1	1
211	0	1	42	1	0	1	1
212	0	1	56	0.2	0	1	1
213	1	1	34	3.5	1	1	0
214	1	1	51	0.7	1	1	1
215	1	1	51	1.8	1	1	1
216	1	0	33	2.6	0	1	1
217	1	1	29	4.6	0	1	0
218	1	0	34	0.8	1	1	1
219	1	1	79	0.9	1	1	1
220	0	1	51	0.4	0	1	1
221	1	1	58	11.1	0	1	1
222	0	0	70	0.7	1	1	1

Table 19.27 Data from a Randomized CTE Brain Tumor Clinical Trial (Cont'd).

Num	Sex	Nitro	Weeks	Event	Path	Grade
187	0	1	5.86	1	1	1
188	1	1	32.43	1	2	1
189	0	0	12.57	1	2	1
190	1	0	18.57	1	1	1
191	0	0	12.29	1	3	.
192	1	0	32.57	1	1	1
193	1	1	19.71	1	3	1
194	0	1	34.29	1	2	1
195	0	1	46.86	1	2	0
196	1	1	6.43	1	2	1
197	0	0	56.14	1	2	1
198	1	1	10.71	1	1	1
199	1	1	28.43	1	1	1
200	1	1	8.14	1	1	1
201	0	1	13.29	1	1	1
202	1	1	19.71	1	1	1
203	1	0	11.86	1	1	1
204	0	0	14.14	1	3	1
205	1	0	14.71	1	2	1
206	1	0	6.86	1	2	1
207	0	0	79.57	1	3	1
208	0	1	39.29	1	1	1
209	1	0	19.00	1	3	1
210	0	1	32.43	1	1	1
211	1	1	12.29	1	1	1
212	1	1	28.00	1	2	.
213	1	1	47.00	1	1	1
214	1	1	51.14	1	1	0
215	1	1	7.29	1	2	1
216	0	1	5.43	1	1	1
217	1	0	27.43	1	2	1
218	1	0	14.43	1	1	1
219	0	0	19.57	1	1	1
220	0	0	19.14	1	1	1
221	0	0	33.14	1	3	1
222	1	1	20.57	1	1	1

19.9 Cross-Over Trial from Chapter 16

The data are listed in Table 19.2. The data are also listed in the following SAS program that performs an analysis using a linear model in addition to the summary of within patient differences.

```
title 'Cross-Over Trial from Chapter 16';
data one;
input group id y treat;
period = treat;
if group = 2 then do;
if treat = 1 then period = 2;
if treat = 2 then period = 1;
end;
cards;
1 1 8 1
1 1 5 2
1 3 14 1
1 3 10 2
1 4 8 1
1 4 0 2
1 6 9 1
1 6 7 2
1 7 11 1
1 7 6 2
1 9 3 1
1 9 5 2
1 11 6 1
1 11 0 2
1 13 0 1
1 13 0 2
1 16 13 1
1 16 12 2
1 18 10 1
1 18 2 2
1 19 7 1
1 19 5 2
1 21 13 1
1 21 13 2
1 22 8 1
1 22 10 2
1 24 7 1
1 24 7 2
1 25 9 1
1 25 0 2
1 27 10 1
1 27 6 2
```

```
1 28 2 1
1 28 2 2
2 2 11 1
2 2 12 2
2 5 8 1
2 5 6 2
2 8 9 1
2 8 13 2
2 10 8 1
2 10 8 2
2 12 9 1
2 12 8 2
2 14 8 1
2 14 4 2
2 15 14 1
2 15 8 2
2 17 4 1
2 17 2 2
2 20 13 1
2 20 8 2
2 23 7 1
2 23 9 2
2 26 10 1
2 26 7 2
2 29 6 1
2 29 7 2
data one;
set one;
by id notsorted;
retain y1;
drop y1;
if first.id then y1=y;
if last.id then d=y1-y;
proc print;
proc sort;
by group period;
proc means;
by group period;
var d;
proc glm data=one;
class id treat period group;
model y = group id(group) period treat;
random id(group);
estimate "drug vs placebo" treat 1 -1;
run;
```

19.10 Design Programs

All of the following programs are provided on the data disk that accompanies this book. They will run on IBM compatible microcomputers running DOS. The programs are written in the C language and are quite fast, but a math coprocessor is required. Source code is not provided, because the programs utilize a proprietary screen manager.

19.10.1 Exact binomial confidence limits

The program to perform these calculations is BCL.exe (Binomial Confidence Limits). The bcl.vvd file is also required. There are 4 input fields, of which any 3 are required. The input fields are the one-sided percentile characterizing the confidence limits (e.g., .975 for two-sided 95% bounds), the numerator of the proportion, the denominator of the proportion, and the value of p at the confidence bound. See Chapter 7. The program assumes that confidence bounds are symmetric with respect to the tail area.

Often, the first three parameters will be specified and the program will solve for p. However, the program can solve for any parameter in terms of the other three by pressing the appropriate function key. The calculations are performed using Beta distributions, so that non-integer values for numerators and denominators are permitted (and are often required to solve the equations exactly). The users is responsible for appropriate rounding. When one side of the confidence bound is specified in this way, the other side is also calculated. Additionally, the program displays a sketch of the point estimate and confidence bounds.

19.10.2 Optimal two-stage designs

The program to perform these calculations is opt.exe. The opt.vvd file is also required. Very little calculation is required in this program, except to determine some factorials and the probability of rejection (Chapter 7). The required inputs are $p0$, $p1$, α, β, a search range (upper and lower total sample sizes to limit the search), and a search method (shortcut or complete). The shortcut method searches only a subset of designs likely to contain optima. For thorough searches, the program is very time consuming, because it enumerates all possible designs within the range specified by the user.

The complete method is highly reliable, provided enough time is available and the search range actually contains an optimum. If the search range contains a global optimum, the algorithm will find it. Unfortunately, there is no simple way to determine if an optimum is local or global except to examine a sufficiently broad search range. This program could require hours on a fast computer for some design problems (e.g., those where $p0$ and $p1$ are close). Others can be solved in a matter of seconds.

19.10.3   Logrank power and sample size

Power and sample size calculations can be performed using the program logrank.exe and the associated file logrank.vvd. Design parameters are input via a single screen and the solution of one parameter in terms of the remaining ones is obtained by pressing the appropriate function key. Type I and II error probabilities can be specified as quantiles of the normal distribution (the usual way) or in terms of the actual probabilities. Although these calculations are not difficult to perform or program, the user should take care to note that the formula is written in terms of the number of events (e.g., deaths or recurrences) and not the "sample size". In the presence of censoring, the sample size will be larger than the number of events.

19.10.4   Blocked stratified randomization

The program to perform blocked stratified randomizations is bsr.exe. The file bsr.vvd is also required. This program generates numbered, blocked, randomized treatment assignments in the form of a logbook for use by a study coordinator. Up to five treatment arms can be specified. The program should be run separately for each stratum with appropriate titles, assignment numbering, and number prefixes. The block size, or a mixture of block sizes, and the allocation ratio are specified by the user. The assignment list generated in this way can be stored as a computer file or printed. The pseudo-random number generator is documented in the printout, and has a user-specified starting seed.

19.10.5   Continual reassessment method

The program to assist with this method is crm.ma, written for *Mathematica* version 2.2 or 3.0 for *Windows* [Wolfram, 1996]. Several CRM methods have been described in the literature. This one is based on a recently proposed implementation [Piantadosi, Fisher, and Grossman, 1997]. The program is internally documented and requires modification to incorporate user data when run.

19.10.6   Conditional power

Conditional power calculations using B-values can be accomplished using the program cpower.exe and the associated screens in cpower.vvd. Limited context-sensitive help is available in this program and the notation differs slightly from that employed in Chapter 10. However, the user can consult the reference and the program should be self-explanatory. Like the interfaces for the other programs, parameters are entered on a single screen. Treatment effects under alternative hypotheses can be calculated with the assistance of a second screen.

Chapter References

Andrews, D.F. and Herzberg, A.M. (1985). Data: A Collection of Problems from Many Fields for the Student and Research Worker. New York: Springer-Verlag.

Civilized Software (1996). MLAB Users Guide. Bethesda, MD: Civilized Software, Inc.

Hand, D.J., Daly, F., Lunn, A.D., McConway, K.J., and Ostrowski, E. (Eds.) (1994). A Handbook of Small Data Sets. London: Chapman & Hall.

Piantadosi, S., Fisher, J.D., and Grossman, S. for the New Approaches to Brain Tumor Therapy Consortium (1997). A practical implementation of a modified continual reassessment method for dose finding trials. J. Clin. Oncol. (submitted).

SAS Institute (1985). SAS User's Guide: Statistics, Version 5 Edition. Cary, NC: SAS Institute, Inc.

Statistical Sciences (1995). S-PLUS Guide to Statistical and Mathematical Analysis, Version 3.3. Seattle: StatSci (MathSoft).

Wolfram, S. (1996). The Mathematica Book, Third Edition. Cambridge: Cambridge University Press.

CHAPTER 20

Notation and Terminology

20.1 Introduction

The purpose of this chapter is twofold: to provide definitions of terms and statistical notations that are commonly used and to provide additional details about some statistical concepts found in the literature related to clinical trials. The definitions provided here are not authoritative in the sense of representing a consensus of experts. However, they are internally consistent and are in accord with common usage. More details and additional references can be found in Everitt [1995], Kotz and Johnson [1988], and Meinert [1996]. In the following, defined terms are in **bold face**. Comments, clarifications, and examples are in *italic face*.

20.2 Notation

Greek and Roman letters are commonly used in two ways in statistical contexts. The first is to represent specific values, functions, or variables. The second is as a shorthand for certain mathematical calculations that would be inconvenient or tedious to write out fully. Almost all symbols are used in the first context, while only a few are typically used in the second. In the following, the explanation offered for each symbol is for the one most frequently encountered. However, usage varies and depends on the specific context.

Frequently, the quantities represented by symbols are a single number or constant (scalars). However, sometimes they represent a vector or matrix. Vectors or matrices are usually denoted by boldface type, although vectors are sometimes denoted by an underscore. The quantities here are not vectors or matrices unless explicitly stated.

515

20.2.1 Greek Letters

- α (alpha): the type I error rate; also used as a model parameter.
- β (beta): the type II error rate; equally often used to denote the coefficient or coefficients that are to be estimated from the data in a regression model.
- B (beta, uppercase): beta function, $B(a, b) = \Gamma(a)\Gamma(b)/\Gamma(a + b)$; or beta distribution function.
- γ (gamma): a variable or model parameter. $\gamma(\cdot)$ is also the incomplete gamma function, a generalization of $\Gamma(\cdot)$, the complete gamma function.
- Γ (gamma, uppercase): gamma or factorial function, $\Gamma(n + 1) = n!$.
- δ (delta): often denotes a difference of two quantities, $\delta = x_1 - x_2$.
- Δ (delta, uppercase): denotes a change in a measurement or a difference between two quantities. Also frequently represents a ratio of hazard rates, $\Delta = \lambda_1/\lambda_2$, where λ_1 and λ_2 are hazard rates of interest.
- ϵ (epsilon): random error term in a model; usually implies an error with a normal distribution.
- ζ (zeta): a variable.
- η (eta): a variable.
- θ (theta): a variable or a statistical parameter to be estimated.
- ι (iota): infrequently used.
- κ (kappa): a statistic measuring rater agreement commonly used for categorical outcomes.
- Λ (lambda, uppercase): cumulative hazard.
- λ (lambda): hazard or failure rate.
- μ (mu): the mean of some normal distribution.
- ν (nu): degrees of freedom, e.g., in a chi-squared or F statistic.
- ξ (xi): a variable.
- o (omricron): infrequently used.
- π (pi): a proportion; also used in the more familiar context $3.14159\ldots$
- $\prod$ (pi, uppercase or larger): product sign, $\prod_{i=1}^{n} x_i = x_1 \cdot x_2 \cdot x_3 \cdot \ldots \cdot x_n$.
- ρ (rho): correlation coefficient.
- σ (sigma): standard deviation of some normal distribution. σ^2 is the variance of a normal distribution.
- Σ (sigma, uppercase): covariance matrix.
- $\sum$ (sigma, uppercase or larger): summation sign, $\sum_{i=1}^{n} x_i = x_1 + x_2 + x_3 + \ldots + x_n$.
- τ (tau): a variable related to time.
- υ (upsilon): infrequently used.
- ϕ (phi): the normal density function, $\phi(x) = \frac{1}{\sqrt{2\pi}}e^{-x^2/2}$. Sometimes same as Φ.
- Φ (phi, uppercase): the cumulative normal distribution function, $\Phi(z) = \int_{-\infty}^{z} \frac{1}{\sqrt{2\pi}}e^{-x^2/2}dx$.
- χ (chi): as in χ^2, the chi-squared statistic, used for goodness of fit.

- ψ (psi): infrequently used.
- Ω (omega, uppercase): the set of all outcomes; the last possible case.
- ω (omega): a point in the set Ω.

20.2.2 Roman Letters

- **B**: beta function or distribution.
- **c**: arbitrary constant.
- **d**: difference or infinitesimal difference. For example, dx is an infinitesimal change in x, as in a derivative; also number of events (deaths) in event time studies.
- **e**: base of the natural logarithms, $e = 2.71828\ldots$ Also, the exponential function (anti-logarithm).
- **E**: expectation or expected value operator.
- **f**: f(x), often a probability density function; sometimes an arbitrary function.
- **F**: F(x), often a cumulative distribution function; sometimes an arbitrary function.
- **g**: g(x), arbitrary function.
- **G**: same as F.
- **h**: h(x), arbitrary function; sometimes the hazard function in survival models.
- **H**: same as F.
- **i**: counting subscript (index) to denote an arbitrary item in a list. In the context of complex numbers such as characteristic functions (not used in this book), $i = \sqrt{-1}$.
- **j**: counting subscript like i.
- **k**: same as j.
- **l** or ℓ: same as j.
- **L,** or $\mathcal{L}$: likelihood or log-likelihood function.
- **m**: similar to n.
- **n**: number of items or a count; sample size.
- **N**: same as n.
- **p**: proportion.
- **P**: probability of an event, e.g., $P[X = 1]$ is the probability that a random variable, x, equals 1. This is also often written $\Pr[X = 1]$.
- **q**: proportion, often 1-p.
- **r**: a counter like n.
- **s**: standard deviation of a sample, often an estimate of σ.
- **t**: variable representing time. Also, the t distribution.
- **T**: time, especially a fixed constant.
- **u**: arbitrary variable, especially for integrals; also a uniform random deviate.
- **U**: uniform distribution function.
- **v**: arbitrary variable.

- **w**: a weight in a weighted average.
- **x**: arbitrary quantity; independent variable in a regression.
- **X**: often a random variable.
- **y**: arbitrary quantity; dependent variable in a regression.
- **Y**: often a random variable.
- **z**: arbitrary quantity; variable which is normally distributed.
- **Z**: often a random variable.

20.2.3 Other Symbols

- $\int$: integral sign, used in two ways. $\int f(x)dx$ is a *function*, i.e., the function whose derivative is $f(x)$. In contrast, $\int_a^b f(x)dx$ is a *number* which can often be thought of as the "area under the curve $f(x)$ between a and b".
- ∂ : infinitesimal difference in a partial derivative.
- |: vertical bar, used to specify quantities given in a conditional probability. For example, $P[A \mid B]$ is the probability of the event A given that B has occurred.
- $\hat{\ }$: hat overscore, denotes an estimate of the quantity covered as opposed to the actual value. For example, $\widehat{\Theta}$ is an estimate of Θ.
- $\tilde{\ }$: tilde overscore, an alternative estimator to the one denoted by $\hat{\ }$.
- —: bar overscore, an average. For example, $\overline{X} = \sum_{i=1}^{n} X_i/n$. Also used to denote the complement of the probability of an event. For example, $P[\overline{A}] = P[not\ A] = 1 - P[A]$.
- __ : underscore, denotes a vector quantity. For example, $\underline{\Theta} = \{\Theta_1, \Theta_2, \Theta_3, \ldots, \Theta_n\}$. Often, boldface type is used instead to represent a vector.
- $\sim$: distributed as or sampled from. For example, if x is a sample from a standard Gaussian distribution, we might write $x \sim N(0, 1)$.
- **exp**: exponential (anti-logarithm) function, $exp(log(x)) = e^{\log(x)} = x$.
- **log**: logarithmic function. *There is only one log function, i.e., that with base e. All others are multiples of it. Sometimes "ln" is used to represent the natural logarithm and "log" is reserved for base 10 logarithms. This is not good notation – a better notation for bases other than e is $\log_b$ where b is the base.*

20.3 Terminology and Concepts

- **adherence**: compliance with treatment assignment or specification.
- **accrual rate:** the rate at which eligible patients are entered onto a clinical trial, measured as persons per unit of time.
- **adjustment**: use of any of several statistical methods to account for the effect of **prognostic factors** or baseline characteristics when estimating differences

attributable to treatments or other prognostic factors. Adjustments may be non-risk adjusted (**stratification**) or risk-adjusted (**multiple regression** equations).

- **alpha error**: type I error.
- **area under the curve (AUC)**: estimated area under a time-concentration curve in pharmacokinetic studies. The AUC may be a predictor of biological effects such as toxicity or efficacy.
- **average**: see **mean**.
- **balanced design**: an experimental design in which the same number of observations is made for each factor. A balanced two-armed trial would employ an equal sample size in each arm.
- **Bayes rule**: theorem or rule of probability that relates the conditional probabilities of two events in the following way. If B_1, B_2, ... B_n are disjoint events and A is any other event,

$$\Pr\{B_i \mid A\} = \frac{\Pr\{A \mid B_i\}\Pr\{B_i\}}{\sum_{j=1}^{n}\Pr\{A \mid B_j\}\Pr\{B_j\}} \, .$$

For two events, A and B,

$$\Pr\{B \mid A\} = \frac{\Pr\{A \mid B\}\Pr\{B\}}{\Pr\{A \mid B\}\Pr\{B\} + \Pr\{A \mid \overline{B}\}\Pr\{\overline{B}\}} \, ,$$

where $\overline{B}$ represents the event not-B. In the special case where B represents the event that a person has a disease and A represents a positive diagnostic test for the disease, Bayes rule yields

$$\Pr\{disease \mid positive\ test\} = $$
$$\frac{sensitivity \times prevalence}{sensitivity \times prevalence + (1 - specificity) \times (1 - prevalence)} \, .$$

- **beta error**: type II error.
- **bias**: systematic (non-random) error in the **estimate** of a **treatment effect** or **parameter** of interest.
- **binary variable**: observations that can take one of only two values (e.g., yes/no; alive/dead; success/failure). Often the possible outcomes or variable values are numerically coded as 0 or 1 for analysis purposes.
- **binomial distribution**: the probability distribution for binary outcome variables that characterizes the number of "successes" in a series of independent trials with a constant probability of success for each trial. If X is a random variable that counts the number of successes in n trials, the distribution is

$$\Pr[X = x] = \binom{n}{x}p^x(1 - p)^{n-x},$$

where $\binom{n}{x} = \frac{n!}{x!(n-x)!}$ is the binomial coefficient. The expected value (mean) of X is np and the variance is $np(1 - p)$.

- **block**: a group of treatment assignments or experimental units arranged to control a particular source of variability. Usually the treatment effect or difference is estimated within each block, thereby eliminating the variability arising from the blocking factor.

- **blocked randomization**: a method of constrained randomization that exactly balances the treatment assignments at the end of each block. This prevents the treatment assignments from becoming very unbalanced. When used with **stratification**, blocked randomization reduces the variability due to the stratifying variable(s).

- **case report:** published report of a detailed clinical case history. Most such histories are published because the very existence of the case, or some aspect of it, is unique or rare.

- **case series:** the clinical results of an informative series of cases. The number of cases in a series may be large or small, depending on the frequency of the condition and the practice experience of the author. Series are usually defined temporally, i.e., based on a practitioner's experience with a consecutive sequence of patients having a particular diagnosis. The purpose of reporting a case series is often to make treatment inferences.

- **clinical trial**: an **experiment** in humans designed to accurately assess the effects of a treatment or treatments by reducing **random error** and **bias**.

- **confidence interval** (informal definition): a range of values calculated from the data in which the investigator believes a true parameter value will lie with some specified probability. Informally (and incorrectly) a confidence interval is a probability statement about the true parameter value.

- **confidence interval** (formal frequentist definition): a range of values calculated from the data that will contain the true parameter with a specified probability if the experiment were repeated a large number of times. Formally, a confidence interval is a probability statement about the range of values or region. *It is customary to report confidence intervals whose coverage probability is 95%, i.e., such an interval would enclose the true parameter value 95% of the time if the experiment were repeated a large number of times. Approximate 95% confidence intervals can be constructed by taking the mean ±2 standard deviations. However, there are many circumstances in which intervals other than 95% are useful.*

- **confounder**: a **prognostic factor** that is associated with both treatment and outcome and can affect both. The term is most often used in an epidemiologic context.

- **correlation coefficient**: a statistic that measures the linear relationship between a pair of variables. The correlation coefficient is a **parameter** in a bivariate normal distribution and has values between -1 and 1. A frequently used estimate is the Pearson correlation coefficient

$$\hat{\rho} = \frac{\sum_{i=1}^{n}(x_i - \bar{x})(y_i - \bar{y})}{\sqrt{\sum_{i=1}^{n}(x_i - \bar{x})^2(y_i - \bar{y})^2}},$$

where n (x, y) pairs have been sampled. *"Correlation" is often used informally to described the degree of association between two variables.*

- **cross-over**: a trial in which patients receive all the study treatments during different periods separated by a "washout" period. This permits estimating the within-patient treatment difference. *Treatment cross-overs are planned, whereas unplanned switching of treatments are called **drop-in**.*

- **CTE (comparative treatment efficacy)**: a type of trial design which assesses the efficacy of a new treatment relative to an alternative, placebo, standard therapy, or no treatment. These studies are often called **phase III**.

- **data**: observations or measurements structured in a way amenable to inspection and/or analysis. *Sometimes the word is used informally as a synonym for "information". However, it will not be used in that fashion here.*

- **data-dependent stopping**: the process of evaluating accumulating data in a clinical trial and making a decision whether the trial should be continued or stopped because the available evidence is already convincing.

- **deterministic**: without randomness.

- **DF (dose-finding)**: a type of drug development trial design that has as a primary objective identifying the optimal dose of drug to administer. Such designs are often called **phase I**.

- **dichotomous**: having only two possible values.

- **dose escalation**: see **DF**.

- **drop-in**: in a comparative trial, a study subject who takes another treatment on the trial instead of the one to which he or she was assigned and remains available for follow-up.

- **drop-outs**: study subjects who stop taking the treatment to which they were assigned but remain available for follow-up.

- **effectiveness**: the effect of a treatment when widely used in practice.

- **efficacy**: the true biological effect of a treatment.

- **endpoint:** a clinical or laboratory outcome that yields the definitive information about the result of treatment for an individual study subject. *For example, death or survival time is a frequently used endpoint in studies of chronic disease progression or recurrence. In theory, the investigator need not follow the subject past the endpoint (if this were even possible), however intermediate endpoints are sometimes used because of their strong association with more definitive outcomes. Examples of intermediate endpoints are CD4+ lymphocyte counts in AIDS, PSA levels in prostate cancer, and blood pressure in cardiovascular disease.*

- **ES (expanded safety)**: a type of surveillance trial design that has a primary objective of estimating the frequency of uncommon side effects from a particular treatment. In drug development, such studies are often called **phase IV**.

- **estimate** (verb): the process of determining the value for an unknown **parameter**. (noun): the numerical value of an estimator when it is evaluated with some specific data.

- **eligibility**: criteria that must be satisfied for each patient before entering them in a clinical trial. Examples include disease type and extent, medical history, and organ system function.
- **evaluability**: criteria that must be satisfied before concluding that the patient has had a legitimate trial on the treatment. Examples include duration of treatment or number of cycles of therapy completed. *Unfortunately, evaluability is partially an outcome of treatment and is therefore not a proper basis for excluding patients from analysis.*
- **experiment**: a study in which the investigator makes a series of careful observations under controlled or arranged conditions. In particular, the investigator controls the treatment or exposure applied to the subject(s) by design and then carefully and thoroughly records outcome measurements. *In nonexperimental studies, the investigator lacks control over exposure or treatment assignment.*
- **experimental unit**: the smallest unit or entity assigned to a particular treatment in an **experiment**. For example, individuals are often the experimental unit. However, groups of individuals such as families or households may all be assigned to receive the same treatment. See **observational unit**.
- **exponential distribution**: a probability distribution that takes on continuous positive values, x, with density function

$$f(x) = \lambda e^{-\lambda x}.$$

This distribution has expected value (mean) $1/\lambda$ and variance $1/\lambda^2$. The exponential distribution is widely used in survival and reliability analysis to model failure times.

- **factor**: a categorical variable or prognostic factor. Usually a factor has only a few levels or categories. *In experimental design, a factor refers to a variable that must be controlled. An example is "treatment" where the factor levels may be different drugs or different doses of the same drug.*
- **fully sequential**: clinical trial designs that permit the evaluation of study results after *every* patient has been accrued. Such designs can provide convincing evidence of efficacy at the earliest possible time, provided the type I error is properly controlled. *To use such a design, endpoints must be ascertained quickly, before the next patient is accrued.*
- **group sequential: clinical trial** designs similar to **fully sequential** ones, except that treatment comparisons are made after groups of patients have been accrued. These designs also terminate early when treatment differences are large.
- **hazard**: the instantaneous risk of failure when time to failure (e.g., survival) is the **endpoint**. If T is the observed failure time, any of three functions can be used to characterize a distribution of failure times: 1) the cumulative failure time distribution

$$F(t) = \Pr[T < t],$$

which is the probability that an individual fails in less than t units of time; 2) the failure density

$$f(t) = F'(t) = \Pr[t = T],$$

which is the probability that an individual fails in the time interval $t < T < t + \Delta t$; or 3) the hazard or instantaneous failure rate

$$h(t) = f(t)/(1 - F(t)),$$

which is the probability of failure in the interval $t < T < t + \Delta t$, given that there was no failure before t. The overall hazard in a cohort can be estimated by

$$\widehat{\lambda} = \frac{d}{\sum_{i=1}^{n} t_i},$$

where d is the number of events during the observation period, n is the number of study subjects, and $\sum t_i$ is the sum of all the observation times of the patients. This is the maximum likelihood estimate of the failure rate assuming an exponential survival model. More generally, the hazard can vary with time or individual characteristics in which case this estimate may not be appropriate. *This estimate of the overall hazard is sometimes termed the "linearized rate". Even when the exponential assumption is not true, this is a useful summary.*

- **hazard function regression**: a method for analysis of a time-related event and its correlates that accounts simultaneously for the distribution of times until the event in terms of a biomathematical **model** and for **prognostic factors** in terms of one or more regression models that modulate parameters of the biomathematical model.

- **hazard ratio**: the **hazard** in one group divided by the hazard in another group. A hazard ratio of 1 implies no difference in risk. *A hazard ratio of 1.8, for example, implies that the numerator group is at persistently higher risk of failure than the denominator group. The clinical significance of an elevated hazard ratio depends on other evidence including the absolute risk, the significance level, and the clinical context.*

- **inference**: drawing conclusions while accounting for **random variability**.

- **intention-to-treat**: the idea that patients assigned to treatments in randomized clinical trials should be analyzed according to the assigned treatment group rather than according to the treatment actually received. *Clinicians sometimes disagree with this perspective, which views clinical trials as tests of treatment policy rather than tests of treatment received. However, the clinical trials literature supports the validity of the intention-to-treat principle, because it yields valid tests of the null hypothesis of no treatment difference. In studies where a large fraction of patients do not receive the assigned treatment, neither the intention-to-treat (ITT) nor the treatment received (TR) analyses necessarily yield the most clinically relevant conclusions. The ITT analysis does not correspond closely to efficacy, because many patients did not*

*receive the intended treatment and the TR analysis is potentially biased, be-
cause patients may switch treatments for reasons associated with outcome.*

- **interim analysis**: an analysis of an ongoing clinical trial, particularly one
where the trial might be stopped if convincing evidence of efficacy is seen.
See **data-dependent stopping**.

- **likelihood** (likelihood function): the probability of observing the data under
an assumed model. The likelihood is an equation that combines **data** with a
probability **model** and **parameters** of interest. If one views the data as fixed,
the parameters of the model can be chosen to yield the maximum value (probability) of the likelihood function. This technique, called "maximum likelihood", is very general and usually yields parameter estimates with desirable
statistical properties. *For example, suppose we have a sample of n independent observations thought to arise from a normal distribution, $\mathbf{X} = \{x_1, x_2,
x_3, \ldots, x_n\}$. Using the normal probability density function and the fact that
independent probabilities multiply to give a joint probability, the probability
of observing the data is*

$$L(\mathbf{X}, \mu, \sigma) = \prod_{i=1}^{n} \frac{1}{\sqrt{2\pi}\sigma} e^{-\frac{(x_i - \mu)^2}{2\sigma}},$$

*where μ is the mean and σ the standard deviation of the distribution from
which the sample came. To maximize $L(\mathbf{X}, \mu, \sigma)$ with respect to μ (for example), we take logarithms (the maximum of the log likelihood will be the
same) to obtain*

$$\mathcal{L}(\mathbf{X}, \mu, \sigma) = \sum_{i=1}^{n} \left(-\log(\sqrt{2\pi}\sigma) - \frac{(x_i - \mu)^2}{2\sigma} \right).$$

The maximum occurs at $\widehat{\mu}$ when the derivative with respect to μ is zero,

$$0 = \frac{\partial \mathcal{L}}{\partial \mu} = \sum_{i=1}^{n} \left(-\frac{x_i - \widehat{\mu}}{\sigma} \right)$$

or multiplying by $-\sigma$,

$$0 = \sum_{i=1}^{n} (x_i - \widehat{\mu}).$$

This yields

$$n\widehat{\mu} = \sum_{i=1}^{n} x_i$$

or

$$\widehat{\mu} = \frac{1}{n} \sum_{i=1}^{n} x_i,$$

which is the familiar estimate of the sample mean.

- **logistic regression**: a statistical **model** in which the log **odds** of the response probability is predicted from a set of **prognostic factors**,

$$\log\left\{\frac{p}{1-p}\right\} = \beta_0 + \beta_1 X_1 + \beta_2 X_2 + \dots ,$$

where p is the probability of response, $X_1, X_2, \dots$ are the predictor (explanatory) variables, and $\beta_1, \beta_2, \dots$ are **parameters** to be estimated from the data. Thus, the effect of each prognostic factor is to multiply the baseline log odds. *Note the similarity of this to proportional hazards.*

- **lost to follow-up**: trial participant who cannot be traced or contacted to determine vital status or other endpoints. *Sometimes the terms "lost to follow-up" and "drop-out" are used synonymously. However, patients lost to follow-up are different from drop-outs in the following ways. Individuals who are lost to follow-up could remain compliant with the assigned treatment. Drop-outs are non-compliant but remain available for follow-up.*

- **LS (large-scale) trials**: studies that randomize thousands of patients, that being an order of magnitude larger than the typical CTE trial.

- **matrix**: a two-dimensional array of numbers or mathematical objects that typically represents an operation on a **vector** or one-dimensional object. *Matrix algebra is a subject of considerable importance to statistics.*

- **maximum tolerated dose**: the highest dose of a drug that can be tolerated with an acceptable or manageable level of toxicity. This is an important dose to be employed in cytotoxic therapy of cancer where the treatment typically produces serious side effects.

- **mean**: the expected value or first central moment of a probability distribution or random variable. Formally, the expected value of a discrete random variable is

$$E\{X\} = \sum x_i f(x_i),$$

where the probability of each x_i is denoted by $f(x_i)$. The mean of a series of n observations usually implies the ordinary arithmetic mean or average

$$\bar{x} = \frac{1}{n}\sum_{i=1}^{n} x_i.$$

There are other means such as the geometric and harmonic. A general form is

$$g(\tilde{x}) = \frac{1}{n}\sum_{i=1}^{n} g(x_i),$$

where the mean is denoted by $\tilde{x}$ and $g(\cdot)$ is a suitable monotonic function. For example, the ordinary mean is obtained when $g(z) = z$, the harmonic mean is obtained for $g(z) = 1/z$, and the geometric mean when $g(z) = \log(z)$.

- **meta-analysis**: see **overview**.

- **minimum effective dose**: the lowest dose of a drug that produces the desired clinical effect.

- **model**: a logical mathematical construct, generally containing **parameters** (β_1 above) and **variables** (X_1 above), (placemarks for data values). *When data have been entered, and the values for parameters have been estimated by statistical techniques, the model, which is generic, becomes a specific equation.*

- **monitoring**: observing the conduct of an ongoing clinical trial according to a set of pre-defined guidelines.

- **multiple comparisons**: performing many hypothesis tests or comparisons in the same study. A problem arises when attempting to interpret the results of numerous tests. By chance, 5% of tests will reject the **null hypothesis** if all tests are performed at the 5% significance level. To preserve the overall **type I error** rate at 5% (assuming this is a worthwhile goal), each test might be performed at a significance level less than 5%.

- **multiple regression**: use of statistical **models** to account for the effects of several **prognostic factors** simultaneously. *Linear* regression relates the response variable to the predictor variables through a linear function of **parameters**:

$$Y = \beta_0 + \beta_1 X_1 + \beta_2 X_2 + \ldots + \epsilon\,,$$

where Y is the response variable, $X_1, X_2, \ldots$ are the predictor variables, β_0, $\beta_1, \beta_2, \ldots$ are the parameters to be estimated from the data, and ϵ is a random error term.

- **multivariable**: analyzing several <u>predictor</u> (explanatory) variables simultaneously. *Suppose that a univariable analysis suggests that treatment A is better than treatment B: the hazard ratio is 2.2 (95% confidence interval 1.5–2.9) and $p = .02$. However, when we simultaneously account for the effects of sex and treatment using multivariable analysis we estimate the adjusted hazard ratio to be 1.35 (95% confidence interval 0.75–1.95) and $p = .45$. We might conclude from these results that the apparent univariable effect of treatment is due to sex and that treatment A is not likely to be of real benefit.*

- **multivariate**: analyzing several <u>outcome</u> variables simultaneously, all as a function of one or more predictor variables. *Note that multivariate does not mean "several predictor variables", as it is often informally used, but refers to several outcome variables. When there are several predictors, the term "multiple" and "multivariable" are probably better descriptors.*

- **nesting**: a design characteristic in which a particular effect lies hierarchically entirely within some other effect. In a simple parallel group comparison, patients receive only one treatment, i.e., patients are nested within treatments. In a simple **cross-over design**, patients receive both treatments, i.e., patients are not nested within treatments.

- **null hypothesis**: in statistical hypothesis tests, the hypothesis of no difference between the comparison groups. It is usually established as a "straw man" to be disproved.

- **observation**: process of study; a datum from an experiment.
- **observational study**: a study design in which the investigator does not control the assignment of treatment to individual study subjects.
- **observational unit**: the entity or unit in an **experiment** on which one observation is made. This may be the same or different from the **experimental unit**. *For example, households may be the experimental unit but individuals could be the observational unit. If so, a household would be randomized so that every member receives the same treatment but a single individual in each would be followed for the outcome.*
- **odds**: the probability of an outcome divided by the probability of not having that outcome. If p is the probability of the outcome, the odds equals $p/(1-p)$. *This is the ordinary betting odds.*
- **odds ratio**: **odds** in one group divided by the odds in another group. The odds ratio is commonly used for categorical data which might be summarized as

		Outcome	
		Yes	No
Exposure	Yes	a	b
	No	c	d

where a, b, c, and d are the counts in the various categories. The odds of outcome when the condition is present is

$$\frac{\frac{a}{a+b}}{\frac{b}{a+b}} = \frac{a}{b} .$$

When the condition is absent, the odds of outcome are

$$\frac{\frac{c}{c+d}}{\frac{d}{c+d}} = \frac{c}{d} .$$

Thus the odds ratio is

$$\frac{ad}{bc} .$$

The odds ratio is related to the risk ratio or relative risk in that when the probability of the outcome is small (i.e., $a \ll b$ and $c \ll d$), the odds ratio approximately equals the risk ratio

$$\frac{\frac{a}{a+b}}{\frac{c}{c+d}} .$$

However, the odds ratio is a useful measure of difference between groups even when it does not approximate the relative risk and arises naturally in important statistical models such as logistic regression. An odds ratio of 1 implies no difference in risk between the groups. An odds ratio of 2.3, for example, implies that the numerator group is at higher risk than the denominator group.

The clinical significance of an elevated odds ratio depends on other evidence including the absolute risk, the significance level, and the clinical setting.

- **overview**: a comprehensive re-analysis of published and unpublished studies, usually based on obtaining individual patient data, to investigate and quantify consistency or lack of consistency among study results.

- **parallel design**: a trial design in which patients receive only one of two or more concurrently administered treatments.

- **parameter**: a constant in a **model,** or a constant that wholly or partially characterizes a function or probability distribution.

- **phase I trial**: a **clinical trial** designed to measure the distribution, metabolism, excretion, and toxicity of a new drug. See **DF.**

- **phase II trial**: a **clinical trial** designed to test the feasibility of, and level of activity of, a new agent or procedure. See **SE.**

- **phase III trial**: a **clinical trial** designed to estimate the relative efficacy of a treatment against a standard, alternative, or placebo. See **CTE.**

- **phase IV trial**: a surveillance trial designed to estimate the frequency of uncommon side effects, toxicity, or interactions. See **ES.** In drug development such trials are sometimes initiated as post-marketing studies.

- **placebo**: a treatment that appears like a comparison treatment but with no true biological effect. Placebos are used to reduce bias in a comparison where assessment of outcome could be affected by patient or investigator knowledge that no treatment was given to one group.

- **power**: the chance of detecting a difference of a specified size as being statistically significant. If the **type II error** probability is β, power $= 1 - \beta$.

- **precision**: the certainty with which a measurement or **estimate** is made. *A precise measurement may not be accurate because of unrecognized bias or other errors in methodology.*

- **probit**: a term used to describe the cumulative normal distribution curve, especially when its sigmoidal shape is used for dose response modeling as in bioassay. The probit curve is given by

$$p = \frac{1}{\sqrt{2\pi}} \int_{-\infty}^{y} e^{-u^2/2} du,$$

where y represents dose or logarithm of dose and p is the probability of response.

- **prognostic factor:** a variable or measurement that carries information about future clinical outcomes. Baseline prognostic factors have values fixed at study onset and never change. Time dependent prognostic factors have values that change over time and are considerably more difficult to model statistically.

- **proportional hazards:** a mathematical assumption used in survival models in which the **hazard ratio** between two groups is assumed to be constant over time although the baseline hazard can fluctuate. For example, the usual assumption is

$$\log\left\{\frac{\lambda(t)}{\lambda_0(t)}\right\} = \beta_1 X_1 + \beta_2 X_2 + \dots,$$

where $\lambda_0(t)$ is the baseline hazard function which can vary over time, $\lambda(t)$ is the hazard function in the test group, $X_1, X_2, \dots$ are the predictor variables, and $\beta_1, \beta_2, \dots$ are **parameters** to be estimated from the data. *Because the covariate terms are additive on a logarithmic scale, we refer to this model as employing multiplicative covariate effects.*

- **protocol**: the logical plans for conducting an **experiment,** clinical study, or **clinical trial**. *Sometimes this term is used to refer to the study or trial itself. However, it is always used here to refer to either the written document or the logical plan of the study.*

- **pseudorandom**: numbers that pass important tests of randomness but are actually generated by a non-random (deterministic) algorithm. Most computer generated "random" numbers are pseudorandom.

- **publication bias**: the tendency for studies with positive results, i.e., those finding significant differences, to be published in journals in preference to those with negative findings. When journals are reviewed for summarizing study results (meta-analysis), a biased impression of treatment efficacy might then result.

- **p-value**: the conditional probability that an observed effect or one larger is due to chance given that the **null hypothesis** is true. *P-values are frequently mis-interpreted as the unconditional probability of an error or the probability that the observed result is due to chance. It is important to recognize that the p-value assumes the null hypothesis is true and accounts for outcomes that have not been observed.*

- **quantile**: in a probability function, the value of the variable that yields a particular probability. For example, the normal quantile that yields a probability of 0.95 is 1.645.

- **random**: the result of chance alone.

- **randomization**: assignment of patients or experimental subjects to two or more treatments by chance alone.

- **rate**: a **ratio** in which the numerator and denominator are incremental differences. Often the rate has dimensions of reciprocal time. For example, an incidence rate is the number of new cases divided by an interval of time.

- **ratio**: a fraction in which the numerator and denominator have clinical or epidemiological importance. The dimensions of the numerator and denominator may be different so that the ratio has dimensions. For example, a mortality ratio might be the number of deaths per 100,000 population.

- **risk ratio**: the probability of a specified outcome in one group divided by the probability of the outcome in another group. A risk ratio of 1 implies no difference in risk.

- **sample size**: the number of patients or experimental subjects on a study. *For studies with event time as an outcome (e.g., survival or disease recurrence), one must distinguish the sample size from the number of events required by the design of the study. Ideally, the sample size is determined as a consequence of the need for precision in the estimate of treatment difference. However, in many cases, the sample size is determined by cost, time, or other mundane practical constraints.*

- **SE (safety and efficacy)**: a type of trial design with safety and efficacy estimation as a primary objective. In drug development, such studies are often called **phase II**.

- **selection bias**: a systematic error or bias that causes a sample to be unrepresentative of the population from which it came.

- **statistic**: any function of the data; a special case is one derived to estimate some parameter which is called an estimator.

- **statistical significance**: the quantitative degree, as measured by the **p-value**, to which a difference is likely to be the result of chance, assuming the **null hypothesis** is true. *Conventionally, p-values less than 0.05 are judged to be "significant". However, p-values are influenced by several factors, making universal criteria impossible.*

- **statistics**: the study of the inferential process, especially the planning and analysis of experiments or surveys. *Statistics deals with numerical data relating to aggregates of individuals. It is the science of collecting, analyzing, and interpreting such data.*

- **stratification:** performing a statistical procedure separately in groups (strata) to reduce the effects of the group factor. *As an adjunct to randomization, stratification can only effectively be used with blocking. As an analysis method, estimates are made within strata and pooled, when possible, across strata to reduce the influence of the stratifying variable.*

- **surrogate outcome**: an outcome measurement in a clinical trial that substitutes for a definitive clinical outcome or disease status. Examples of possible surrogate outcomes include prostatic specific antigen (PSA) in prostate cancer, blood pressure in cardiovascular disease, and CD4 positive lymphocyte count in AIDS. *To be useful, a surrogate outcome must be strongly (even causally) related to a definitive outcome like disease progression or length of survival but manifest relatively early after treatment. Trials designed using ideal surrogate outcomes, if they exist, may be shorter, more efficient, and as equally valid as ones using definitive endpoints.*

- **Taylor series**: a method of expanding a function as a polynomial using successive derivatives. For x in the region of a, the Taylor series is

$$
\begin{aligned}
f(x) \;=\; & f(a) + f^{(1)}(a)(x-a) \\
& + f^{(2)}(a)(x-a)^2/2! \\
& + f^{(3)}(a)(x-a)^3/3! \\
& + \ldots
\end{aligned}
$$

$$+f^{(n-1)}(a)(x-a)^{n-1}/(n-1)! + R_n,$$

where $f^{(n)}$ is the nth derivative of the function f with respect to x and R_n is a remainder that can be expressed in various forms. The utility of the formula usually comes from employing only the first two terms,

$$f(x) \approx f(a) + (x-a)f^{(1)}(a),$$

which yields an approximation for $f(x)$ in the region of the point a.

- **therapeutic ratio**: the ratio of efficacy response over toxicity response. High values indicate that a treatment is beneficial without causing much chance of toxicity. Low values indicate that the chance of benefit is low compared with the chance of toxicity. For drugs, the therapeutic ratio may depend on dose such that one dose may yield the best chance of benefit with the least chance of toxicity.

- **TM (treatment mechanism)**: a type of early developmental trial design that tests the mechanism of delivering treatment to the patient. Treatment mechanisms include device function, drug bioavailability, and surgical technique. **Phase I** drug trials usually have treatment mechanism objectives, but the terms are not equivalent. See **DF**.

- **trial**: a study in which the investigator controls three elements of design: 1) the treatment assigned to the subject(s), 2) ascertainment of outcomes, and 3) analysis of results. *We have carefully chosen the word "assigned" rather than using "applied" because, at least in humans, if not in all trials and experiments, the investigator cannot guarantee the application of an intended treatment.*

- **type I error**: concluding that a **treatment effect** or difference exists when, in reality, it does not (false positive).

- **type II error**: concluding that a **treatment effect** or difference does not exist when, in reality, it does (false negative).

- **univariable**: analyzing one *explanatory* variable at a time.

- **univariate**: analyzing one *outcome* variable at a time.

- **variability**: unaccounted for fluctuation (random error) in the **estimate** of a **treatment effect** or measurement of a variable.

- **variable**: a measurement which can take on different values for each experimental subject or observation.

- **vector**: a one-dimensional array of numbers or mathematical objects usually representing a point or direction in space.

20.4 Abbreviations

ABMF: Advisory Board of the Medical Faculty

ACAPS: Asymptomatic Carotid Artery Plaque Study

ACE: angiotensin converting enzyme

ACS: American Cancer Society

AIDS: Acquired Immunodeficiency Syndrome

AMA: American Medical Association

ANCOVA: analysis of covariance

ASA: acetylsalicylic acid (aspirin)

ASA: American Statistical Association

AUC: area under the curve

AZT: zidovudine

BCNU: 1,3-bis (2-chloroethyl)-1-nitrosourea (carmustine)

BEMAC: Biometric and Epidemiology Methods Advisory Committee

CALGB: Cancer and Leukemia Group B

CAP: cytoxan, Adriamycin (doxorubicin), and platinum

CARET: Carotene and retinol efficacy trial

CAST: Cardiac Arrythmia Supression Trial

CDC: Centers for Disease Control

CDP: Coronary Drug Project

CEA: carcinoembryonic antigen

CIOMS: Council for International Organizations of Medical Sciences

COMMIT: Community Intervention Trial (for smoking cessation)

COPD: chronic obstructive pulmonary disease

CRM: continual reassessment method

CTE: comparative treatment efficacy

DHHS: Department of Health and Human Services

DF: dose-finding

DLT: dose limiting toxicity

DSMC: Data and Safety Monitoring Committee

DSMB: Data and Safety Monitoring Board

EBCTCG: Early Breast Cancer Trialists Collaborative Group

ECMO: extracorporeal membrane oxygenation

EGRET: Epidemiology, Graphics, Estimation, and Testing

EORTC: European Organization for Research on the Treatment of Cancer

EPP: extrapleural pneumonectomy

ER: estrogen receptor

ES: expanded safety

FAP: familial adenomatous polyposis

FDA: Food and Drug Administration

GAO: General Accounting Office

HIV: human immunodeficiency virus

HPB: Health Protection Branch

IARC: Internation Agency for Research on Cancer

ICH: International Conference on Harmonisation

ICU: intensive care unit

IEC: Independent Ethics Committee

IND: investigational new drug

IOM: Institute of Medicine

IRB: Institutional Review Board

ITT: intention to treat

IV: intravenous

LREC: Local Research Ethics Committee

LST: large-scale trials

LVR: lung volume reduction

MACS: Multi-Center AIDS Cohort Study

MLAB: Modeling LABoratory

MLE: maximum likelihood estimate

MSE: mean squared error

MTD: maximum tolerated dose

NAS: National Academy of Sciences

NCCTG: North Central Cancer Treatment Group

NHLBI: National Heart Lung and Blood Institute

NIH: National Institutes of Health

NLM: National Library of Medicine

NSABP: National Surgical Adjuvant Breast and Bowel Project

NSC: National Service Center

NSF: National Science Foundation

OIG: Office of the Inspector General

ORI: Office of Research Integrity

OSI: Office of Scientific Integrity

OSIR: Office of Scientific Integrity Review

PASS: Power and Sample Size

PCP: personal care principle

PDQ: Physician Data Query

PFA: prognostic factor analyses

PH: proportional hazards

PHS: Public Health Service

PI: principal investigator

PK: pharmacokinetic

PS: performance status

PSA: prostatic specific antigen

RCP: Royal College of Physicians

RPA: recursive partitioning and amalgamation

RSS: Royal Statistical Society

SAS: Statistical Analysis System

SE: safety and efficacy

SERC: Statistics and Epidemiology Research Corporation

SPRT: sequential probability ratio test

SSD: sum of squared deviations

TDC: time dependent covariates

TM: treatment mechanism

TR: treatment received

VOD: veno-occlusive disease

WHO: World Health Organization

WMA: World Medical Association

Chapter References

Everitt, B.S. (Ed.) (1995). The Cambridge Dictionary of Statistics in the Medical Sciences. Cambridge: Cambridge University Press.

Kotz, S. and Johnson, N.L. (Eds.) (1988). Encyclopedia of Statistical Sciences. New York: John Wiley & Sons.

Meinert, C.L. (Ed.) (1996). Clinical Trials Dictionary. Baltimore: C.L. Meinert.

Comprehensive Bibliography

ACAPS Group. (1992). Rationale and design for the Asymptomatic Carotid Artery Plaque Study (ACAPS). Controlled Clinical Trials 13: 293-314.

ASA (1995). Ethical Guidelines for Statistical Practice.

Abby, M., Massey, M.D., Galandiuk, S., and Polk, H.C., Jr. (1994). Peer review is an effective screening process to evaluate medical manuscripts. JAMA 272: 105-107.

Achenwall, G. (1748). Vorbereitung zur Staatswissenschaft. This became the introduction to: Staatsverfassung der heutigen vornehmsten europäischen Reiche und Völker im Grundrisse. Göttingen, 1749.

Ad Hoc Working Group for Critical Appraisal of the Medical Literature. (1987). A proposal for more informative abstracts of clinical articles. Ann. Intern. Med. 106: 598-604.

Advisory Committee on Human Radiation Experiments, Final Report (1995). Washington, DC: Government Printing Office.

Agresti, A. (1996). An Introduction to Categorical Data Analysis. New York: John Wiley & Sons.

Ahrens, E.H. (1992). The Crisis in Clinical Research: Overcoming Institutional Obstacles. New York: Oxford University Press.

Albain, K.S., Green, S., LeBlanc, M., Rivkin, S., O'Sullivan, J., and Osborne, C.K. (1992). Proportional hazards and recursive partitioning and amalgamation analyses of the Southwest Oncology Group node-positive adjuvant CMFVP breast cancer data base: A pilot study. Breast Cancer Research Treat. 22: 273-284.

Altman, D.G., Gore, S., Gardner, M., and Pocock, S. (1983). Statistical guidelines for contributors to medical journals. Brit. Med. J. 286: 1489-1493.

Altman, D.G. and Bland, J.M. (1995). Absence of evidence is not evidence of absence. BMJ 311: 485.

Amberson, J.B., Jr., McMahon, B.T., and Pinner, M. (1931). A clinical trial of sanocrysin in pulmonary tuberculosis. Am. Rev. Tuberc. 24: 401-404.

American Cancer Society (ACS) (1990). Questionable cancer practices in Tijuana and other Mexican border clinics. Statement approved by the Committee on Questionable Methods of Cancer Management.

American Cancer Society (ACS) (1993). Questionable methods of cancer management: "nutritional" therapies. CA Cancer Journal for Clinicians 43(5): 309-319.

Andersen, B. (1990). Methodological Errors in Medical Research. Oxford: Blackwell Scientific Publications.

Andersen, P.K. (1987). Conditional power calculations as an aid in the decision whether to continue a clinical trial. Controlled Clinical Trials 8: 67-74.

Anderson, J.R., Cain, K.C., Gelber, R.D., and Gelman, R.S. (1985). Analysis and interpretation of the comparison of survival by treatment outcome variables in cancer clinical trials. Cancer Treat. Rep. 69: 1139-1144.

Andrews, D.F. and Herzberg, A.M. (1985). Data: A Collection of Problems from Many Fields for the Student and Research Worker. New York: Springer-Verlag.

Angell, M. and Kassire, J.P. (1994). Setting the record straight in the breast cancer trials (editorial). New Engl. J. Med. 330: 1448-1450.

Annas, G.J. and Grodin, M.A. (1992). The Nazi Doctors and the Nuremberg Code: Human Rights in Human Experimentation. New York: Oxford University Press.

Anscombe, F.J. (1963). Sequential medical trials. J. Am. Stat. Assoc. 58: 365-383.

Ansell, S.M., Rapoport, B.L., Falkson, G., Raats, J.I., and Moeken, C.M. (1993). Survival determinants in patients with advanced ovarian cancer. Gyn. Oncol. 50: 215-220.

Appelbaum, P.S., Lidz, C.W., and Meisel, A. (1987). Informed Consent: Legal Theory and Clinical Practice. New York: Oxford University Press.

Appleton, D.R. (1995). What do we mean by a statistical model? Statistics in Med. 14: 185-197.

Armitage, P. (1981). Importance of prognostic factors in the analysis of data from clinical trials. Controlled Clinical Trials 1: 347-353.

Armitage, P., and Berry, G. (1994). Statistical Methods in Medical Research, 3rd Edition. Oxford: Blackwell.

Assaf, A.R. and Carleton, R.A. (1994). The Women's Health Initiative clinical trial and observational study: History and overview. Rhode Island Medicine 77: 424-427.

ATBC Cancer Prevention Study Group (1994a). The alpha-tocopherol beta-carotene lung cancer prevention study: Design, methods, participant characteristics, and compliance. Ann. Epidemiol. 4: 1-9.

ATBC Cancer Prevention Study Group (1994b). The effect of vitamin E and beta carotene on the incidence of lung cancer and other cancers in male smokers. New Engl. J. Med. 330: 1029-1034.

Aulas, J.J. (1996). Alternative cancer treatments. Scientific American 275(3): 162-163.

Babbage, C. (1830, 1970). Reflections on the Decline of Science in England. New York: Augustus Kelley.

Bailar, J. and Mosteller, F. (1988). Guidelines for statistical reporting for medical journals: Amplifications and explanations. Ann. Int. Med. 108: 266-273.

Bailar, J.C. (1995). The practice of meta-analysis. J. Clin. Epidemiol. 48: 149-157.

Bailar, J.C.I., Louis, T.A., Lavori, P.W., and Polansky, M. (1984). Studies without internal controls. New Engl. J. Med. 311: 156-162.

Bakke, O.M., Manocchia, M., de Abajo, F., Kaitin, K.I., and Lasagna, L. (1995). Drug safety discontinuations in the United Kingdom, the United States, and Spain from 1974 through 1993: A regulatory perspective. Clin. Pharmacol. Ther. 58(1): 108-117.

Balke, A.A. and Pearl, J. (1994). Universal formulas for treatment effects from noncompliance data. Technical Report R-199-A, Cognitive Systems Laboratory, UCLA.

Barnett, V. (1982). Comparative Statistical Inference, 2nd edition. New York: John Wiley & Sons.

Barrett, S. (1993). "Alternative" Cancer Treatment. Chapter 6 in S. Barrett and W.T. Jarvis (Eds.). The Health Robbers. Buffalo, NY: Prometheus Books.

Barrow, J.D. (1991). Theories of Everything. Oxford: Clarendon Press.

Bartlett, R.H., Roloff, D.W. Cornell, R.G., Andrews, A.F., Dillon, P.W., and Zwischenberger, J.B. (1985). Extracorporeal circulation in neonatal respiratory failure: A prospective randomized study. Pediatrics 76: 479-487.

Baum, M, Houghton, J., and Abrams, K. (1994). Early stopping rules – clinical perspectives and ethical considerations. Statistics in Med. 13: 1459-1469.

Bayes, T. (1763). An essay towards solving a problem in the doctrine of chances. Phil. Trans. Roy. Soc. Lond. 53: 370-418.

Bayes, T. (1958). Reprint of the 1763 paper. Biometrika 45: 298-315.

Beach, M.L. and Meier, P. (1989). Choosing covariates in the analysis of clinical trials. Controlled Clinical Trials 10: 161S-175S.

Beauchamp, T.L. and Childress, J.F. (1989). Principles of Biomedical Ethics. 3rd Ed., New York: Oxford University Press.

Becker, N., Chambliss, C., Marsh, C., and Montemayor, R. (1995). Effects of mellow and frenetic music and stimulating and relaxing scents on walking by seniors. Perceptual & Motor Skills 80: 411-415.

Beecher, H.K. (1955). The powerful placebo. J.A.D.A. 159: 1602-1606.

Beecher, H.K. (1966). Ethics and clinical research. New Engl. J. Med. 274: 1354-1360.

Beecher, H.K. (1970). Research and the Individual: Human Studies. Boston: Little, Brown.

Begg, C.B. and Berlin, J.A. (1988). Publication bias: A problem in interpreting medical data. J. R. Stat. Soc. A 151: 419-463.

Begg, C.D. and Iglewicz, B.A. (1980). A treatment allocation procedure for sequential clinical trials. Biometrics 36: 81-90.

Berry, D.A. (1985). Interim analyses in clinical trials: Classical vs. Bayesian approaches. Statistics in Med. 4: 521-526.

Berry, D.A. (1993). A case for Bayesianism in clinical trials. Statistics in Med. 12: 1377-1393.

Berson, E.L., Rosner, B., Sandberg, M.A., Hayes, K.C., Nicholson, B.W., Weigel-DiFranco, C., and Willet, W. (1993). A randomized trial of vitamin A and vitamin E supplementation for retinitis pigmentosa. Arch. Ophthalmol. 111: 761-772.

Bertram, J.F., Kolonel, L.N., and Meyskens, F.L. Jr. (1987). Strategies and rationale for chemoprevention of cancer in humans. Cancer Research 47: 3012-3031.

Bhasin, S., Storer, T.W., Berman, N., et al. (1996). The effects of supraphysiologic doses of testosterone on muscle size and strength in normal men. New Engl. J. Med. 335: 1-7.

Biros, M.H., Lewis, R.J., Olson, C.M., et al. (1995). Informed consent in emergency research. JAMA 273: 1283-1287.

Bivens, L.V. and Macfarlane, D.K. (1994). Fraud in breast cancer trials. New Engl. J. Med. 330: 1461.

Bobbio, M., Demichelis, B., and Giustetto, G. (1994). Completeness of reporting trial results: Effect on physicians' willingness to prescribe. Lancet 343: 1209-1211.

Bock, R.D. (1975). Multivariate Statistical Methods in Behavioral Research. New York: McGraw-Hill.

Boden, W.E. (1992). Meta-analysis in clinical trials reporting: Has a tool become a weapon? (editorial). Am. J. Cardiology 69: 681-686.

Bogoch, S. and Bogoch, E.S. (1994). A checklist for suitability of biomarkers as surrogate endpoints in chemoprevention of breast cancer. J. Cellular Biochemistry, Supplement 19: 173-185.

Boissel, J.-P., Collet, J.-P., Moleur, P., and Haugh, M. (1992). Surrogate endpoints: A basis for a rational approach. Eur. J. Clin. Pharmacol. 43: 235-244.

Bonita, R. and Beaglehole, R. (1996). The enigma of the decline in stroke deaths in the United States. Stroke 27: 370-372.

Borgen, P.I. (1991). Reviewing peer review: The NCI clinical alert three years later. J. LA. State Med. Soc. 143(3): 39-41.

Box, J.F. (1980). R. A. Fisher and the design of experiments, 1922-1926. Am. Statistician 34: 1-7.

Brandt, A.M. (1978). Racism and research: The case of the Tuskegee syphilis study. Hastings Center Report 8: 21-29.

Brem, H., Piantadosi, S., Burger, P.C. et al. (1995). Placebo-controlled trial of safety and efficacy of intraoperative controlled delivery by biodegradable polymers of chemotherapy for recurrent gliomas. Lancet 345: 1008-1012.

Brett, A.S. (1981). Sounding board – hidden ethical issues in clinical decision analysis. New Engl. J. Med. 5: 1150-1152.

Bridgen, M.L. (1995). Unproven (questionable) cancer therapies. Western J. Med. 163(5): 463-469.

Broad, W. and Wade, N. (1982). Betrayers of the Truth. New York: Simon and Schuster.

Broder, S. (1994). Fraud in breast cancer trials. New Engl. J. Med. 330: 1460-1461.

Bross, I.D. (1990). How to eradicate fraudulent statistical methods: Statisticians must do science. Biometrics 46: 1213-1225.

Brown, B.W., Jr. (1980). The cross-over experiment for clinical trials. Biometrics 36: 69-79.

Brown, R.D., Whisnant, J.P., Sicks, J.D., O'Fallon, W.M., and Wiebers, D.O. (1996). Stroke incidence, prevalence, and survival: Secular trends in Rochester, Minnesota, through 1989. Stroke 27: 373-380.

Bulger, R.E. (1994). Toward a statement of the principles underlying responsible conduct in biomedical research. Academic Medicine 69(2): 102-107.

Bull, J.P. (1959). The historical development of clinical therapeutic trials. J. Chron. Dis. 10: 218-248.

Burish, T.G. and Jenkins, R.A. (1992). Effectiveness of biofeedback and relaxation training in reducing the side effects of cancer chemotherapy. Health Psychol. 11: 17-23.

Burton, P.R. (1994). Helping doctors to draw appropriate inferences from the analysis of medical studies. Statistics in Med. 13: 1699-1713.

Buyse, M.E., Staquet, M.J., and Sylvester, R.J. (Eds.) (1984). Cancer Clinical Trials. Methods and Practice. Oxford: Oxford University Press.

Byar, D.A., Schoenfeld, D.A., Green, S.B., et al. (1990). Design considerations for AIDS trials. New Engl. J. Med. 323: 1343-1348.

Byar, D.P. (1980). Why data bases should not replace randomized clinical trials. Biometrics 36: 337-342.

Byar, D.P. (1982). Analysis of Survival Data: Cox and Weibull Models With Covariates. Chapter 12 in Valerie Mike and Kenneth Stanley (Eds.) Statistics in Medical Research, New York: John Wiley & Sons.

Byar, D.P. (1984). Identification of Prognostic Factors. Chapter 24 in M.J. Buyse, M.J. Staquet, and R.J. Sylvester (Eds.), Cancer Clinical Trials. Oxford: Oxford University Press.

Byar, D.P. (1991). Problems with using observational databases to compare treatments. Statistics in Med. 10: 663-666.

Byar, D.P., Green, S.B., Dor, P., Williams, E.D., Colon, J., van Gilse, H.A., Mayer, M., Sylvester, R.J., and Van Glabbeke, M. (1979). A prognostic index for thyroid carcinoma. A study of the EORTC Thyroid Cancer Cooperative Group. European J. Cancer 15: 1033-1041.

Byar, D.P. (1978). On combining information: Historical controls, overviews, and comprehensive cohort studies. Recent Results in Cancer Research 111: 95-98.

Byar, D.P. (1985). Assessing apparent treatment–covariate interactions in randomized clinical trials. Statistics in Med. 4: 255-263.

Byar, D.P. (1990). Factorial and reciprocal control designs. Statistics in Med. 9: 55-64.

Byar, D.P., Herzberg, A.M., and Tan, W.-Y. (1993). Incomplete factorial designs for randomized clinical trials. Statistics in Med. 12: 1629-1641.

Byar, D.P., Simon, R.M., Friedewald, W.T., et al. (1976). Randomized clinical trials. Perspectives on some recent ideas. New Engl J Med. 295: 74-80.

Byar, D.P., and Piantadosi, S. (1985). Factorial designs for randomized clinical trials. Cancer Treatment Rep. 69: 1055-1063.

Carroll, R.J., Ruppert, D., and Stefanski, L.A. (1995). Measurement Error in Nonlinear Models. London: Chapman-Hall.

Campbell, M.J. and Machin, D. (1990). Medical Statistics. Chichester: John Wiley & Sons.

Carlin, B.P. and Sargent, D.J. (1996). Robust Bayesian approaches for clinical trial monitoring. Statistics in Med. 15: 1093-1106.

Carson, E.R., Cobelli, C., and Finkelstein, L. (1983). The Mathematical Modeling of Metabolic and Endocrine Systems. New York: John Wiley & Sons.

Carter, R.L., Scheaffer, R.L., and Marks, R.G. (1986). The role of consulting units in statistics departments. Am. Stat. 40: 260-262.

Casey, A.T.H., Crockard, H.A., Bland, J.M. et al. (1996). Surgery on the rheumatoid cervical spine for the non-ambulant myelopathic patient – too much, too late? Lancet 347: 1004-1007.

Casselith, B.R. and Chapman, C.C. (1996). Alternative cancer medicine: A ten-year update. Cancer Invest. 14(4) 396-404.

CAST Investigators (1989). Preliminary report: Effect of encainide and flecainide on mortality in a randomized trial of arrythmia suppression after myocardial infarction. New Engl. J. Med 312: 406-412.

Centers for Disease Control. (1997). Paralytic poliomyelitis – United States, 1980-1994. MMWR 46(4): 79-83.

Challis, G.B. and Stam, H.J. (1990). The spontaneous regression of cancer: A review of cases from 1900 to 1987. Acta Oncologica 29: 545-550.

Chalmers, I. (1990). Underreporting research is scientific misconduct. JAMA 263: 1405-1408.

Chalmers, I. (1993). The Cochrane Collaboration: Preparing , maintaining, and disseminating systematic reviews of the effects of health care. Ann. N. Y. Acad. Sci. 703: 156-165.

Chalmers, I., and Silverman, W.A. (1987). Professional and public double standards on clinical experimentation. Controlled Clin. Trials 8: 388-391.

Chalmers, T.C. (1975a). Ethical aspects of clinical trials. Am. J. Ophthalmol. 79: 753-758.

Chalmers, T.C. (1975b). Randomization of the first patient. Med. Clin. North Am. 59: 1035-1038.

Chalmers, T.C. (1989). A belated randomized control trial. Pediatrics 85: 366-368.

Chalmers, T.C. (1991). Problems induced by meta-analyses. Statistics in Med. 10: 971-980.

Chalmers, T.C. (1993). Meta-analytic stimulus for changes in clinical trials. Statist. Methods in Med. Research 2: 161-172.

Chalmers, T.C., Matta, R.J., Smith, H., Jr., and Kunzler, A.M. (1977). Evidence favoring the use of anticoagulants in the hospital phase of acute myocardial infarction. New Engl. J. Med. 297: 1091-1096.

Chastang, C., Byar, D.P., and Piantadosi, S. (1988). A quantitative study of the bias in estimating the treatment effect caused by omitting a balanced covariate in survival models. Statistics in Med. 7(12): 1243-1255.

Chlebowski, R.T., Bulcavage, L., Grosvenor, M. et al. (1990). Hydrazine sulfate influence on nutritional status and survival in non-small cell lung cancer. J. Clin. Oncol. 8: 9-15.

Cho, M.K. and Bero, L.A. (1994). Instruments for assessing the quality of drug studies published in the medical literature. JAMA 272: 101-104.

Chop, R.M. and Silva, M.C. (1991). Scientific fraud: definitions, policies, and implications for nursing research. J. Prof. Nursing 7: 166-171.

Chow, S.C. and Ki, F.Y.C. (1994). On statistical characteristics of quality of life assessment. J. Biopharmaceutical Statistics 1: 1-17.

Chow, S.C. and Ki, F.Y.C. (1996). Statistical issues in quality of life assessment. J. Biopharmaceutical Statistics 6: 37-48.

Chowdhury, A.M., Karim, F., Rohde, J.E., Ahmed, J., and Abed, F.H. (1991). Oral rehydration therapy: A community trial comparing the acceptability of homemade sucrose and cereal-based solutions. Bull. World Health Organ. 69: 229-234.

Civilized Software (1996). MLAB Users Guide. Bethesda, MD: Civilized Software.

Clark, G.M., Hilsenbeck, S.G., Ravdin, P.M., De Laurentiis, M., and Osborne, C.K. (1994). Prognostic factors: Rationale and methods of analysis and integration. Breast Cancer Research Treat. 32: 105-112.

Cleophas, T.J.M. and Tavenier, P. (1995). Clinical trials in chronic diseases. J. Clin. Pharmacol. 35: 594-598.

Cochran, W.G. and Cox, G.M. (1957). Experimental Designs, 2nd Edition. New York: John Wiley & Sons.

Cochrane, A.L. (1972). Effectiveness and Efficiency. London: Nuffield Provincial Hospital Trust.

Coffey, D.S. (1978). General summary remarks (regarding the Workshop in Genitourinary Cancer Immunology, Iowa City, 1976). Department of Health, Education, and Welfare. National Cancer Institute Monograph 49. Publication No. (NIH) 78-1467.

Cohen, J. (1994). Clinical trial monitoring: Hit or miss? Science 264: 1534-1537.

Cohen, J., Marshall, E., and Taubes, G. (1995). Conduct in science. Science 268: 1705-1720.

Cohn, I. (1994). Whither NCI and NSABP? (editorial). Arch. Surg. 129: 1005-1009.

Cole, W.H. (1976). Opening address: Spontaneous regression of cancer and the importance of finding its cause. NCI Monograph No. 44: 5-9.

Collett, D. (1994). Modelling Survival Data in Medical Research. London: Chapman and Hall.

Colvin, L.B. (1969). Metabolic fate of hydrazines and hydrazides. J. Pharm. Sci. 58: 1433-1443.

COMMIT (1995a). Community intervention trial for smoking cessation (COMMIT): I. Cohort results from a four-year community intervention. Am. J. Public Health 85: 183-192.

COMMIT (1995b). Community intervention trial for smoking cessation (COMMIT): II. Changes in adult cigarette smoking prevalence. Am. J. Public Health 85: 193-200.

Cook, D.J., Guyatt, G.H., Ryan, G., et al. (1993). Should unpublished data be included in meta-analyses? Current convictions and controversies. JAMA 269: 2749-2753.

Cook, D.J., Sackett, D.L., and Spitzer, W.O. (1995). Methodologic guidelines for systematic reviews of randomized control trials in health care from the Pottsdam Consultation on Meta-Analysis. J. Clin. Epidemiol. 48: 167-171.

Cooper, J.E. (1991). Balancing the scales of public interest: Medical research and privacy. Med. J. Austr. 155: 556-560.

Cornfield, J. (1966a). Sequential trials, sequential analysis, and the likelihood principle. Am. Statistician. 20: 18-23.

Cornfield, J. (1966b). A Bayesian test of some classical hypotheses with applications to sequential clinical trials. J. Am. Stat. Assoc. 61: 577-594.

Cornfield, J. (1969). The Bayesian outlook and its application. Biometrics 25: 617-657.

Cornfield, J. (1978). Randomization by group: A formal analysis. Am J Epidem. 108: 100-102.

Coronary Drug Project Research Group (1980). Influence of adherence to treatment and response of cholesterol on mortality in the Coronary Drug Project. New Engl. J. Med. 303: 1038-1041.

Coughlin, S.S. (Ed.) (1995). Ethics in Epidemiology and Clinical Research. Newton, MA: Epidemiology Resources.

Council for International Organizations of Medical Sciences (CIOMS) (1993). International Ethical Guidelines for Biomedical Research Involving Human Subjects. Geneva.

Cournand, A. (1977). The code of the scientist and its relationship to ethics. Science 198: 699-705.

Cowley, A.J., McEntegart, D.J., Hampton, J.R., et al. (1994). Long-term evaluation of treatment for chronic heart failure: A 1 year comparative trial of flosequinan and captopril. Cardiovascular Drugs & Therapy 8(6): 829-836.

Cox, D.R. (1972). Regression models and life-tables (with discussion). J. Roy. Statist. Soc. (B) 34: 187-220.

Cox, D.R. and Hinkley, D.V. (1974). Theoretical Statistics. London: Chapman and Hall.

Cox, D.R. (1953). Some simple tests for Poisson variates. Biometrika 40: 354-360.

Cox, D.R. (1992). Planning of Experiments. New York: John Wiley & Sons.

Cox, D.R. and Oakes, D. (1984). Analysis of Survival Data. London: Chapman and Hall.

Culliton, B.J. (1983). Coping with fraud: The Darsee case. Science 220: 31-35.

Cureton, E.E. (1968). Unbiased estimation of the standard deviation. Am. Statistician. 22: 22.

Curran, W.J., Jr., Scott, C.B., Horton, J., Nelson, J.S., Weinstein, A.S., Fischbach, A.J., Chang, C.H., Rotman, M., Asbell, S.O., Krisch, R.E., et al. (1993). Recursive partitioning analysis of prognostic factors in three Radiation Therapy Oncology Group malignant glioma trials. J. Nat. Cancer Instit. 85: 704-710.

Cuschieri, A., Fayers, P., Fielding, J. et al. (1996). Postoperative morbidity and mortality after D_1 and D_2 resections for gastric cancer: Preliminary results of the MRC randomised controlled surgical trial. Lancet 347: 995-999.

Cytel Software Corporation (1992). EaSt. A Software Package for the Design and Interim Monitoring of Group Sequential Clinical Trials. Cambridge, MA: Cytel Software.

Dalal, S.R., Fowlkes, E.B., and Hoadley, B. (1989). Risk analysis of the space shuttle: Pre-Challenger prediction of failure. J. Am. Statist. Assoc. 84: 945-957.

Danforth, W.H. and Schoenhoff, D.M. (1992). Fostering integrity in scientific research. Academic Medicine 67: 351-356.

Darsee, J.R. and Heymsfield, S.B. (1981). Decreased myocardial taurine levels and hypertaurinuria in a kindred with mitral valve-valve prolapse and congestive cardiomyopathy. New Engl. J. Med. 304: 129-135.

Davis, S., Wright, P.W., Schulman, S.F. et al. (1985). Participants in prospective, randomized clinical trials for resected non-small cell lung cancer have improved survival compared with nonparticipants in such trials. Cancer 56: 1710-1718.

Day, N.E. and Walter, S.D. (1984). Simplified models of screening for chronic disease: Estimation procedures from mass screening programmes. Biometrics 40: 1-14.

Dear, K.B.G. and Begg, C.B. (1992). An approach for assessing publication bias prior to performing a meta-analysis. Stat. Sci. 7: 237-245.

DeMets, D.L. (1990). Data monitoring and sequential monitoring – An academic perspective. Journal of Acquired Immune Deficiency Syndrome 3(suppl. 2): S124-S133.

DeMets, D.L. and Lan, K.K.G. (1994). Interim analysis: The alpha spending function approach. Statistics in Med. 13: 1341-1352.

Deming, W.E. (1986). Principles of professional statistical practice. In S. Kotz, N.L. Johnson, and C.B. Read (Eds.), Encyclopedia of Statistical Sciences. New York: John Wiley & Sons.

Denham, S.A. (1993). Stemming the tide of disreputable science: Implications for nursing. Nursing Forum 28: 11-18.

Denzin, N. and Lincoln, Y. (1994). Handbook of Qualitative Research. Newbury Park, CA: Sage Publications.

Department of Health and Human Services (1993). NIH Guideline for the Study and Evaluation of Gender Differences in the Clinical Evaluation of Drugs; Notice. Federal Register: 58: 39406-39416.

Department of Health and Human Services (1994). NIH Guidelines on the Inclusion of Women and Minorities as Subjects in Clinical Research. Federal Register: 59: 14508-14513.

Department of Health and Human Services (DHHS) (1993). Findings of scientific misconduct: Roger Poisson, M.D., St. Luc Hospital, Montreal, Canada. Fed. Regist. 58(117): 33831.

Department of Health and Human Services (DHHS) (1989). Responsibilities of PHS awardee and applicant institutions for dealing with and reporting possible misconduct in science: Final rule. Federal Register 54 (August 8): 32446-32451.

Department of Health, Education, and Welfare (1973). Final Report of the Tuskegee Syphilis Study Ad Hoc Advisory Panel. Washington, DC: Government Printing Office.

DerSimonian, R. Charette, L.J., McPeek, B., and Mosteller, F. (1982). Reporting on methods in clinical trials. New Engl. J. Med. 306: 1332-1337.

Detsky, A.S. and Sackett, D.L. (1985). When was a "negative" clinical trial big enough? Arch. Int. Med. 145: 709-712.

DeVita, V.T. (1991). Is a mechanism such as the NCI's clinical alert ever an appropriate alternative to journal peer review? Important Advances in Oncology : 241-246.

Dickersin, K. and Berlin, J.A. (1992). Meta-analysis: State-of-the-science. Epidemiologic Reviews 14: 154-176.

Diem, K. and Lentner, C. (Eds.) (1970). Scientific Tables, 7th Edition. Basel: CIBA-Geigy.

Diggle, P.J., Liang, K.Y., and Zeger, S.L. (1994). Analysis of Longitudinal Data. Oxford: Oxford University Press.

Dixon, W.J. and Mood, A.M. (1948). A method for obtaining and analyzing sensitivity data. J. Am. Statist. Assoc. 43: 109-126.

Dobson, A.J. (1983). An Introduction to Statistical Modelling. London: Chapman and Hall.

Dodge, Y. and Afsarinejad, K. (1985). Minimal 2 connected factorial experiments. Comput Stat and Data Analysis 3: 187-200.

Doll, R. (1994). The use of meta-analysis in epidemiology: Diet and cancers of the breast and colon. Nutr. Rev. 52: 233-237.

Donner, A. (1984). Approaches to sample size estimation in the design of clinical trials – A review. Statistics in Med. 3: 199- 214.

Donner, A. and Klar, N. (1994). Methods for comparing event rates in intervention studies when the unit of allocation is a cluster. Am. J. Epidemiol. 140: 279-289.

Dorland's Medical Dictionary, 28th Edition (1994). Philadelphia: W. B. Saunders.

Draper, N.R. and Smith, H. (1981). Applied Regression Analysis, Second Edition. New York: John Wiley & Sons.

Duan-Zheng, X. (1990). Computer Analysis of Sequential Medical Trials. New York: Ellis Horwood.

Dupont, W.D. (1985). Randomized vs. historical clinical trials: Are the benefits worth the cost? Am. J. Epid. 122: 940-946.

Durrleman, S. and Simon, R. (1991). When to randomize? J. Clin. Oncol. 9: 116-122.

Dyson, F.J. (1993). Science in trouble. American Scholar 62: 513-525.

Early Breast Cancer Trialists' Collaborative Group (1990). Treatment of Early Breast Cancer, Vol. 1: Worldwide Evidence 1985-1990. Oxford: Oxford University Press.

Edwards, A.W.F. (1972). Likelihood. Cambridge: Cambridge University Press.

Efron, B. (1971). Forcing a sequential experiment to be balanced. Biometrika 58: 403-417.

Efron, B. and Feldman, D. (1991). Compliance as an explanatory variable in clinical trials. J. Am. Stat. Assoc. 86: 9-17.

Eisenberg, D.M., Kessler, R.C., Foster, C., Norlock, F.E., Calkins, D.R., and Delbanco, T.L. (1993). Unconventional medicine in the United States: Prevalence, costs, and patterns of use. New Engl. J. Med. 328(4): 246-252.

Eisenberg, L. (1977). The social imperatives of medical research. Science 198: 1105-1110.

Eisenhut, L.P. (1990). Universität prüft Anschuldigungen gegen Professorin. Kolner Stadtanzeiger (October 24).

Elashoff, J.D. (1995). nQuery Advisor User's Manual. Los Angeles: Dixon Associates.

Elks, M.L. (1993). The right to participate in research studies. J. Lab. Clin. Med. 122: 130-136.

Ellenberg, S.S. and Hamilton, J.M. (1989). Surrogate endpoints in clinical trials: Cancer. Statistics in Med. 8: 405-413.

Ellison, N.M., Byar, D.P., and Newell, G.R. (1978). Special report on Laetrile: The NCI Laetrile review. New Engl. J. Med. 229: 549-552.

Elting, L.S. and Bodey, G.P. (1991). Is a picture worth a thousand medical words? A randomized trial of reporting formats for medical research data. Methods Inf. Med. 30: 145-150.

Emerson, S.S. and Banks, P.L.C. (1994). Interpretation of a Leukemia Trial Stopped Early, Chapter 14 in Nicholas Lange et al. (Eds.), Case Studies in Biometry, New York: John Wiley & Sons.

Endophthalmitis Vitrectomy Study Group (1995). Results of the Endophthalmitis Vitrectomy Study. A randomized trial of immediate vitrectomy and of intravenous antibiotics for the treatment of postoperative bacterial endophthalmitis. Archives Ophthalmol. 113: 1479-1496.

Engler, R.L., Covell, J.W., Friedman, P.J., Kitcher, P.S., and Peters, R.M. (1987). Misrepresentation and responsibility in medical research. New Engl. J. Med. 317: 1383-1389.

Ensign, L.G., Gehan, E.A., Kamen, D.S., and Thall, P.F. (1994). An optimal three-stage design for phase II clinical trials. Statistics in Med. 13: 1727-1736.

Epstein, B. and Sobel, M. (1953). Life testing. J. Am. Statist. Assoc. 48: 486-502.

Everitt, B.S. (1989). Statistical Methods for Medical Investigations. New York: Oxford University Press.

Everitt, B.S. (1995). The Cambridge Dictionary of Statistics in the Medical Sciences. Cambridge: Cambridge University Press.

Faden, R.R. and Beauchamp, T.L. (1986). A History and Theory of Informed Consent. New York: Oxford University Press.

Fang, J. (1972). Mathematicians from Antiquity to Today. Hauppage, NY: Paideia Press.

Faraggi, D. and Simon, R. (1995). A neural network model for survival data. Statistics in Med. 14: 73-82.

Faries, D. (1994). Practical modifications of the continual reassessment method for phase I cancer clinical trials. J. Biopharmaceutical Statistics 4: 147-164.

Farrington, C.P. and Manning, G. (1990). Test statistics and sample size formulae for comparative binomial trials with null hypothesis of non-zero risk difference or non-unity relative risk. Statistics in Med. 9: 1447-1454.

Fayerweather, W.E., Higginson, J., and Beauchamp, T.L. (Eds.) (1991). Ethics in Epidemiology. Journal of Clinical Epidemiology (suppl.) 44: 1S-151S.

Feingold, M. and Gillespie, B.W. (1996). Cross-over trials with censored data. Statistics in Med. 15: 953-967.

Feinstein, A.R. (1991). Intention-to-treat policy for analyzing randomized trials: Statistical distortions and neglected clinical challenges. Chapter 28 in Patient Compliance in Medical Practice and Clinical Trials, edited by J.A. Cramer and B. Spilker. New York: Raven Press, Ltd.

Feinstein, A.R. (1995). Meta-analysis: Statistical alchemy for the 21st century. J. Clin. Epidemiol. 48: 71-79.

Feurer, I.D., Becker, G.J., Picus, D., Ramirez, E., Darcy, M.D., and Hicks, M.E. (1994). Evaluating peer reviews: Pilot testing of a grading instrument. JAMA 272: 98-100.

Finkelstein, D.M. and Schoenfeld, D.A. (Eds.) (1995). AIDS Clinical Trials. New York: Wiley-Liss.

Finney, D.J. (1995). A statistician looks at met-analysis. J. Clin. Epidemiol. 48: 87-103.

Fisher, B., Costantino, J., Redmond, C., et al. (1989). A randomized clinical trial evaluating tamoxifen in the treatment of patients with node-negative breast cancer who have estrogen-receptor-positive tumors. New Engl. J. Med. 320: 479-484.

Fisher, C.J., Agosti, J.M., Opal, S.M., et al., (1996). Treatment of septic shock with the tumor necrosis factor receptor: Fc fusion protein. New Engl. J. Med. 334: 1697-1702.

Fisher, L.D., Dixon, D.O., Herson, J., Frankowski, R.K., Hearron, M.S., and Peace, K.E. (1990). Intention-to-treat in clinical trials, in K.E. Peace (Ed.), Statistical Issues in Drug Research and Development. New York: Marcel Dekker.

Fisher, R.A. (1935). The Design of Experiments. Edinburgh: Oliver and Boyd.

Fisher, R.A. (1936). Has Mendel's work been rediscovered? Annals of Science 1: 115-137.

Fisher, R.A. (1935). The Design of Experiments. London: Collier Macmillan.

Fisher, R.A. (1960). The Design of Experiments, 8th Edition. New York: Hafner.

Flather, M., Pipilis, A., Collins, R. et al. (1994). Randomized controlled trial of oral captopril, of oral isosorbide mononitrate and of intravenous magnesium sulphate started early in acute myocardial infarction: Safety and haemodynamic effects. Eur. Heart J. 15: 608-619.

Fleiss, J.L. (1986). The Design and Analysis of Clinical Experiments. New York: John Wiley & Sons.

Fleiss, J.L. (1989). A critique of recent research on the two-treatment cross-over design. Controlled Clin. Trials 10: 237-243.

Fleming T.R., Green S.J., and Harrington D.P. (1984). Considerations for monitoring and evaluating treatment effects in clinical trials. Controlled Clin. Trials 5: 55-66.

Fleming, T.R. and DeMets, D.L. (1993). Monitoring of clinical trials: Issues and recommendations. Conrolled Clin. Trials 14: 183-197.

Fleming, T.R. (1994). Surrogate markers in AIDS and cancer trials. Statistics in Med. 13: 1423-1435.

Fleming, T.R., Prentice, R.L., Pepe, M.S., and Glidden, D. (1994). Surrogate and auxiliary endpoints in clinical trials with potential applications in cancer and AIDS research. Statistics in Med. 13: 955-968.

Fleming, T.R. and DeMets, D.L. (1996). Surrogate end points in clinical trials: Are we being misled? Ann. Intern. Med. 125: 605-613.

Foesling, A. (1984). Der Mogelfaktor. Hamburg, 20-21.

Food and Drug Administration (1977). A report on the two-period crossover design and its applicability in trials of clinical effectiveness. Minutes of the Biometric and Epidemiology Methodology Advisory Committee (BEMAC) meeting.

Forrow, L., Taylor, W.C., and Arnold, R.M. (1992). Absolutely relative: How research results are summarized can affect treatment decisions. Am. J. Med. 92: 121-124.

Fox, R.C. and Swazey, J.P. (1992). Spare Parts: Organ Replacement in American Society. New York: Oxford University Press.

Freedman, B. (1987). Equipoise and the ethics of clinical research. N. Engl. J. Med. 317: 141-145.

Freedman, B. (1992). A response to a purported ethical difficulty with randomized clinical trials involving cancer patients. J. Clinical Ethics 3(3): 231-234.

Freedman, L.S. (1982). Tables of the number of patients required in clinical trials using the logrank test. Statistics in Med. 1: 121-129.

Freedman, L.S., Spiegelhalter, D.J., and Parmar, M.K.B. (1989). Comparison of Bayesian with group sequential methods for monitoring clinical trials. Controlled Clinical Trials 10: 357-367.

Freedman, L., Sylvester, R., and Byar, D.P. (1989). Using permutation tests and bootstrap confidence limits to analyze repeated events data from clinical trials. Controlled Clinical Trials 10: 129-141.

Freedman, L.S and Green, S.B. (1990). Statistical designs for investigating several interventions in the same study: Methods for cancer prevention trials. JNCI 82(11): 910-914.

Freedman, L.S. (1989). The size of clinical trials in cancer research: What are the current needs? Br. J. Cancer 59: 396-400.

Freedman, L.S. and Schatzkin, A. (1992). Sample size for studying intermediate endpoints within intervention trials or observational studies. Am. J. Pub. Health 136: 1148-1159.

Freeman, P.R. (1989). The performance of the two-stage analysis of two-treatment, two-period crossover trials. Statistics in Medicine 8: 1421-1432.

Frei, E. III (1982). Clinical cancer research: An embattled species. Cancer 50: 1979-1992.

Frei, E. III and Freireich, E. (1993). The clinical cancer researcher – still an embattled species. J. Clin. Oncol. 11: 1639-1651.

Freidman, L.M., Furberg, C.D., and DeMets, D.L. (1985). Fundamentals of Clinical Trials, Second Edition. Littleton, MA: PSG Publishing.

Freiman, J.A., Chalmers, T.C., Smith, H., and Kuebler, R.R. (1978). The importance of beta, the type II error, and sample size in the design and interpretation of the randomized controlled trial: Survey of 71 "negative" trials. New Engl. J. Med. 299: 690-694.

Freund, P.A. (1972). Experimentation with Human Subjects. Great Britain: Clarke Doble and Brendon Ltd.

Fried, C. (1974). Medical experimentation: Personal integrity and social policy. Vol. 5 [A.G. Bearn, D.A.K. Black, and H.H. Hiatt (Eds.)], Amsterdam: North-Holland.

Friedlander, M.W. (1995). At the Fringes of Science. Boulder, CO: Westview Press.

Friedman, M.A. (1990). If not now, when? JNCI 82: 106-108.

Fuchs, S. and Westervelt, S.D. (1995). Fraud and trust in science. Perspectives in Biology and Medicine 39: 248-269.

Furberg, C.D., Psaty, B.M., and Meyer, J.V. (1995). Nifedipine: Dose-related increase in mortality in patients with coronary heart disease. Circulation 92: 1326-1331.

GAO (1995). Cancer Drug Research: Contrary to Allegation, NIH Hydrazine Sulfate Studies Were Not Flawed. Washington, DC: General Accounting Office. Publication GAO/HEHS-95-141.

Gail, M.H. (1974). Power computations for designing comparative Poisson trials. Biometrics 30: 231-237.

Gail, M.H. (1984). Nonparametric frequentist proposals for monitoring comparative survival studies. Handbook of Statistics 4: 791-811.

Gail, M.H. (1982). Monitoring and Stopping Clinical Trials. Chapter 15 in Valerie Miké and Kenneth Stanley (Eds.), Statistics in Medical Research. New York: John Wiley & Sons.

Gail, M.H. (1985). Eligibility exclusions, losses to follow-up, removal of randomized patients, and uncounted events in cancer clinical trials. Cancer Treat. Rep. 69(10): 1107-1112.

Gail, M.H. (1996). Use of observational data, including surveillance studies, for evaluating AIDS therapies. Statistics in Medicine 15: 2273-2288.

Gail, M.H., Tan, W.-Y., and Piantadosi, S. (1988). The size and power of tests for no treatment effect in randomized clinical trials when needed covariates are omitted. Biometrika 75: 57-64.

Gail, M.H., Wieand, H.S., and Piantadosi, S. (1984). Biased estimates of treatment effect in randomized experiments with non-linear regressions and omitted covariates. Biometrika 71(3): 431-444.

Gail, M.H., Mark, S.D., Carroll, R.J., Green, S.B., and Pee, D. (1996). On design considerations and randomization-based inference for community intervention trials. Statistics in Med. 15: 1069-1092.

Garceau, A.J., Donaldson, R.M., O'Hara, E.T., Callow, A.D., Muench, H., Chalmers, T.C., and the Boston Inter-Hospital Liver Group. (1964). A controlled trial of prophylactic porta-caval shunt surgery. N. Engl. J. Med. 270: 496-500.

Gardiner, B. and Currant, A. (1996).

Gardner, M.J., Machin, D., and Campbell, M.J. (1986). Use of checklists in assessing the statistical content of medical studies. BMJ 292: 810-812.

Gatsonis, C. and Greenhouse, J.B. (1992). Bayesian methods for phase I clinical trials. Statistics in Med. 11: 1377-1389.

Gavarret, J. (1840). Principes Généraux de Statistique Médicale, ou, Dévelopement des Règles Qui Doivent Présider à Son Emploi. Bechet jeune et Labé, Paris.

Gehan, E.A. (1961). The determination of the number of patients required in a preliminary and follow-up trial of a new chemotherapeutic agent. J. Chron. Dis. 13: 346-353.

Gehan, E.A. and Lemak, N.A. (1994). Statistics in Medical Research: Developments in Clinical Trials. New York: Plenum.

Gehan, E.A. and Schneiderman, M.A. (1990). Historical and methodological developments in clinical trials at the National Cancer Institute. Statistics in Med. 9: 871-880.

Gehlbach, S.H. (1988). Interpreting the Medical Literature: Practial Epidemiology for Clinicians (Second Edition). New York: Macmillan.

Gelber, R.D. (1996). Gemcitabine for pancreatic cancer: How hard to look for clinical benefit? An American perspective. Annals of Oncology 7: 335-337.

Geller, N.L. (1987). Planned interim analysis and its role in cancer clinical trials. J. Clinical Onc. 5: 1485-1490.

George, S.L. and Desu, M.M. (1974). Planning the size and duration of a clinical trial studying the time to some critical event. J. Chron. Dis. 27: 15-24.

George, S.L. (1988). Identification and assessment of prognostic factors. Sem. Onc. 15: 462-471.

Giardiello, F.M., Hamilton, S.R., Krush, A.J., Piantadosi, S., Hylind, L.M., Celano, P., Booker, S.V., Robinson, C.R., and Offerhaus, G.J.A. (1993). Treatment of Colonic and Rectal Adenomas with Sulindac in Familial Adenomatous Polyposis. N. Engl. J. Med. 328: 1313-1316.

Gilbert, J.P., McPeek, B., and Mosteller, F. (1977). Statistics and ethics in surgery and anesthesia. Science 198: 684-689.

Gillings, D. and Koch, G. (1991). The application of the principle of intention-to-treat in the analysis of clinical trials. Drug Inf. J. 25: 411-424.

Gilpin, A.K. and Meinert, C.L. (1994). Gender bias in clinical trials? Proceedings of the Society for Clinical Trials, Houston, Texas.

Glass, G.V. (1976). Primary, secondary, and meta-analysis of research. Educ. Research 5: 3-8.

Gold, J. (1975). Use of hydrazine sulfate in terminal and preterminal cancer patients: Results of investigational new drug (IND) study in 84 evaluable patients. Oncology 32: 1-10.

Goldberg, K.B. and Goldberg, P. (Eds.) (1994). NCI apologizes for mismanagement of NSABP, says Fisher resisted criticism. Cancer Letter 20 (16): April 22.

Goldstein, R. (1989). Power and sample size via MS/PC-DOS computers. Am. Statistician 43: 253-260.

Good, P. (1994). Permutation Tests. New York: Springer Verlag.

Goodman, S.N., Zahurak, M.L., and Piantadosi, S. (1995). Some practical improvements in the continual reassessment method for phase I studies. Statistics in Med. 14: 1149-1161.

Gordon, N.H. and Wilson, J.K. (1992). Using toxicity grades in the design and analysis of cancer phase I clinical trials. Statistics in Med. 11: 2063-2075.

Gore, S.M., Jones, G., and Thompson, S.G. (1992). The Lancet's statistical review process: Areas for improvement by authors. Lancet 340: 100-102.

Gotay, C.C. (1991). Accrual to cancer clinical trials: directions from the research literature. Soc. Sci. Med. 33: 569-577.

Gøtzsche, P.C. (1989). Methodology and overt and hidden bias in reports of 196 double-blind trials of nonsteroidal anti-inflammatory drugs in rheumatoid arthritis. Controlled Clinical Trials 10: 31-56. Correction (1989) 10: 356.

Govindarajulu, Z. (1988). Statistical Techniques in Bioassay. Basel: Karger.

Graham, N.M.H., Park, L.P., Piantadosi, S., Phair, J.P., Mellors, J., Fahey, J.L., and Saah, A.J. (1994). Prognostic value of combined response markers among human immunodeficiency virus infected persons: Possible aid in the decision to change zidovudine monotherapy. Clinical Infect. Dis. 20: 352-362.

Grant, A. (1989). Reporting controlled trials. Br. J. Obstet. Gynaecol. 96: 397-400.

Gray, J.N., Lyons, P.M., Jr., and Melton, G.B. (1995). Ethical and Legal Issues in AIDS Research. Baltimore: Johns Hopkins University Press.

Greco, D., Salmaso, S., and Mastrantonio, P. (1994). The Italian pertussis vaccine trial: Ethical issues (letter). JAMA 272: 1898-1899.

Green, A., Battistitta, D., Hart, V., et al. (1994). The Nambour skin cancer and actinic eye disease prevention trial: Design and baseline characteristics of participants. Controlled Clinical Trials 15: 512-522.

Green, S.B., and Byar, D.P. (1984). Using observational data from registries to compare treatments: The fallacy of omnimetrics. Statistics in Med. 3: 361-370.

Green, S.J., Fleming, T.R., and O'Fallon, J.R. (1987). Policies for study monitoring and interim reporting of results. J. Clinical Onc. 5: 1477-1484.

Greenberg, E.R., Baron, J.A., Tosteson, T.D., et al. (1994). A clinical trial of antioxidant vitamins to prevent colorectal adenoma. New Engl. J. Med. 331: 142-147.

Greenberg, E.R., Baron, J.A., Tosteson, T.D., et al. (1994). A clinical trial of antioxidant vitamins to prevent colorectal adenoma. New Engl. J. Med. 331: 141-147.

Greenhouse, S.W. (1990). Some historical and methodological developments in early clinical trials at the National Institutes of Health. Statistics in Med. 9: 893-901.

Greenland, S. (1987). Quantitative methods in the review of the epidemiologic literature. Epidem. Reviews 9: 1-30.

Greenland, S. (1994). A critical look at some popular meta-analytic methods (with discussion). Am. J. Epidemiol. 140: 290-296.

Greenland, S., and Salvan, A. (1990). Bias in the one-step method for pooling study results. Statist. in Med. 9: 247-252.

Greenwald, P. (1985). Prevention of Cancer. Chapter 10 in DeVita, V.T., Hellman, S., and Rosenberg, S.A. (Eds.) Cancer: Principles and Practice of Oncology. 2nd Edition. Philadelphia: JB Lippincott.

Greenwald, P. and Cullen, J.W. (1985). The new emphasis in cancer control. J. Nat. Cancer Inst. 74: 543-551.

Greenwood, M. (1926). The errors of sampling of the survivorship tables, in Reports on Public Health and Statistical Subjects, no. 33. London: HMSO, Appendix 1.

Grender, J.M. and Johnson, W.D. (1993). Analysis of crossover designs with multivariate response. Statistics in Med. 12: 69-89.

Grieve, A.P. (1985). A Bayesian analysis of the two period cross-over design for clinical trials. Biometrics 42: 979-990. Corrigenda 42: 459 (1986).

Grizzle, J.E. (1965). The two-period change-over design and its use in clinical trials. Biometrics 21: 467-480. Corrigenda 30: 727, (1965).

Gross, A.J. and Clark, V.A. (1975). Survival Distributions: Reliability Applications in the Biomedical Sciences. New York: John Wiley & Sons.

Grossman, S.A., Sheidler, V.A., Swedeen, K., Mucenski, J., and Piantadosi, S. (1991). Correlation of patient and caregiver ratings of cancer pain. J. Pain Symptom Manage. 6(2): 53-7.

Guttentag, O.E. (1953). The problem of experimentation on human beings: II The physician's point of view. Science 117: 207-210.

Haaland, P.D. (1989). Experimental Design in Biotechnology. New York: Marcel Dekker.

Hadorn, D.C., Draper, D., Rogers, W.H., Keeler, E.B., and Brook, R.H. (1992). Cross-validation performance of mortality prediction models. Statistics in Med. 11: 475-489.

Halpern, D.F. and Coren, S. (1991). Handedness and life span (letter). New Engl. J. Med. 324: 998. See also letters in 325: 1041-1043.

Halperin, M. (1952). Maximum likelihood estimation in truncated samples. Ann. Math. Stat 23: 226-238.

Halperin, M., DeMets, D.L., and Ware, J.H. (1990). Early methodological developments for clinical trials at the National Heart, Lung, and Blood Institute. Statistics in Med. 9: 881-892.

Hand, D.J. (1992). Statistical methods in diagnosis. Stat. Methods in Med. Research 1: 49-67.

Hand, D.J., Daly, F., Lunn, A.D., McConway, K.J., and Ostrowski, E. (Eds.) (1994). A Handbook of Small Data Sets. London: Chapman & Hall.

Hankins, F.H. (1930). Gottfried Achenwall. In E.R.A. Seligman and A. Johnson (Eds.), Encyclopaedia of the Social Science, New York: Macmillan.

Hansen, B.C. and Hansen, K.D. (1995). Academic and scientific misconduct: Issues for nursing educators. J. Prof. Nursing 11: 31-39.

Hansen, K.D. and Hansen, B.C. (1991). Scientific fraud and the Public Health Service Act: A critical analysis. News 5: 2512-2515.

Harrell, F.E., Jr., Lee, K.L., and Mark, D.B. (1996). Multivariable prognostic models: Issues in developing models, evaluating assumptions and adequacy, and measuring and reducing errors. Statistics in Medicine 15: 361-387.

Harris, E.K. and Albert, A. (1991). Survivorship Analysis for Clinical Studies. New York: Marcel Dekker.

Harris, N., Gang, D.L., Quay, S.C., Poppmea, S., Zamecnik, P.C., Nelson-Rees, W.A., and O'Brien, S.J. (1981). Contamination of Hogdkin's disease cell cultures. Nature 289: 228-230.

Hawkins, B.S. (1991). Controlled clinical trials in the 1980s: A bibliography. Controlled Clin. Trials 12: 5-272.

Haynes, R.B., Mulrow, C.D., Huth, E.J., Altman, D.G., and Gardner, M.J. (1990). More informative abstracts revisited. Ann. Intern. Med. 113: 69-76.

Healy, B. (1996). The dangers of trial by Dingell. New York Times, July 3.

Hedges, L.V. (1992). Modeling publication selection effects in meta-analysis. Stat. Sci. 7: 246-255.

Hedges, L.V. and Olkin, I. (1985). Statistical Methods for Meta-Analysis. Orlando, FL: Academic Press.

Heiberger, R.M. (1989). Computation for the Analysis of Designed Experiments. New York: John Wiley & Sons.

Heinonen, O.P., Virtamo, J., Albanes, D. et al. (1987). Beta carotene, alpha-tocopherol lung cancer intervention trial in Finland. In Proceedings of the XI Scientific Meeting of the International Epidemiologic Association, Helsinki, August, 1987. Helsinki: Pharmy.

Heiss, M.M., Mempel, W., Delanoff, C. et al. (1994). Blood transfusion-modulated tumor recurrence: First results of a randomized study of autologous versus allogeneic blood transfusion in colorectal cancer surgery. J. Clin. Oncol. 12: 1859-1867.

Heitjan, D.F., Houts, P.S., and Harvey, H.A. (1992). A decision-theoretic evaluation of early stopping rules. Statistics in Medicine 11: 673-683.

Hellman, S. (1991). Clinical alert: A poor idea prematurely used. Important Advances in Oncology : 255-257.

Hellman, S. and Hellman, D.S. (1991). Of mice but not men: problems of the randomized clinical trial. New Engl. J. Med. 324: 1585-1589.

Henderson, I.C. (1995). Using clinical trial information in the practice of medicine. Cancer Journal 1: 101-103.

Henderson, I.C. (1990). Shouldn't we see the white flag before we cry victory? JNCI 82: 103-109.

Hennekens, C.H. and Eberlein, K. (1985). A randomized trial of aspirin and beta-carotene among U.S. physicians. Prev. Med. 14: 165-168.

Herbert, V. (1977). Acquiring new information while retaining old ethics. Science 198: 690-693.

Herbert, V. (1994). Three stakes in hydrazine sulfate's heart, but questionable cancer remedies, like vampires, always rise again (editorial). J. Clin. Oncol. 12: 1107-1108.

Herdan, G. (1955). Statistics of Therapeutic Trials. Amsterdam: Elsevier.

Herson, J. (1984). Statistical Aspects in the Design and Analysis of Phase II Clinical Trials, Chapter 15 in M.J. Buyse, M.J. Staquet, and R.J. Sylvester (Eds.), Cancer Clinical Trials. Oxford: Oxford University Press.

Herson, J. (1989). The use of surrogate endpoints in clinical trials (an introduction to a series of four papers). Statistics in Medicine 8: 403-404.

Herson, J., and Wittes, J. (1993). The use of interim analysis for sample size adjustment. Drug Info. J. 27: 753-760.

Herxheimer, A. (1993). Clinical trials: Two neglected ethical issues. J. Med. Ethics 19: 211 and 218.

Hill, A.B. (1961). Principles of Medical Statistics, Seventh Edition. London: The Lancet.

Hill, A.B. (1963). Medical ethics and controlled trials. British Med. J. April 20: 1043-1049.

Hill, T.P. (1995). The significant-digit phenomenon. Am. Math. Monthly 102: 322-327.

Hillis, A. and Seigel, D. (1989). Surrogate endpoints in clinical trials: Ophthalmologic disorders. Statistics in Med. 8: 427-430.

Hills, M. and Armitage, P. (1979). The two-period cross-over clinical trial. British J. Clin. Pharmacol. 8: 7-20.

Hinkelmann, K., and Kempthorne, O. (1994). Design and Analysis of Experiments: Vol. I: Introduction to Experimental Design. New York: Johns Wiley & Sons.

Hintze, J.L. (1996). PASS User's Guide: Power Analysis and Sample Size for Windows. Kaysville, UT: NCSS.

Hoel, D.G., Sobel, M., and Weiss, G.H. (1975). A Survey of Adaptive Sampling for Clinical Trials. In: Elashoff, R.M. (Ed.), Perspectives in Biometrics. New York: Academic Press.

Holtzman, W.H. (1950). The unbiased estimate of the population variance and standard deviation. Am. J. Psychology 63: 615-617.

Homans, G. (1965). Group factors in worker productivity. In H. Proshansky and B. Seidenberg (Eds.). Basic Studies in Social Psychology (pp. 592-604). New York: Holt, Rinehart, and Winston.

Horton, R. (1996). Surgical research or comic opera: Questions, but few answers. Lancet 347: 984.

Hubard, S.M., Martin, N.B., and Thurn, A.L. (1995). NCI's cancer information systems – bringing medical knowledge to clinicians. Oncology 9: 302-314.

Hughes, M.D. (1993). Stopping guidelines for clinical trials with multiple treatments. Statistics in Med. 12: 901-915.

Hulstaert, F., Van Belle, S., Bleiberg, H., et al. (1994). Optimal combination therapy with tropisetron in 445 patients with incomplete control of chemotherapy-induced nausea and vomiting. J. Clin. Oncol. 12: 2439-2446.

Humphrey, G.F. (1992). Scientific fraud: The McBride case. Med. Sci. Law 32: 199-203.

Hurley, F.L. (1991). Statistical approach to subgroup analyses: Patient compliance data and clinical outcomes, in J.A. Cramer and B. Spilker (Eds.), Patient Compliance in Medical Practice and Clinical Trials. New York: Raven Press.

Hwang, I.K. and Shih, W.J. (1990). Group sequential designs using a family of type I error probability spending functions. Statistics in Med. 9: 1439-1445.

Hyman, N.H., Foster, R.S., DeMeules, J.E., Costanza, M.C. (1985). Blood transfusions and survival after lung cancer resection. Am. J. Surg. 149: 502-507.

ISIS-2 Collaborative Group (1988). Randomized trial of intravenous streptokinase, oral aspirin, both, or neither among 17,187 cases of suspected acute myocardial infarction. Lancet, ii, 349-360.

ISIS-4 Collaborative Group (1995). ISIS-4: A randomized factorial trial assessing early captopril, oral mononitrate, and intravenous magnesium sulphate in 58,050 patients with suspected acute myocardial infarction. Lancet 345: 669-685.

Inspector General Act Amendments (1988). Public Law 100-504 (102 Stat. 2515).

Institute of Medicine (IOM) (1989). The Responsible Conduct of Research in the Health Sciences. Washington, DC: National Academy Press.

International Agency for Research on Cancer (IARC) (1974). Evaluation of carcinogenic risk of chemicals to man: Some aromatic amines, hydrazine and related substances, N-nitroso compounds and miscellaneous alkylating agents. Vol. 4. Lyon: IARC.

International Chronic Granulomatous Disease Cooperative Study Group (1991). A controlled trial of interferon gamma to prevent infection in chronic granulomatous disease. New Engl. J. Med 324: 509-516.

International Committee of Medical Journal Editors. (1993). Uniform requirements for manuscripts submitted to biomedical journals. JAMA 269: 2282-6.

International Conference on Harmonisation (1994). Good Clinical Practice Guideline for Essential Documents for the Conduct of a Clinical Trial. Geneva: ICH Secretariat (c/o IFPMA).

International Conference on Harmonisation (1995). Structure and Content of Clinical Study Reports. Draft Consensus Guideline. Geneva: ICH Secretariat (c/o IFPMA).

Ivy, A.C. (1948). The history and ethics of the use of human subjects in medical experiments. Science 108: 1-5.

Iyengar, S. and Greenhouse, J.B. (1988). Selection models and the file drawer problem (with discussion). Stat. Sci. 3: 109-135.

Jabs, D., Enger, C., and Bartlett, J.G. (1989). Cytomegalovirus retinitis and acquired immunodeficiency syndrome. Arch. Ophthal. 107: 75-80.

Jayaraman, K.S. (1991). Gupta faces suspension. Nature 349: 645.

Jenks, S. and Volkers, N. (1992). Razors and refrigerators and reindeer – oh my! J. National Cancer Institute 84: 1863.

Johns Hopkins University School of Medicine (1995). Procedures for Dealing With Issues of Professional Misconduct, in Faculty Policies, p. 15-23. Baltimore: Johns Hopkins University School of Medicine.

Johnson, N.L. and Kotz, S. (1969). Distributions in Statistics, Discrete Distributions. New York: John Wiley & Sons.

Johnson, N.L. and Kotz, S. (1970). Continuous Univariate Distributions. Boston: Houghton Mifflin.

Jones, B. and Donev, A.N. (1996). Modelling and design of cross-over trials. Statistics in Med. 15: 1435-1446.

Jones, B. and Kenward, M.G. (1989). Design and Analysis of Cross-Over Trials. London: Chapman and Hall.

Jones, D.R. (1995). Meta-analysis: Weighing the evidence. Statistics in Med. 14: 137-149.

Jones, J.H. (1981). Bad Blood: The Tuskegee Syphilis Experiment. New York: Free Press.

Judicial Council of the American Medical Association (1946). Supplementary Report. J. Am. Medical Assoc. 132: 1090.

Judson, H.F. (1994). Structural transformation of the sciences and the end of peer review. JAMA 272: 92-94.

Judson, H.F. (1994). Structural transformations of the sciences and the end of peer review. JAMA 272: 92-95.

Kadane, J.B. (Ed.) (1996). Bayesian Methods and Ethics in a Clinical Trial Design. New York: John Wiley & Sons.

Kalbfleisch, J.D. and Prentice, R.L. (1980). The Statistical Analysis of Failure Time Data. New York: John Wiley & Sons.

Kalish, L.A., and Begg, C.B. (1985). Treatment allocation methods in clinical trials: A review. Statistics in Med. 4: 129-144.

Kamen, J. (1993). Medical Genocide, Part 26: Hope, Heartbreak, and Horror. Penthouse, April.

Kamen, J. (1994). Stonewalled in the U.S.A. Penthouse, July.

Kaplan, E.L., and Meier, P. (1958). Nonparametric estimation from incomplete observations. Am. Stat. Assoc. J. 53: 457-480.

Karlstrom, P.O., Bergh, T., and Lundkvist, O. (1993). A prospective randomized trial of artificial insemination versus intercourse in cycles stimulated with human menopausal gonadotropin or clomiphene citrate. Fertil. Steril. 59: 554-559.

Kaslow, R.A., Ostrow, D.G., Detels, R., et al. (1987). The Multicenter AIDS Cohort Study: Rationale, organization, and selected characteristics of the participants. Am. J. Epidemiol. 126: 310-318.

Kassaye, M., Larson, C., and Carlson, D. (1994). A randomized community trial of prepackaged and homemade oral rehydration therapies. Arch. Ped. Adolesc. Med. 148: 1288-1292.

Kassirer, J.P. and Campion, E.W. (1994). Peer review: crude and understudied but indispensable. JAMA 272: 96-97.

Katz, J. (1972). Experimentation with Human Beings. New York: Russell Sage Foundation.

Keller, S.M., Groshen, S., Martini, N., and Kaiser, L.R. (1988). Blood transfusion and lung cancer recurrence. Cancer 62(3): 606-610.

Kelloff, G.J., Boone, C.W., Crowell, J.A., Steele, V.E., Lubet, R., and Doody, L.A. (1994). Surrogate endpoint biomarkers for phase II cancer chemoprevention trials. J. Cellular Biochemistry, Supplement 19: 1-9.

Kelloff, G.J., Johnson, J.R., Crowell, J.A., et al. (1995). Approaches to the development and marketing approval of drugs that prevent cancer. Cancer Epidemiol. Biomarkers & Prevention 4: 1-10.

Kemper, K.J. (1990). Pride and prejudice in peer review. J. Clin. Epidemiol. 44: 343-345.

Kendall, M.G. (1960). Where shall the history of statistics begin? Biometrika 47: 447-449.

Kenward, M.G. and Jones, B. (1987). A log linear model for binary cross-over data. Appl. Statist. 36: 192-204.

Kessler, D.A., Rose, J.L., Temple, R.J., Schapiro, R., and Griffin, J.P. (1994). Therapeutic-class wars – drug promotion in a competitive marketplace. New Engl. J. Med. 331: 1350-1353.

Kevles, D.J. (1996). The assault on David Baltimore. New Yorker, May 27, 1996.

Khan, K.S., Daya, S., and Jadad, A.R. (1996). The importance of quality of primary studies in producing unbiased systematic reviews. Arch. Intern. Med. 156: 661-666.

Klein D.F. (1993). Should the government assure scientific integrity? Academic Med. 68 (Suppl.): S56-S59.

Kleinbaum, D.G. (1996). Survival Analysis: A Self-Learning Text. New York: Springer.

Kloner, R.A. (1995). Nifedipine in ischemic heart disease. Circulation 92: 1074-1078.

Knox, R.A. (1983). Deeper problems for Darsee: Emory probe. JAMA 249: 2867-2874.

Knuth, D. (1981). Seminumerical Algorithms, 2nd Edition, Vol. 2 of The Art of Computer Programming. Reading, MA: Addison-Wesley.

Kohn, A. (1986). False Prophets. Oxford: Basil Blackwell.

Korn, E.L., Midthune, D., Chen, T.T., Rubinstein, L.V., Christian, M.C., and Simon, R.M. (1994). A comparison of two phase I trial designs. Statistics in Med. 13: 1799-1806.

Kosty, M.P., Fleishman, S.B., Herndon II, J.E., et al. (1994). Cisplatin, vinblastine, and hydrazine sulfate in advanced, non-small cell lung cancer: A randomized placebo controlled, double blind phase III study of the Cancer and Leukemia Group B. J. Clin. Oncol. 12: 1113-1120.

Kosty, M.P., Herndon, J.E., Green, M. R., and McIntyre, O.R. (1995). Placebo-controlled randomized study of hydrazine sulfate in lung cancer (letter). J. Clin. Oncol. 13: 1529.

Kotz, S. and Johnson, N.L. (1988). Encyclopedia of Statistical Sciences. New York: John Wiley & Sons.

Kraemer, H.C. and Thiemann, S. (1987). How Many Subjects? Newbury Park, CA: Sage Publications.

Kuznetsov, D.A. (1989). In vitro studies of interactions between frequent and unique mRNAs and cytoplasmic factors from brain tissue of several species of wild timber voles of Northern Eurasia, Clethrionomys glareolus, Clethrionomys fratter, and Clethrionomys gapperi : A new criticism to a modern molecular-genetic concept of biological evolution. International J. Neuroscience 49: 43-59.

Lachin, J.M. (1981). Introduction to sample size determination and power analysis for clinical trials. Controlled Clin. Trials 2: 93-113.

Lachin, J.M. (1988a). Properties of simple randomization in clinical trials. Controlled Clin. Trials 9: 312-326.

Lachin, J.M. (1988b). Statistical properties of randomization in clinical trials. Controlled Clin. Trials 9: 289- 311.

Lachin, J.M., Matts, J.P., and Wei, L.J. (1988). Randomization in clinical trials: Conclusions and recommendations. Controlled Clin. Trials 9: 365-374.

Lacourciere, Y., Lefebvre, J., Poirier, L., Archambault, F., and Arnott, W. (1994). Treatment of ambulatory hypertensives with nebivolol or hydrochlorthiazide alone and in combination. A randomized, double-blind, placebo-controlled, factorial-design trial. Am. J. Hypertension 7: 137-145.

Lad, T., Rubinstein, L., Sadeghi, A. et al. (1988). The benefit of adjuvant treatment for resected locally advanced non-small cell lung cancer. J. Clin. Oncol. 6: 9-17.

Lagakos, S.W., Lim, L., and Robins, J.M. (1990). Adjusting for early treatment termination in comparative clinical trials. Statistics in Medicine 9: 1417-1424.

Laird, N. (1983). Further comparative analyses of pretest posttest research designs. Amer. Statistician 37: 329-330.

Laird, N. and Ware, J.H. (1982). Random effects models for longitudinal data. Biometrics 38: 963-974.

Lan, K.K.G. and DeMets, D.L. (1983). Discrete sequential boundaries for clinical trials. Biometrika 70: 659-663.

Lan, K.K., DeMets, D.L., and Halperin, M. (1984). More flexible sequential and non-sequential designs in long-term clinical terms. Commun. Statist.-Theor. Meth. 13: 2339-2353.

Lan, K.K.G., Simon, R., and Halperin, M. (1982). Stochastically curtailed tests in long-term clinical trials. Commun. Stat.-Sequential Analysis 1: 207-219.

Lan, K.K.G. and Wittes, J. (1988). The B-value: A tool for monitoring data. Biometrics 44: 579-585.

Lancaster, H.O. (1994). Quantitative Methods in Biological and Medical Sciences: A Historical Essay. New York: Springer-Verlag.

Lantos, J. (1993). Informed consent. The whole truth for patients? Cancer (suppl.) 72: 2811-2815.

Lantos, J. (1994). Ethics, randomization, and technology assessment. Cancer (suppl.) 74: 2653-656.

Larhammar, D. (1994). Lack of experimental support for Kuznetsov's criticism of biological evolution (letter). International J. Neuroscience 77: 199-201.

Larhammar, D. (1995). Severe flaws in scientific study criticizing evolution. Skeptical Inquirer 19: 30-31.

Laska, E., Meisner, M., and Kushner, H.B. (1983). Optimal crossover designs in the presence of carryover effects. Biometrics 39: 1087-1091.

Layard, M.W.J. and Arvesen, J.N. (1978). Analysis of Poisson data in crossover trials. Biometrics 34: 421-428.

LeBlanc, M. and Crowley, J. (1992). Relative risk trees for censored survival data. Biometrics 48: 411-425.

Leary, W.E. (1994). Critics question ethics of U.S.-sponsored vaccine tests in Italy and Sweden. New York Times (Sunday, March 13).

Leber, P. (1991). Is there an alternative to the randomized controlled trial? Psychopharm. Bull. 27: 3-8.

Lechmacher, W. (1991). Analysis of the cross-over design in the presence of residual effects. Statistics in Med. 10: 891-899.

Lee, E.T. (1992). Statistical Methods for Surival Data Analysis, Second Edition. New York: John Wiley & Sons.

Lee, Y.J., Ellenberg, J.H., Hirtz, D.G., and Nelson, K.B. (1991). Analysis of clinical trials by treatment actually received: Is it really an option? Statistics in Med. 10: 1595-1605.

Lehmann, E.L. (1989). Testing Statistical Hypotheses, Second Edition. New York: John Wiley & Sons.

Leventhal, B.G. and Wittes, R.E. (1988). Research Methods in Clinical Oncology. New York: Raven Press.

Levine, R.J. (1986). Ethics and Regulation of Clinical Research. Second Edition, New Haven and London: Yale University Press.

Levine, R.J. (1992). Clinical trials and physicians as double agents. Yale J. Biology Med. 65: 65-74.

Levinsky, N.G. (1996). Social, institutional, and economic barriers to the exercise of patients' rights. New Engl. J. Med. 334: 532-534.

Lewis, J.A. and Machin, D. (1993). Intention-to-treat – who should use ITT? Br. J. Cancer 68: 647-650.

Lewis, R.J. and Berry, D.A. (1994). Group sequential clinical trials: A classical evaluation of Bayesian decision-theoretic designs. J. Am. Statist. Assoc. 89: 1528-1534.

Li, B, Taylor, P.R., Li, J.Y. et al. (1993). Linxian nutrition intervention trials. Design, methods, participant characteristics, and compliance. Ann. Epidemiol. 3: 577-585.

Li, D., German, D., Lulla, S., Thomas, R.G., and Wilson, S.R. (1995). Prospective study of hospitalization for asthma. A preliminary risk factor model. Am. J. Respir. Crit. Care Med. 151: 647-655.

Liang, K.Y., and Zeger, S.L. (1986). Longitudinal data analysis using generalized linear models. Biometrika 73: 13-22.

Light, R.J. and Smith, P.V. (1971). Accumulating evidence: procedures for resolving contradictions among different research studies. Harvard Educ. Rev. 41: 429-471.

Lilencron, F. von (Ed.). (1967). Achenwall, in Allgemeine Deutsche Biographie, Second Edition. Berlin: Duncker & Humblot.

Lindley, D.V. (1965). Introduction to Probability and Statistics from a Bayesian Viewpoint. Cambridge: Cambridge University Press.

Lindley, D.V. and Scott, W.F. (1995). New Cambridge Statistical Tables, Second Edition. Cambridge: Cambridge University Press.

Liu, G. and Piantadosi, S. (1997). Ridge estimation in generalized linear models and proportional hazards regressions. Statistics in Medicine, submitted.

Lock, S. (1988). Scientific misconduct. Brit. Med. J. 297: 1531-1535.

Lock, S. (1990). Medical Misconduct: A Survey in Britain. In J. Bailar et al. (Eds.).In Ethics and Policy in Scientific Publication. Bethesda, MD: Council of Biology Editors.

Lock, S. (1995). Lessons from the Pearce affair: Handling scientific fraud. BMJ 310: 1547-1548.

Loprinzi, C.L. Kuross, S.A., O'Fallon, J.R., et al. (1994). Randomized placebo controlled evaluation of hydrazine sulfate in patients with advanced colorectal cancer. J. Clin. Oncol. 12: 1121-1125.

Loprinzi, C.L., Goldberg, R.M., Su, J.Q., et al. (1994). Placebo controlled trial of hydrazine sulfate in patients with newly diagnosed non-small cell lung cancer. J. Clin. Oncol. 12: 1126-1129.

Lorenzen, T.J. and Anderson, V.L. (1993). Design of Experiments: A No-name Approach. New York: Marcel Dekker.

Lubsen, J. and Pocock, S.J. (1994). Factorial trials in cardiology (editorial). Eur. Heart. J. 15: 585-588.

Lunn, A.D. and McNeil, D.R. (1991). Computer-Interactive Data Analysis. Chichester: John Wiley & Sons.

Macdonald, J.S. (1990). Sometimes a great notion. JNCI 82: 102-104.

Machin, D. and Campbell, M.J. (1987). Statistical Tables for the Design of Clinical Trials. Oxford: Blackwell.

Magner, L.N. (1979). A History of the Life Sciences. New York-Basel: Marcel Dekker.

Mahfouz, A.A., Abdel-Moneim, M., al-Erian, R.A., and al-Amari, O.M. (1995). Impact of chlorination of water in domestic storage tanks on childhood diarrhoea: A community trial in the rural areas of Saudi Arabia. J. Trop. Med. Hyg. 98: 126-130.

Mahon, W.A. and Daniel, E.E. (1964). A method for the assessment of the reports of drug trials. Can. Med. Assoc. J. 90: 565-569.

Majeed, A.W., Troy, G., Nicholl, J.P. et al. (1996). Randomised, prospective, single-blind comparison of laparoscopic versus small-incision cholecystectomy. Lancet 347: 989-994.

Manski, C.F. (1990). Nonparametric bounds on treatment effects. American Economic Review, Papers and Proceedings 80: 319-323.

Manson, J.E., Gaziano, J.M., Spelsberg, A., Ridker, P.M., Cook, N.R., Buring, J.E., Willett, W.C., and Hennekens, C.H. (1995). A secondary prevention trial of antioxidant vitamins and cardiovascular disease in women. Rationale, design, and methods. Annals of Epidemiology 5: 261-269.

Mantel, N., and Haenszel, W. (1959). Statistical aspects of the analysis of data from retrospective studies of disease. JNCI 22: 719-748.

Markman, M. (1992). Ethical difficulties with randomized clinical trials involving cancer patients: Examples from the field of gynecologic oncology. J. Clinical Ethics 3(3): 193-195.

Marshall, E. (1993). Women's Health Initiative draws flak. Science 262: 838.

Marshall, E. (1994). The politics of alternative medicine. Science 265: 2000-2002.

Martz, H.F. and Waller, R.A. (1982). Bayesian Reliability Analysis. New York: John Wiley & Sons.

Marubini, E., Mariani, L., Salvadori, B. et al. (1996). Results of a breast-cancer-surgery trial compared with observational data from routine practice. Lancet 347: 1000-1003.

Marubini, E. and Valsecchi, M.G. (1995). Analysing Survival Data from Clinical Trials and Observational Studies. Chichester: John Wiley & Sons.

Marwick, C. (1994). Ethicist faults human research protection. JAMA 271: 1228-1229.

Mason, R.L. and Gunst, R.L (1989). Statistical Design and Analysis of Experiments. New York: John Wiley & Sons.

Mastroianni, A.C., Faden R., and Federman, D. (Eds.) (1994). Women and Health Research: Ethical and Legal Issues of Including Women in Clinical Studies. Washington, DC: National Academy Press.

Matthews, J.N.S. (1988). Recent developments in crossover designs. International Statistical Review 56: 117-127.

Matthews, J.R. (1995). Quantification and the Quest for Medical Certainty. Princeton: Princeton University Press.

Matthews, L.H. (1981). Piltdown Man: The missing kinks. New Scientist, April 30, 1981: 282-282 (ten-part series).

Matts, J.P., and Lachin, J.M. (1988). Properties of permuted-block randomization in clinical trials. Controlled Clin. Trials 9: 327-344.

Max, M.B., Zeigler, D., Shoaf, S.E. et al. (1992). Effects of a single oral dose of desipramine on postoperative morphine analgesia. J. Pain Symptom Manage. 7: 454-462.

McConnochie, K.M., Roghmann, K.J., and Pasternack, J. (1993). Developing prediction rules and evaluating patterns using categorical clinical markers: Two complementary procedures. Med. Decis. Making 13: 30-42.

McCullagh, P. and Nelder, J.A. (1989). Generalized Linear Models. London: Chapman and Hall.

McCutchen, C.W. (1991). Peer review: Treacherous servant, disastrous master. Technol. Rev. October 1991: 28-36.

McGinnis, L.S. (1990). Alternative therapies, 1990. Cancer 67: 1788-1792.

McIntyre, O.R., Kornblith, A.B., and Coburn, J. (1996). Pilot survey of opinions on data falsification in clinical trials. Cancer Invest. 14(4): 392-395.

McKean, K. (1981). A scandal in the laboratory. Discover (November, 1981): 18-23.

McKnight, B. and Van Den Eeden, S.K. (1993). A conditional analysis for two-treatment multiple-period crossover designs with binomial or Poisson outcomes and subjects who drop out. Statistics in Med. 12: 825-834.

McLean, R.A., Sanders, W.L., and Stroup, W.W. (1991). A unified approach to mixed linear models. Am. Statistist. 45: 54-64.

McNeill, P.M. (1993). The Ethics and Politics of Human Experimentation. Cambridge: Press Syndicate of the University of Cambridge.

McNeill, P.M. (1993). The Ethics and Politics of Human Experimentation. Cambridge: Press Syndicate of the University of Cambridge.

McPeek, B., Mosteller, F., and McKneally, M. (1989). Randomized clinical trials in surgery. Int. J. Technology Assessment in Health Care 5: 317-332.

Meier, P. (1991). Comment (on a paper by Efron and Feldman). J. Am. Stat. Assoc. 86: 19-22.

Meinert, C.L. (1986). Clinical Trials: Design, Conduct, and Analysis. Oxford: Oxford University Press.

Meinert, C.L. (1996). A Dictionary of Clinical Trials. Baltimore: Johns Hopkins Center for Clinical Trials.

Meinert, C.L. (1989). Extracorporeal membrane oxygenation trials (commentary). Pediatrics 85: 365-366.

Meinert, C.L. (1989). Meta-analysis: Science or religion? Controlled Clin. Trials 10: 257S-263S.

Meyer, L., Job-Spira, N., Bouyer, J., Bouvet, E., and Spira, A. (1991). Prevention of sexually transmitted diseases: A randomised community trial. J. Epidemiol. Community Health 45: 152-158.

Meyers, A.H., Rosner, B., Abbey, H., Willet, W., Stampfer, M.J., and Bain, C. (1995). The Women Physicians' Health Study: Background, objectives, and methods. J. Am. Med. Womens Assoc. 50: 64-66.

Miettinen, O. (1983). The need for randomization in the study of intended effects. Statistics in Med. 2: 267-271.

Miké, V., Krauss, A.N., and Ross, G.S. (1993). Neonatal extracorporeal membrane oxygenation (ECMO): Clinical trials and the ethics of evidence. J. Med. Ethics 19: 212-218.

Miller, D.J (1992). Personality Factors in Scientific Fraud and Misconduct. Chapter 7 in D.J. Miller and M. Hersen (Eds.), Research Fraud in the Behavioral and Biomedical Sciences. New York: John Wiley & Sons.

Miller, T.P., Crowley, J., Mira, J., Schwartz, J.G., Hutchins, L., Baker, L., Natale, R., Chase, E.M., and Livingston, R. (1995). A randomized trial of treatment for localized inoperable non-small cell lung cancer comparing radiation alone to radiation plus chemotherapy and testing the efficacy of prophylactic whole brain radiation. International Journal of Radiation Oncology, Biology, Physics (submitted).

Mills, J.L. (1993). Data torturing. New Engl. J. Med. 329: 1196-1199.

Minor, J.M. and Namini, H. (1996). Analysis of clinical data using neural nets. J. Biopharmaceutical Statistics 6: 83-104.

Moertel, C.G., Schutt, A.J., Hahn, R.G., and Reitemeier, R.S. (1974). Effects of patient selection on results on phase II chemotherapy trials in gastrointestinal cancer. Cancer Chemother. Rep. 58: 257-260.

Moertel, C.G. and Rebibitemreier, R.J. (1969). Advanced Gastrointestinal Cancer. Clinical Management and Chemotherapy. New York: Harper and Row.

Moertel, C.G. and Thynne, G.S. (1982). Large Bowel. In: Cancer Medicine, edited by J.F. Holland and E. Frei III, pp.1830-1859, 2nd Edition. Philadelphia: Lea and Febiger.

Moertel, C.G., Fleming, T.R., Rubin, J. et al. (1982). A clinical trial of amygdalin (Laetrile) in the treatment of human cancer. New Engl. J. Med. 306: 201-206.

Moher, D., Dulberg, C.S., and Wells, G.A. (1994). Statistical power, sample size, and their reporting in randomized controlled trials. JAMA 272: 122-124.

Moher, D., Fortin, P., Jada, A.R., et al. (1996). Completeness of reporting of trials published in languages other than English: Implications for conduct and reporting of systematic reviews. Lancet 347: 363-366.

Moore, R.D., Hidalgo, J., and Sugland, B.W. (1991). Zidovudine and the natural history of the acquired immunodeficiency syndrome. New Engl. J. Med. 324: 1412-1416.

Moores, D.W.O., Piantadosi, S., and McKneally, M.F. (1989). Effect of perioperative blood transfusion on outcome in patients with surgically resected lung cancer. Ann. Thorac. Surg. 47: 346-351.

Morrison, R.S. (1990). Disreputable science: Definition and detection. J. Adv. Nursing 15: 911-913.

Moss, A.J., Hall, W.J., Cannom, D.S, et al. (1996). Improved survival with an implanted defibrillator in patients with coronary disease at high risk for ventricular arrhythmia. New Engl. J. Med. 335: 1933-1940.

Mosteller, F., Gilbert, J., and McPeek, B. (1980). Reporting standards and research strategies for controlled clinical trials; agenda for the editor. Cont. Clin. Trials 1: 37-58.

Mountain, C.F. and Gail, M.H. (1981). Surgical adjuvant intrapleural BCG treatment for stage I non-small cell lung cancer. Preliminary report of the National Cancer Institute Lung Cancer Study Group. J. Thorac. Cardiovasc. Surg. 82: 649-657.

Murray, G.D. (1991). Statistical aspects of research methodology. Br. J. Surg. 78: 777-781.

Murray, G.D. (1991). Statistical guidelines for the British Journal of Surgery. Br. J. Surg. 78: 782-784.

National Academy of Sciences (NAS) (1992a). Responsible Science: Ensuring the Integrity of the Research Process, Vol. I. Washington, DC: National Academy Press.

National Academy of Sciences (NAS) (1992b). Responsible Science: Ensuring the Integrity of the Research Process, Vol. II. Washington, DC: National Academy Press.

National Cancer Institute (1993). Final Report to the Food and Drug Administration: Hydrazine Sulfate, NSC 150014, IND 33233. Private communication.

NCI Press Office (1994a). Press release. March 24.

NCI Press Office (1994b). Press release. March 29.

NCI Press Office (1994c). Press release. April 12.

NCI Press Office (1994d). Press release. April 21.

NCI Press Office (1994e). Press release. April 22.

NCI Press Office (1994f). Press release. May 2.

National Cancer Institute (1996). NCI Cooperative Group Data Monitoring Committee Policy (unpublished).

National Commission for Protection of Human Subjects of Biomedical and Behavioral Research (1978). The Belmont Report: Ethical Principles and Guidelines for the Protection of Human Subjects of Research. Washington, DC: DHEW Publication Number (OS) 78-0012. Appendix I, DHEW Publication No. (OS) 78-0013; Appendix II, DHEW Publication No. (OS) 78-0014.

National Science Foundation (NSF) (1987). Misconduct in science and engineering research: Final regulations. Fed. Reg. 52 (July 1): 24466-24470.

National Science Foundation (NSF) (1991). Misconduct in science and engineering research: Final rule. Fed. Reg. 56 (May 14): 22286-22290.

National Science Foundation (NSF) (1990). Semiannual Report to the Congress. Number 3. Washington, DC: Office of the Inspector General, NSF.

Naylor, C.D., Chen, E., and Strauss, B. (1992). Measured enthusiasm: Does the method of reporting trial results alter perception of therapeutic effectiveness? Ann. Intern. Med. 117: 916-921.

Nelder, J.A. and Weddeburn, R.W.M. (1972). Generalized linear models. JRSS A 135: 370-384.

Newell, D.J. (1992). Intention-to-treat analysis: implications for quantitative and qualitative research. Int. J. Epidemiol. 21: 837-841.

Neyman, J. and Pearson, E.S. (1933). On the problem of the most efficient tests of statistical hypotheses. Phil. Trans. Roy. Soc. A. 231: 289-337.

NHLBI (1994a). NHLBI Guidelines for Data Quality Assurance in Clinical Trials and Large Epidemiologic Studies (unpublished).

NHLBI (1994b). NHLBI Guide for Data and Safety Monitoring Boards (unpublished).

NIH (1993). Final findings of scientific misconduct: Roger Poisson, M.D., St. Luc Hospital, Montreal, Canada. NIH Guide for Grants and Contracts. Vol. 22, No. 23, June 25, 1993: 3.

Non-Small Cell Lung Cancer Collaborative Group (1995). Chemotherapy in non-small cell lung cancer: A meta-analysis using updated data on individual patients from 52 randomised clinical trials. BMJ 311: 899-909.

Noseworthy, J.H., Ebers, G.C., Vandervoort, M.K., et al. (1994). The impact of blinding on the results of a randomized, placebo-controlled multiple sclerosis clinical trial. Neurology 44: 16-20.

NSABP (1992). NSABP Protocol P-1 (Breast Cancer Prevention Trial). Pittsburg, PA: NSABP Center Headquarters.

Oakes, M. (1993). The logic and role of meta-analysis in clinical research. Stat. Methods in Med. Research 2: 147-160.

O'Brien, P.C., and Fleming, T.R. (1979). A multiple testing procedure for clinical trials. Biometrics 35: 549-556.

O'Bryan, T. and Walter, G. (1979). Sankhyā A, 41: 95-108.

O'Fallon, J.R. (1985). Policies for interim analysis and interim reporting of results. Cancer Treat. Rep. 69(10): 1101-1106.

Office of Research Integrity (ORI) (1993). Office of Research Integrity: An Introduction. Rockville: Department of Health and Human Services.

Office of Research Integrity (ORI) (1993). Case Summary: Fabricated and falsified clinical trial data. Office of Research Integrity Newsletter Vol. 1, No. 2. April, 1993: 2.

Office of Research Integrity (ORI) (1995). Annual Report 1995. Rockville, MD: Office of Research Integrity.

Office of Technology Assessment (1983). Factors affecting the impact of RCTs on medical practice, in The Impact of Randomized Clinical Trials on Health Policy and Medical Practice. Washington, DC: Government Printing Office, OTA-BP-H-22.

Office of Technology Assessment (1990). Unconventional Cancer Treatments. Washington, DC: Government Printing Office, OTA-H-405.

O'Hagan, A. (1994). Kendall's Advanced Theory of Statistics, Volume 2B, Bayesian Inference. London: Edward Arnold.

Ohashi, Y. (1990). Randomization in cancer clinical trials: Permutation test and development of computer program. Environmental Health Perspectives 87: 13-17.

Oliver, S.G., van der Aart, Q.J.M., Agostoni-Carbone, M.L., et al. (1992). The complete DNA sequence of yeast chromosome III. Nature 357: 38-46.

Olkin, I. (1994). Invited commentary re: A critical look at some popular meta-analytic methods. Am. J. Epidemiol. 140: 297-299.

Olkin, I. (1995a). Statistical and theoretical considerations in meta-analysis. J. Clin. Epidemiol. 48: 133-146.

Olkin, I. (1995b). Meta analysis: Reconciling the results of independent studies. Statistics in Med. 14: 457-472.

O'Neill, R.T. (1978). Subjects-own-control designs in clinical drug trials: Overview of the issues with emphasis on the two treatment problem. Presented at the Annual NCDEU Meeting, Key Biscayne, Florida.

Opie, L.H. and Messerli, F.H. (1995). Nifedipine and mortality: Grave defects in the dossier. Circulation 92: 1068-1073.

O'Quigley, J. (1992). Estimating the probability of toxicity at the recommended dose following a phase I clinical trial in cancer. Biometrics 48: 853-862.

O'Quigley, J. and Shen, L.Z. (1996). Continual reassessment method: A likelihood approach. Biometrics 52: 673-684.

O'Quigley, J., Pepe, M., and Fisher, L. (1990). Continual reassessment method: A practical design for phase I clinical trials in cancer. Biometrics 46: 33-48.

O'Quigley, J., and Chevret, S. (1991). Methods for dose finding studies in cancer clinical trials: A review and results of a Monte Carlo study. Statistics in Med. 10: 1647-1664.

O'Regan, B. and Hirshberg, C. (1993). Spontaneous Remission: An Annotated Bibliography. Sausalito, CA.: Institute of Noetic Sciences.

O'Rourke, P.P. (1991). ECMO: Where have we been? Where are we going? Respiratory Care 36: 683-694.

O'Rourke, P.P., Crone, R.K., Vacanti, J.P., Ware, J.H., Lillehei, C.W., Parad, R.B., and Epstein, M.F. (1989). Extracorporeal membrane oxygenation and conventional medical therapy in neonates with persistent pulmonary hypertension of the newborn: A prospective randomized study. Pediatrics 84: 957-963.

Osler, W. (1910). Man's Redemption of Man. London: Constable.

Packer, M., Carver, J.R., Rodeheffer, R.J., et al. (1991). Effect of oral milrinone on mortality in severe chronic heart failure. New Engl. J. Medicine 325: 1468-1475.

Palafox, N., Schatz, I., Lange, R., et al. (1997). Intravenous 20% mannitol versus intravenous 5% dextrose for the treatment of acute ciguatera: A randomized, placebo controlled, double masked trial. JAMA (submitted).

Palta, M. (1985). Investigating maximum power losses in survival studies with nonstratified randomization. Biometrics 41: 497-504.

Parkinson Study Group (1993). Effects of tocopherol and deprenyl on the progression of disability in early Parkinson's Disease. New Engl. J. Med. 328: 176-183.

Parmar, M.K.B. (1992). Randomization Before Consent. Ch. 14 in C.J. Williams (Ed.). Introducing New Treatments for Cancer: Practical, Ethical, and Legal Problems. Chichester: John Wiley & Sons.

Parmar, M.K.B. and Machin, D. (1995). Survival Analysis: A Practical Approach. New York: John Wiley & Sons.

Passamani, E. (1991). Clinical trials – Are they ethical? New Engl. J. Med. 324: 1589-1592.

Patterson, B. and Piantadosi, S. (1989). Identification of endpoints: Selection and ascertainment. Chapter 19 in T. Moon, and M. Micozzi (Eds.), Nutrition and Cancer Prevention: The Role of Micronutrients. New York: Dekker.

Peduzzi, P., et al. (1991). Intention-to-treat analysis and the problem of crossovers: An example from the Veterans Administration coronary bypass surgery study. J. Thorac. Cardiovasc. Surg. 101: 481-487.

Peduzzi, P., et al. (1993). Analysis as-randomized and the problem of non-adherence: An example from the Veterans Affairs randomized trial of coronary artery bypass surgery. Statistics in Med. 12: 1185-1195.

Pena, C.M., Rice, T.W., Ahmad, M., and Medendorp, S.V. (1992). Significance of perioperative blood transfusions in patients undergoing resection of stage I and II non-small cell lung cancers. Chest 102: 84-88.

Petitti, D.B. (1994). Meta-Analysis, Decision Analysis, and Cost-Effectiveness Analysis. Synthesis in Medicine. New York: Oxford University Press.

Peto, J. (1984). The Calculation and Interpretation of Survival Curves. Chapter 21, in Cancer Clinical Trials, edited by M.J. Buyse, M.J. Staquet, and R.J. Sylvester. Oxford: Oxford University Press.

Peto, R. (1987). Why do we need systematic overviews of randomized trials? Statistics in Med. 6: 233-240.

Peto, R., Collins, R., and Gray, R. (1995) Large-scale randomized evidence: Large simple trials and overviews of trials. J. Clin. Epidemiol. 48: 23-40.

Peto, R., Pike, M.C., Armitage, P., Breslow, N.E., Cox, D.R., Howard, S.V., Mantel, N., McPherson, K., Peto, J., and Smith, G. (1977a). Design and analysis of randomized clinical trials requiring prolonged observation of each patient. I. Introduction and design. Br. J. Cancer. 34: 585-612.

Peto, R., Pike, M.C., Armitage, P., Breslow, N.E., Cox, D.R., Howard, S.V., Mantel, N., McPherson, K., Peto, J., and Smith, G. (1977b). Design and analysis of randomized clinical trials requiring prolonged observation of each patient. II. Analysis and examples. Br. J. Cancer. 35: 1-39.

Piantadosi, S. (1990). Clinical Trials Design Program. Cambridge, UK: BIOSOFT.

Piantadosi, S. (1990). Hazards of Small Clinical Trials (editorial). J. Clin. Oncol. 8(1): 1-3.

Piantadosi, S. (1992). The adverse effect of blood transfusion in lung cancer (editorial). Chest 102: 608.

Piantadosi, S., Fisher, J.D., and Grossman, S. for the New Approaches to Brain Tumor Therapy Consortium (1997). A practical implementation of a modified continual reassessment method for dose finding trials. J. Clin. Oncol. (submitted).

Piantadosi, S. and Gail, M.H. (1995). Statistical Issues Arising in Thoracic Surgery Clinical Trials. Chapter 71 in F.G. Pearson, J. Deslauriers, R.J. Ginsberg, et al. (Eds.), Thoracic Surgery. New York: Churchill Livingstone.

Piantadosi, S., Graham, N.M.H., Park, L., Saah, A., Kaslow, R., Detels, R. Rinaldo, C., and Phair, J. for the Multicenter AIDS Cohort Study (MACS). Risk sets for time to AIDS and survival based on pre- and post-treatment prognostic markers. First National Conference on Human Retroviruses and Related Infections, Am. Soc. Microbiology, December 12–16, 1993.

Piantadosi, S. and Liu, G. (1996). Improved designs for phase I studies using pharmacokinetic measurements. Statistics in Med. 15: 1605-1618.

Piantadosi, S., and Patterson, B. (1987). A method for predicting accrual, cost, and paper flow in clinical trials. Controlled Clin. Trials 8: 202-215.

Pocock, S. (1993). Statistical and ethical issues in monitoring clinical trials. Statistics in Med. 12: 1459-1469. (See also the discussion that follows.)

Pocock, S. and Simon, R. (1975). Sequential treatment assignment with balancing for prognostic factors in the controlled clinical trial. Biometrics 31: 103-115.

Pocock, S.J. (1996). Clinical Trials: A Practical Approach. New York: John Wiley & Sons.

Pocock, S.J., Hughs, M.D., and Lee, R.J. (1987). Statistical problems in the reporting of clinical trials. New Engl. J. Med. 317: 426-432.

Polanyi, M. (1957). Personal Knowledge. Chicago: University of Chicago Press.

Poloniecki, J.D. and Pearce, A.C. (1983). Letter to the editor. Biometrics 39: 789.

Popper, K.R. (1959). The Logic of Scientific Discovery. London: Hutchinson.

Pordy, R.C. (1994). Cilazapril plus hydrochlorthiazide: improved efficacy without reduced safety in mild to moderate hypertension. A double-blind placebo-controlled multicenter study of factorial design. Cardiology 85: 311-322.

Prentice, R.L. (1989). Surrogate endpoints in clinical trials: Definition and operational criteria. Statistics in Med. 8: 431-440.

Press, W.H., Teukolsky, S.A., Vetterling, W.T., and Flannery, B.P. (1992). Numerical Recipes in C: The Art of Scientific Computing. Second Edition. Cambridge: University Press.

Proschan, M.A., Follmann, D.A., and Geller, N.L. (1994). Monitoring multi-armed trials. Statistics in Med. 13: 1441-1452.

Prostate Cancer Trialists' Collaborative Group (1995). Maximum androgen blockade in advanced prostate cancer: An overview of 22 randomised trials with 3283 deaths in 5710 patients. Lancet 346: 265-269.

Public Law 103-43 (1993). Clinical Research Equity Regarding Women and Minorities. Public Law 103-43, Subtitle B, Sec. 131.

Pyros Education Group (1996). Current Clinical Trials: Oncology. Green Brook, NJ: Thomas J. Timko.

RSS (1993). The Royal Statistical Society: Code of Conduct.

Racker, E. and Spector, M. (1981). The Warburg effect revisited: Merger of biochemistry and molecular biology. Science 213: 303-307.

Ramsey, P. (1975). The Ethics of Fetal Research. New Haven, CT and London: Yale University Press.

Ratain, M.J., Mick, R., Schilsky, R.L., and Siegler, M. (1993). Statistical and ethical issues in the design and conduct of phase I and II clinical trials of new anticancer agents. JNCI 85: 1637-1643.

Ravdin, P.M. and Clark, G.M. (1992). A practical application of neural network analysis for predicting outcome of individual breast cancer patients. Breast Cancer Research Treat. 22: 285-293.

Reich, W.T. (Ed.) (1995). Encyclopedia of Bioethics. New York: Simon & Schuster/Macmillan.

Reiser, S.J. (1993). The ethics movement in the biological sciences: A new voyage of discovery. Overview in R.E. Bulger, E. Heitman, and S.J. Reiser (Eds.), The Ethical Dimensions of the Biological Sciences. Cambridge: Cambridge University Press.

Relman, A.S. (1983). Lessons from the Darsee affair. New Engl. J. Med. 308: 1415-1417.

Relman, A.S. (1984). Dealing with conflicts of interest. New Engl. J. Med. 311: 405.

Rennie, D., Flanagin, A., and Glass, R.M. (1991). Conflicts of interest in the publication of science. JAMA 266: 266-267.

Resampling Stats, Inc. (1995). Resampling Stats User's Guide. Arlington, VA: Resampling Stats.

Resnick, R.H., Ishihara, A., Chalmers, T.C., Schimmel, E.M., and the Boston Inter-Hospital Liver Group. (1968). A controlled trial of colon bypass in chronic hepatic encephalopathy. Gastroenterology 54: 1057-1069.

Riggs, B.L., Hodgson, S.F., O'Fallon, W.M., et al. (1990). Effect of fluoride treatment on the fracture rate in postmenopausal women with osteoporosis. New Engl. J. Med. 322: 802-809.

Robbins, H. and Monro, S. (1951). A stochastic approximation method. Annals Math. Stat. 22: 400-407.

Roberson, N.L. (1994). Clinical trial participation. Cancer 74: 2687-2691.

Roberts, A.H., Kewman, D.G., Mercier, L., and Hovell, M. (1993). The power of nonspecific effects in healing: Implications for psychosocial and biological treatments. Clin. Psychol. Rev. 13: 375-391.

Robins, J.M. (1989). The analysis of randomized and non-randomized AIDS treatment trials using a new approach to causal inference in longitudinal studies. In L. Sechrest, H. Freeman, and A. Mulley (Eds.) Health Service Research Methodology: A Focus on AIDS. NCHSR, U.S. Public Health Service.

Rochon, P.A., Gurwitz, J.H., Cheung, M., Hayes, J.A., and Chalmers, T.C. (1994). Evaluating the quality of articles published in journal supplements compared with the quality of those published in the parent journal. JAMA 272: 108-113.

Roebruck, P. and Kühn, A. (1995). Comparison of tests and sample size formulae for proving therapeutic equivalence based on the difference of binomial probabilities. Statistics in Med. 14: 1583-1594.

Rondel, R.K., Varley, S.A., and Webb, C.F. (Eds.) (1993). Clinical Data Management. Chichester: John Wiley & Sons.

Rosell, R., Gomez-Codina, J., Camps, C., et al. (1994). A randomized trial comparing preoperative chemotherapy plus surgery with surgery alone in patients with non-small-cell lung cancer. New Engl. J. Med. 330: 153-158.

Rossiter, E.J.R. (1992). Reflections of a whistle-blower. Nature 357: 434-436.

Rothenberg, M.L., Moore, M.J., Cripps, M.C. et al. (1996). A phase II trial of gemcitabine in patients with 5-FU-refractory pancreas cancer. Annals of Oncology 7: 347-353.

Rothman, K.J. and Michels, K.B. (1994). The continuing unethical use of placebo controls. New Engl. J. Med. 331: 394-398.

Roy, D.J. (1986). Controlled clinical trials: An ethical imperative. J. Chron. Dis. 39: 159-162.

Royal College of Physicians (1991). Fraud and misconduct in medical research. J Royal College Physicians London 25: 89-94.

Royall, R.M. (1986). The effect of sample size on the meaning of significance tests. Am. Statistician 40: 313-315.

Royall, R.M. (1991). Ethics and statistics in randomized clinical trials. Statistical Science 6: 52-88.

Royall, R.M. (1992). Ignorance and altruism. Journal of Clinical Ethics 3(3): 229-230.

Royall, R.M. (1997). Statistical Evidence (A Likelihood Primer). London: Chapman and Hall (in press).

Rozovsky, F.A. (1990). Consent to Treatment, A Practical Guide. Boston: Little, Brown.

Ruberg, S.J. (1995a). Dose response studies. I. Some design considerations. J. Biopharmaceutical Statistics 5: 1-14.

Ruberg, S.J. (1995b). Dose response studies. II. Analysis and interpretation. J. Biopharmaceutical Statistics 5: 15-42.

Rubinow, S.I. (1975). Introduction to Mathematical Biology. New York: John Wiley & Sons.

Rubinstein, L.V., Gail, M.H., and Santner, T.J. (1981). Planning the duration of a comparative clinical trial with loss to follow-up and a period of continued observation. J. Chron. Dis. 34: 469-479.

Rubinstein, L.V., and Gail, M.H. (1982). Monitoring rules for stopping accrual in comparative survival studies. Controlled Clinical Trials 3: 325-343.

Rusch, V.W., Piantadosi, S., and Holmes, E.C. (1991). The role of extrapleural pneumonectomy in malignant pleural mesothelioma. J. Thoracic. Cardiovasc. Surg. 102: 1-9.

Rutstein, D. (1969). Daedalus 98: 523.

Rutter, C.M. and Elashoff, R.M. (1994). Analysis of longitudinal data: Random coefficient regression modeling. Statistics in Medicine 13: 1211-1231.

SAS Institute (1985). SAS User's Guide: Statistics, Version 5 Edition. Cary, NC: SAS Institute.

Sackett, D.L. (1979). Bias in analytic research. J. Chron. Dis. 32: 51-63.

Sackett, D.L. (1983). On some prerequisites for a successful clinical trial. In S.H. Shapiro and T.A. Louis (Eds.) Clinical Trials. New York: Marcel-Dekker.

Sackett, D.L. and Gent, M. (1979). Controversy in counting and attributing events in clinical trials. New Engl. J. Med. 301(26): 1410-1412.

Sadeghi, A., Lad, T., Payne, D., Rubinstein, L., and the Lung Cancer Study Group (1988). Combined modality treatment for resected advanced non-small cell lung cancer: Local control and local recurrence. Int. J. Radiat. Oncol. Biol. Phys. 15: 89-97.

Sahai, H. and Khurshid, A. (1996). Formulae and tables for the determination of sample sizes and power in clinical trials for testing differences in proportions for the two-sample design: A review. Statistics in Med. 15: 1-21.

Salsburg, D. (1990). Hypothesis versus significance testing for controlled clinical trials: A dialogue. Statistics in Med. 9: 201-211.

Savage, L.J. (1954). The Foundations of Statistics. New York: John Wiley & Sons.

Schaefer, A. (1982). The ethics of the randomized clinical trial. N. Engl. J. Med. 307: 719-724.

Schechtman, K.B. and Gordon, M.O. (1994). The effect of poor compliance and treatment side effects on sample size requirements in randomized clinical trials. J. Biopharmaceutical Statistics 4: 223-232.

Schellhammer, P., Sharifif, R., Block, N., Soloway, M., Venner, P., Patterson, A.L., Sarosdy, M., Vogelzang, N., Jones, J., and Kiovenbag, G. (1995). A controlled trial of bicalutamide versus flutamide, each in combination with lutenizing hormone-releasing hormone analogue therapy, in patients with advanced prostate cancer. Casodex Combination Study Group. Urology 45(5): 745-752.

Schmucker, D.L. and Vesell, E.S. (1993). Underrepresentation of women in clinical drug trials. Clin. Pharmacol. Ther. 54: 11-15.

Schulz, K.F. (1995). Subverting randomization in controlled trials. JAMA 274: 1456-1458.

Schulz, K.F., Chalmers, I., Hayes, R.J., and Altman, D.G. (1995). Empirical evidence of bias: Dimensions of methodologic quality associated with estimates of treatment effects in controlled trials. JAMA 273: 408-412.

Schuman, S.H., Olansky, S., Rivers, E., Smith, C.A., and Rambo, D.S. (1955). Untreated syphilis in the male negro. J. Chron. Dis. 2: 543-558.

Schwartz, D. and Lellouch, J. (1967). Explanatory and pragmatic attitudes in therapeutic trials. J. Chron. Dis. 20: 637-648.

Schwartz, D., Flamant, R., and Lellouch, J. (1980). Clinical Trials. London: Academic Press.

Schwartz, R.P. (1991). Maintaining integrity and credibility in industry-sponsored clinical research. Controlled Clin. Trials 12: 753-760.

Sechzer, J.A., Rabinowitz, V.C., Denmark, F.L., McGinn, M.F., Weeks, B.M., and Wilkens, C.L. (1994). Sex and gender bias in animal research and in clinical studies of cancer, cardiovascular disease, and depression. Ann. N.Y. Acad. Sci. 736: 21-.

Segal, M.R. (1988). Regression trees for censored data. Biometrics 44: 35-47.

Selby, C. and Scheiber, B. (1996). Science or pseudoscience? Pentagon grant funds alternative health study. Skeptical Inquirer 20: 15-17.

Seleznick, M.J. and Fries, J.F. (1991). Variables associated with decreased survival in systemic lupus erythematosus. Sem. Arthritis Rheum. 21: 73-80.

Senn, S. (1993). Cross-over Trials in Clinical Research. Chichester: John Wiley & Sons.

Shapiro, M.F. and Charrow, R.P. (1989). The role of data audits in detecting scientific misconduct. JAMA 261: 2505-2511.

Shapiro, S. (1994). Meta-analysis/shmeta-analysis. Am. J. Epidemiol. 140: 771-778.

Sheiner, L.B. and Rubin, D.B. (1995). Intention-to-treat analysis and the goals of clinical trials. Clinical Pharmacol. & Therapeutics 57(1): 6-15.

Shimkin, M.B. (1953). The problem of experimentation on human beings: I The research worker's point of view. Science 117: 205-207.

Shuster, J.J. (1990). Handbook of Sample Size Guidelines for Clinical Trials. Boca Raton, FL: CRC Press.

Shuster, J.J., McWilliams, N.B., Castleberry, R., Nitschke, R., Smith, E.I., Altshuler, G., Kun, L., Brodeur, G., Joshi, V., Vietti, T., and Hayes, F.A. (1992). Serum lactate dehydrogenase in childhood neuroblastoma. Am. J. Clin. Oncol. 15: 295-303.

Sieber, J.E. (1993). Ethical considerations in planning and conducting research on human subjects. Academic Medicine (suppl.) 68: S9-S13.

Siegler, M. (1982). Confidentiality in medicine – A decrepit concept. New Engl. J. Med. 307: 1518-1521.

Silverman, W.A. (1985) Human Experimentation: A Guided Step Into the Unknown. Oxford: Oxford University Press.

Simon, R. (1984). Use of Regression Models: Statistical Aspects, Chapter 25, in Cancer Clinical Trials, edited by M.J. Buyse, M.J. 7 Staquet, and R.J. Sylvester. Oxford: Oxford University Press.

Simon, R. (1989). Optimal two-stage designs for phase II clinical trials. Controlled Clinical Trials 10: 1-10.

Simon, R. (1991). A decade of progress in statistical methodology for clinical trials. Statistics in Med. 10: 1789-1817.

Simon, R., Wittes, R.E., and Ellenberg, S.S. (1985). Randomized phase II clinical trials. Cancer Treatment Reports 69: 1475-1381.

Simons, J.W., Jaffee, E.M., Weber, C. et al. (1997). Bioactivity of human GM-CSF gene transfer in autologous irradiated renal cell carcinoma vaccines. Cancer Research, in press.

Singer, M. (1996). Assault on science. Washington Post, June 26.

Skolnick, A. (1990). Key witness against morning sickness drug faces scientific fraud charges. JAMA 263: 1468-1473.

Slud, E.V. (1994). Analysis of factorial survival experiments. Biometrics 50; 25-38.

Snedecor, G.W. and Cochran, W.G. (1980). Statistical Methods. Seventh Edition. Ames, IA: Iowa State University Press.

Society of University Surgeons (1991). Misconduct and fraud in research: Social and legislative issues symposium of the Society of University Surgeons. Surgery 110: 1-7.

Sokal, A.D. (1996a). Transgressing the boundaries: Toward a transformative hermeneutics of quantum gravity. Social Text 14: 217-251.

Sokal, A.D. (1996b). A physicist experiments with cultural studies. Lingua Franca: May/June.

Sommer, A. Tarwotjo, I., Djunaedi, E., West, K.P., Jr., and Loeden, A.A. (1986). Impact of vitamin A supplementation on childhood mortality: A randomized controlled community trial. Lancet, i, 1169-1173.

Sommer, A. and Zeger, S.L. (1991). On estimating efficacy from clinical trials. Statistics in Med. 10: 45-52.

Souhami, R.(1992). Large-Scale Studies. Chapter 13 in C.J. Williams (Ed.), Introducing New Treatments for Cancer: Practical Ethical and Legal Problems. Chichester: John Wiley & Sons.

Souhami, R.L. and Whitehead, J. (Eds.) (1994). Workshop on Early Stopping Rules in Cancer Clinical Trials, Robinson College, Cambridge, U.K., 13-15 April, 1993. Statistics in Med. 13: 1289-1500.

Spector, S.A., McKinley, G.F., Lalezari, J.P., et al., (1996). Oral ganciclovir for the prevention of cytomegalovirus disease in persons with AIDS. Roche Cooperative Oral Ganciclovir Study Group. New Engl. J. Med. 334(23): 1491-1497.

Sperduto, R.D., Hu, T.S., Milton, R.C., et al. (1993). The Linxian cataract studies. Two nutrition intervention trials. Arch. Ophthalmol. 111: 1246-1253.

Spiegelhalter, D.J., Freedman, L.S., and Parmar, M.K.B. (1994). Bayesian approaches to randomized trials. J. R. Statist. Soc. A 157: 357-416.

Spilker, W.A. (1991) Guide to Clinical Trials. New York: Raven Press.

Spitzer, W.O. (1995). The challenge of meta-analysis. J. Clin. Epidemiol. 48: 1-4.

Spodick, D.H. (1983). Randomize the first patient: scientific, ethical, and behavioral bases. Am. J. Cardiol. 51: 916-917.

Sposto, R., and Krailo, M.D. (1987). Use of unequal allocation in survival trials. Statistics in Medecine 6: 119-25.

Stampfer, M.J., Buring, J.E., Willett, W. et al. (1985). The 2×2 factorial design: Its application to a randomized trial of aspirin and carotene in U.S. physicians. Statistics in Med. 4: 111- 116.

Standards of Reporting Trials Group. (1994). A proposal for structured reporting of randomized controlled trials. JAMA 272: 1926-1931. Correction: 273: 776.

Stansfield, S.K., Pierre-Louis, M., Lerebours, G., and Augustin, A. (1993). Vitamin A supplementation and increased prevalence of childhood diarrhoea and acute respiratory infections. Lancet 341: 578-582.

Statistical Sciences (1995). S-PLUS Guide to Statistical and Mathematical Analysis, Version 3.3. Seattle: StatSci, a division of MathSoft.

Statistics and Epidemiology research Corporation (SERC). (1993). EGRET SIZ Reference Manual. Seattle: SERC.

Stebbing, L.S. (1961). Philosophy and the Physicist. Middlesex, England: Penguin Books.

Steering Committee of the Physicians' Health Study Research Group (1989). Final report on the aspirin component of the ongoing physicians' health study. New Engl. J. Med. 321(3): 129-135.

Stewart, L.A. and Clarke, M.J. (1995). Practical methodology of meta-analyses (overviews) using updated individual patient data. Statistics in Med. 14: 2057-2079.

Stigler, S. (1986). The History of Statistics. Cambridge, MA: Belknap Press.

Storer, B.E. (1989). Design and analysis of phase I clinical trials. Biometrics 45: 925-937.

Strauss, M.B. (1968). Familiar Medical Quotations. Boston: Little, Brown, p. 492.

Stuart, A. and Ord, J.K. (1987). Kendall's Advanced Theory of Statistics, Volume 1: Distribution Theory. Fifth Edition. New York: Oxford University Press.

Swazey, J.P., Anderson, M.S., and Lewis, K.S. (1993). Ethical problems in academic research. Am. Sci. 81: 542-553.

Tartter, P.I., Burrows, L., Kirschner, P. (1984). Perioperative blood transfusion adversely affects prognosis after resection of stage I (subset N0) non-oat cell lung cancer. J. Thorac. Cardvasc. Surg. 88: 659-662.

Task Force of the Working Group on Arrhythmias of the European Society of Cardiology (1994). The early termination of clinical trials: Causes, consequences, and control – with special reference to trials in the field of arrhythmias and sudden death. Circulation 89: 2892-2907.

Taylor, J.M.G., Cumberland, W.G., and Sy, J.P. (1994). A stochastic model for longitudinal AIDS data. J. Am. Statist. Assoc. 89: 727-736.

Taylor, K.M., Margolese, R.G., and Soskolne, C.L. (1984). Physicians' reasons for not entering eligible patients in a randomized clinical trial of surgery for breast cancer. New Engl. J. Med. 310: 1363-1367.

ten Bokkel Huinink, W.W, Eisenhaur, E., and Swenerton, K. (1993). Preliminary evaluation of a multicenter, randomized comparative study of TAXOL (paclitaxel) dose and infusion length in platinum-treated ovarian cancer. Cancer Treat. Rev. 19 (Suppl. C): 79-86.

Terrin, M.L. (1990). Efficient use of endpoints in clinical trials: A clinical perspective. Statistics in Med. 9: 155-160.

Testa, M.A. and Simonson, D.C. (1996). Assessment of quality of life outcomes. New Engl. J. Med. 334: 835-840.

Thall, P.F. and Simon, R. (1994). A Bayesian approach to establishing sample size and monitoring criteria for phase II clinical trials. Controlled Clin. Trials 15: 463-481.

Thall, P.F., Simon, R., and Estey, E.H. (1995). Bayesian sequential monitoring designs for single-arm clinical trials with multiple outcomes. Statistics in Med. 14: 357-379.

Thall, P.F., Simon, R., and Estey, E.H. (1996). A new statistical strategy for monitoring safety and efficacy in single-arm clinical trials. J. Clin. Oncology 14: 296-303.

Thelen, M.H. and DiLorenzo, T.M. (1992). Academic Pressures. Chapter 9 in D.J. Miller and M. Hersen (Eds.), Research Fraud in the Behavioral and Biomedical Sciences. New York: John Wiley & Sons.

Thomas, L. (1977). Biostatistics in medicine. (Editorial). Science 198(4318): 675.

Thornquist, M.D., Owenn, G.S., Goodman, G.E., et al. (1993). Statistical design and monitoring of the carotene and retinol efficacy trial (CARET). Controlled Clin. Trials 14: 308-324.

Toronto Leukemia Study Group (1986). Results of chemotherapy for unselected patients with acute myeloblastic leukaemia: effect of exclusions on interpretation of results. Lancet 1: 786-788.

Tukey, J.W. (1977). Some thoughts on clinical trials, especially problems of multiplicity. Science 198: 670-684.

Turner, J.G. (1994). The Effect of Therapeutic Touch on Pain and Infection in Burn Patients (N94-020A1). Grant No. MDA 905-94-Z-0080, Uniformed Services University of the Health Sciences.

Tygstrup, N., Lachin, J.M., and Juhl, E. (Eds.) (1982). The Randomized Clinical Trial and Therapeutic Decisions. New York: Marcel Dekker.

U.S. Congress (Aug., 1980). The Forgotten Guinea Pigs; A Report on the Health Effects of Low Level Radiation Sustained as a Result of the Nuclear Weapons Testing Program Conducted by the United States Government. Washington, DC: Government Printing Office.

USA Today (1996). Nationline: Full Disclosure. Monday, December 16.

Valtonen, S., Timonen, U., Toivanen, P., et al. (1997). Interstitial chemotherapy with carmustine-loaded polymers for high grade gliomas: A randomized, double-blind study. Neurosurgery, in press.

Verweij, J. (1996). The benefit of clinical benefit: A European perspective. Annals of Oncology 7: 333-334.

Villanueva, C., Balanzo, J., Novella, M.T., et al., (1996). Nadolol plus isosorbide mononitrate compared with sclerotherapy for the prevention of variceal rebleeding. New Engl. J. Med. 334: 1624-1629.

Vollset, S.E. (1993). Confidence intervals for a binomial proportion. Statistics in Med. 12: 809-824.

Wachter, K.W. (1988). Disturbed by meta-analysis? Science 241: 1407-1408.

Wade, N. (1981). A diversion of the quest for truth. Science 211: 1022-1025.

Wald, A. (1947). Sequential Analysis. New York: John Wiley & Sons.

Waldhausen, J.A. and Localio, A.R. (1996). Notes from the editors. J. Thorac. Cardiovasc. Surg. 112: 209-220.

Walter, S.D. and Day, N.E. (1983). Estimation of the duration of a preclinical state using screening data. Am. J. Epidemiol. 118: 865-886.

Walter, S.D. (1995). Methods of reporting statistical results from medical research studies. Am. J. Epidemiol. 141: 896-906.

Walter, S.D. (1995). Methods of reporting statistical results from medical research studies. Am. J. Epidemiol. 141: 896-906.

Ware, J.H. and Epstein, M.F. (1985). Extracorporeal circulation in neonatal respiratory failure: A prospective randomized study (commentary). Pediatrics 76: 849-851.

Warner, B. and Misra, M. (1996). Understanding neural networks as statistical tools. Am. Statistscian 50(4): 284-293.

Weber, W.W. (1987). The Acetylator Genes and Drug Response. New York: Oxford University Press.

Wei, L.J. and Lachin, J.M. (1988). Properties of the urn randomization in clinical trials. Controlled Clin. Trials 9: 345-364.

Wei, L.J. and Durham, S. (1978). The randomized play-the-winner rule in medical trials. J. Am. Stat. Assoc. 73: 840-843.

Weijer, C. and Fuks, A. (1994). The duty to exclude: excluding people at undue risk from research. Clin. Invest. Med. 17: 115-122.

Weiss, R. (1996). Proposed shifts in misconduct reviews unsettle many scientists. Washington Post, June 30.

Weiss, R.B., Vogelzang, N.J., Peterson, B.A. et al. (1993). A successful system of scientific data audits for clinical trials. JAMA 270: 459-464.

Wells, F. (1992) Good Clinical Research Practice. Chapter 19 in Introducing New Treatments for Cancer: Practical, Ethical, and Legal Problems, edited by C.J. Williams. New York: John Wiley & Sons.

Wetherill, G.B. (1963). Sequential estimation of quantal response curves (with discussion). JRSS B 25: 1-48.

Weymuller, E.A. and Goepfert, H. (1991). Uniformity of results reporting in head and neck cancer (editorial). Head & Neck, July/August: 275-277. Reprinted in Laryngoscope 104: 784-785.

Whitehead, J. (1992). The Design and Analysis of Sequential Clinical Trials, Second Edition. New York: Ellis Horwood.

Whitehead, J. (1993). The case for frequentism in clinical trials. Statistics in Med. 12: 1405-1413.

Whitehead, J. (1994). Sequential methods based on the boundaries approach for the clinical comparison of survival times. Statistics in Med. 13: 1357-1368.

Whitehead, J., Brunier, H., and Facey, K. (1992) PEST: Planning and Evaluation of Sequential Trials, User's Manual. Reading, UK: The PEST Project.

Whitworth, J.A., Morgan, D., Maude, G.H., Luty, A.J., and Taylor, D.W. (1992). A community trial of ivermectin for onchocerciasis in Sierra Leone: Clinical and parisitological responses to four doses given at six-monthly intervals. Trans. R. Soc. Trop. Med. Hyg. 86: 277-280.

Wilde, D.J. (1964). Optimum Seeking Methods. Englewood Cliffs, NJ: Prentice-Hall.

Willan, A. and Pater, J. (1986). Carryover and the two-period cross-over clinical trial. Biometrics 42: 593-599.

Willan, A. and Pater, J. (1986). Using baseline measurements in the two-period cross-over clinical trial. Controlled Clin. Trials 7: 282-289.

Williams, C.J. (Ed.) (1992). Introducing New Treatments for Cancer: Practical, Ethical, and Legal Problems. Chichester: John Wiley & Sons.

Williams, D.H. and Davis, C.E. (1994). Reporting of treatment assignment methods in clinical trials. Controlled Clin. Trials 15: 294-298.

Wilson, E.O. (1992). The Diversity of Life. New York: W. W. Norton.

Winer, B.J. (1962). Statistical Principles in Experimental Design, 2nd Edition. New York: McGraw Hill.

Winer, B.J. (1971). Statistical Principles in Experimental Design, Second Edition. New York: McGraw-Hill.

Winget, M.D. (1996). Selected Issues Related to the Conduct, Reporting, and Analysis of Phase I Trials. Ph.D. Dissertation, Johns Hopkins University.

Wittes, J., Lakatos, E., and Probstfield, J. (1989). Surrogate endpoints in clinical trials: Cardiovascular diseases. Statistics in Medicine 8: 415-425.

Wittes, R.E. (1988). Of clinical alerts and peer review (editorial). JNCI 80: 984-985.

Wolfram, S. (1996). The Mathematica Book, Third Edition. Cambridge: Cambridge University Press.

Wong, W.K. and Lachenbruch, P.A. (1996). Designing studies for dose response. Statistics in Med. 15: 343-359.

Wooding, W.M. (1994). Planning Pharmaceutical Clinical Trials. New York: John Wiley & Sons.

Woolf, P.K. (1981). Fraud in science: How much, how serious? Hastings Center Report 11 (October): 9-14.

Woolf, P.K. (1986). Pressure to publish and fraud in science. Annals of Internal Medicine 104: 254-256.

Woolf, P.K. (1988). Deception in scientific research. Jurimetrics Journal 29: 67-95.

Working Group on Recommendations for Reporting Clinical Trials in the Biomedical Literature (1994). Call for comments on a proposal to improve reporting of clinical trials in the biomedical literature: position paper. Ann. Intern. Med. 121: 894-895.

World Medical Association (1964). Declaration of Helsinki: recommendations guiding medical doctors in biomedical research involving human subjects. (Revised 1975, 1983, and 1989.) Helsinki: World Medical Association. See also British Med. J. 2: 177, 1964.

Wu, M., Fisher, M., and DeMets, D. (1980). Sample sizes for long-term medical trial with time-dependent dropout and event rates. Controlled Clinical Trials 1: 109-121.

Yates, F. (1935). Complex experiments (with discussion). J. Roy. Statist. Soc. B. 2: 181-247.

Yates, F. (1984). Tests of significance for 2×2 contingency tables (with discussion). J. Roy. Statist. Soc. (A) 147: 426-463.

Yusuf, S., Collins, R., and Peto, R. (1984). Why do we need some large, simple, randomized trials? Statistics in Med. 3: 409-420.

Yusuf, S., Held, P., Teo, K.K., and Toretsky, E.R. (1990). Selection of patients for randomized controlled trials: Implications of wide or narrow eligibility criteria. Statistics in Med. 9: 73-86.

Yusuf, S. (1995). Calcium antagonists in coronary artery disease and hypertension: Time for reevaluation? Circulation 92: 1079-1082.

Zeger, S.L., Liang, K.Y., and Albert, P. (1988). Models for longitudinal data: A generalized estimating equation approach. Biometrics 44: 1049-1060.

Zeger, S.L., and Liang, K.Y. (1986). Longitudinal data analysis for discrete and continuous outcomes. Biometrics 42: 121-130.

Zelen, M. (1969). Play the winner rule and the controlled clinical trial. J. Am. Stat. Assoc. 64: 131-146.

Zelen, M. (1979). A new design for randomized clinical trials. N. Engl. J. Med. 300: 1242-1245.

Zelen, M. (1983). Guidelines for publishing papers on cancer clinical trials: Responsibilities of editors and authors. J. Clin. Oncol. 1: 164-169.

Zelen, M. (1990). Randomized consent designs for clinical trials: An update. Statistics in Med. 9: 645-656.

Subject Index

577

WILEY SERIES IN PROBABILITY AND STATISTICS

ESTABLISHED BY WALTER A. SHEWHART AND SAMUEL S. WILKS

Editors
Vic Barnett, Ralph A. Bradley, Nicholas I. Fisher, J. Stuart Hunter,
J. B. Kadane, David G. Kendall, David W. Scott, Adrian F. M. Smith,
Jozef L. Teugels, Geoffrey S. Watson

*Now available in a lower priced paperback edition in the Wiley Classics Library.

*Now available in a lower priced paperback edition in the Wiley Classics Library.

*Now available in a lower priced paperback edition in the Wiley Classics Library.

*Now available in a lower priced paperback edition in the Wiley Classics Library.

*Now available in a lower priced paperback edition in the Wiley Classics Library.

*Now available in a lower priced paperback edition in the Wiley Classics Library.